Posterior Cruciate Ligament Injuries

Gregory C. Fanelli, MD
Editor

Posterior Cruciate Ligament Injuries

A Practical Guide to Management

Second Edition

Springer

Editor
Gregory C. Fanelli, MD
GHS Orthopaedics
Danville
Pennsylvania
USA

ISBN 978-3-319-30774-9 ISBN 978-3-319-12072-0 (e-Book)
DOI 10.1007/978-3-319-12072-0

Springer Cham Heidelberg New York Dordrecht London

Softcover reprint of the hardcover 2nd edition 2015

Printed on acid-free paper

Springer is part of Springer Science+Business Media (www.springer.com)

To my wife Lori, and my children Matthew, David, and Megan who all have a tireless work ethic, and are a never-ending source of inspiration to me.

To my wife Lori, and my children Matthew, David, and Megan, who all endured my tireless work effort and are a never-ending source of inspiration to me.

Preface

Our practice environment largely determines the pathways that our individual orthopedic careers take. It has been a blessing to be in a position that enabled me to expand my surgical techniques and research interest in the evaluation and treatment of posterior cruciate ligament (PCL) injuries and the multiple-ligament-injured knee. I believe the same situation exists for other contributors to this book. We all share a passion and a commitment to the treatment of complex knee ligament instabilities. The purpose of this book is to provide experienced knee surgeons, general orthopedic surgeons, fellows, residents, medical students, and other health care professionals with an interest in PCL injuries and the PCL-based multiple ligament injured knee, a useful tool for the management of these complex injuries.

Posterior Cruciate Ligament Injuries: A Practical Guide to Management, Second Edition, is expanded from 19 chapters in the *First Edition* to 29 chapters in the *Second Edition*. The *Second Edition* is composed of eight functional segments with each segment having a number of chapters. New topics in the *Second Edition* include chapters addressing osteotomy, mechanical graft tensioning, articular cartilage restoration, meniscus transplantation, new cutting edge surgical techniques of PCL reconstruction, outcomes data, selected case studies, and the editor's 25-year evolutionary experience in the evaluation and treatment of PCL injuries and the PCL-based multiple-ligament-injured knee. The chapters were organized and written so that they build upon each other, and also so that they are able to stand alone. This will enable the reader to leisurely explore the topic of the PCL injured knee, or to use the text as a quick, practical reference when the need arises.

Chapter 1 presents the editor's 25-year experience in evaluation and treatment of PCL injuries and the PCL-based multiple-ligament injured knee. Chapters 2 and 3 address anatomy and biomechanics of the knee, while Chaps. 4 through 7 address diagnosis, clinical examination, instrumented measurement, MRI imaging, and nonsurgical treatment of the PCL injured knee. Chapters 8 through 20 provide multiple authors' advanced surgical techniques for PCL reconstruction. Topics in these chapters include graft selection, arthroscopic PCL primary repair, arthroscopic PCL reconstruction techniques, tibial inlay PCL reconstruction surgical techniques, PCL-based multiple knee ligament surgical techniques, PCL reconstruction in patients 18 years of age and younger, and revision PCL reconstruction.

Chapters 21 through 27 address topics that are often encountered when treating PCL injuries. These include mechanical graft tensioning, the role of osteotomy, articular cartilage restoration, meniscus transplantation, postoperative rehabilitation, functional bracing, and complications in PCL injuries and reconstruction.

Chapter 28 presents the results of treatment of PCL surgery from an outcomes data perspective. The final chapter, 29, presents nine case studies in the management of PCL injuries and the PCL-based multiple-ligament-injured knee. Each case study presents a different knee instability problem, and then takes the reader through the decision making process, the surgical treatment, and the final outcome.

The PCL injured knee and the PCL based multiple ligament injured knee are extremely complex pathologic entities. I believe that through research, improved surgical techniques, the use of allograft tissue, advancement in surgical equipment, careful documentation, and experience, we are progressively improving our outcomes in treating this devastating knee injury. It is my personal hope that this book will serve as a catalyst for new ideas to further develop treatment plans and surgical techniques for PCL and related injuries, and that God and His Son Jesus Christ will continue to guide us in the care and treatment of these patients.

Danville, PA

Gregory C. Fanelli, M.D.

Acknowledgements

I want to acknowledge the following people who have directly and indirectly contributed to this textbook. Connie Walsh (Developmental Editor) at Springer-Verlag, New York for her help in creating this book. Craig J. Edson, M.S., P.T./A.T.C., friend, colleague, and outstanding clinician and teacher. The Orthopedic Surgery Team at Geisinger Woodbine Lane and Geisinger Medical Center are the best orthopedic support staff in the world. Their dedication and drive for excellence are unequaled. To my patients and their referring doctors who have entrusted their care to me, and to my orthopedic colleagues and friends who have taken time out of their busy schedules to contribute chapters to this book.

Danville, PA Gregory C. Fanelli, M.D.

Contents

Part I Editor's Experience

1 **Posterior Cruciate Ligament Injuries and Reconstruction: What I Have Learned** 3
Gregory C. Fanelli

Part II Anatomy and Biomechanics

2 **Anatomy and Biomechanics of the Posterior Cruciate Ligament and Their Surgical Implications** 19
Christopher G. Stevens, Keith Jarbo, Kostas Economopoulos and Anikar Chhabra

3 **Anatomy and Biomechanics of the Posterolateral and Posteromedial Corners of the Knee and Their Surgical Implications** 33
Evan W. James, Christopher M. LaPrade, Adam M. Johannsen and Robert F. LaPrade

Part III Diagnosis and Evaluation

4 **Clinical and Arthroscopic Evaluation of the Posterior-Cruciate-Ligament-Injured Knee** 49
Brian M. Devitt and Daniel B. Whelan

5 **Instrumented Measurement of the Multiple-Ligament-Injured Knee: Arthrometry, Stress Radiography, Rotationometry, and Computer Navigation** 65
Sasha Carsen, Robert Timothy Deakon and Don Johnson

6 **MRI of PCL, Posteromedial, and Posterolateral Corner Injuries of the Knee** 75
W. James Malone, Satre Stuelke, Robert R. Snowden and Joel S. Salesky

Part IV Non-Surgical Treatment

7 **Nonoperative Treatment and Natural History of Posterior Cruciate Ligament Injuries** 89
K. Donald Shelbourne

Part V Surgical Treatment

8 **Graft Selection in Posterior Cruciate Ligament Surgery** 101
Natalie L. Leong, Nima Kabir and David R. McAllister

9 **Arthroscopic Transtibial Tunnel Posterior Cruciate Ligament Reconstruction** 111
Gregory C. Fanelli

10 **Open Tibial Inlay Graft for Posterior Cruciate Ligament Reconstruction** 123
S. Mark Heard and Meagan Heard

11 **All-Arthroscopic Tibial Inlay Double-Bundle Posterior Cruciate Ligament Reconstruction** 137
Alexander E. Weber and Jon K Sekiya

12 **All-Inside Posterior Cruciate Ligament Reconstruction** 147
William M. Engasser, Paul L. Sousa, Michael J. Stuart and Bruce A. Levy

13 **The All-Inside Technique: Surgical Technique and Outcomes** 157
Ranjodh Dhami, Robby S. Sikka, Ryan P. Dunlay and Joel L. Boyd

14 **Arthroscopic Primary Repair of Posterior Cruciate Ligament Injuries** 165
Dominique D. Nieves, Micah J. Lissy and Gregory S. DiFelice

15 **Combined PCL, ACL, Posteromedial, and Posterolateral Reconstruction** 173
Gregory C. Fanelli

16 **Surgical Treatment of Combined PCL/Lateral-Sided Injuries** 189
Christopher J. Wahl and Paul C. Chin

17 **Combined Posterior Cruciate Ligament and Posteromedial Reconstruction** 209
Adnan Saithna and Peter B. MacDonald

18 **Combined PCL, Posteromedial Corner, and Posterolateral Corner Reconstruction** 219
Clayton W. Nuelle and James P. Stannard

19 **Posterior Cruciate Ligament Reconstruction in Patients 18 Years of Age and Younger** 231
Gregory C. Fanelli and David G. Fanelli

20 **Revision Surgery in Posterior Cruciate Ligament Reconstruction** 245
Kevin N. Jiang, Scott R. Kling, Timothy L. Miller and Christopher D. Harner

Part VI Other Considerations

21 **Mechanical Graft Tensioning in Posterior Cruciate Ligament Reconstruction** 263
Gregory C. Fanelli

22 **The Role of Osteotomy in the Treatment of Posterior Cruciate Ligament (PCL) Injuries** ... 271
Jonathan A. Godin, Kathryne J. Stabile and Claude T. Moorman, III

23 **Articular Cartilage Restoration in the PCL-Injured Knee** ... 281
Clay G. Nelson and Kevin F. Bonner

24 **Meniscus Transplant in the PCL-Injured Knee** ... 295
Chad A. Haley, Steven J. Svoboda and Brett D. Owens

25 **Rehabilitation Following PCL Reconstruction: Scientific and Theoretical Basis** ... 311
Craig J. Edson

26 **Brace Considerations for Posterior Cruciate Ligament Injuries of the Knee** ... 321
Eileen A. Crawford and Edward M. Wojtys

27 **Complications and PCL Reconstruction** ... 329
Matthew S. Marcus and Jason L. Koh

Part VII Outcomes of Treatment

28 **Results of Treatment of Posterior Cruciate Ligament Surgery** ... 337
Iftach Hetsroni, Samuel A. Taylor and Robert G. Marx

Part VIII Clinical Case Studies

29 **Selected Case Studies in Posterior Cruciate Ligament Reconstruction** ... 349
Gregory C. Fanelli

Index ... 359

Contributors

Kevin F. Bonner, MD Jordan-Young Institute, Sentara Leigh Hospital, Virginia Beach, VA

Joel L. Boyd, MD Orthopaedic Surgery, University of Minnesota, Bloomington, MN

Sasha Carsen, MD, CM, MBA, FRCSC Orthopaedic Surgery, Division of Sports Medicine, Boston Children's Hospital, Boston, MA

Anikar Chhabra, MD, MS Orthopedics Sports Medicine, Banner Good Samaritan Orthopedic Residency; Orthopedic Surgery, Arizona State University; Phoenix, AZ

Paul C. Chin, MD, PhD San Diego Arthroscopy and Sports Medicine Fellowship, San Diego, CA

Eileen A. Crawford, MD Sports Medicine, Orthopedic Surgery, University of Michigan, Ann Arbor, MI

Robert Timothy Deakon, MD, FRCSC Oakville Sports Injury Clinic, Deakon Medicine Professional Corporation; Orthopaedic Surgery, Halton Healthcare Services, Oakville Trafalgar Site; Oakville, Ontario, Canada

Brian M. Devitt, MD, FRCS Orthopaedic Surgery, Sports Surgery Clinic, Dublin, Ireland

Ranjodh Dhami, BS Penn State Hershey Medical Center, Hershey, PA

Gregory S. DiFelice, MD Orthopaedics, Hospital for Special Surgery, New York, NY

Ryan P. Dunlay, MD Orthopaedic Surgery, ORA Orthopedics, Bettendorf, IA

Kostas Economopoulos, MD Orthopaedic Surgeon, Phoenix, AZ

Craig J. Edson, MHS, PT Sports Medicine, Geisinger / Healthsouth, Danville, PA

William M. Engasser, MD Sports Medicine, Orthopedic Surgery, Mayo Clinic, Rochester, MN

David G. Fanelli, BS Orthopaedic Surgery, Geisinger Health Systems, Danville, PA

Jonathan A. Godin, MD, MBA Department of Orthopaedic Surgery, Duke University Hospital, Durham, NC

Chad A. Haley, MD Department of Surgery, Keller Army Community Hospital, West Point, NY

Christopher D. Harner, MD Blue Cross of Western Pennsylvania; Orthopaedic Surgery, University of Pittsburgh Medical Center; Pittsburgh, PA

Meagan Heard BSc, SSP Kine Banff Sport Medicine, Canmore, Alberta, Canada

S. Mark Heard, BPE, MD, FRCS(C) Sport Medicine Orthopaedic Surgery, Banff Mineral Springs Hospital, Banff, Alberta, Canada

Iftach Hetsroni, MD Department of Orthopedic Surgery, Meir General Hospital, Sapir Medical Center, Kfar Saba, Israel, and Sackler Faculty of Medicine, Tel Aviv University, Tel Aviv, Israel

Evan W. James, BS Department of BioMedical Engineering, Steadman Philippon Research Institute, Vail, CO

Keith Jarbo, MD Orthopaedic Surgery, Banner Good Samaritan Medical Center, Phoenix, AZ

Kevin N. Jiang, MD Orthopaedic Sports, Department of Orthopaedic Surgery, University of Pittsburgh Medical Center, Pittsburgh, PA

Adam M. Johannsen, BS Department of BioMedical Engineering, Steadman Philippon Research Institute, Vail, CO

Don Johnson, MD, FRCSC Department of Orthopaedics, The Ottawa Hospital, Ottawa, Ontario, Canada

Nima Kabir, MD Department of Orthopaedic Surgery, David Geffen School of Medicine at UCLA, Los Angeles, CA

Scott R. Kling, MD UPMC Center for Sports Medicine, Department of Orthopaedic Surgery, University of Pittsburgh, Pittsburgh, PA

Jason L. Koh, MD University of Chicago Pritzker School of Medicine; Department of Orthopaedic Surgery, NorthShore University HealthSystem; Evanston, IL

Christopher M. LaPrade, BA Department of BioMedical Engineering, Steadman Philippon Research Institute, Vail, CO

Robert F. LaPrade, MD, PhD Department of BioMedical Engineering, Steadman Philippon Research Institute, Vail, CO

Natalie L. Leong, MD Department of Orthopaedic Surgery, University of California Los Angeles, Los Angeles, CA

Bruce A. Levy, MD Orthopedic Surgery, Mayo Clinic, Rochester, MN

Micah J. Lissy, MD, MS PT, ATC, CSCS Sports Medicine, UHS, Binghamton, NY

Peter B. MacDonald, MD FRCS(C) Orthopaedics, Pan Am Clinic, Winnipeg, Manitoba, Canada

David R. McAllister, MD Sports Medicine, Clinical Operations, Department of Orthopaedic Surgery, David Geffen School of Medicine at UCLA, Los Angeles, CA

W. James Malone, DO Musculoskeletal Radiology, Geisinger Health System, Geisinger Medical Center, Danville, PA

Matthew S. Marcus, MD Department of Orthopaedics, Division of Sports Medicine, University of Illinois at Chicago, Chicago, IL

Robert G. Marx, MD, MSc, FRCSC Sports Medicine and Shoulder Service, Hospital for Special Surgery, New York, NY

Timothy L. Miller, MD Orthopaedic Surgery, Sports Medicine Division, The Ohio State University Wexner Medical Center, Granville, OH

Claude T. Moorman III, MD Department of Orthopaedic Surgery, Duke University Hospital, Durham, NC

Clay G. Nelson, BSc Eastern Virginia Medical School, Norfolk, VA

Dominique D. Nieves, BA Orthopaedics, Hospital for Special Surgery, New York, NY

Clayton W. Nuelle, MD Orthopaedics, University of Missouri-Columbia, Columbia, MO

Brett D. Owens, MD Orthopaedic Surgery, USUHS, Keller Army Hospital, West Point, NY

Adnan Saithna, MBChB, Dip SEM, MSc, FRCS (T&O) Sports Medicine and Upper Extremity Reconstruction, Pan Am Clinic, Winnipeg, Manitoba, Canada

Joel S. Salesky, MD Radiology, Geisinger Wyoming Valley Medical Center, Wilkes-barre, PA

Jon K. Sekiya, MD Orthopaedic Surgery, University of Michigan, Ann Arbor, MI

K. Donald Shelbourne, MD Orthopaedic Surgery, Shelbourne Knee Center, Indianapolis, IN

Robby S. Sikka, MD TRIA Orthopaedic Center, Minneapolis, MN

Robert R. Snowden, MD Radiology, Geisinger Medical Center, Danville, PA

Paul L. Sousa, BA Sports Medicine, Orthopedic Surgery, Mayo Clinic, Rochester, MN

Kathryne J. Stabile, MD, MS Department of Orthopaedic Surgery, Duke University Hospital, Durham, NC

James P. Stannard, MD Missouri Orthopaedic Institute; Department of Orthopaedic Surgery, University of Missouri; Columbia, MO

Christopher G. Stevens, MD Orthopaedic Sports Medicine, Orthopaedic Surgery, Banner Good Samaritan, Phoenix, AZ

Michael J. Stuart, MD Orthopedic Surgery, Mayo Clinic, Rochester, MN

Satre Stuelke, MD, MFA Radiology Department, Geisinger Medical Center, Danville, PA

Steven J. Svoboda, MD John A. Feagin Jr. Sports Medicine Fellowship, Department of Surgery, Keller Army Community Hospital, West Point, NY

Samuel A. Taylor, MD Hospital for Special Surgery, Weill Medical College of Cornell University, New York, NY

Christopher J. Wahl, MD Department of Orthopaedic Surgery, Division of Sports Medicine, UC San Diego Health System, San Diego, CA

Alexander E. Weber, MD Department of Orthopaedic Surgery, University of Michigan Hospital, Ann Arbor, MI

Daniel B. Whelan, MD, MSc, FRCSC Division of Orthopaedic Surgery, St. Michael's Hospital, Toronto, Ontario, Canada

Edward M. Wojtys, MD Sports Medicine, Orthopedic Surgery, University of Michigan, Ann Arbor, MI

Part I
Editor's Experience

Posterior Cruciate Ligament Injuries and Reconstruction: What I Have Learned

1

Gregory C. Fanelli

Introduction

This chapter is a compilation of my experience treating posterior cruciate ligament (PCL) injuries and PCL-based multiple ligament knee injuries over the past 25 years. Departing from the style of most text books, this chapter is written in the first person, and is intended to be a conversation between the reader and myself about one of the most complex and interesting topics in orthopedic surgery—PCL injuries and the multiple ligament-injured knee. The goal of this chapter is to maximize success, avoid complications, and help the surgeon stay out of trouble treating these complex and difficult cases. This chapter is organized to present brief sections of information that will help the orthopedic surgeon and other health care professionals to make treatment decisions in PCL and multiple ligament knee injury cases. Topics addressed include incidence of PCL injuries, three-zone arthroscopic evaluation of the PCL, diagnosis and classification of posterolateral and posteromedial instability, multiple knee ligament injury evaluation protocol, surgical timing, concepts of repair and/or reconstruction, graft preparation, arthroscopic or open surgical procedures, surgical technique highlights, mechanical graft tensioning, postoperative rehabilitation, PCL knee injuries in patients 18 years of age and younger, and results of treatment. Specific surgical procedures are discussed in various chapters throughout this text book.

Incidence

I live in rural central Pennsylvania in the USA. This is both a farming and industrial area located among multiple interstate highway systems, and I work in a level one trauma hospital. This combination of location, patient population, and hospital facility creates an environment where PCL knee injuries occur with some frequency. PCL injuries in trauma patients with acute knee injuries range between 38 and 44 % in our hospital [1, 2]. These injuries are related to higher-energy trauma in approximately 56 %, and to sports-related injuries in approximately 32 %. Isolated PCL tears occur 3.5 % of the time in this population, while PCL tears combined with other ligaments (the PCL-based multiple ligament-injured knee) occur in 96.5 % of PCL injuries in our series. The combined PCL and anterior cruciate ligament (ACL) tears, 45.9 %, and the combined PCL posterolateral instability, 41.2 %, are the most common posterior cruciate-based combined injuries that have been seen in our series [2]. The purpose of reviewing these data is to emphasize the point that PCL tears that occur in a higher-energy trauma population will most likely be PCL-based multiple ligament knee injuries. It is also important to realize that PCL injuries in high-energy sports are also at risk of being a combined ligament injury [1–3].

Arthroscopic Evaluation of the Posterior Cruciate Ligament

Arthroscopic evaluation of the PCL has been reported by Lysholm and Guillquist and by Fanelli et al. [4–6]. Arthroscopic evaluation of the PCL is a very helpful adjunct to physical examination and imaging studies especially with respect to surgical planning. We have developed and published the three-zone concept of arthroscopic PCL evaluation, and used this method in our treatment of PCL injuries [5, 6]. In this concept, the PCL is divided into three distinct zones. Zone 1 extends from the femoral insertion of the PCL to where the PCL disappears behind the ACL. Zone 2 of the PCL is where the PCL lies behind the ACL which is the middle section of the PCL. Zone 3 is the PCL tibial insertion site.

Arthroscopic PCL evaluation is performed with the surgical leg draped free using a lateral post for extremity control. A 25° or 30° arthroscope is used through the anterior inferior lateral patellar portal to visualize zone 1 of the PCL. The posterior medial portal is used to visualize zone 2 and zone

G. C. Fanelli (✉)
303 Kaseville Road, Danville, PA 17821, USA
e-mail: gregorycfanelli@gmail.com

G. C. Fanelli (ed.), *Posterior Cruciate Ligament Injuries*,
DOI 10.1007/978-3-319-12072-0_1, © Springer International Publishing Switzerland 2015

3 also using the 25° or 30° arthroscope. These two portal-viewing combinations enable complete visualization of the PCL.

Arthroscopic findings in the PCL-injured knee are either direct or indirect [5, 6]. Direct findings include damage to the PCL itself such as midsubstance tears, interstitial tears with ligament stretching, hemorrhage within the synovial sheath, and avulsion of bony insertions. Indirect arthroscopic findings occur as a result of the PCL injury and include the sloppy ACL sign, altered contact points, and degenerative changes of the patellofemoral joint and medial compartment.

The sloppy ACL sign demonstrates relative laxity of the ACL secondary to posterior tibial drop back with the knee at 90° of knee flexion because of the PCL insufficiency. When the tibia is reduced, the normal ACL tension is restored. Altered contact points occur secondary to tibial drop back with the knee flexed 90°. Clinically, this is the posterior sag sign [7]. Placing the arthroscope in the anterolateral inferior patellar portal shows closer proximity of the anterior horn of the medial and lateral menisci to the distal femoral condyle articular surfaces. This altered tibiofemoral relationship allows abnormal stress distribution in the tibiofemoral and patellofemoral compartments, and may promote degenerative joint disease [8, 9].

Arthroscopic visualization of the posterolateral and posteromedial corners of the knee is helpful in diagnosis and surgical planning in these complex knee ligament injuries. Posterolateral and posteromedial instability will often result in widening of the affected compartment with the respective varus or valgus stress. The widening indicates damage to the posteromedial or posterolateral structures, and the position of the menisci relative to the femur and tibia indicates the location of the capsular injury. In my experience, when the meniscus stays with the tibia, the capsular damage is on the femoral side, and when the meniscus stays with the femur, the capsular damage is on the tibial side. When the meniscus is floating in the middle of the affected compartment gap, there is structural damage on both the femoral and tibial sides. Axial rotation instability can occur without medial or lateral compartment widening which is seen with posterolateral and posteromedial instability type A [10, 11]. Arthroscopic visualization is helpful to make the diagnosis by seeing the tibia rotates under the medial or lateral meniscus with the knee at 90° of knee flexion and internal and external axial rotation applied to the tibia.

Arthroscopic evaluation of the PCL and related structures in the PCL-injured knee is a useful adjunct to the history, physical examination, arthrometer testing, and imaging studies. Arthroscopic PCL evaluation aids in surgical decision making and planning of reparative or reconstructive surgical procedures. A standard 25° or 30° arthroscope placed in the inferior lateral patellar and posteromedial arthroscopic portals provides excellent visualization of all three zones of the PCL, and the posterolateral and posteromedial corners of the knee.

Correct Diagnosis

Isolated PCL injuries are uncommon in my experience. The patients that I see most commonly have PCL-based multiple ligament knee injuries. Identifying the multiple planes of instability in these complex knee ligament injuries is essential for successful treatment of the PCL-based multiple ligament-injured knee, and the ACL-based multiple ligament-injured knee. The posterior and ACL disruptions will lead to increased posterior and anterior laxity at 90° and 30° of knee flexion. The difficulty arises in recognizing the medial- and lateral-side instability patterns in the multiple ligament-injured knee. Recognition and correction of the medial- and lateral-side instabilities is the key to successful posterior and ACL surgery.

There are three different types of instability patterns that I have observed in medial- and lateral-side knee injuries [10–12]. These are, type A (axial rotation instability only), type B (axial rotation instability combined with varus and/or valgus laxity with a firm end point), and type C (axial rotation instability combined with varus and/or valgus laxity with little or no end point). In my experience, the axial rotation instability (type A) medial or lateral side is most frequently overlooked. It is also critical to understand that combined medial- and lateral-side instabilities of different types occur with bicruciate and unicruciate multiple ligament knee injuries. Examples include PCL, ACL, lateral-side type C, and medial-side type A, or PCL, medial-side type B, and lateral-side type A instability patterns.

A combination of careful clinical examination, radiographs, and MRI studies aids in making the correct diagnosis of multiple ligament knee injuries. Knee examination under anesthesia combined with fluoroscopy, stress radiography, and diagnostic arthroscopy also contribute to accurately diagnosing the multiple planes of instability [5, 6, 13]. Once again, recognition and correction of the medial- and lateral-side instabilities is the key to successful posterior and ACL surgery.

Considerations in the PCL-Based Multiple Ligament-Injured Knee

Respect the Anatomy

As orthopedic knee surgeons, we focus on the knee ligaments, menisci, articular cartilage, and extensor mechanism. In multiple ligament knee injuries, it is critically important to be aware of arterial and venous injuries, skin trauma, and peroneal and tibial nerve injuries. Bony injuries to the tibia, femur, patella, pelvis, and spine may also occur in patients with multiple knee ligament injuries. Head injuries also occur in this patient population placing these patients at risk for heterotopic ossification and lower-extremity spasticity complicating the treatment and postoperative course in these patients with multiple knee ligament injuries. Multiple system injuries can affect the outcomes of treatment in multiple ligament knee injuries, and must be considered in the treatment plans in these complex knee injuries.

The incidence of vascular injuries in multiple knee ligament injuries may occur in 32–50 % of cases with bicruciate tears having the same incidence as frank tibiofemoral dislocations [14–16]. Hyperextension mechanisms of injury may result in anterior tibial displacement with subsequent popliteal artery stretch and rupture, while a direct impact to the proximal tibia in the 90° flexed knee leads to posterior tibial displacement with potential arterial contusion and intimal damage [17]. I have also seen posttraumatic deep venous thrombosis in these severe knee injuries.

Vascular Assessment

Evaluation of the acute multiple ligament-injured knee includes careful physical examination of the injured and uninjured lower extremities, and an ankle-brachial index measurement. If there are abnormal or asymmetric pulses or an ankle-brachial index of less than 0.9, more advanced vascular evaluation and vascular surgical consultation is indicated [18]. The absence of pulses distal to the knee requires prompt vascular surgical intervention. It is very important to evaluate the popliteal artery for intimal flap tears that could potentially cause delayed vascular occlusion. Clinical examination suggesting deep venous thrombosis indicates the need for further vascular evaluation.

External Fixation

External fixation is a useful tool in the management of the multiple ligament-injured knee. Preoperative indications for the use of spanning external fixation include open dislocations, vascular repair, and inability to maintain reduction [19]. The advantages of using spanning external fixation include skin assessment, compartment pressure observation, and monitoring the neurovascular status of the affected limb. Preoperative use of external fixation compared to brace immobilization may lead to less terminal flexion postoperatively; however, this may be more dependent on injury severity of the involved extremity than the use of the spanning external fixation device [20]. According to some clinicians, postoperative protection of multiple knee ligament reconstructions in a hinged external fixation device has led to more favorable static stability than postoperative brace immobilization [21]. My opinion regarding the use of spanning external fixation in treatment of the multiple ligament-injured knee preoperatively and postoperatively is that if I can control the knee in a brace, I use a brace. If I cannot control the knee in a brace, I use an external fixation device. Occasionally, I have used a spanning external fixator for treatment of the multiple ligament-injured knee in patients who are not surgical candidates.

Surgical Treatment

Over the past two decades, technical advancements in the use of allograft tissue, arthroscopic surgical instruments, graft fixation methods, improved surgical techniques and postoperative rehabilitation programs, and an improved understanding of knee ligament structure and biomechanics have, in my experience, led to more predictable and successful results with multiple knee ligament reconstructions documented with physical examination, arthrometer measurements, knee ligament rating scales, stress radiography, and return to function [22–31].

Surgical Timing

Surgical timing in the acute multiple ligament-injured knee is dependent on the vascular status of the extremity, collateral ligament injury severity, and the degree of reduction stability. My experience and that of others demonstrates that a delayed or staged reconstruction of 2–3 weeks has resulted in less motion loss and arthrofibrosis [22–35]. My preferred surgical approach is a single-stage arthroscopic posterior and ACL reconstruction using allograft tissue, and medial- and/or lateral-side primary repair combined with allograft augmentation reconstruction within 2–4 weeks of the initial injury. Some medial-side injuries may be successfully treated with bracing [23, 24, 26].

There are surgical timing modifiers or considerations that may occur in the evaluation and treatment of the acute multiple ligament-injured knee. These modifiers may adversely affect the timing of surgery creating a situation where the surgical procedure may need to be performed earlier or later than desired by the surgeon. These modifiers include vascular status of the extremity, open injuries, reduction stability of the knee, severe medial- or lateral-side injuries, skin conditions, multiple system injuries, other orthopedic injuries, and meniscus and articular surface injuries. It is important to recognize and understand that in complex multiple knee ligament injuries, ideal surgical timing is not always possible.

The Chronic Multiple Ligament-Injured Knee

Chronic multiple knee ligament injuries typically present to my clinic with progressive functional instability. These patients may or may not have some degree of posttraumatic arthrosis depending upon their time from injury. It is important to identify both the structural injuries and the planes of instability in these chronic knee ligament injuries. The structural injuries may include meniscus damage, malalignment, articular surface defects, and gait abnormalities in addition to the chronic knee ligament instability. Surgical options under consideration include osteotomies to correct malalignment and gait abnormalities, ligament reconstruction, meniscus surgery (repair, resection, transplantation), and osteochondral grafting. My preference is to perform staged surgeries in these complex injury patterns beginning with correction of malalignment.

Repair or Reconstruction

Since beginning my treatment of multiple knee ligament injuries, my preference has been to reconstruct the cruciate ligaments and to perform a combined repair and reconstruction of the medial- and lateral-side injuries. Allograft tissue is preferred for these surgeries, however, we have had successful results with both allograft and autograft tissue [22–26]. Large PCL tibial bony avulsions are treated with reduction and fixation of the bony fragment. Small PCL tibial bony avulsions are evaluated with the arthroscopic three-zone PCL surgical technique to determine the condition of the PCL before proceeding with fixation of the small bony fragment [5]. Several studies have shown high rates of medial- and lateral-side surgical failures with primary repair alone [36–38]. We have had consistently successful results with combined primary repair and reconstruction with allograft or autograft tissue for medial- and lateral-side injuries [22–31, 39, 40]. The important point is that medial- and lateral-side-combined primary repair and reconstruction is more successful than primary repair alone in our experience, and in the recent literature. Allograft and autograft tissue both provide successful results.

Posterior Cruciate Ligament and Multiple Knee Ligament Reconstruction Surgical Technique

Graft Preparation

Intraoperative graft preparation is a very important part of the surgical procedure, and can enhance or destroy the flow of the operation. I have always prepared my allograft and autograft tissue personally with the help of an assistant. When allograft tissue is used, this tissue is prepared in the sterile operating room prior to bringing the patient into the operating room to minimize general anesthesia time for the patient. Cases where autograft tissue is used, the autografts are harvested, and then I personally prepare them with an assistant. During the graft preparation, the surgeon "gets a feel for the graft" which provides insight into optimal tunnel size, and how the graft will behave during graft passage. This attention to detail facilitates the flow of the surgical procedure by maximizing the probability of uneventful graft passage leading to successful tensioning and final graft fixation. It is not recommended to delegate graft preparation responsibility to the lowest-ranking member of the surgical team.

Arthroscopic or Open Surgical Procedure

How do I decide to perform an open or arthroscopic combined posterior and ACL reconstruction in these multiple ligament-injured knees, and whether or not to do a single- or two-stage procedures? My preference is to perform a single-stage arthroscopic posterior and ACL reconstruction using allograft tissue combined with medial- and/or lateral-side-combined primary repair and reconstruction with allograft tissue within 2–4 weeks of the initial injury. Severe medial- and/or lateral-side injuries with significant capsular damage that do not allow arthroscopic fluid to be maintained safely in the knee joint are treated as two-stage surgical procedures. The medial- and/or lateral-side surgery will be performed within the first week following the injury. The knee will be immobilized in full extension, and the arthroscopic combined posterior and ACL reconstruction will be performed approximately 4–5 weeks after the initial medial- or lateral-side surgery. When necessary, all ligament repairs and reconstructions are performed as a single-stage open surgical procedure. As always, surgical timing modifiers such as skin condition, vascular status, reduction stability, fractures, and other systemic injuries may alter the course of treatment.

Patient Positioning and Operating Room Preparation

The patient is positioned on the fully extended operating room table [28, 41–45]. A lateral post is used and the well leg is supported by the fully extended operating room table. The Biomet Sports Medicine PCL/ACL System (Biomet Sports Medicine, Warsaw, Indiana) are the surgical instruments used for this surgical procedure. Intraoperative radiography and C-arm image intensifier are not routinely used for this surgical procedure.

My preferred surgical technique is an arthroscopic PCL reconstruction using an Achilles tendon allograft to reconstruct the anterolateral bundle of the PCL. When I perform a double-bundle PCL reconstruction, an Achilles tendon allograft is used to reconstruct the anterolateral bundle of the PCL, and a tibialis anterior allograft for the posteromedial bundle of the PCL reconstruction. The ACL is reconstructed using an Achilles tendon allograft. Lateral-side surgery is a combined primary repair and fibular head-based figure-of-eight reconstruction using a semitendinosus or other soft-tissue allograft. The addition of a tibialis anterior allograft through a drill hole in the proximal tibia is added for knees with severe hyperextension external rotation recurvatum deformity and revision posterolateral reconstruction when needed. Lateral-side surgeries also have a posterolateral capsular shift or capsular reattachment performed as indicated. Medial-side injuries are treated with primary repair combined with allograft augmentation/reconstruction, and posteromedial capsular shift as indicated.

The allograft tissue used is from the same tissue bank with the same methods of tissue procurement and preservation that provide a consistent graft of high quality. It is very important for the surgeon to "know the tissue bank" and to obtain high-quality allograft tissue that will maximize the probability of surgical success. These multiple knee ligament reconstruction procedures are routinely performed in an outpatient setting unless specific circumstances indicate the necessity of an inpatient environment. The same experienced surgical teams are assembled for these complex surgical procedures. Experienced and familiar teams provide for a smoother operation, shorter surgical times, enhanced patient care, and a greater probability of success in these difficult surgical procedures. Preoperative and postoperative prophylactic antibiotics are routinely used in these complex and time-consuming surgical procedures to decrease the probability of infection. The specific details of my surgical procedure, including intraoperative photographs and diagrams, are presented in Chaps. 9 and 15 of this text book. The following sections in this chapter will address specific points that contribute to the success of this complex surgical procedure.

Posteromedial Safety Incision

Three factors that contribute to PCL reconstruction surgical failures are failure to address associated ligamentous instabilities, varus osseous malalignment, and incorrect tunnel placement [5, 41–44]. My PCL reconstruction principles are to identify and treat all pathology, protect the neurovascular structures, accurately place tunnels to approximate the PCL anatomic insertion sites, use strong graft material, minimize graft bending, restore the anatomic tibial step-off, utilize a mechanical graft-tensioning device, use primary and backup fixation, and to use a slow and deliberate postoperative rehabilitation program.

My PCL reconstruction surgical technique since 1990 has been an arthroscopic transtibial tunnel PCL reconstruction using a posteromedial safety incision to protect the neurovascular structures, confirm the accuracy of the tibial tunnel placement, and to facilitate the flow of the surgical procedure [5, 41, 43, 44]. An extracapsular extra-articular posteromedial safety incision is made by creating an incision approximately 2–3 cm long at the posteromedial border of the tibia near the diaphyseal–metaphyseal junction of the proximal medial aspect of tibia. Dissection is carried down to the crural fascia, which is incised longitudinally, and as always, the neurovascular structures are protected. An interval is developed between the medial head of the gastrocnemius muscle and the nerves and vessels posterior to the surgeon's finger, and the capsule of the knee joint anterior to the surgeon's finger. The posteromedial safety incision enables the surgeon to protect the neurovascular structures, confirm the accuracy of the PCL tibial tunnel, and to facilitate the flow of the surgical procedure. The neurovascular structures of the popliteal fossa are in close proximity to the posterior capsule of the knee joint, and are at risk during transtibial PCL reconstruction. The posteromedial safety incision is very important for the protection of these structures.

PCL Tibial Tunnel Creation

The arm of the PCL/ACL guide (Biomet Sports Medicine, Warsaw, Indiana) is inserted through the inferior medial patellar portal. The tip of the guide is positioned at the inferior lateral aspect of the PCL anatomic insertion site. This is below the tibial ridge posterior and in the lateral aspect of the PCL anatomic insertion site. The bullet portion of the guide contacts the anteromedial surface of the proximal tibia at a point midway between the posteromedial border of the tibia, and the tibial crest anterior at or just below the level of the tibial tubercle. This will provide a relatively vertically oriented PCL tibial tunnel, and an angle of graft orientation such that the graft will turn two very smooth 45° angles on the posterior aspect of the tibia. The tip of the guide, in the posterior aspect of the tibia, is confirmed with the surgeon's finger through the extracapsular extra-articular posteromedial safety incision. Intraoperative anteroposterior and lateral X-ray may also be used, however, I do not routinely use intraoperative X-ray. When the PCL/ACL guide is positioned in the desired area, a blunt spade-tipped guide wire is drilled from anterior to posterior. The surgeon's finger confirms the position of the guide wire through the posterior medial safety incision. The critical posteromedial safety incision protects the neurovascular structures, confirms the accuracy of the PCL tibial tunnel placement, and enhances the flow of the surgical procedure.

The appropriately sized standard cannulated reamer is used to create the tibial tunnel. The surgeon's finger through the extracapsular extraarticular posteromedial incision is monitoring the position of the guide wire. When the drill is engaged in bone, the guide wire is reversed, blunt end pointing posterior, for additional patient safety. The drill is advanced until it comes to the posterior cortex of the tibia. The chuck is disengaged from the drill, and completion of the tibial tunnel is performed by hand. The position and orientation of the PCL reconstruction transtibial tunnel creates a trough in the back of the tibia that mimics the tibial inlay technique, and provides a very smooth transition for the PCL grafts from the back of the tibia into the joint.

PCL Femoral Tunnel Creation

The PCL single- or double-bundle femoral tunnels are made from inside out using the double-bundle aimers, or using an endoscopic reamer as an aiming device (Biomet Sports Medicine, Warsaw, Indiana). With the knee in approximately 100–110° of flexion, the appropriately sized double-bundle aimer or endoscopic reamer is inserted through a low anterior lateral patellar arthroscopic portal to create the PCL anterior lateral bundle femoral tunnel. The double-bundle aimer or endoscopic reamer is positioned directly on the footprint of the femoral anterior lateral bundle PCL insertion site. The appropriately sized guide wire is drilled through the aimer or endoscopic reamer, through the bone, and out from a small skin incision. Care is taken to prevent any compromise of the articular surface. The double-bundle aimer is removed, and the endoscopic reamer is used to drill the anterior lateral PCL femoral tunnel from inside to outside. When the surgeon chooses to perform a double-bundle double-femoral tunnel PCL reconstruction, the same process is repeated for the posterior medial bundle of the PCL. Care must be taken to ensure that there will be an adequate bone bridge (approximately 5 mm) between the two femoral tunnels prior to drilling. This is accomplished using the calibrated probe, and direct arthroscopic visualization of the PCL femoral anatomic insertion sites.

I have evolved from outside-to-inside PCL femoral tunnel creation to inside-to-outside PCL femoral tunnel creation for two reasons. There is a greater distance and margin of safety between the PCL femoral tunnels and the medial femoral condyle articular surface using the inside-to-outside method. Additionally, a more accurate placement of the PCL femoral tunnel(s) is possible because I can place the double-bundle aimer or endoscopic reamer on the anatomic foot print of the anterior lateral and posterior medial PCL insertion sites under direct visualization.

ACL Reconstruction

With the knee in approximately 90° of flexion, the ACL tibial tunnel is created using a drill guide. My preferred method of ACL reconstruction is the transtibial femoral tunnel endoscopic surgical technique. The arm of the drill guide enters the knee joint through the inferior medial patellar portal. The bullet of the drill guide contacts the anterior medial proximal tibia externally at a point midway between the posterior medial border of the tibia, and the anterior tibial crest just above the level of the tibial tubercle. A 1-cm bone bridge or greater exists between the PCL and ACL tibial tunnels. This will reduce the possibility of tibial fracture. The guide wire is drilled through the guide and positioned so that after creating the ACL tibial tunnel, the graft will approximate the tibial anatomic insertion site of the ACL. A standard cannulated reamer is used to create the tibial tunnel.

With the knee in approximately 90–100° of flexion, an over-the-top femoral aimer is introduced through the tibial tunnel, and used to position a guide wire on the medial wall of the lateral femoral condyle to create a femoral tunnel approximating the anatomic insertion site of the ACL. The ACL graft is positioned, and fixation achieved on the femoral side using a bioabsorbable interference screw, and cortical suspensory backup fixation with a polyethylene ligament fixation button. The endoscopic transtibial femoral tunnel ACL reconstruction surgical technique enables reliable tunnel creation which allows the ACL graft tissue to approximate the tibial and femoral anatomic insertion sites of the ACL. Proper tunnel position increases the probability of successful results.

Mechanical Graft Tensioning and Fixation

The cyclic dynamic method of graft tensioning using the Biomet graft-tensioning boot (Biomet Sports Medicine, Warsaw, Indiana) is used to tension the posterior and ACL grafts [44, 45]. During this surgical technique, the posterior and/or ACL grafts are secured on the femoral side first with the surgeon's preferred fixation method. The technique described is a tibial-sided tensioning method. I routinely use polyethylene ligament fixation buttons for cortical suspensory fixation, and aperture-opening interference fixation with bioabsorbable interference screws for femoral side posterior and ACL fixation. In combined PCL–ACL reconstructions, the PCL graft is tensioned first, followed by final PCL graft(s) tibial fixation. The ACL graft tensioning and fixation follows that of the PCL.

The tensioning boot is applied to the foot and leg of the surgical extremity, and tension is placed on the PCL graft(s) distally using the Biomet graft-tensioning boot (Biomet Sports Medicine, Warsaw, Indiana). Tension is gradually applied with the knee in 0° of flexion (full extension) reducing the tibia on the femur. This restores the anatomic tibial step-off. Although there are numbers on the torque wrench dial, these numbers are not used to set the tension. The numbers on the torque wrench serve as a reference point during the cycling process, and readjustment process, and are not indicators of final tension in the graft. The tension is determined by reduction of the tibia on the femur in 0° of knee flexion (full extension), the restoration of the anatomic tibial step-offs, a negative posterior drawer on intraoperative examination of the knee, and full range of motion of the knee. The knee is cycled through a full range of motion multiple times to allow pretensioning and settling of the graft. The process is repeated until there is no further change on the torque setting on the graft tensioner with the knee at 0° of flexion (full extension). When there are no further changes or adjustments necessary in the tension applied to the graft, the knee is placed in 70–90° of flexion, and fixation is achieved on the tibial side of the PCL graft with a bioabsorbable interference screw for interference fit fixation, and back-up cortical suspensory fixation with a bicortical screw and spiked ligament washer or polyethylene ligament fixation button.

The cyclic dynamic method of tensioning of the ACL graft is performed using the Biomet graft-tensioning boot (Biomet Sports Medicine, Warsaw, Indiana) after tensioning and final fixation of the PCL graft(s) have been performed. Traction is placed on the ACL graft sutures with the knee in 0° of flexion (full extension), and tension is gradually applied reducing the tibia on the femur. The knee is then cycled through multiple full flexion and extension cycles to allow settling of the graft. The Lachman and pivot shift tests are performed. The process is repeated until there is no further change in the torque setting on the graft tensioner at full extension (0° of knee flexion), and the Lachman and pivot shift tests are negative. Although there are numbers on the torque wrench dial, these numbers are not used to set the tension. The numbers on the torque wrench serve as a reference point during the cycling process, and readjustment process, and are not indicators of final tension in the graft. Final ACL graft tension is determined by the Lachman and pivot shifts becoming negative, and achieving full range of motion of the knee. The knee is placed in approximately 30° of flexion, and fixation is achieved on the tibial side of the ACL graft with a bioabsorbable interference screw, and backup fixation with a polyethylene ligament fixation button.

I have found it very important to use primary and backup fixation. During cruciate ligament reconstruction, primary aperture fixation is achieved with bioabsorbable interference screws, and backup fixation is performed with a screw and spiked ligament washer, and ligament fixation buttons. Secure fixation is critical to the success of this surgical procedure. Mechanical tensioning of the cruciates at 0° of knee flexion (full extension), and restoration of the normal anatomic tibial step-off at 70–90° of flexion has provided the most reproducible method of establishing the neutral point of the tibia–femoral relationship in my experience. Full range of motion is confirmed on the operating table to assure the knee is not "captured" by the reconstruction.

Posterolateral Reconstruction

My most commonly utilized surgical technique for posterolateral reconstruction is the free graft figure-of-eight technique utilizing semitendinosus allograft, or other soft-tissue allograft material. This procedure requires an intact proximal tibiofibular joint, and the absence of a severe hyperextension external rotation recurvatum deformity. This technique combined with capsular repair and posterolateral capsular shift procedures mimics the function of the popliteofibular ligament and lateral collateral ligament, tightens the posterolateral capsule, and provides a post of strong allograft tissue to reinforce the posterolateral corner. When there is a disrupted proximal tibiofibular joint, or severe hyperextension external rotation recurvatum deformity, a two-tailed (fibular head, proximal tibia) posterior lateral reconstruction is performed in addition to the posterolateral capsular shift procedure [28, 41, 43, 44].

In acute cases, primary repair of all lateral-side-injured structures is performed with suture anchors, screws and washers, and permanent sutures through drill holes as indicated. The primary repair is then augmented with an allograft tissue reconstruction. Posterolateral reconstruction with the free graft figure-of-eight technique utilizes semitendinosus or other soft-tissue allograft. A curvilinear incision is made in the lateral aspect of the knee extending from the interval between Gerdy's tubercle and the fibular head to the lateral epicondyle and then proximal following the course of the iliotibial band. A peroneal nerve neurolysis is performed, and the peroneal nerve is protected throughout the procedure. The fibular head is identified and a tunnel is created in an anterior lateral to posterior medial direction at the area of maximal fibular head diameter. The tunnel is created by passing a guide pin followed by a standard cannulated drill 7 mm in diameter. The peroneal nerve is protected during tunnel creation, and throughout the procedure. The free tendon graft is passed through the fibular head drill hole. An incision is made in the iliotibial band in line with the fibers exposing the lateral femoral epicondyle area of the distal femur. The graft material is passed medial to the iliotibial band for the fibular collateral ligament limb, and medial to the common biceps tendon and iliotibial band for the popliteus tendon popliteofibular ligament limb. The limbs of the graft are crossed to form a figure of eight with the fibular collateral ligament component being lateral to the popliteus tendon component. A 3.2-mm drill hole is made to accommodate a

6.5-mm-diameter fully threaded cancellous screw that is approximately 30–35 mm in length. The drill hole is positioned in the lateral epicondylar region of the distal lateral femur so that after seating a 17–20-mm-spiked ligament fixation washer with the aforementioned screw, the spiked ligament fixation washer will precisely secure the two limbs of the allograft tissue at the respective anatomic insertion sites of the fibular collateral ligament and popliteus tendon on the distal lateral femoral condyle. This drill hole is approximately 1 cm anatomically anterior to the fibular collateral ligament femoral insertion. A longitudinal incision is made in the lateral capsule just posterior to the fibular collateral ligament, and the posterolateral capsular shift is performed with number 2 ethibond suture with the knee in 90° of knee flexion to correct posterolateral capsular redundancy. The graft is tensioned at approximately 30–40° of knee flexion, secured to the lateral femoral epicondylar region with a screw and spiked ligament washer at the above mentioned point. Number 2 ethibond suture is used to sew the tails of the graft together proximal to the washer to prevent slipping, and also to sew the allograft to the deep capsular layers for additional reinforcement. The anterior and posterior limbs of the figure-of-eight graft material are sewn to each other and to the deep capsular layer to reinforce and tighten the construct. The final graft-tensioning position is approximately 30–40° of knee flexion with a slight valgus force applied to the knee, and slight internal tibial rotation, while the posterior lateral capsular shift and reinforcing suture placement is performed at 90° of knee flexion. The iliotibial band incision is closed. The procedures described are designed to eliminate pathologic posterolateral axial rotation and varus rotational instability.

When there is a disrupted proximal tibiofibular joint, or hyperextension external rotation recurvatum deformity, a two-tailed (fibular head, proximal tibia) posterior lateral reconstruction is utilized combined with a posterolateral capsular shift. A 7- or 8-mm drill hole is made over a guide wire approximately 2 cm below the lateral tibial plateau. A tibialis anterior or other soft-tissue allograft is passed through this tibial drill hole and follows the course of the popliteus tendon to its anatomic insertion site on the lateral femoral epicondylar region. Nerves and blood vessels must be protected. The tibialis anterior or other soft-tissue allograft is secured with a suture anchor, and multiple number 2 braided nonabsorbable sutures at the popliteus tendon anatomic femoral insertion site. The knee is cycled through multiple sets of full flexion and extension cycles, placed in 90° of flexion, the tibia slightly internally rotated, slight valgus force applied to the knee, and the graft tensioned, and secured in the tibial tunnel with a bioabsorbable interference screw, and polyethylene ligament fixation button. The fibular-head-based reconstruction and posterolateral capsular shift procedures are then carried out as described above. Number 2 ethibond suture is used to sew the tails of the graft together proximal to the washer to prevent slipping, and also to sew the allograft to the deep capsular layers for additional reinforcement.

When local autogenous tissue is preferred for posterolateral reconstruction, we have had successful results controlling posterolateral instability types A and B using the split biceps tendon transfer [22–25, 40]. I have found that the split biceps tendon transfer is not as effective at controlling posterolateral instability type C as a fibular-head-based free graft [24, 26].

Posteromedial Reconstruction

The surgical leg positioned on the extended operating room table in a supported flexed knee position. Posteromedial and medial reconstructions are performed through a medial curved incision taking care to maintain adequate skin bridges between incisions [28, 41, 43, 44]. In acute cases, primary repair of all medial-side-injured structures is performed with suture anchors, screws, and washers, and permanent sutures through drill holes as indicated. The primary repair is then augmented with an allograft tissue reconstruction. In chronic cases of posteromedial reconstruction, the sartorius fascia is incised and retracted exposing the superficial medial collateral ligament (MCL) and the posterior medial capsule. Nerves and blood vessels are protected throughout the procedure. A longitudinal incision is made just posterior and parallel to the posterior border of the superficial MCL. Care is taken not to damage the medial meniscus during the capsular incision. Avulsed capsular structures are primarily repaired using bioabsorbable suture anchors and permanent braided number 2 ethibond sutures. The interval between the posteromedial capsule and medial meniscus is developed. The posteromedial capsule is shifted in an anterior and superior direction. The medial meniscus is repaired to the new capsular position, and the shifted capsule is sewn into the MCL using three number 2 permanent braided ethibond sutures in horizontal mattress fashion, and that suture line is reinforced using a running number 2 ethibond suture.

When superficial MCL reconstruction is indicated, this is performed using allograft tissue after completion of the primary capsular repair, and posteromedial capsular shift procedures are performed as outlined above. This graft material is attached at the anatomic insertion sites of the superficial MCL on the femur and tibia using a screw and spiked ligament washer, suture anchors, or looped around the adductor magnus tendon on the femoral side and sewn back on itself. The final graft-tensioning position is approximately 30–40° of knee flexion. It is my preference to secure the tibial insertion site first, and to perform the final tensioning and fixation of the allograft tissue on the femoral side. Number 2 ethibond suture is used to sew the tails of the graft together proximal to the washer to prevent slipping, and also to sew the allograft to the deep capsular layers for additional reinforcement.

Postoperative Rehabilitation

The knee is maintained in full extension for 3–5 weeks nonweight bearing. This initial period of immobilization is followed by progressive range of motion and progressive weight bearing. Progressive closed kinetic chain strength training, proprioceptive training, and continued motion exercises are initiated very slowly beginning at postoperative week 11. The long leg range of motion brace is discontinued after the 10th week and the patient may wear a global laxity functional brace for all activities for additional protection if necessary. Return to sports and heavy labor occurs after the 9th–12th postoperative month when sufficient strength, range of motion, and proprioceptive skills have returned [46–49]. It is very important to carefully observe these complex knee ligament injury patients, and get a feel for the "personality of the knee." The surgeon may need to make adjustments and individualize the postoperative rehabilitation program as necessary. Careful and gentle range of motion under general anesthesia is a very useful tool in the treatment of these complex cases, and is utilized as necessary. Our postoperative rehabilitation program is discussed in more detail in Chap. 25 of this book.

Posterior Cruciate Ligament Injuries in Patients 18 Years of Age and Younger

My experience with PCL injuries and multiple ligament knee injuries in children ranges from 6 to 18 years of age. These patients have varying degrees of open growth plates, and their injury mechanisms include trampoline, motorcycle, gymnastics, soccer, automobile, and farming accidents. The principles of reconstruction in the PCL-injured knee and the multiple ligament-injured knee are to identify and treat all pathology, accurate tunnel placement, anatomic graft insertion sites, utilize strong graft material, mechanical graft tensioning, secure graft fixation, and a deliberate postoperative rehabilitation program [27, 28, 41, 43–45, 49–55]. The concern in the 18 years of age and younger patient population with open growth plates is the potential for growth arrest and resultant angular deformity about the knee after surgical intervention. This risk can be decreased by insuring that no fixation devices or bone blocks cross or damage the physis during ligament reconstruction. Therefore, in patients with open physes, soft-tissue allografts without the bone plugs are used, and no fixation devices cross the physis. Patients with closed or nearly closed growth plates may be treated with the same surgical techniques as adults. Our preference is to perform single-bundle PCL reconstruction in patients with open growth plates, while single- or double-bundle PCL reconstructions have both been successful in patients with closed or nearly closed growth plates. Medial- and lateral-side reconstructions have been performed with combined primary repair, capsular shift, and allograft augmentation as indicated. The goal of each surgical technique is growth plate preservation. Results evaluated with arthrometer measurements, stress radiography, and knee ligament rating scales demonstrate results similar to those we have achieved in adult patient populations. I have had no patients with growth arrest and resultant angular deformity about the knee after surgical intervention. These severe knee injuries do occur in children, and can be a source of significant instability. Surgical reconstruction of the PCL-injured and the multiple ligament-injured knee in children using surgical techniques to preserve the growth plates results in functionally stable knees, and no growth plate arrest in my experience.

Outcomes and Results of Treatment

Combined PCL Posterolateral Reconstruction

Fanelli and Edson, in 2004, published the 2–10-year (24–120 months) results of 41 chronic arthroscopically assisted combined PCL–posterolateral reconstructions evaluated pre- and postoperatively using Lysholm, Tegner, and Hospital for Special Surgery (HSS) knee ligament rating scales, KT 1000 arthrometer testing, stress radiography, and physical examination [25]. PCL reconstructions were performed using the arthroscopically assisted single femoral tunnelsingle-bundle transtibial tunnel PCL reconstruction technique using fresh-frozen Achilles tendon allografts in all 41 cases. In all 41 cases, posterolateral instability reconstruction was performed with combined biceps femoris tendon tenodesis, and posterolateral capsular shift procedures. Postoperative physical exam revealed normal posterior drawer/tibial step off for the overall study group in 29/41 (70 %) of knees. Normal posterior drawer and tibial step offs were achieved in 91.7 % of the knees tensioned with the Biomet Sports Medicine mechanical graft tensioner. Posterolateral stability was restored to normal in 11/41 (27 %) of knees, and tighter than the normal knee in 29/41 (71 %) of knees evaluated with the external rotation thigh foot angle test. Thirty degrees varus stress testing was normal in 40/41 (97 %) of knees, and grade 1 laxity in 1/41 (3 %) of knees. Postoperative KT 1000 arthrometer testing mean side-to-side difference measurements were: 1.80 mm (PCL screen), 2.11 mm (corrected posterior), and 0.63 mm (corrected anterior). This is a statistically significant improvement from preoperative status for the PCL screen and the corrected posterior measurements ($p = 0.001$).

The postoperative stress radiographic mean side-to-side difference measurement measured at 90° of knee flexion, and 32 lb. of posterior directed force applied to the proximal tibia using the Telos device was 2.26 mm. This is a statistically significant improvement from preoperative measurements ($p=0.001$). Postoperative Lysholm, Tegner, and HSS knee ligament rating scale mean values were 91.7, 4.92, and 88.7, respectively, demonstrating a statistically significant improvement from preoperative status ($p=0.001$). The authors concluded that chronic combined PCL–posterolateral instabilities can be successfully treated with arthroscopic PCL reconstruction using fresh-frozen Achilles tendon allograft combined with posterolateral corner reconstruction using biceps tendon tenodesis combined with posterolateral capsular shift procedure. Statistically significant improvement is noted ($p=0.001$) from the preoperative condition at the 2–10-year follow-up using objective parameters of knee ligament rating scales, arthrometer testing, stress radiography, and physical examination.

Combined PCL–ACL Reconstruction Without Mechanical Graft Tensioning

Our results of multiple ligament-injured knee treatment without mechanical graft tensioning are outlined below [24]. This study presented the 2–10-year (24–120 months) results of 35 arthroscopically assisted combined ACL–PCL reconstructions evaluated pre- and postoperatively using Lysholm, Tegner, and HSS knee ligament rating scales, KT 1000 arthrometer testing, stress radiography, and physical examination.

This study population included 26 males, 9 females, 19 acute, and 16 chronic knee injuries. Ligament injuries included 19 ACL–PCL–posterolateral instabilities, 9 ACL–PCL–MCL instabilities, 6 ACL–PCL–posterolateral–MCL instabilities, and 1 ACL–PCL instability. All knees had grade III preoperative ACL–PCL laxity, and were assessed pre- and postoperatively with arthrometer testing, three different knee ligament rating scales, stress radiography, and physical examination. Arthroscopically assisted combined ACL–PCL reconstructions was performed using the single-incision endoscopic ACL technique, and the single femoral tunnel-single-bundle transtibial tunnel PCL technique. PCLs were reconstructed with allograft Achilles tendon (26 knees), autograft BTB (7 knees), and autograft semitendinosus/gracilis (2 knees). ACLs were reconstructed with autograft BTB (16 knees), allograft BTB (12 knees), Achilles tendon allograft (6 knees), and autograft semitendinosus/gracilis (1 knee). MCL injuries were treated with bracing or open reconstruction. Posterolateral instability was treated with biceps femoris tendon transfer, with or without primary repair, and posterolateral capsular shift procedures as indicated. No Biomet Sports Medicine graft-tensioning boot was used in this series of patients Biomet Sports Medicine, Warsaw, Indiana).

Postoperative physical examination results revealed normal posterior drawer/tibial step off in 16/35 (46%) of knees. Normal Lackman and pivot shift tests in 33/35 (94%) of knees. Posterolateral stability was restored to normal in 6/25 (24%) of knees, and tighter than the normal knee in 19/25 (76%) of knees evaluated with the external rotation thigh foot angle test. Thirty degrees varus stress testing was normal in 22/25 (88%) of knees, and grade 1 laxity in 3/25 (12%) of knees. Thirty degrees valgus stress testing was normal in 7/7 (100%) of surgically treated MCL tears, and normal in 7/8 (87.5%) of brace-treated knees. Postoperative KT 1000 arthrometer testing mean side-to-side difference measurements were: 2.7 mm (PCL screen), 2.6 mm (corrected posterior), and 1.0 mm (corrected anterior), a statistically significant improvement from preoperative status ($p=0.001$). Postoperative stress radiographic side-to-side difference measurements measured at 90° of knee flexion, and 32 lb. of posteriorly directed proximal force were 0–3 mm in 11/21 (52.3%), 4–5 mm in 5/21 (23.8%), and 6–10 mm in 4/21 (19%) of knees. Postoperative Lysholm, Tegner, and HSS knee ligament rating scale mean values were 91.2, 5.3, and 86.8, respectively, demonstrating a statistically significant improvement from preoperative status ($p=0.001$). No Biomet graft-tensioning boot was used in this series of patients.

The conclusions drawn from the study were that combined ACL–PCL instabilities could be successfully treated with arthroscopic reconstruction and the appropriate collateral ligament surgery. Statistically significant improvement was noted from the preoperative condition at the 2–10-year follow-up using objective parameters of knee ligament rating scales, arthrometer testing, stress radiography, and physical examination.

Combined PCL–ACL Reconstruction with Mechanical Graft Tensioning

Our results of multiple ligament-injured knee treatment using mechanical graft tensioning are outlined below [26]. These data present the 2-year follow-up of 15 arthroscopic-assisted ACL–PCL reconstructions using the Biomet graft-tensioning boot (Biomet Sports Medicine, Warsaw, Indiana). This study group consists of 11 chronic and 4 acute injuries. These injury patterns included six ACL–PCL–PLC injuries, four ACL–PCL–MCL injuries, and five ACL–PCL–PLC–MCL injuries. The Biomet graft-tensioning boot was used during the procedures as in the surgical technique described above. All knees had grade III preoperative ACL–PCL laxity, and were assessed pre- and postoperatively using Lysholm, Tegner, and HSS knee ligament rating scales, KT 1000 arthrometer testing, stress radiography, and physical examination.

Arthroscopically assisted combined ACL–PCL reconstructions was performed using the single-incision endoscopic ACL technique, and the single femoral tunnelsingle-bundle transtibial tunnel PCL technique. PCLs were reconstructed with allograft Achilles tendon in all 15 knees. ACLs were reconstructed with Achilles tendon allograft in all 15 knees. MCL injuries were treated surgically using primary repair, posteromedial capsular shift, and allograft augmentation as indicated. Posterolateral instability was treated with allograft semitendinosus free graft, with or without primary repair, and posterolateral capsular shift procedures as indicated. The Biomet graft-tensioning boot was used in this series of patients.

Postreconstruction physical examination results revealed normal posterior drawer/tibial step off in 13/15 (86.6%) of knees. Normal Lackman test in 13/15 (86.6%) knees, and normal pivot shift tests in 14/15 (93.3%) knees. Posterolateral stability was restored to normal in all knees with posterolateral instability when evaluated with the external rotation thigh foot angle test (nine knees equal to the normal knee, and two knees tighter than the normal knee). Thirty degrees varus stress testing was restored to normal in all 11 knees with posterolateral lateral instability. Thirty degrees and 0° valgus stress testing was restored to normal in all nine knees with medial-side laxity. Postoperative KT-1000 arthrometer testing mean side-to-side difference measurements were 1.6 mm (range 3–7 mm) for the PCL screen, 1.6 mm (range 4.5—9 mm) for the corrected posterior, and 0.5 mm (range 2.5–6 mm) for the corrected anterior measurements, a significant improvement from preoperative status. Postoperative stress radiographic side-to-side difference measurements measured at 90° of knee flexion, and 32 lb. of posteriorly directed proximal force using the Telos stress radiography device were 0–3 mm in 10/15 knees (66.7%), 0–4 mm in 14/15 (93.3%), 4 mm in 4/15 knees (26.7%), and 7 mm in 1/15 knees (6.67%). Postoperative Lysholm, Tegner, and HSS knee ligament rating scale mean values were 86.7 (range 69–95), 4.5 (range 2–7), and 85.3 (range 65–93), respectively, demonstrating a significant improvement from preoperative status. The study group demonstrates the efficacy and success of using a mechanical graft-tensioning device in posterior and ACL reconstruction procedures.

Double-Bundle Compared to Single-Bundle PCL Reconstruction

Our comparison of single- and double-bundle PCL reconstruction in the PCL based multiple ligament-injured knee using allograft tissue revealed the following [29]. Ninety consecutive arthroscopic transtibial PCL reconstructions were performed by a single surgeon (GCF). Forty-five single- and double-bundle reconstructions were performed using fresh-frozen Achilles tendon allograft for the anterolateral bundle, and tibialis anterior allograft for the posteromedial bundle. Postoperative comparative results were assessed using Telos stress radiography, KT 1000, Lysholm, Tegner, and HSS knee ligament rating scales. Postoperative period ranged from 15 to 72 months.

Three groups of data were analyzed: Single- and double-bundle all; single- and double-bundle PCL collateral; and single- and double-bundle PCL–ACL collateral.

Mean postoperative side-to-side difference values for Telos, KT PCL screen, and KT-corrected posterior and KT-corrected anterior measurements for the overall single-bundle group in millimeters were 2.56, 1.91, 2.11, and 0.23, respectively. Mean postoperative side-to-side difference values for Telos, KT PCL screen, and KT-corrected posterior and KT-corrected anterior measurements for the overall double-bundle group in millimeters were 2.36, 2.46, 2.94, and 0.15, respectively. Mean postoperative values for Tegner, Lysholm, and HSS knee ligament rating scales for the single-bundle group was 5.0, 90.3, and 86.2, respectively. Mean postoperative values for Tegner, Lysholm, and HSS knee ligament rating scales for the double-bundle group was 4.6, 87.6, and 83.3, respectively.

Mean postoperative side-to-side difference values for Telos, KT PCL screen, and KT-corrected posterior and KT-corrected anterior measurements for the PCL-collateral single-bundle group in millimeters were 2.59, 1.63, 2.03, and 0.25, respectively. Mean postoperative side-to-side difference values for Telos, KT PCL screen, and KT-corrected posterior and KT-corrected anterior measurements for the PCL-collateral double-bundle group in millimeters were 1.85, 2.03, 2.83, and −0.17, respectively. Mean postoperative values for Tegner, Lysholm, and HSS knee ligament rating scales for the single-bundle PCL-collateral group was 5.4, 90.9, and 87.7, respectively. Mean postoperative values for Tegner, Lysholm, and HSS knee ligament rating scales for the double-bundle PCL-collateral group was 4.9, 89.0, and 86.5, respectively.

Mean postoperative side-to-side difference values for Telos, KT PCL screen, and KT-corrected posterior and KT-corrected anterior measurements for the PCL–ACL-collateral single-bundle group in millimeters were 2.53, 2.19, 2.19, and 0.22, respectively. Mean postoperative side-to-side difference values for Telos, KT PCL screen, and KT-corrected posterior and KT-corrected anterior measurements for the PCL–ACL-collateral double-bundle group in millimeters were 3.16, 2.86, 3.09, and 0.41, respectively. Mean postoperative values for Tegner, Lysholm, and HSS knee ligament rating scales for the PCL–ACL-collateral single-bundle group was 4.7, 89.6, and 84.6, respectively. Mean postoperative values for Tegner, Lysholm, and HSS knee ligament rating scales for the PCL–ACL-collateral double-bundle group was 4.3, 86.0, and 79.4, respectively. There was no statistically significant difference between the single- and the double-bundle PCL reconstruction in any of the groups compared ($p > 0.05$).

Return to preinjury level of activity was evaluated between the single- and double-bundle PCL reconstruction groups. The bicruciate single-bundle reconstruction group return to pre-injury level of activity was 73.3 %, and the bicruciate double-bundle reconstruction group return to pre-injury level of activity was 84.0 %. There was no statistically significant difference ($p = 0.572$) between the single- and double-bundle group in the PCL-based multiple ligament-injured knee. Both single- and double-bundle arthroscopic transtibial tunnel PCL reconstructions provide excellent results in these complex multiple ligament-injured knee instability patterns. Our results did not indicate that one PCL reconstruction surgical procedure was clearly superior to the other.

PCL Reconstruction in Knees with Global Laxity with 2–18-Year Follow-Up

Our 2–18-year postsurgical results in combined PCL, ACL, medial- and lateral-side knee injuries (global laxity) revealed the following information [30]. Forty combined PCL–ACL-lateral–medial-side (global laxity reconstructions were performed by a single surgeon (GCF). Twenty-eight of 40 were available for the 2–18-year follow-up (70 % follow-up rate). The patients were evaluated postoperatively with three different knee ligament rating scales for physical examination and functional capacity (Hospital for Special Surgery, Lysholm, Tegner). Static stability was assessed postoperatively comparing the normal to the injured knee using the KT 1000 knee ligament arthrometer (PCL screen, corrected posterior, corrected anterior, and 30° posterior to anterior translation), and stress radiography at 90° of flexion to assess PCL static stability using the Telos device. All measurements are reported as a side-to-side difference in millimeters comparing the normal to the injured knee. Range of motion, varus and valgus stability, and axial rotation stability of the tibia relative to the femur using the dial test are reported comparing the injured to the normal knee. Incidence of degenerative joint disease and return to pre-injury level of function are also reported.

Knee ligament rating scale mean scores were: HSS 79.3/100 (range 56–95), Lysholm 83.8/100 (range 58–100), and Tegner 4/10 (range 2–9). KT 1000 mean side-to-side difference measurements in millimeters were: PCL screen at 90° of knee flexion 2.02 mm (range 0–7 mm), corrected posterior at 70° of knee flexion 2.48 mm (range 0–9 mm), corrected anterior at 70° of knee flexion 0.28 mm (range −3 to 7 mm), and the 30° of knee flexion posterior to anterior translation 1.0 mm (range −6 to 6 mm). Telos stress radiography at 90° of knee flexion with a posterior displacement force applied to the area of the tibial tubercle mean side-to-side difference measurements in millimeters were 2.35 mm (range—2 to 8 mm).

Range of motion side-to-side difference mean flexion loss comparing the normal to the injured knee was 14.0° (range 0–38°). There were no flexion contractures. Varus and valgus stability were evaluated on physical examination at hyperextension, zero, and 30° of knee flexion comparing the injured to the normal knee. Symmetrical varus stability was achieved in 93.3 % of knees, and symmetrical valgus stability was achieved in 92.6 % of knees. The dial test performed at 30° of knee flexion to evaluate axial rotation posterolateral stability comparing the injured to the normal knee was symmetrical in 85.2 %, tighter than the normal knee (less external rotation) in 11.1 %, and more lax (greater external rotation) in 3.7 % of knees. Thus, posterior lateral axial rotation instability was corrected or over corrected in 96.3 % of knees.

Radiographic posttraumatic degenerative joint disease occurred in 29.6 % of injured knees. No degenerative joint disease was found in 70.4 % of the injured knees. Postoperatively, patients were able to return to their pre-injury level of activity in 59.3 % of cases, and returned to decreased level of postoperative activity in 40.7 % of cases.

Summary

The goals leading to successful PCL reconstruction surgery include identification and treatment of associated pathology such as posterolateral instability, posteromedial instability, and lower extremity malalignment. The use of strong graft material, properly placed tunnels to approximate the PCL insertion sites, and minimization of graft bending also enhances the probability of PCL reconstruction success. In addition, mechanical graft tensioning, primary and back-up PCL graft fixation, and the appropriate postoperative rehabilitation program are also necessary ingredients for the PCL reconstruction success. Both single- and double-bundle PCL reconstruction surgical techniques are successful when evaluated with stress radiography, KT 1000 arthrometer measurements, and knee ligament rating scales. Indications for double-bundle PCL reconstruction as of this writing include severe hyperextension of the knee and revision PCL reconstruction.

The multiple ligament-injured knee is a severe injury subgroup of PCL injuries that may also involve neurovascular injuries, fractures, skin compromise, and other systemic injuries. Abnormal pulses and/or an ankle-brachial index less than 0.9 indicate the need for more advanced vascular evaluation or intervention. Correct diagnosis of the multiple planes of instability is essential to maximize successful surgical results. The severity of the medial- and lateral-side injuries determines whether the procedure will be done arthroscopically, open, single stage, or in two stages.

Selective external fixation for preoperative and postoperative control of the injured extremity may be used if control of the injured knee cannot be maintained with bracing. Surgical timing in acute multiple ligament-injured knee cases depends upon the ligaments injured, injured extremity vascular status, skin condition of the extremity, degree of instability, and the patients overall health. Delayed reconstruction of 2–3 weeks may decrease the incidence of arthrofibrosis. It is important to address all components of the instability. Surgical treatment, in my experience, offers good functional results documented in the literature by physical examination, arthrometer testing, stress radiography, and knee ligament rating scales. Some low-grade MCL complex injuries may be amenable to brace treatment, while high-grade medial-side injuries require repair reconstruction. Lateral posterolateral injuries are most successfully treated with surgical repair reconstruction. Allograft tissue is my preference for these complex surgical procedures. A slow, deliberately progressive postoperative rehabilitation program is utilized to avoid overloading healing tissues.

PCL and multiple knee ligament injuries also occur in children with open growth plates. Surgical reconstruction of the PCL-injured and the multiple ligament-injured knee in children using surgical techniques to preserve the growth plates results in functionally stable knees, and no growth plate arrest in my experience.

References

1. Fanelli GC. PCL injuries in trauma patients. Arthroscopy. 1993;9:291–4.
2. Fanelli GC, Edson CJ. PCL injuries in trauma patients, part II. Arthroscopy. 1995;11:526–9.
3. Fanelli GC. The multiple ligament injured knee: what I have learned. In: Fanelli GC, editor. The multiple ligament injured knee. A practical guide to management. 2nd ed. New York: Springer; 2013. pp. 3–14.
4. Lysholm J, Gillquist J. Arthroscopic examination of the posterior cruciate ligament. J Bone Joint Surg. 1981;63A:363–6.
5. Fanelli GC, Giannotti B, Edson CJ. Current concepts review. The posterior cruciate ligament: arthroscopic evaluation and treatment. Arthroscopy. 1994 Dec;10(6):673–88.
6. Fanelli GC. Arthroscopic evaluation of the PCL. In: Fanelli GC, editor. Posterior cruciate ligament injuries. A practical guide to management. New York: Springer; 2001. pp. 95–105.
7. Hughston JC, Baker CL, Norwood LA. Acute combined posterior cruciate and posterolateral instability of the knee. Am J Sports Med. 1983;12:204–8.
8. Clancy WG, Shelbourne KD, Zoellner GB, Keene JS, Reider B, Rosenberg TD. Treatment of knee joint instability secondary to rupture of the posterior cruciate ligament. Report of a new procedure. J Bone Joint Surg. 1983;65A:310–22.
9. Clancy WG. Repair and reconstruction of the posterior cruciate ligament. In: Chapman M, editor. Operative orthopaedics. Philadelphia: JB Lippincott; 1988. pp. 1651–65.
10. Fanelli GC, Feldman DD. Management of combined anterior cruciate ligament/posterior cruciate ligament/posterolateral complex injuries of the knee. Oper Tech Sports Med. 1999;7(3):143–9.
11. Fanelli GC, Harris JD. Late MCL (medial collateral ligament) reconstruction. Tech Knee Surg. 2007;6(2):99–105.
12. Fanelli GC, Harris JD. Surgical treatment of acute medial collateral ligament and posteromedial corner injuries of the knee. Sports Med Arthrosc Rev. 2006 May;14(2):78–83.
13. LaPrade RF. Arthroscopic evaluation of the lateral compartment of knees with grade 3 posterolateral knee complex injuries. Am J Sports Med. 1997;25(5):596–602.
14. Green NE, Allen BL. Vascular injuries associated with dislocation of the knee. J Bone Joint Surg. 1977;59A:236–9.
15. Welling RE, Kakkasseril J, Cranley JJ. Complete dislocations of the knee with popliteal vascular injury. J Trauma. 1981;21(6):450–3.
16. Wascher DC, Dvirnik PC, Decoster TA. Knee dislocation: Initial assessment and implications for treatment. J Orthop Trauma. 1997;11:525–9.
17. Kennedy JC. Complete dislocations of the knee joint. J Bone Joint Surg. 1963;45:889–904.
18. Mills WJ, Barei DP, McNair P. The value of the ankle-brachial index for diagnosing arterial injury after knee dislocation: a prospective study. J Trauma. 2004;56(6):1261–5.
19. Stuart MJ. Evaluation and treatment principles of knee dislocations. Oper Tech Sports Med. 2001;9(2):91–5.
20. Levy B, Fanelli GC, Whalen D, Stannard J, MacDonald P, Boyd J, Marx R, Stuart M. Modern perspectives for the treatment of knee dislocations and multiligament reconstruction. J Am Acad Orthop Surg. 2009 April;17(4):197–206.
21. Stannard JP. Stabilization of knee dislocations using a hinged external fixator: a prospective randomized study. In: Proceedings of the 73rd annual meeting of the American Academy of Orthopaedic Surgeons; 2006. Chicago, IL.
22. Fanelli GC, Gianotti BF, Edson CJ. Arthroscopically assisted combined posterior cruciate ligament/posterior lateral complex reconstruction. Arthroscopy. 1996;12(5):521–30.
23. Fanelli GC, Gianotti BF, Edson CJ. Arthroscopically assisted combined anterior and posterior cruciate ligament reconstruction. Arthroscopy. 1996;12(1):5–14.
24. Fanelli GC, Edson CJ. Arthroscopically assisted combined ACL/PCL reconstruction. 2–10 year follow-up. Arthroscopy. 2002;18(7):703–14.
25. Fanelli GC, Edson CJ. Combined posterior cruciate ligament–posterolateral reconstruction with Achilles tendon allograft and biceps femoris tendon tenodesis: 2–10 year follow-up. Arthroscopy. 2004;20(4):339–45.
26. Fanelli GC, et al. Treatment of combined anterior cruciate-posterior cruciate ligament-medial-lateral side knee injuries. J Knee Surg. 2005;18(3):240–8.
27. Fanelli GC, Beck JD, Edson CJ. Double bundle posterior cruciate ligament reconstruction. Surgical technique and results. Sports Med Arthrosc Rev. 2010;18(4):242–8.
28. Fanelli GC, Beck JD, Edson CJ. Combined PCL ACL lateral and medial side injuries: treatment and results. Sports Med Arthrosc Rev. 2011;19(2):120–30.
29. Fanelli GC, Beck JD, Edson CJ. Single compared to double bundle PCL reconstruction using allograft tissue. J Knee Surg. 2012;25(1):59–64.
30. Fanelli GC, Edson CJ. Surgical treatment of combined PCL, ACL, medial, and lateral side injuries (global laxity): surgical technique and 2–18 year results. J Knee Surg. 2012;25(4):307–16.
31. Fanelli GC, Sousa P, Edson CJ. Long term follow-up of surgically treated knee dislocations: stability restored, but arthritis is common. Clin Orthop Relat Res. 2014;472(9):2712–7.
32. Fanelli GC, Orcutt DR, Edson CJ. The multiple-ligament injured knee: evaluation, treatment, and results. Arthroscopy. 2005;21(4):471–86.

33. Fanelli GC, Beck JD, Edson CJ. How I manage the multiple ligament injured (dislocated) knee. Oper Tech Sports Med. 2010 Dec;18(4):198–210.
34. Wascher DC. High-velocity knee dislocation with vascular injury. Treatment principles. Clin Sports Med. 2000;19(3):457–77.
35. Mook WR, Miller MD, Diduch DR, Hertel J, Boachie-Adjei Y, Hart JM. Multiple-ligament knee injuries: a systematic review of the timing of operative intervention and postoperative rehabilitation. J Bone Joint Surg. 2009;91(12):2946–57.
36. Stannard JP, et al. The posterolateral corner of the knee: repair versus reconstruction. Am J Sports Med. 2005;33(6):881–8.
37. Levy BA, Dajani KA, Morgan JA, Shah JP, Dahm DL, Stuart MJ. Repair versus reconstruction of the fibular collateral ligament and posterolateral corner in the multiligament-injured knee. Am J Sports Med. 2010;38(4):804–9.
38. Levy BA, Dahm DL, Herrera DA, MacDonald PB, Dajani KA, Stuart MJ. Acute repair of posteromedial and posterolateral corners in multiligament knee injury is not indicated. Presented at the 27th Annual Meeting of the Arthroscopy Association of North America, Washington, DC, April 24–27; 2008.
39. Fanelli GC, Fanelli DG, Edson CJ, Fanelli MG. Combined anterior cruciate ligament and posterolateral reconstruction of the knee using allograft tissue in chronic knee injuries. J Knee Surg. 2014;27(5):353–8.
40. Fanelli GC, Fanelli DG. Fibular head based posterolateral reconstruction of the knee combined with capsular shift procedure. Sports Med Arthrosc Rev. In press.
41. Fanelli GC. Rationale and surgical technique for PCL and multiple knee ligament reconstruction. 3rd ed. Warsaw: Biomet Sports Medicine; 2012.
42. Noyes FR, Barber-Westin SD. Posterior cruciate ligament revision reconstruction, part 1. Causes of surgical failure in 52 consecutive operations. Am J Sports Med. 2005;33(5):646–54.
43. Fanelli GC. The multiple ligament injured knee: what I have learned. In: Fanelli GC, editor. The multiple ligament injured knee. A practical guide to management. 2nd ed. New York: Springer; 2013. pp. 3–14.
44. Fanelli GC. Surgical treatment of combined PCL ACL medial and lateral side injuries (global laxity): acute and chronic. In: Fanelli GC, editor. The multiple ligament injured knee. A practical guide to management. 2nd ed. New York: Springer; 2013. pp. 281–301.
45. Fanelli GC. Mechanical graft tensioning in multiple ligament knee surgery. In: Fanelli GC, editor. The multiple ligament injured knee. A practical guide to management. 2nd ed. New York: Springer; 2013. pp. 323–30.
46. Edson CJ, Fanelli GC, Beck JD. Postoperative rehabilitation of the posterior cruciate ligament. Sports Med Arthrosc Rev. 2010;18(4):275–9.
47. Edson CJ, Fanelli GC, Beck JD. Rehabilitation after multiple ligament reconstruction of the knee. Sports Med Arthrosc Rev. 2011;19(2):162–6.
48. Edson CJ, Fanelli GC. Postoperative rehabilitation of the multiple ligament injured knee. In: Fanelli GC, editor. The multiple ligament injured knee. A practical guide to management. 2nd ed. New York: Springer; 2013. pp. 437–42.
49. Fanelli GC, Feldmann DD. Arthroscopically assisted combined anterior cruciate ligament/posterior cruciate ligament reconstruction. In: Fanelli GC, editor. Posterior cruciate ligament injuries: a practical guide to management. New York: Springer; 2001. pp. 215–36.
50. Fanelli GC. Arthroscopic PCL reconstruction: transtibial technique. In: Fanelli GC, editor. Posterior cruciate ligament injuries. A guide to practical management. New York: Springer; 2001. pp. 141–56.
51. Fanelli GC. Combined ACL PCL medial lateral side injuries of the knee. In: Fanelli GC, editor. The multiple ligament injured knee. A practical guide to management. New York: Springer; 2004. pp. 111–31.
52. Fanelli GC, Edson CJ, Reinheimer KN. Evaluation and treatment of the multiple ligament injured knee. Am Acad Orthop Surg Instr Course Lect. 2009;58:389–95.
53. Levy B, Dajani KA, Whalen DB, Stannard JP, Fanelli GC, Stuart MJ, Boyd JL, MacDonald PA, Marx RG. Decision making in the multiple ligament injured knee: an evidence based systematic review. Arthroscopy. 2009 April;25(4):430–8.
54. Levy B, Fanelli GC, Whalen D, Stannard J, MacDonald P, Boyd J, Marx R, Stuart M. Modern perspectives for the treatment of knee dislocations and multiligament reconstruction. J Am Acad Orthop Surg. 2009 April;17(4):197–206.
55. Fanelli GC, Stannard JP, Stuart MJ, MacDonald PB, Marx RG, Whelan DB, Boyd JL, Levy BA. Management of complex knee ligament injuries. J Bone Joint Surg. 2010 Sept 15;92-A(12):2235–46.

Recommended Reading

56. Fanelli GC, editor. Posterior cruciate ligament injuries: a practical guide to management. New York: Springer; 2001.
57. Fanelli GC, editor. The multiple ligament injured knee. A practical guide to management. New York: Springer; 2004.
58. Fanelli GC, editor. The multiple ligament injured knee. A practical guide to management. 2nd ed. New York: Springer; 2013.

Part II

Anatomy and Biomechanics

Anatomy and Biomechanics of the Posterior Cruciate Ligament and Their Surgical Implications

2

Christopher G. Stevens, Keith Jarbo, Kostas Economopoulos and Anikar Chhabra

Anatomy

The knowledge and understanding of the complex anatomy and biomechanical function of the native posterior cruciate ligament (PCL) is vitally important when evaluating PCL injury and possible reconstruction. Many studies have been performed looking specifically at the PCL and its unique relationships to the surrounding structures in the knee. The first section of this chapter serves as a foundation for understanding the complex origin and insertional anatomy, the relationships of the distinct bundles of the PCL within the knee, as well as detailing the neurovascular anatomy as it pertains to the PCL. Advanced imaging of the PCL is also covered in detail.

Gross Anatomy

The PCL is the largest of the intraarticular ligaments and travels from the lateral aspect of the medial femoral condyle to the posterior tibia. The PCL plays an integral role in knee joint stability. The PCL is named due to its insertion on the posterior aspect of the proximal tibia. The PCL originates from a broad, concave, semicircular area along the medial femoral condyle within the intracondylar notch. The PCL inserts into a depression just inferior to joint line, between the two tibial plateaus, and posterior to the tibial spine (Figs. 2.1 and 2.2). This depression is known as the posterior intercondyloid fossa or PCL fossa [1]. The PCL consists of longitudinally oriented collagen fibers which is narrowest in its middle portion and fans out superiorly and to a lesser extent inferiorly [2]. The fibers of the PCL attach to the femoral footprint in a lateral to medial orientation and to the tibial footprint in an anterior to posterior orientation. The average length of the PCL as measured in 44 cadaver knees was 38 mm and the average width within the middle portion was 11 mm [2, 3]. The range of PCL width measurements was higher than that of the PCL length measurements due to variation in intercondylar notch size. Utilizing comparative data from anatomic dissection with radiologic correlation, an Austrian group obtained geometric anatomic data characterizing the dimensions of the anterolateral and posteromedial bundles and their footprints. Using 15 cadaver specimens, they found the overall average length and diameter of the PCL was 37 and 11 mm, respectively [4].

The PCL has a wide variation in shape and size of its femoral attachments, whereas the tibial attachments size and shape are more consistent [5]. The substance of the ligament is made up of two distinct but inseparable bundles that allow for resistance of posterior translation in both extension and flexion. The bundles are named by their position within the femoral footprint/attachment: anterolateral bundle and posteromedial bundle (Fig. 2.3).To help identify these bundles during dissection or arthroscopy, other anatomical landmarks have been identified.

On the femoral side, the medial intercondylar ridge defines the proximal limit of the insertion of the PCL, whereas the medial bifurcate ridge separates the insertion sites of the two bundles (Figs. 2.4 and 2.5) [6]. There is a change in slope as each bundle approaches the femoral insertion site, putting the bundles in different planes when the knee is flexed. The PCL footprint on the femur is made up of approximately

A. Chhabra (✉)
The Orthopedic Clinic Association, PC, 2222 E. Highland Ave., #300, Phoenix, AZ 85016, USA
e-mail: phoenixsportsdoc@hotmail.com

Orthopedics Sports Medicine, Banner Good Samaritan Orthopedic Residency, Phoenix, AZ, USA

Orthopedic Surgery, Arizona State University, Phoenix, AZ, USA

C. G. Stevens
Orthopaedic Sports Medicine, Orthopaedic Surgery, Banner Good Samaritan Medical Center, Phoenix, AZ, USA

K. Jarbo
Orthopaedic Surgery, Banner Good Samaritan Medical Center, Phoenix, AZ, USA

K. Economopoulos
The Orthopedic Clinic Association, PC
Phoenix, AZ, USA

G. C. Fanelli (ed.), *Posterior Cruciate Ligament Injuries*,
DOI 10.1007/978-3-319-12072-0_2, © Springer International Publishing Switzerland 2015

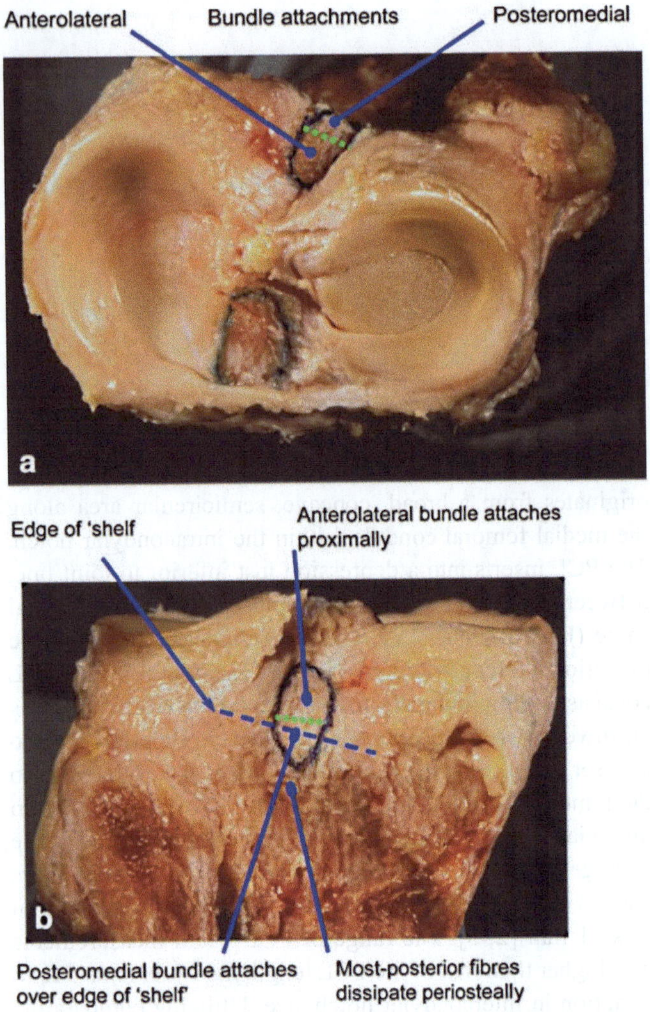

Fig. 2.1 **a** Posterior–anterior view of tibial plateau with PCL attachment marked. Note how the attachment area passes 'over the back. **b** Proximal-distal view of tibial plateau with PCL attachment marked [62]. *PCL* posterior cruciate ligament

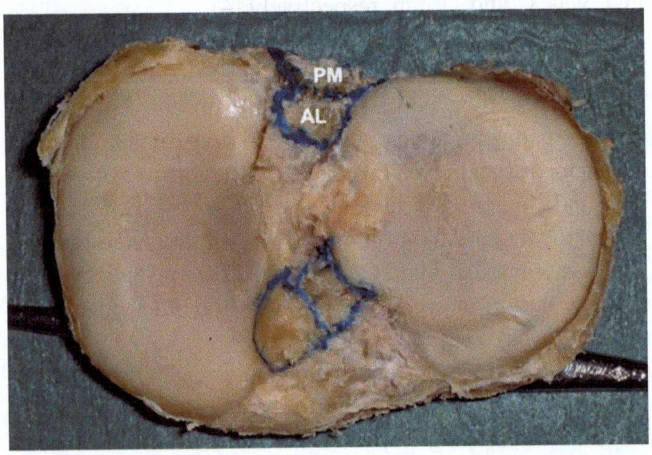

Fig. 2.2 Tibial footprints of the insertions of anterolateral (AL) and posteromedial (PM) bundles of the PCL [63]. *PCL* posterior cruciate ligament

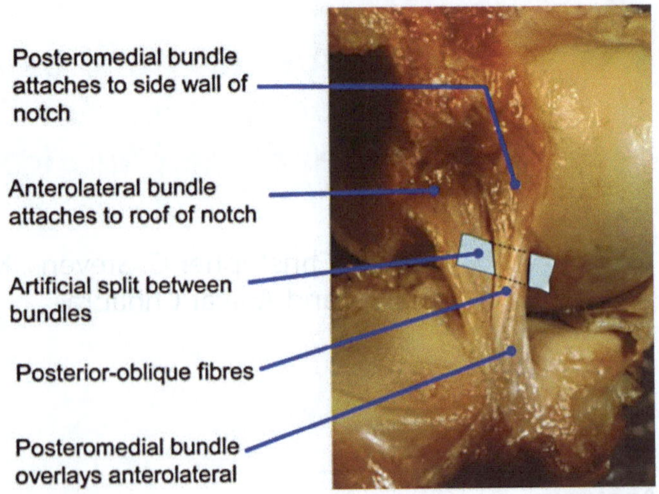

Fig. 2.3 The PCL fibers have been separated into the ALB and the PMB. Posterolateral view of left knee after removal of the lateral femoral condyle [62]. *PCL* posterior cruciate ligament, ALB anterolateral bundle, PMB posteromedial bundle

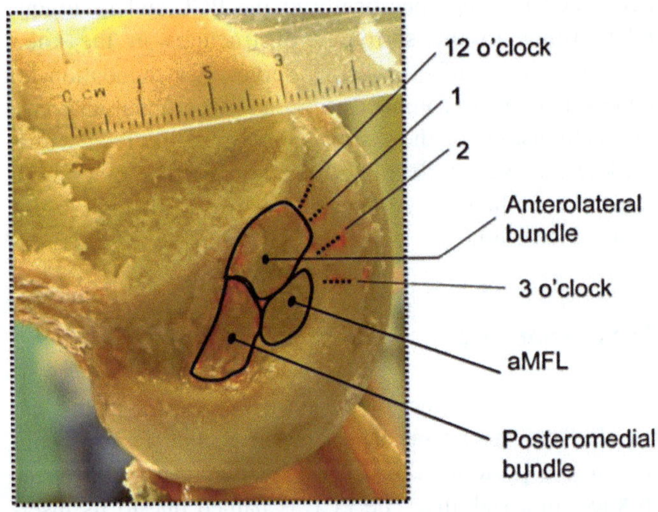

Fig. 2.4 The femoral attachment of the PCL. Lateral–medial view in a left knee after removal of the lateral femoral condyle. The anterolateral and posteromedial bundles of the PCL, plus anterior meniscofemoral ligament attachments are outlined [62]. PCL posterior cruciate ligament

55 % anterolateral bundle and 45 % posteromedial bundle. The mean distance between the centers of the anterolateral and posteromedial bundles on the femur is 12.1 mm. The distal margins of the anterolateral and posteromedial bundles are a mean 1.5 and 5.8 mm proximal to the notch articular cartilage, respectively [7]. While the femoral footprint size is nearly equal between the two bundles (Fig. 2.6), the anterolateral bundle's crosssectional area is significantly larger than the posteromedial bundle. The anterolateral bundle is the major contributor to PCL strength.

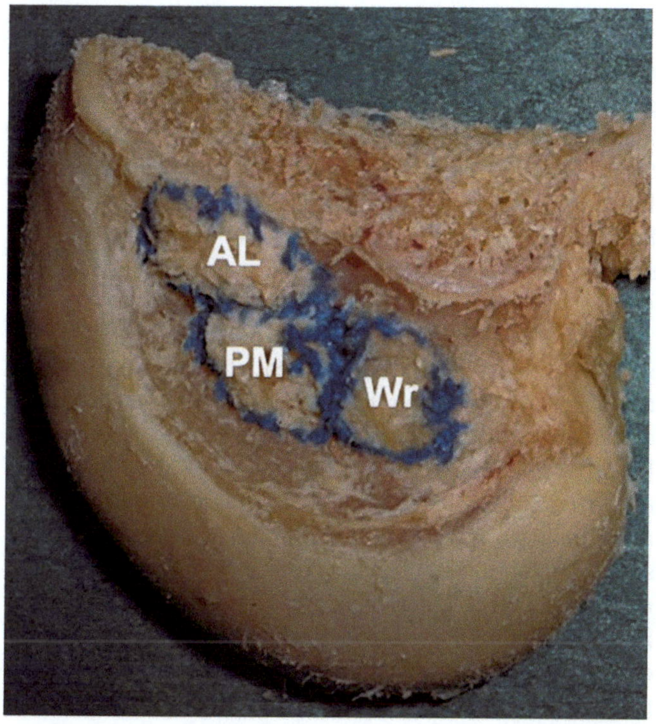

Fig. 2.5. Femoral footprints of the insertions of anterolateral (AL), posteromedial (PM) bundles of the PCL, and Wrisberg ligament (Wr) [63]. *PCL* posterior cruciate ligament

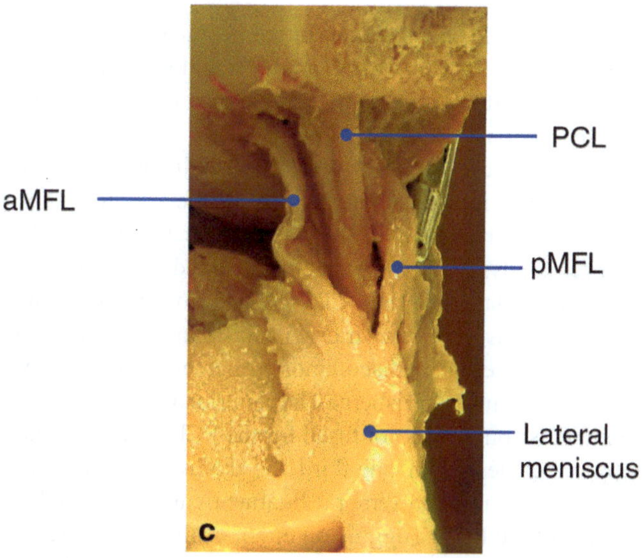

Fig. 2.7 Posterior view of knee showing the PCL attachment on the tibia and accessory ligaments located posteriorly [65]. *PCL* posterior cruciate ligament

The tibial insertions of the anterolateral and posteromedial bundle occur within the PCL fossa which is trapezoidal in shape and becomes wider inferiorly. The anterolateral bundle is attached at the superolateral aspect of the footprint and the posteromedial bundles are seen in the inferomedial portion of the fossa. The identification of each bundle is made easier with each bundle attachment having separate slopes. Across 21 knees, this change in slope angle was found to be an average of 14.5°. Also, an extensive portion of the posteromedial bundle is below the posterior part of the tibial rim, whereas none of the anterolateral bundle attachment is below the tibial rim. The superolateral and superomedial corners of the footprint were both represented by depressions and a reproducible ridge represented the inferior border, all of which could be identified with arthroscopy [8].

Johannsen et al. analyzed the posterior root attachments of the medial and lateral menisci, quantifying their position in relation to the PCL (Fig. 2.7). The lateral meniscus posterior root attachment center was 4.3 mm medial to the lateral tibial plateau articular cartilage edge and directly 12.7 mm to the most anterior edge of the PCL tibial attachment. The medial meniscus posterior root attachment center was 9.6 mm posterior and 0.7 mm lateral from the medial

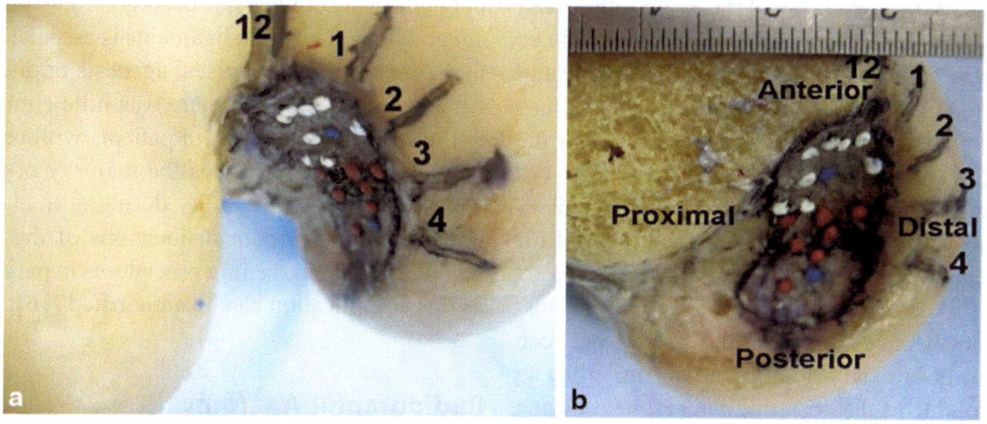

Fig. 2.6. **a** Positions of the anterolateral bundles (*white*) and the posteromedial bundles (*red*) and the anatomical centers of the two bundles of the PCL (*blue*) when viewed from anterior to lateral direction into the intercondylar notch in the knee flexed to 90°. **b** Positions of the anterolateral bundles (*white*) and the posteromedial bundles (*red*) and the anatomical centers of the two bundles of the PCL (*blue*) as seen in the sagittal section to view the medial femoral condyle [64]. *PCL* posterior cruciate ligament

tibial eminence, and 8.2 mm anteromedial from the PCL. This anatomy is very important during PCL reconstruction as nonanatomic tunnel placement may compromise the meniscal root attachment.

The meniscofemoral ligaments are two distinct structures with variable incidence that run from the posterior horn of the lateral meniscus to the lateral aspect of the medial femoral condyle. The ligaments are named based on their location in relation to the PCL. The anterior meniscofemoral ligament is also known as the ligament of Humphrey, while the posterior meniscofemoral ligament is also known as the ligament of Wrisberg. The anterior meniscofemoral ligament is sometimes confused for the PCL during arthroscopy, albeit less than one-third the diameter of the PCL. The posterior meniscofemoral ligament can be nearly half the size of the PCL. Tugging on either of the meniscofemoral ligaments should reveal obvious motion of the lateral meniscus and thus will help you to identify it from the PCL. Multiple research studies looking at cadaver knees found the presence of either the anterior or posterior meniscofemoral ligaments in ~70% of the time. Anderson et al. found that in those knees where both meniscofemoral ligaments were present, the posterior meniscofemoral ligament, posteromedial bundle, and anterior meniscofemoral ligament were aligned parallel to each other, proximally to distally [7]. The posterior meniscofemoral ligament is located directly proximal to the medial intercondylar ridge, proximal to the posteromedial bundle. There are no attachments from the PCL to the medial meniscus.

The posterior joint capsule runs in near continuation with the PCL. The posterior joint capsule originates above the femoral condyles and extends distally to the posterior margin of the tibial plateau. The posterior capsule is within 1–2 mm of the posterior aspect of the tibial attachment of the PCL. The anterior wall of the popliteal artery lies approximately 7–10 mm from the posterior border of the PCL at 90° of flexion [3]. Matava et al. found the distance between the PCL and popliteal artery was maximal at 100° of knee flexion, with measurements of 9.9 mm in the axial plane and 9.3 mm in the sagittal plane, using magnetic resonance imaging (MRI) [9]. There is an anterior septum between the capsule and PCL that is made up of fatty tissue wrapped in a thin synovial membrane which creases a triangular thickening. In the upper third of this tissue is the entry point for the bundle of the middle genicular artery, above the oblique popliteal ligament. Ahn et al. advocate for release of the posterior capsule. They believe it increases the distance between the insertion of the PCL and the popliteal artery, providing an increase in the volume of the posterior compartment during arthroscopy through expansion of this septal tissue. Greater posterior compartment volume enables better viewing of the insertion of the PCL and lowers the risk of neurovascular complication [10].

The blood supply to the PCL comes from the middle genicular artery, a branch of the popliteal artery. The middle genicular artery shows variations in its origin off the popliteal artery. The thin synovial sheath vessels that surround the cruciate ligaments are also seen in the fat pad have been found to be major contributors. These end arteries appear to branch from the middle genicular artery [11]. Capsular vessels supply distal portions of the PCL via branches from the inferior genicular and popliteal arteries [12].

Nerve fibers from the popliteal plexus supply the PCL and its synovial sleeve. The popliteal plexus is derived from the posterior articular nerve and the terminal branches of the obturator nerve [13]. The posterior articular nerve branches from the tibial nerve. A histologic study of mechanoreceptors performed by Katonis et al. observed three types of nerve endings in the PCL: Ruffini corpuscles (type I, pressure receptors), Vater–Pacini corpuscles (type II, velocity receptors), and free nerve endings (type IV, pain receptors) [14]. Golgi tendon organlike structures are found in the PCL origins beneath the synovial sheath and likely play a role in proprioceptive function in the knee [13]. Thus, injury to the PCL creates not only a mechanical disturbance but also a neurologic one by severing the afferent signals to the central nervous system [1].

Congenital deficiency of the PCL is described in association with various congenital longitudinal deficiencies of the lower limb. Albeit rare, PCL deficiency is often seen in conjunction with ACL deficiency. Congenital absence of the cruciate ligaments can result in anterior or posterior dislocation, specifically when undergoing surgery for leg length discrepancy. It is not uncommon for these patients to complain of retropatellar pain as they lock the knee in extension to help provide stability during gait increasing patellofemoral pressure during ambulation [15]. Arthroscopy of these patients often finds a shallow, hypoplastic intercondylar notch, poorly developed or absent tibial spines, and in some, fibular hypoplasia. There has not been good evidence to show that agenesis of the cruciate ligaments is associated with changes in the menisci (i.e., meniscal agenesis or discoid meniscus). Chomiak et al. reported there was little clinical significance to the cruciate deficiency in patients with proximal femoral focal deficiency (PFFD) as the majority of patients did not complain of knee instability during normal daily activities. Prevention of posterior dislocations of the knee is recommended in all lengthening procedures in patients with PFFD, as this complication can be anticipated [16].

Radiographic Anatomy

MRI is widely used to image internal derangements of the knee. To obtain good quality images, an appropriately sized field of view should be used to maximize the resolution. The

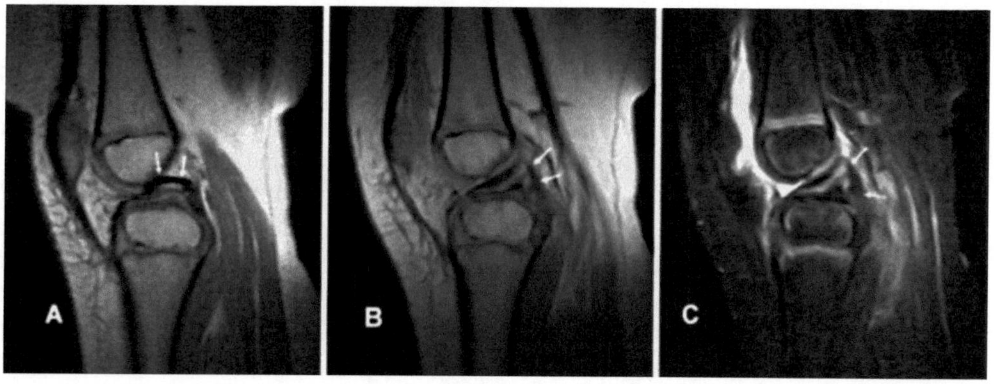

Fig. 2.8 **a** Normal PCL (*arrows*) in the left knee on TSE PD sagittal MR image (TR/TE 1840/21 ms). **b** TSE PD (TR/TE 1840/21 ms) and **c** fat-suppressed TSE T2-weighted sagittal MR images (TR/TE 4430/27, TI 90 ms) shows a thickened, poorly defined PCL with abnormal internal high signal intensity (*arrows*) [66]. PCL posterior cruciate ligament, TSE PD turbo spin-echo proton density

knee should be imaged in three orthogonal planes: axial, coronal, and sagittal planes (Fig. 2.8). On sagittal T2-weighted images, the normal PCL appears as a well-defined uniform band of very low signal intensity. When the knee is in extension, the PCL is lax and it has a gentle posterior convex curvature (Fig. 2.9). The PCL should be found near the midline of the joint in at least 2–3 consecutive images. The meniscofemoral ligaments can often be seen as a small round or oval structure of low signal intensity just anterior or posterior to the PCL. On coronal images, the posterior vertical portion of the PCL is seen in the intercondylar notch, adjacent to the lateral aspect of the medial femoral condyle. The ligament curves forward anteriorly and the horizontal portion appears as a circular or ovoid area of low signal intensity within the intercondylar notch. Axial images are useful in visualizing the vertical portion of the PCL from its tibial insertion [15]. Coronal and axial images can be complementary in the evaluation of the femoral and tibial attachments of the PCL.

The majority of PCL tears are associated with other injuries due to the high level of force necessary to tear the strong PCL fibers. Tears occur most frequently at the middle portion of the PCL. Uncommonly, the PCL may avulse from its tibial attachment. Injuries are best evaluated using sagittal T2-weighted images. A normal intact PCL is a well-defined continuous band of low signal intensity in all pulse sequences. In a complete tear of the PCL, the fibers are discontinuous, with high-intensity fluid signal completely traversing the fibers (Fig. 2.10). Amorphous high signal intensity would also be seen on T1-weighted imaging. In a partial tear, the PCL is thickened, with an increased signal (Fig. 2.11). Avulsion fracture of the PCL is uncommonly seen but would reveal increased signal on T2-weighted images through the posterior portion of the tibia at the level of the PCL attachment. Common associated injuries with PCL tear include ACL tear, anterior bone contusion, collateral ligament injury, and menisci tears [17]. T1-weighted or short tau inversion recovery (STIR) images are valuable in the assessment of associated bone marrow injury [18]. The

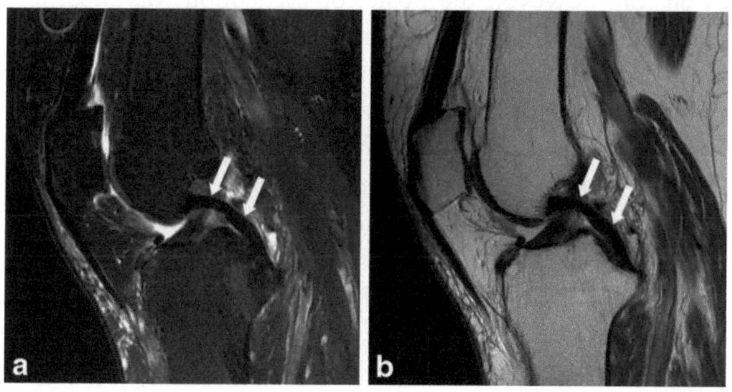

Fig. 2.9 **a** and **b** Demonstrate the normal appearance of the PCL (*arrows*) on T2 and PD images, respectively. Note the normal curved appearance and the homogeneously low signal on both sequences [67]. PCL posterior cruciate ligament, PD proton density

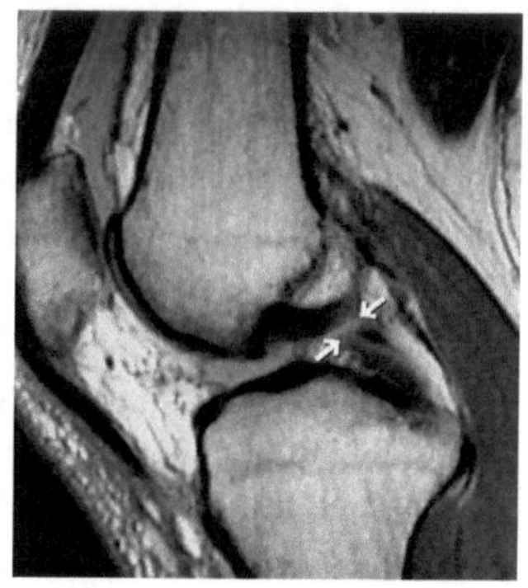

Fig. 2.10 Complete PCL tear. PDWI of a woman in her thirties shows complete tear of PCL at its mid-portion (*arrow*) [68]. PCL posterior cruciate ligament, PDWI proton-density-weighted image

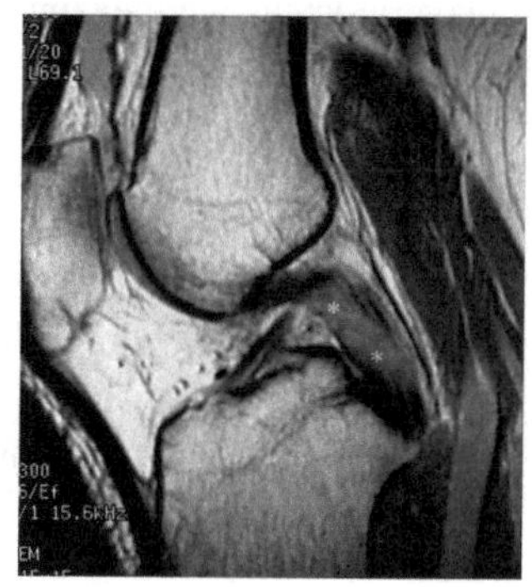

Fig. 2.11 Partial tear of PCL (intrasubstance injury) (1). PDWI of a man in his thirties shows partially torn PCL, which is swollen and shows hyperintensity (*) for the entire length, representing intrasubstance injury. Periphery of the PCL retains continuity of fibers [68]. PCL posterior cruciate ligament, PDWI proton-density-weighted image

sensitivity and specificity for diagnosing a PCL tear by MRI approaches 100%. MRI has proven to be an accurate modality for evaluating the integrity of the PCL [19].

Biomechanics

Over the past 30 years, the biomechanical role of the PCL has been investigated by many authors. Cadaveric sectioning studies of the PCL, comparison studies with PCL deficiency in one knee and a normal contralateral knee, as well as contact pressure studies and kinematic analysis have all been performed, yielding insight into the multitude of functions the PCL provides in the normal and pathologic knee. We have found that attempting to understand the literature available is best done by collating the studies based on their findings to specific questions. As such, this chapter has been subdivided into various subtopics of PCL biomechanics, each of which examines the present literature and based upon the best available evidence attempts to draw conclusions. The subdivisions are as follows: posterior tibial translation, rotational and medial/lateral stability, joint contact pressure studies, morphological/meniscal/chondral degeneration, strength, proprioception, and compensatory mechanisms: electromyography and muscle activation.

Posterior Tibial Translation

In vitro studies reaffirm the role the PCL has in preventing posterior tibial translation; however, controversy still exists as to the relative translational stability provided by the PCL at varying angles of knee flexion. Kumagai et al. conducted translational measurements in the anterior to posterior plane on five cadaveric specimens before and after PCL sectioning [20]. They found no difference in posterior translation below 25° of knee flexion, while displacement increased significantly between 25° and 90° of flexion, averaging >10 mm of posterior translation at 90° of flexion [20]. In contrast, Li et al. examined eight cadaveric knees and found that in PCL-deficient knees, posterior tibial translation only occurred above 60°; this was reaffirmed by Pearsall et al. where eight cadaveric knees were examined with strain gauges in either meniscus to measure strain in the menisci in varying degrees of flexion in the PCL intact, ruptured, and reconstructive states [21, 22]. They found that in scenarios where the PCL was cut, the total anterior–posterior translation was >18 mm and was statistically significant compared to the intact and reconstructive PCL states at knee flexion angles of 60° and 90° [22].

However, other authors have shown increased posterior tibial displacement in PCL-deficient knees throughout the arc of motion (0–120°) [23–28]. Gollehon et al. published their work in the *Journal of Bone and Joint Surgery* (JBJS) in 1987 where they tested the static stability of the PCL and the posterolateral corner structures in a sectioning study of 17 human cadaveric knees at knee flexion angles between 0° and 90° [23]. They found that at all angles of flexion, the PCL was the principle restraint to posterior translation and that at all angles tested, isolated sectioning of the PCL did not affect varus or external rotation stability [23]. Similarly, Li et al. examined 12 fresh-frozen cadaveric knees using a robotic testing system and applied a 130 N posteriorly directed load at 30° increments between 0° and 150°; they found statistically significant posterior tibial translation at all knee flexion angles except 150°, indicating the role of the PCL in posterior stability except for at extreme flexion angles [24]. Hagemeister et al. reaffirmed the importance of the PCL in providing posterior stability at low flexion angles when they looked at five pairs of fresh-frozen cadaveric knees with a mean age of 73.2 years and used electromagnetic sensors to effectively examine the translation caused by sectioning of the PCL and posterolateral corner structures [25]. Statistically significant differences in anterior–posterior translation existed at all 15° intervals measured from 0° to 75° [25]. Furthermore, Harner et al. examined the effect of the popliteus tendon in conjunction with the PCL in ten cadaveric specimens and found that with a simulated posterior drawer test of 110 N and a simulated popliteus contraction of 44 N in the PCL-intact knees did not result in increased posterior tibial translation; however, when the PCL was sectioned, not only did the posterior tibial translation increase at knee flexion angles of 0°/30°/60°/75°/90° but also a statistically significant decrease in posterior tibial translation was found with the addition of a simulated popliteus muscle contraction [26]. As such, they concluded that the popliteus muscle is an important stabilizer against posterior tibial translation in the PCL-deficient knee [26]. Grood et al. also looked at the effect of tibial translation at low flexion angles of the knee using 15 whole lower limb cadavera and found that sectioning of the PCL did produce posterior tibial sag even at full extension; however, the posterior translation was most apparent at 90° of flexion (the highest flexion angle they measured) where it averaged 11.4 mm of posterior displacement [27]. Finally, Hoher et al. examined eight cadaveric knees using a universal force-moment sensor (UFS) testing system to apply a 110-N load to the knee at 0°/30°/60°/75°/90° [28]. They found that with the application of the load, even at full extension there was a difference in posterior tibial translation of 3.0 mm, which progressively increased to 14.1 mm at 90° of knee flexion [28].

In addition, in vivo studies examining the posterior tibial translation of PCL-deficient knees also exist. Castle et al. examined posterior tibial translation at varying degrees of knee flexion in ten patients with unilateral PCL deficiency using lateral radiographs [29]. They found that at knee flexion angles between 70 ° and 90°, the mean displacement of the tibia posteriorly was 7.4 mm, while knee flexion angles between 30 ° and 50 ° resulted in a mean displacement of just 2.1 mm [29]. Furthermore, displacement at lower flexion angles was not uniform. Logan et al. also looked at in vivo analysis of the PCL in their series of six patients with unilateral PCL deficiency who underwent MRI evaluation while squatting as well as while a posterior drawer test was performed [30]. Their findings were suggestive of altered kinematics in the medial compartment, with approximately 5 mm of posterior tibial translation measured on the sagittal image throughout all weight-bearing flexion angles [30]. Additionally, in the stress sagittal images obtained at 90° of flexion, a mean of 10.1 mm of posterior tibial translation occurred [30].

Assimilation of the data available in all of these studies would suggest that the PCL is the primary restraint to posterior translation of the knee and that although it likely has an effect throughout the functional arc of motion, its effect is likely greatest at high angles of knee flexion (60–120°). Additionally, the popliteus muscle may act as a restraint to posterior translation in the PCL-deficient knee.

Rotational and Medial/Lateral Stability

The role that the PCL plays in providing rotational stability to the knee is still unclear. Many reports exist throughout the literature that show isolated sectioning of the PCL does not significantly affect tibial external rotation. Gollehon et al. sectioned the PCL in 17 cadaveric specimens and showed that external rotation or varus stress did not increase at any position of knee flexion [23]. Grood et al. performed sectioning of the PCL and posterolateral structures in 15 cadaveric specimens and measured displacement in varying degrees of knee flexion with a electrogoniometer [27]. Their results showed no increased tibial external rotation or varus/valgus angulation compared to the intact state [27]. Nielsen et al. evaluated 25 osteoligamentous-intact cadaveric knees and performed sectioning of the PCL along with the medial and lateral structures [31]. They found that axial rotatory instability was only detectable when the PCL lesion was combined with either a medial or lateral side ligamentous injury; furthermore, a reverse pivot shift was only elicited when the PCL/lateral collateral ligament (LCL)/popliteus tendon were sectioned [31]. Finally, Kaneda et al. looked at 15 cadaveric fresh-frozen knees and performed sequential sectioning of the PCL, LCL, and posterolateral structures and found that in isolated sectioning of the PCL, there was no increase in tibial external rotation; however, they did find that isolated sectioning of just the anterolateral bundle of the PCL shifted the axis of external rotation of the knee [32].

This is in contrast to four other studies, all which showed that isolated sectioning of the PCL does lead to increased tibial rotation. Li et al. examined eight cadaveric knees using a robotic testing system with applied simulated quadriceps and hamstring loads (400 and 200 N, respectively) at knee flexion angles from 0° to 120° and found that at angles above 60° significant external tibial rotation occurred [21]. Harner et al. performed an investigation using ten cadaveric knee specimens where simulated popliteus muscle contraction was performed in both the presence and absence of the PCL [26]. They found that simulated popliteus muscle contraction resulted in an internal tibial rotation of 2° and 4° at 60° and 90° of knee flexion, regardless of whether or not the PCL was intact [26]. Gupte et al. used eight cadaveric knees to evaluate the role of the meniscofemoral ligaments in providing sagittal plane and rotational stability in the posterior cruciate ligament-deficient knee [33]. They found that although isolated sectioning of the PCL does increase rotational instability between 60° and 90°, further sectioning of the meniscofemoral ligaments still does not lead to increased rotational instability [33]. Finally, Ogata et al. performed sequential sectioning of the PCL and collateral ligaments and found increasing posterior sag and internal rotation of the tibia with increasing degrees of knee flexion in specimens in which only the PCL was deficient [34].

Additionally, three in vivo studies examined the varus/valgus and rotational stability provided by the PCL. Fontbote et al. examined ten patients with unilateral grade II (6–10 mm posterior displacement) PCL insufficiency and found objective clinical and radiographic evidence of posterior tibial displacement; however, although differences in gait and vertical landing existed, they concluded that minimal biomechanical and neuromuscular differences were found between PCL-intact and PCL-insufficient knees [35]. Hooper et al. examined nine patients with PCL deficiency compared to a control group in walking and ascending and descending stairs [36]. They found a direct correlation between subjective patient outcome measures (Flandry) and higher peak knee extensor torque during stance phase [36]. Finally, Jonsson and Karrholm looked at eight patients with unilateral PCL deficiency and performed radiostereometric measurements in patients performing a step-up test while a posterior stress test was applied to the tibia at 30° of flexion; this study was unable to show any kinematic differences in the knee during the step-up test [37]. In addition, the study suggested that of the eight patients with known isolated PCL deficiency, six of them were found to show abnormalities in the other ligaments of the knee [37].

In conclusion, the role the PCL plays in the rotational control of the knee is still unclear, with many contradictory studies published in the literature. It may act as a secondary stabilizer to rotational forces when other ligaments are compromised and other ligaments may provide control to rotation when the PCL is deficient. Further work both in the in vivo and biomechanical arenas may provide further insight into the exact role the PCL plays in providing rotational stability to the knee.

Joint Contact Pressure Studies

To further delineate the biomechanical alterations in the medial compartment after PCL injury, two in vitro studies have been performed to look specifically at this. In the first study, Skyhar et al., in their 1993 paper, looked at the contact pressures using pressure-sensitive film in ten cadaveric knees with sequential sectioning of the PCL and posterolateral corner structures (posterolateral capsule, popliteus muscle and tendon, and the lateral collateral ligament) [38]. They found a mean pressure increase of 52% in the medial compartment, regardless of the angle of knee flexion in specimens with isolated PCL deficiency [38]. Furthermore, pressure increases were also noted in the patellofemoral compartment with progressive sectioning of the PCL and posterolateral corner from an intact state measurement of 23.2 Pa to measurements of 28.0 and 34.8 Pa with subsequent sectioning of the PCL and posterolateral corner, respectively [38]. In the second study, MacDonald et al. used nine fresh-frozen cadavers under the age of 45 years to study the biomechanical changes that occur in the absence of the PCL under physiologic loads [39]. They used pressure-sensitive film inserted into the medial and lateral compartments and measured loads up to 1.5 kN at angles of 0°/30°/60° of knee flexion. Their results did show significant posterior subluxation of the tibia at 60° of flexion in the PCL-deficient specimen, which resulted in increased contact pressure and pressure concentration in the medial compartment [39]. They concluded that this increased contact pressure in the medial compartment of PCL-deficient knees might explain the long-term degenerative changes observed in the medial compartment in PCL-deficient states [39].

Based on these studies, it appears that the deficiency of the PCL results in increased joint contact pressures in the medial and patellofemoral compartments. This contact pressure increase correlates with natural history studies of untreated PCL deficiency where over time, greater incidence of medial and patellofemoral compartment degeneration has been observed.

Morphological/Meniscal/Chondral Degeneration

Hamada et al. looked at 61 patients with acute, isolated PCL tears characterized as grade 2+ or higher and found that 28% of these patients had meniscal tears (with the anterior horn of the lateral meniscus being the most common site of pathology) and 52% of these patients had chondral injuries (most commonly in the medial femoral condyle) [40]. They recommended for the clinician to have a high index of suspicion for concomitant pathology in the menisci or cartilage when evaluating patients with presumed isolated, high-grade PCL injuries.

Ochi et al. have evaluated the ultrastructural changes that occur in the anterior cruciate ligament (ACL) in response to chronic PCL deficiency. They examined 14 patients at a mean of 22.1 months from their isolated PCL injury by obtaining biopsy specimens from the anteromedial and proximal one-third of their knees arthroscopically and compared these via electron microscopy to PCL-intact knees that were obtained secondary to amputation [41]. Interestingly, they found that in the PCL-deficient knees, the ACL had decreased number of collagen fibrils, increased collagen fibril diameter, and decreased collagen packing density compared to controls (PCL-intact knees) [41]. They concluded that isolated PCL deficiency can have adverse effects on other ligamentous structures of the knee.

Shelbourne et al. examined the natural history of the isolated PCL-deficient knees in 68 patients with a mean age at the time of injury of 25.2 years, and obtained subjective, objective, functional, and radiographic data at a mean of 5.4 years postinjury [42]. They found no difference in subjective knee scores and the amount of time from the initial injury; furthermore, laxity did not increase with time and laxity did not correlate with radiographic changes [42]. In addition, regardless of laxity, 50% of this cohort returns to sports at the same level or higher [42]. Radiographic interpretation suggested that medial tibiofemoral compartment arthrosis was more prevalent in the PCL-injured knee compared to the contralateral (normal) knee; however, this did not quite reach statistical significance in this series ($p=0.077$) [42]. Shelbourne et al. most recently provided longer-term follow-up (minimum 10 years) in their 2013 paper published in the *American Journal of Sports Medicine* (AJSM) [43]. Here, they had subjective and objective outcomes data on 44 patients at a mean follow-up of 14.3 years (range 10–21) from the time of injury [43]. Although radiographic changes and progressive degeneration of the knee was seen in 41% of patients, patients maintained quadriceps strength compared to the contralateral side (97% of normal), and had subjective knee scores in the form of International Knee Documentation Committee (IKDC) and modified Cincinnati Knee Rating System (CKRS) scores of 73.4 and 81.3, respectively [43].

Parolie et al. treated 25 patients with isolated PCL tears without surgical reconstruction and followed them up for a mean of 6.2 years (range 2.2–16 years); they found that although 36% had radiographic changes, 80% of patients were satisfied with their knees and 84% had returned to their previous sport [44]. In their study, quadriceps strength seemed to correlate with patient satisfaction [44]. They concluded that the majority of athletes with PCL-deficient knees who maintain strength in their quadriceps can predictably return to sports without disability.

Keller et al. examined 40 patients with isolated PCL injuries (75 % were sports related) who were treated nonoperatively at a mean of 6 years from the initial injury [45]. On the modified Noyes knee questionnaire, 65 % of patients noted limitations in their activities and 49 % noted that their knee had not fully recovered despite adequate rehabilitation [45]. In contrast to other studies, they did find a correlation between the length of time since the injury and worse knee score and progression of radiographic degenerative changes [45]. Furthermore, 90 % of patients complained of activity-associated knee pain and 43 % had pain with basic activities such as walking—despite having strength measurements essentially the same as the contralateral, uninjured extremity [45].

Boynton et al. examined 38 patients with isolated PCL injuries both subjectively (questionnaire) and objectively (physical exam and radiographs of both knees) at a mean follow-up of 13.4 years (range 5–38 years) [46]. They found that 21 % of patients had to have additional surgery for meniscal pathology and that those patients had statistically significant worse subjective scores than those without meniscal pathology [46]. In addition, 81 % of patients with normal menisci had at least occasional knee pain and 56 % had occasional swelling [46]. Radiographic examination did demonstrate articular degeneration which seemed to increase with time from the injury [46]. They concluded that a bimodal distribution of patients exists, with some having significant symptoms and radiographic degeneration and others remaining essentially asymptomatic with no loss of function.

Strobel et al. published their series of 181 patients with a known PCL injury who had undergone arthroscopy to assess chondral damage in the Arthroscopy journal in 2003 [47]. They found that patients with a duration of PCL deficiency greater than 5 years had an incidence of nearly 78 % for lesions of the medial femoral condyle and nearly 47 % had chondral damage of the patella [47]. Furthermore, they also found that degenerative changes in the medial femoral condyle set in fairly quickly with a threefold increase in the number of lesions within the first year of becoming PCL-deficient; they also found that medial degeneration increased significantly with the presence of a combined PCL/PLC injury [47]. They recommended that the early and continuous increase in both medial compartment and patellofemoral degeneration be taken into account when counseling patients about options for conservative versus reconstructive treatments.

Assimilation of the literature on both acute and chronic PCL tears would suggest that clinicians examining the acute, high-grade PCL tear should have a high index of suspicion for concurrent diagnosis of lateral meniscus tear or medial femoral condyle chondral injury and that failure to diagnose these conditions may miss an opportunity for potentially natural history-altering intervention. Furthermore, deficiency of the PCL may lead to ultrastructural changes in other knee ligaments as they are required to assume additional roles as posterior stabilizers. Predictable sequences of degeneration occur in both the medial and patellofemoral compartments with untreated PCL deficiency. With regard to the outcomes of nonoperative treatment, the literature is mixed with some series providing very compelling evidence for nonoperative treatment of PCL deficiency with high subjective outcomes and return to sports, and other series showing activity-associated knee pain in 90 % of patients with PCL deficiency. We believe that patients with PCL deficiency should be evaluated for concomitant injuries and counseled about the natural history of nonsurgical treatment so that the patient can make an informed decision regarding their care.

Strength

Many authors have examined the effect that PCL injury has on strength of the ipsilateral and contralateral knee. Both Inoue et al. in 1998 and Fontbote et al. in 2005 examined patients with PCL deficiency and found no difference in strength compared to the contralateral, uninjured extremity [35, 48]. In contrast, Hooper et al. in their study on gait adaptations in patients with chronic PCL deficiency showed that peak knee extension torque at 60°/s was significantly less in both the PCL-deficient and contralateral uninjured knee than the control group, leading one to believe that the loss of the strength in the PCL-deficient knee also leads to decreased strength in the contralateral knee [36]. Shirakura et al. have also examined the effect of strength on the PCL-deficient knee and found that a significant decrease in quadriceps eccentric and concentric torque in the PCL-deficient knee occurred only above 36° of flexion [49]. Additionally, MacLean et al. examined 17 patients with isolated PCL injuries that were treated conservatively and found that the PCL-deficient limb was weaker for both the quadriceps and hamstrings compared to the contralateral, normal side [50]. Finally, Tibone et al. looked at isokinetic and isometric quadriceps strength of patients with conservatively treated PCL injuries and found that the PCL-deficient knees exhibited significantly lower quadriceps peak torque at 60°/s but not at 120°/s [51].

However, there have been many prospective studies on quadriceps strength of conservatively treated PCL-deficient knees which found no difference compared to the contralateral, uninjured side [42, 44, 45, 52]. Still, Torg et al. examined 43 patients who had either isolated PCL deficiency or multidirectional knee ligament injuries at a mean of 6.3 years after the injury and did find that 53 % of subjects had quadriceps strength deficits between 22 and 30 % compared to their contralateral, uninjured limb [53].

In conclusion, the present data regarding strength in the PCL-deficient and contralateral normal knee is mixed in the literature, with some studies suggesting significant differences in both lower extremities compared with controls and others suggesting no difference in strength between the PCL-deficient and normal contralateral knee. Further studies will likely need to be performed to draw any definitive conclusions regarding strength.

Proprioception

It has long been postulated that both of the cruciate ligaments play a role in the proprioception of the lower extremity. Clark et al. sought to further delineate the role the PCL has in this when they examined eight patients with PCL deficiency using a motorized apparatus that flexed or extended the knee at a rate of 0.5°/s in a randomized fashion, using the contralateral normal knee as a control [54]. Subjectively, all eight patients noted greater difficulty in perceiving movement in the PCL-deficient knee. In addition, significant differences were found in the threshold of perception to passive movement (TPPM) with the normal knee exhibiting values of 0.93°±0.32° and the PCL-deficient knees having mean values of 1.19°±2.7° [54]. They concluded that this loss of proprioception may play a role in knee instability and be part of the constellation of degenerative changes that occur as part of the natural history of the PCL-deficient knee.

Safran et al. also examined the role that the PCL has in proprioception of the knee. They examined 18 patients with isolated PCL deficiency between 1 month and 19.5 years after injury and evaluated kinesthesia and joint position sense using the threshold to detect passive motion (TTDPM) and the ability to reproduce passive positioning (RPP) [55]. They did find statistically significant differences in TTDPM and RPP between the PCL-deficient and PCL-intact knees; however, this was dependent on the starting position of each joint and whether the knee was flexed or extended [55]. They concluded that there may be proprioceptive mechanoreceptors within the PCL that play a role in proprioception.

In conclusion, there is some evidence that the PCL has a minor role in proprioception of the knee, with small but statistically significant differences noted in the above studies. Although the loss of proprioception has been postulated to be a potential etiology leading to the predictable pattern of medial compartment and patellofemoral degeneration, this has not yet been substantiated in the literature. Finally, to our knowledge there are no studies suggesting that the reconstruction of the PCL-deficient knee restores this proprioceptive role.

Compensatory Mechanisms: Electromyography and Muscle Activation

Inoue et al. performed electromyogram (EMG) studies on the quadriceps, hamstrings, and gastrocnemius muscles on both the PCL-deficient side and the contralateral normal side in 12 patients, while having them perform concentric isokinetic contractions at 30°/s and 60°/s [48]. There were no differences observed in either the quadriceps or hamstring activation between the deficient and control knees; however, prior to generation of flexion torque, EMG revealed a significantly earlier activation of the gastrocnemius muscle at each velocity in the PCL-deficient knees, suggesting that the gastrocnemius may play a role in compensatory stabilization during flexion in PCL-deficient knees [48].

Cain and Schwab published a case study of a football player with PCL deficiency that was subjected to EMG evaluation while running [56]. Their findings suggested that quadriceps contraction occurs 20 % earlier in the gait cycle in the lower extremity with PCL deficiency [56]. Tibone et al. also evaluated the compensatory mechanisms involved in a PCL-deficient knee by examining 20 patients (10 with PCL deficiency and 10 with PCL reconstructions) during activities such as walking, running and stair climbing; although they did observe differences such as early activation of the gastrocnemius–soleus complex, the results were not statistically tested [51]. Although relevant to the discussion, it is difficult to draw conclusions from case reports and studies where statistical analysis was not performed.

Finally, Fontbote et al. used surface EMG on ten patients with unilateral PCL deficiency to obtain data on six muscles (vastus medialis and lateralis, medial and lateral hamstring, and both heads of the gastrocnemius) during gait (ten trials) and vertical drop landing on one leg from a height of 30 cm (five trials performed) [35]. The contralateral, normal extremity was used as the control. They found no difference in EMG values for either activity on all of the muscles tested [35].

The relative compensatory contributions from other muscles in the setting of PCL deficiency remain an area where further study needs to be performed to draw any real conclusions. Although one study did show earlier activation in the gastrocnemius muscle during walking, this has not yet been validated by other studies.

Clinical Relevance

Although the biomechanical function of the PCL is known to be primary as a restraint to posterior tibial translation, the true clinical relevance lies in the assessment of whether or not operative reconstruction will allow for more predictable improvement in criteria such as return to sports/normal activity, as well as whether residual posterior laxity will negatively affect subjective and functional outcomes. This has been examined with some authors reporting return to sports/activity at a similar level in 76–85 % of patients treated non-operatively for high-grade PCL tears [57, 58]. Still, other authors have noted deficiencies in players returning to sports with PCL-deficient extremity, including players believing they had limitations and decreased performance with high-speed running [46, 59]. Several authors have attempted to discern whether or not the degree of laxity correlates directly to subjective and functional outcomes and were unable to do so [42, 44, 57, 60, 61]. However, at least two other authors have shown correlations between posterior laxity and decreases in functionality scores [45, 46]. Definitive answers to these questions will improve surgeon–patient communication, allowing patients to make well-informed decisions regarding their care.

Future Directions

Future experimental designs will likely focus on using advanced motion analysis and computer programs to further analyze the role of the PCL in both the athlete and nonathlete. Furthermore, a sports-specific analysis may also lend further insight into the exact functional role the PCL plays within the demands of each sport.

References

1. Fanelli GC, Beck JD, Edson CJ. Current concepts review: the posterior cruciate ligament. J Knee Surg. 2010 Jun;23(2):61–72.
2. Girgis FG, Marshall JL, Monajem A. The cruciate ligaments of the knee joint. Anatomical, functional and experimental analysis. Clin Orthop. 1975 Feb;(106):216–31.
3. Bowman KF Jr, Sekiya JK. Anatomy and biomechanics of the posterior cruciate ligament, medial and lateral sides of the knee. Sports Med Arthrosc Rev. 2010 Dec;18(4):222–9.
4. Osti M, Tschann P, Kunzel KH, Benedetto KP. Anatomic characteristics and radiographic references of the anterolateral and posteromedial bundles of the posterior cruciate ligament. Am J Sports Med. 2012 Apr 26;40(7):1558–63.
5. Moorman CT 3rd, Murphy Zane MS, Bansai S, Cina SJ, Wickiewicz TL, Warren RF, et al. Tibial insertion of the posterior cruciate ligament: a sagittal plane analysis using gross, histologic, and radiographic methods. Arthrosc J Arthrosc Relat Surg Off Publ Arthrosc Assoc N Am Int Arthrosc Assoc. 2008 Mar;24(3):269–75.
6. Forsythe B, Harner C, Martins CAQ, Shen W, Lopes OV Jr, Fu FH. Topography of the femoral attachment of the posterior cruciate ligament. Surgical technique. J Bone Joint Surg Am. 2009 Mar 1;91(Suppl 2 Pt 1):89–100.
7. Anderson CJ, Ziegler CG, Wijdicks CA, Engebretsen L, LaPrade RF. Arthroscopically pertinent anatomy of the anterolateral and posteromedial bundles of the posterior cruciate ligament. J Bone Joint Surg Am. 2012 Nov 7;94(21):1936–45.
8. Sheps DM, Otto D, Fernhout M. The anatomic characteristics of the tibial insertion of the posterior cruciate ligament. Arthrosc J Arthrosc Relat Surg Off Publ Arthrosc Assoc N Am Int Arthrosc Assoc. 2005 Jul;21(7):820–5.
9. Matava MJ, Sethi NS, Totty WG. Proximity of the posterior cruciate ligament insertion to the popliteal artery as a function of the knee flexion angle: implications for posterior cruciate ligament reconstruction. Arthrosc J Arthrosc Relat Surg Off Publ Arthrosc Assoc N Am Int Arthrosc Assoc. 2000 Nov;16(8):796–804.
10. Ahn JH, Wang JH, Lee SH, Yoo JC, Jeon WJ. Increasing the distance between the posterior cruciate ligament and the popliteal neurovascular bundle by a limited posterior capsular release during arthroscopic transtibial posterior cruciate ligament reconstruction: a cadaveric angiographic study. Am J Sports Med. 2007 May;35(5):787–92.
11. Scapinelli R. Studies on the vasculature of the human knee joint. Acta Anat (Basel). 1968;70(3):305–31.
12. Scapinelli R. Vascular anatomy of the human cruciate ligaments and surrounding structures. Clin Anat N Y. 1997;10(3):151–62.
13. Kennedy JC, Alexander IJ, Hayes KC. Nerve supply of the human knee and its functional importance. Am J Sports Med. 1982 Dec;10(6):329–35.
14. Katonis PG, Assimakopoulos AP, Agapitos MV, Exarchou EI. Mechanoreceptors in the posterior cruciate ligament. Histologic study on cadaver knees. Acta Orthop Scand. 1991 Jun;62(3):276–8.
15. Kaelin A, Hulin PH, Carlioz H. Congenital aplasia of the cruciate ligaments. A report of six cases. J Bone Joint Surg Br. 1986 Nov;68(5):827–8.
16. Chomiak J, Podškubka A, Dungl P, Ošt'ádal M, Frydrychová M. Cruciate ligaments in proximal femoral focal deficiency: arthroscopic assessment. J Pediatr Orthop. 2012 Feb;32(1):21–8.
17. Kam CK, Chee DWY, Peh WCG. Magnetic resonance imaging of cruciate ligament injuries of the knee. Can Assoc Radiol J J Assoc Can Radiol. 2010 Apr;61(2):80–9.
18. Sonin AH, Fitzgerald SW, Hoff FL, Friedman H, Bresler ME. MR imaging of the posterior cruciate ligament: normal, abnormal, and associated injury patterns. Radiogr Rev Publ Radiol Soc N Am Inc. 1995 May;15(3):551–61.
19. Gross ML, Grover JS, Bassett LW, Seeger LL, Finerman GA. Magnetic resonance imaging of the posterior cruciate ligament. Clinical use to improve diagnostic accuracy. Am J Sports Med. 1992 Dec;20(6):732–7.
20. Kumagai M, Mizuno Y, Mattessich SM, Elias JJ, Cosgarea AJ, Chao EY. Posterior cruciate ligament rupture alters in vitro knee kinematics. Clin Orthop. 2002 Feb;(395):241–8.
21. Li G, Gill TJ, DeFrate LE, Zayontz S, Glatt V, Zarins B. Biomechanical consequences of PCL deficiency in the knee under simulated muscle loads–an in vitro experimental study. J Orthop Res Off Publ Orthop Res Soc. 2002 Jul;20(4):887–92.
22. Pearsall AW 4th, Hollis JM. The effect of posterior cruciate ligament injury and reconstruction on meniscal strain. Am J Sports Med. 2004 Nov;32(7):1675–80.
23. Gollehon DL, Torzilli PA, Warren RF. The role of the posterolateral and cruciate ligaments in the stability of the human knee. A biomechanical study. J Bone Joint Surg Am. 1987 Feb;69(2):233–42.
24. Li G, Most E, DeFrate LE, Suggs JF, Gill TJ, Rubash HE. Effect of the posterior cruciate ligament on posterior stability of the knee in high flexion. J Biomech. 2004 May;37(5):779–83.
25. Hagemeister N, Duval N, Yahia L, Krudwig W, Witzel U, de Guise JA. Computer-based method for the 3-D kinematic analysis of posterior cruciate ligament and postero-lateral corner lesions. Knee. 2002 Dec;9(4):301–8.
26. Harner CD, Höher J, Vogrin TM, Carlin GJ, Woo SL. The effects of a popliteus muscle load on in situ forces in the posterior cruciate ligament and on knee kinematics. A human cadaveric study. Am J Sports Med. 1998 Oct;26(5):669–73.

27. Grood ES, Stowers SF, Noyes FR. Limits of movement in the human knee. Effect of sectioning the posterior cruciate ligament and posterolateral structures. J Bone Joint Surg Am. 1988 Jan;70(1):88–97.
28. Höher J, Harner CD, Vogrin TM, Baek GH, Carlin GJ, Woo SL. In situ forces in the posterolateral structures of the knee under posterior tibial loading in the intact and posterior cruciate ligament-deficient knee. J Orthop Res Off Publ Orthop Res Soc. 1998 Nov;16(6):675–81.
29. Castle TH Jr, Noyes FR, Grood ES. Posterior tibial subluxation of the posterior cruciate-deficient knee. Clin Orthop. 1992 Nov;(284):193–202.
30. Logan M, Williams A, Lavelle J, Gedroyc W, Freeman M. The effect of posterior cruciate ligament deficiency on knee kinematics. Am J Sports Med. 2004 Dec;32(8):1915–22.
31. Nielsen S, Helmig P. Posterior instability of the knee joint. An experimental study. Arch Orthop Trauma Surg Arch Für Orthop Unf-Chir. 1986;105(2):121–5.
32. Kaneda Y, Moriya H, Takahashi K, Shimada Y, Tamaki T. Experimental study on external tibial rotation of the knee. Am J Sports Med. 1997 Dec;25(6):796–800.
33. Gupte CM, Bull AMJ, Thomas RD, Amis AA. The meniscofemoral ligaments: secondary restraints to the posterior drawer. Analysis of anteroposterior and rotary laxity in the intact and posterior-cruciate-deficient knee. J Bone Joint Surg Br. 2003 Jul;85(5):765–73.
34. Ogata K, McCarthy JA, Dunlap J, Manske PR. Pathomechanics of posterior sag of the tibia in posterior cruciate deficient knees. An experimental study. Am J Sports Med. 1988 Dec;16(6):630–6.
35. Fontboté CA, Sell TC, Laudner KG, Haemmerle M, Allen CR, Margheritini F, et al. Neuromuscular and biomechanical adaptations of patients with isolated deficiency of the posterior cruciate ligament. Am J Sports Med. 2005 Jul;33(7):982–9.
36. Hooper DM, Morrissey MC, Crookenden R, Ireland J, Beacon JP. Gait adaptations in patients with chronic posterior instability of the knee. Clin Biomech Bristol Avon. 2002 Mar;17(3):227–33.
37. Jonsson H, Kärrholm J. Three-dimensional knee kinematics and stability in patients with a posterior cruciate ligament tear. J Orthop Res Off Publ Orthop Res Soc. 1999 Mar;17(2):185–91.
38. Skyhar MJ, Warren RF, Ortiz GJ, Schwartz E, Otis JC. The effects of sectioning of the posterior cruciate ligament and the posterolateral complex on the articular contact pressures within the knee. J Bone Joint Surg Am. 1993 May;75(5):694–9.
39. MacDonald P, Miniaci A, Fowler P, Marks P, Finlay B. A biomechanical analysis of joint contact forces in the posterior cruciate deficient knee. Knee Surg Sports Traumatol Arthrosc Off J ESSKA. 1996;3(4):252–5.
40. Hamada M, Shino K, Mitsuoka T, Toritsuka Y, Natsu-Ume T, Horibe S. Chondral injury associated with acute isolated posterior cruciate ligament injury. Arthrosc J Arthrosc Relat Surg Off Publ Arthrosc Assoc N Am Int Arthrosc Assoc. 2000 Feb;16(1):59–63.
41. Ochi M, Murao T, Sumen Y, Kobayashi K, Adachi N. Isolated posterior cruciate ligament insufficiency induces morphological changes of anterior cruciate ligament collagen fibrils. Arthrosc J Arthrosc Relat Surg Off Publ Arthrosc Assoc N Am Int Arthrosc Assoc. 1999 Apr;15(3):292–6.
42. Shelbourne KD, Davis TJ, Patel DV. The natural history of acute, isolated, nonoperatively treated posterior cruciate ligament injuries. A prospective study. Am J Sports Med. 1999 Jun;27(3):276–83.
43. Shelbourne KD, Clark M, Gray T. Minimum 10-year follow-up of patients after an acute, isolated posterior cruciate ligament injury treated nonoperatively. Am J Sports Med. 2013 Jul;41(7):1526–33.
44. Parolie JM, Bergfeld JA. Long-term results of nonoperative treatment of isolated posterior cruciate ligament injuries in the athlete. Am J Sports Med. 1986 Feb;14(1):35–8.
45. Keller PM, Shelbourne KD, McCarroll JR, Rettig AC. Nonoperatively treated isolated posterior cruciate ligament injuries. Am J Sports Med. 1993 Feb;21(1):132–6.
46. Boynton MD, Tietjens BR. Long-term followup of the untreated isolated posterior cruciate ligament-deficient knee. Am J Sports Med. 1996 Jun;24(3):306–10.
47. Strobel MJ, Weiler A, Schulz MS, Russe K, Eichhorn HJ. Arthroscopic evaluation of articular cartilage lesions in posterior-cruciate-ligament-deficient knees. Arthrosc J Arthrosc Relat Surg Off Publ Arthrosc Assoc N Am Int Arthrosc Assoc. 2003 Mar;19(3):262–8.
48. Inoue M, Yasuda K, Yamanaka M, Wada T, Kaneda K. Compensatory muscle activity in the posterior cruciate ligament-deficient knee during isokinetic knee motion. Am J Sports Med. 1998 Oct;26(5):710–4.
49. Shirakura K, Kato K, Udagawa E. Characteristics of the isokinetic performance of patients with injured cruciate ligaments. Am J Sports Med. 1992 Dec;20(6):754–60.
50. MacLean CL, Taunton JE, Clement DB, Regan W. Eccentric and concentric isokinetic moment characteristics in the quadriceps and hamstrings of the chronic isolated posterior cruciate ligament injured knee. Br J Sports Med. 1999 Dec;33(6):405–8.
51. Tibone JE, Antich TJ, Perry J, Moynes D. Functional analysis of untreated and reconstructed posterior cruciate ligament injuries. Am J Sports Med. 1988 Jun;16(3):217–23.
52. Fowler PJ, Messieh SS. Isolated posterior cruciate ligament injuries in athletes. Am J Sports Med. 1987 Dec;15(6):553–7.
53. Torg JS, Barton TM, Pavlov H, Stine R. Natural history of the posterior cruciate ligament-deficient knee. Clin Orthop. 1989 Sep;(246):208–16.
54. Clark P, MacDonald PB, Sutherland K. Analysis of proprioception in the posterior cruciate ligament-deficient knee. Knee Surg Sports Traumatol Arthrosc Off J ESSKA. 1996;4(4):225–7.
55. Safran MR, Allen AA, Lephart SM, Borsa PA, Fu FH, Harner CD. Proprioception in the posterior cruciate ligament deficient knee. Knee Surg Sports Traumatol Arthrosc Off J ESSKA. 1999;7(5):310–7.
56. Cain TE, Schwab GH. Performance of an athlete with straight posterior knee instability. Am J Sports Med. 1981 Aug;9(4):203–8.
57. Shelbourne KD, Muthukaruppan Y. Subjective results of nonoperatively treated, acute, isolated posterior cruciate ligament injuries. Arthrosc J Arthrosc Relat Surg Off Publ Arthrosc Assoc N Am Int Arthrosc Assoc. 2005 Apr;21(4):457–61.
58. Cross MJ, Powell JF. Long-term followup of posterior cruciate ligament rupture: a study of 116 cases. Am J Sports Med. 1984 Aug;12(4):292–7.
59. Toritsuka Y, Horibe S, Hiro-Oka A, Mitsuoka T, Nakamura N. Conservative treatment for rugby football players with an acute isolated posterior cruciate ligament injury. Knee Surg Sports Traumatol Arthrosc Off J ESSKA. 2004 Mar;12(2):110–4.
60. Dandy DJ, Pusey RJ. The long-term results of unrepaired tears of the posterior cruciate ligament. J Bone Joint Surg Br. 1982;64(1):92–4.
61. Shelbourne KD, Gray T. Natural history of acute posterior cruciate ligament tears. J Knee Surg. 2002;15(2):103–7.
62. Amis AA, Gupte CM, Bull AM, Edwards A. Anatomy of the posterior cruciate ligament and the meniscofemoral ligaments. Knee Surg Sports Traumatol Arthrosc. 2006 Mar;14(3):257–63. (Reprinted with permission from Springer).
63. Takahashi M, Matsubara T, Doi M, Suzuki D, Nagano A. Anatomical study of the femoral and tibial insertions of the anterolateral and posteromedial bundles of human posterior cruciate ligament. Knee Surg Sports Traumatol Arthrosc. 2006 Nov;14(11):1055–9. (Reprinted with permission from Springer).

64. Apsingi S, Bull AM, Deehan DJ, Amis AA. Review: femoral tunnel placement for PCL reconstruction in relation to the PCL fibre bundle attachments. Knee Surg Sports Traumatol Arthrosc. 2009 Jun;17(6):652–9. (Reprinted with permission from Springer).
65. Kweon C, Lederman ES, Chhabra A. Anatomy and biomechanics of the cruciate ligaments and their surgical implications. In: Fanelli G, editor. The multiple ligament injured knee. 2nd ed. New York. Springer; 2013.
66. Karabay N, Sugun TS, Toros T. Ultrasonographic diagnosis of the posterior cruciate ligament injury in a 4-year-old child: a case report. Emerg Radiol. 2009 Sep;16(5):415–7. (Reprinted with permission from Springer).
67. Malone WJ, Syed FI, Bolos PR. MRI Imaging in the Multiple-Ligament-Injured Knee. In: Fanelli G, editor. The multiple ligament injured knee. 2nd ed. New York. Springer; 2013.
68. Niitsu M, editor. Magnetic resonance imaging of the knee. Berlin: Springer; 2013. (Reprinted with permission).

Anatomy and Biomechanics of the Posterolateral and Posteromedial Corners of the Knee and Their Surgical Implications

3

Evan W. James, Christopher M. LaPrade, Adam M. Johannsen and Robert F. LaPrade

Posterolateral Corner Anatomy

Introduction

Injury to the posterolateral corner (PLC) of the knee is common; however, it may often be missed during a diagnostic workup due to the lack of understanding of PLC anatomy. The PLC consists of three primary static stabilizers: the fibular collateral ligament (FCL), popliteus tendon (PLT), and popliteofibular ligament (PFL; Fig. 3.1) [1, 2]. In addition, the iliotibial band, biceps femoris, and peroneal nerve are important surgical landmarks (Fig. 3.2). The common peroneal nerve is located approximately 2–3 cm posterior to the long head of the biceps femoris and must be protected during any PLC surgical procedure (Fig. 3.3). Recent advances in PLC anatomy have facilitated the development of anatomic-based repair and reconstruction techniques, which in turn have led to improved outcomes in patients following anatomic PLC repair and reconstruction procedures [3–7].

Fibular (Lateral) Collateral Ligament

The FCL courses proximal to distal along the lateral aspect of the knee and averages 69.6 mm in length [1]. The FCL proximal attachment is located on the femur in a small bony depression approximately 1.4 mm proximal and 3.1 mm posterior to the lateral epicondyle [1]. On anteroposterior radiographs, Pietrini et al. reported that the FCL femoral attachment was located 27.1 mm proximal to the femoral condylar line [8]. LaPrade et al. reported that the average distance between the FCL and PLT femoral attachments was 18.5 mm (Figs. 3.4 and 3.5). At its distal insertion, the FCL inserts 28.4 mm distal to the tip of the fibular styloid in a small bony depression that can be accessed through an incision in the biceps bursa (Fig. 3.6) [1]. On anteroposterior radiographs, the FCL was reported to attach 34.7 mm distal to the tibial plateau [8]. Supplemental FCL fibers have also been described and extend distally along the peroneus longus fascia.

Popliteus Tendon

The PLT emerges from the popliteus muscle in the lateral third of the popliteal fossa before becoming intra-articular and coursing proximolaterally around the lateral femoral condyle through the popliteal sulcus [1]. The PLT attaches on the anterior fifth and proximal half of the popliteal sulcus, deep and anterior to the FCL (Fig. 3.7). On radiographic anteroposterior views, the PLT has been reported to attach 14.5 mm proximal to the femoral condylar line [8]. On lateral radiographic views, the PLT attached 14.2 mm anterior to the femoral attachment of the FCL. As the knee cycles through flexion, LaPrade et al. reported that the PLT disengaged from the popliteal sulcus near extension and reengaged with the sulcus at 112° of flexion (Fig. 3.8) [1]. The length of the tendon was also measured to be 54.5 mm from the popliteus musculotendinous junction to the femoral attachment.

Popliteofibular Ligament

The PFL originates at the musculotendinous junction of the popliteus muscle and consists of an anterior and posterior division [1]. The PFL extends distolaterally before inserting onto the fibular head. The anterior division inserts 2.8 mm distal to the tip of the fibular styloid on the anteromedial downslope. By contrast, the posterior division inserts 1.6 mm distal to the tip of the fibular styloid on the posteromedial downslope. The width of the posterior division is larger than the anterior division at 5.8 and 2.6 mm, respectively. On anteroposterior radiographic views, the PFL was reported to insert

R. F. LaPrade (✉) · E. W. James · C. M. LaPrade · A. M. Johannsen
Department of BioMedical Engineering, Steadman Philippon Research Institute, 181 W. Meadow Dr., Suite 1000, Vail, CO 81657, USA
e-mail: drlaprade@sprivail.org

G. C. Fanelli (ed.), *Posterior Cruciate Ligament Injuries*,
DOI 10.1007/978-3-319-12072-0_3, © Springer International Publishing Switzerland 2015

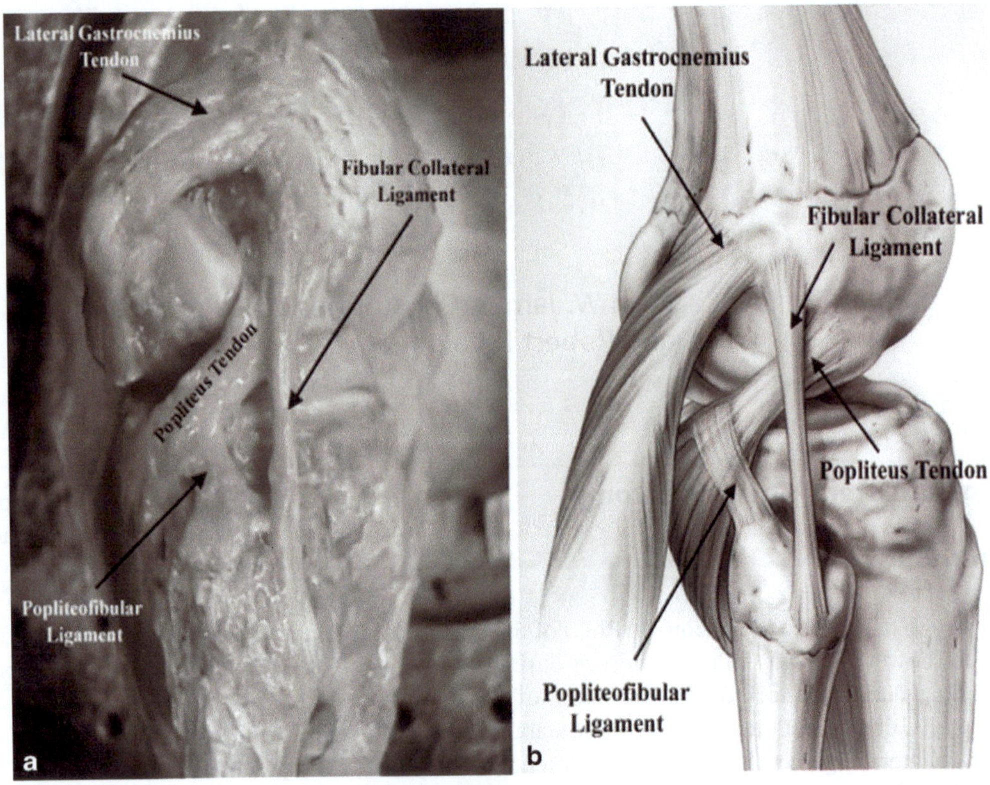

Fig. 3.1 A cadaveric photograph (**a**) and illustration (**b**) of the fibular collateral ligament, lateral gastrocnemius tendon, popliteofibular ligament, and popliteus tendon. (From LaPrade et al. 2003 [1]. Reproduced with permission)

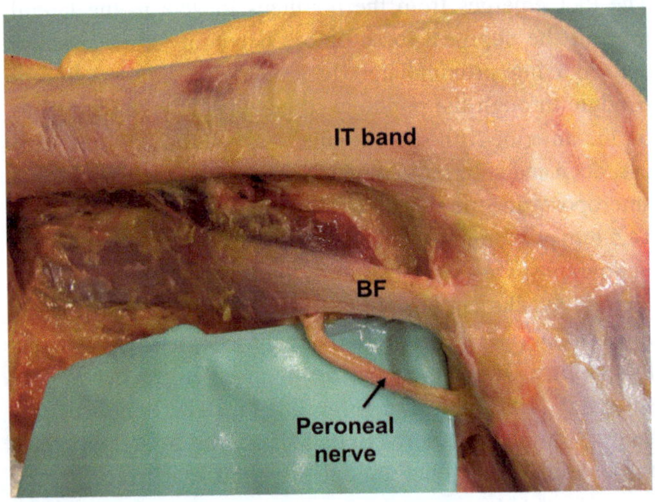

Fig. 3.2 A gross anatomic view of the lateral knee including the iliotibial band, biceps femoris, and peroneal nerve. *BF* biceps femoris, *IT band* iliotibial band

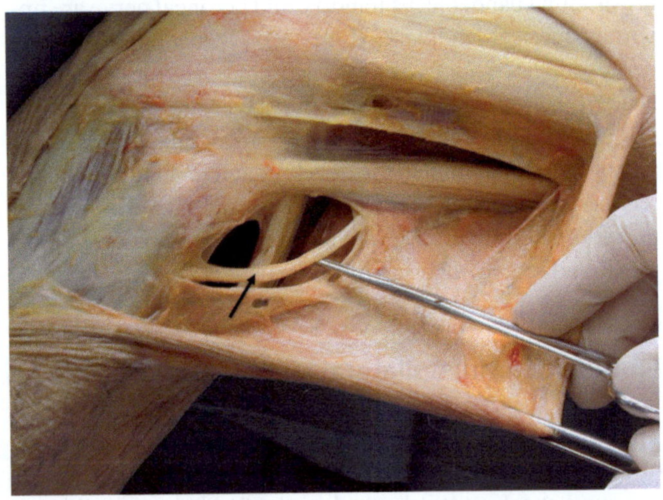

Fig. 3.3 The common peroneal nerve is located approximately 2–3 cm posterior to the long head of the biceps femoris and courses distally along the lateral aspect of the fibular head

21.0 mm distal to the tibial plateau joint line on the fibular head and 14.1 mm proximal to the fibular insertion of the FCL [8].

Summary

The primary PLC structures include the FCL, PLT, and PFL. Improved quantitative understanding of PLC anatomy has been essential for developing improved diagnostic techniques and anatomic-based repair and reconstruction techniques.

PLC Biomechanics

Introduction

In addition to basic anatomy, the biomechanics of PLC structures have been extensively studied. A comprehensive understanding of PLC biomechanics is necessary to understand the functional consequences of injury, develop improved diagnostics, and validate repair and reconstruction techniques. While the PLC consists of numerous static and

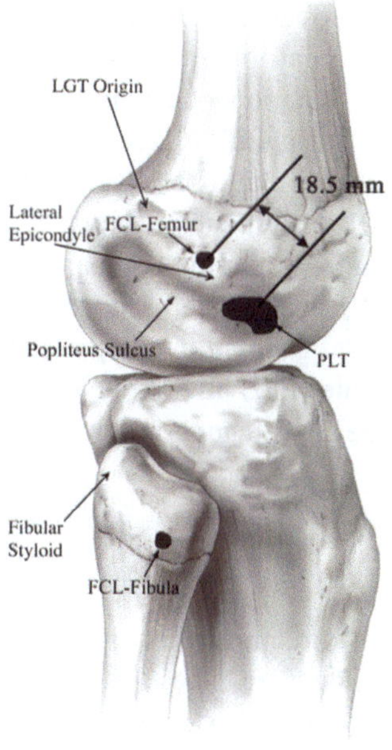

Fig. 3.4 The popliteus tendon and fibular collateral ligament femoral attachments are spaced by an average of 18.5 mm. (From LaPrade et al. 2003 [1]. Reproduced with permission)

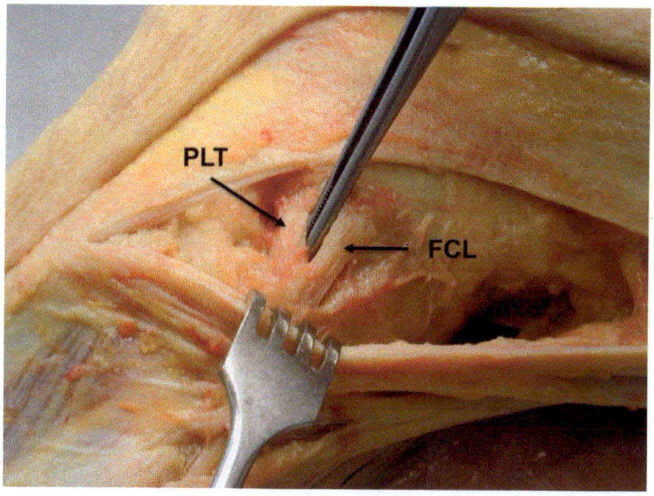

Fig. 3.5 The femoral attachment of the fibular collateral ligament is located through a longitudinal incision in the iliotibial band and is separated from the popliteus tendon attachment by 18.5 mm. *FCL* fibular collateral ligament, *PLT* popliteus tendon

dynamic components, this section highlights the biomechanical properties of the primary static stabilizers, including the FCL, PLT, and PFL.

Fibular (Lateral) Collateral Ligament

The FCL functions as the primary static varus stabilizer in the knee at 0 and 30° of knee flexion and a secondary stabilizer to external rotation [2, 9, 10]. When the FCL is injured, static varus stability is compromised, leading to a varus thrust gait pattern, medial compartment osteoarthritis, and medial meniscus tears [11]. LaPrade et al. reported that a clinician-applied varus stress resulted in an increase of 2.7 mm of side-to-side lateral compartment gapping after an isolated FCL tear [12]. In addition, Coobs et al. reported significantly increased varus rotation and internal rotation at 0, 15, 30, 60, and 90° of knee flexion and external rotation at 60 and 90° after sectioning of the FCL in comparison to the intact knee [13].

Popliteus Tendon

While the popliteus complex combines both static and dynamic functional components, the PLT functions in a ligament-like manner. Under a clinician-applied varus stress, sectioning of the PLT and FCL increased the lateral compartment by 0.8 mm in comparison to the isolated FCL sectioning [12]. The sectioning of both structures resulted in 3.5 mm of lateral gapping in comparison to the intact knee. Isolated sectioning of the PLT has also been reported to result in significant increases in external rotation at 30, 60, and 90° of knee flexion; internal rotation at 0, 20, 30, 60, and 90°; varus angulation at 20, 30, and 60°; and anterior translation at 0, 20, and 30° [7]. No significant differences were noted for posterior translation at any angle. These results lead the

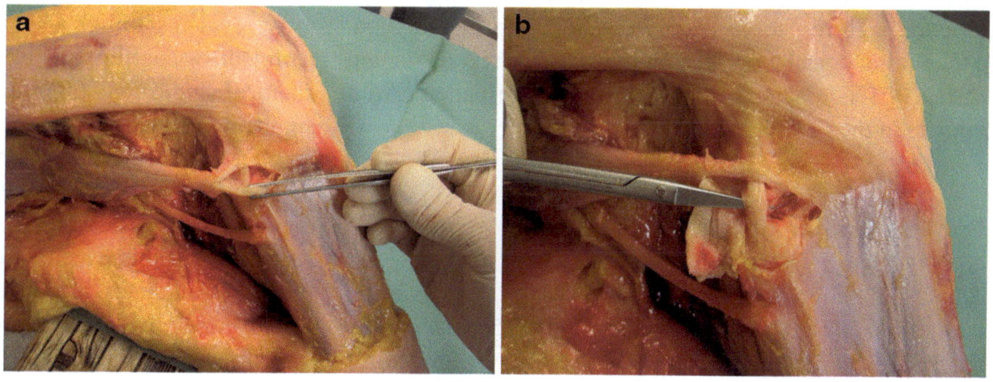

Fig. 3.6 Visualization of the distal FCL attachment is made through the biceps bursa (**a**) (*forceps*) and attaches along the lateral aspect of the fibular head (**b**) (*scissors*). *FCL* fibular collateral ligament

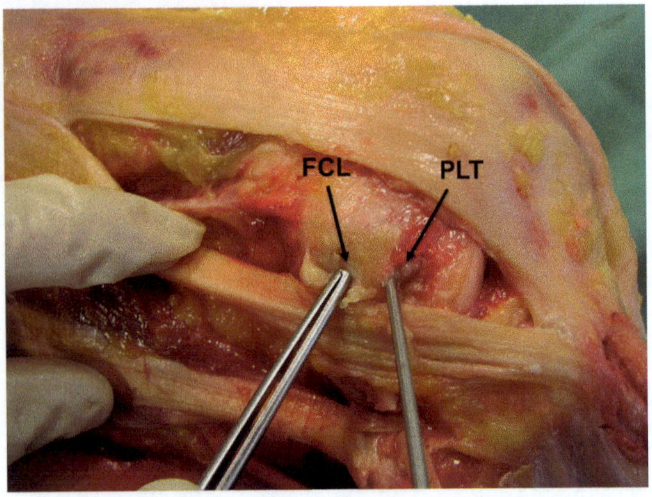

Fig. 3.7 A cadaveric photograph showing the relationship of the fibular collateral ligament and popliteus tendon footprints with both structures removed. *FCL* fibular collateral ligament, *PLT* popliteus tendon

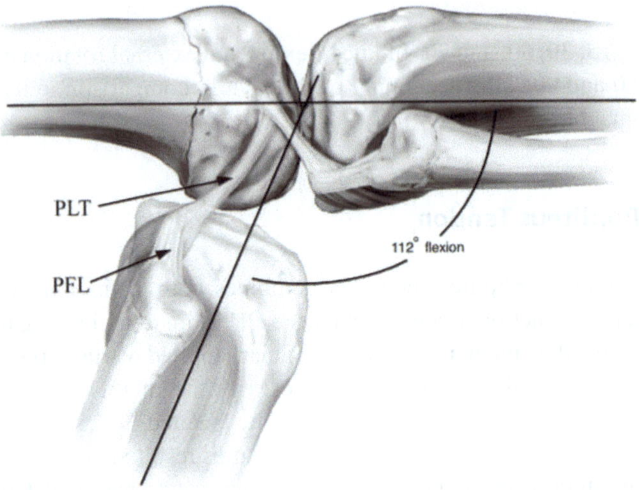

Fig. 3.8 The popliteus tendon engages with the popliteal sulcus at an average of 112° of flexion. (From LaPrade et al. 2003 [1]. Reproduced with permission)

authors to propose that the PLT functions as the "fifth ligament" of the knee by providing primary static stability to external rotation and performing a smaller but significant function with respect to internal rotation, varus angulation, and anterior translation. Therefore, repair or reconstruction of the PLT is essential to restore stability to patients with injuries in the PLC of the knee.

Popliteofibular Ligament

The PFL functions as a stabilizer for external rotation, especially from 30 to 60° of knee flexion [2, 14, 15]. In addition, the PFL functions as a secondary stabilizer against varus gapping with the most pronounced effect at 30° of knee flexion [15]. In light of these functional contributions, McCarthy et al. demonstrated that a PFL tibial component is required to reproduce native knee kinematics during a PLC reconstruction. LaPrade et al. reported that sectioning of the PFL, PLT, and FCL, representing a grade III posterolateral injury, resulted in increased lateral gapping of 4.0 mm in comparison to the intact knee [12]. A grade III posterolateral injury resulted in 0.4 mm of increased lateral gapping in comparison to the FCL- and PLT-sectioned state (PFL intact); however, this increase was not deemed to be significant.

Summary

Together, these three posterolateral structures function as essential stabilizers for the PLC of the knee. These structures limit varus laxity, tibial internal rotation, external rotation, and posterior translation. By understanding the biomechanics of posterolateral knee structures, the diagnosis of injuries is improved. In particular, the use of varus stress radiographs has been shown to yield reproducible results that may aid diagnosis of these injuries. Lastly, by understanding native knee biomechanics, repair and reconstruction techniques can be compared to the functional properties of various intact and sectioned states.

PLC Surgical Implications

Introduction

The PLC of the knee consists of both static and dynamic stabilizers that together provide stability to the lateral compartment of the knee. Injuries to the PLC structures are commonly associated with damage to numerous structures. It has been reported that 56% of PLC injuries include two or more of the major PLC structures, while 70% of PLC injuries are combined with an anterior cruciate ligament (ACL) tear [16]. Untreated PLC injuries often do not heal due to the convex-on-convex contours of the lateral femoral condyle articulating on the lateral tibial plateau, leading to residual instability and increased risk for medial compartment osteoarthritis (Fig. 3.9) [17]. In addition, biomechanical studies have reported that simulated PLC injuries significantly increase the forces on both ACL and posterior cruciate ligament (PCL) grafts [18, 19]. These increased forces after PLC injury have, therefore, been validated as contributors to graft failure after cruciate ligament reconstruction. For this reason, proper diagnosis is imperative to optimize outcomes in patients with isolated or combined PLC injuries to prevent secondary complications to other structures in the knee.

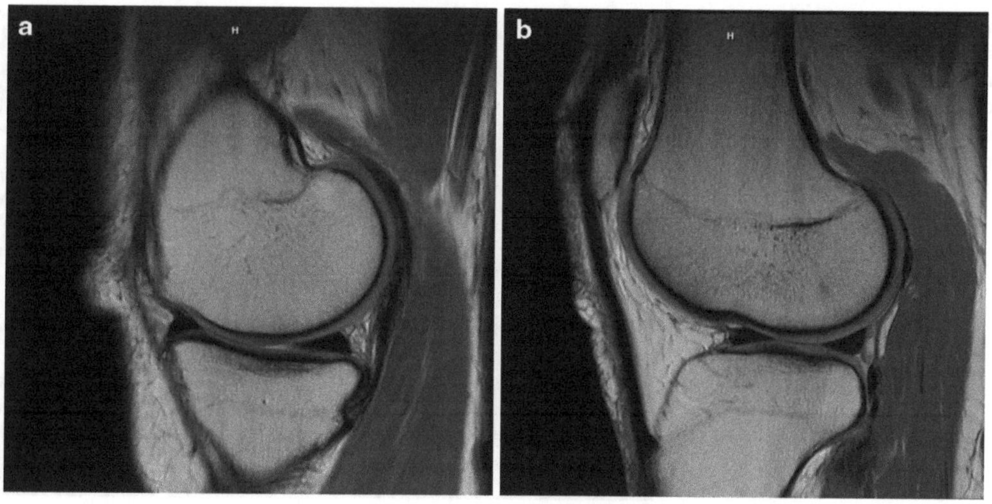

Fig. 3.9 **a** The medial tibiofemoral compartment has convex-on-concave articulating surfaces, providing increased stability to the medial compartment. **b** The lateral tibiofemoral compartment has convex-on-convex articulating surfaces creating an inherent degree of instability (**b**)

Physical Exam

A thorough physical examination of both the injured knee and uninjured knee is essential to diagnose PLC injuries. Inspection and palpation of the PLC should be performed followed by passive and active range-of-motion testing. Special tests include the posterolateral drawer test, dial test, varus stress test, reverse pivot shift test, and standing apprehension test [11]. The external rotation recurvatum test is used to assess for combined PLC and cruciate ligament injuries [20, 21]. Peroneal nerve dysfunction has been reported in 15 % of PLC injuries and must always be considered [22]. Nerve function is evaluated by looking for numbness in the first dorsal web space and weakness to dorsiflexion, foot eversion, and great toe extension. Two widely accepted classification systems for posterolateral knee injury include the Fanelli scale based on the location of injury [23] and the Hughston scale based on the grade of instability [24]. Finally, the results of physical examination can be used to determine injury patterns and develop a treatment plan.

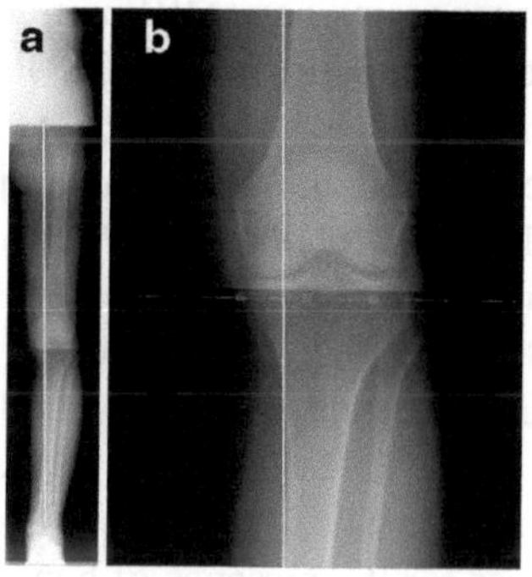

Fig. 3.10 A long-leg radiograph demonstrating a varus weight-bearing axis (**a**); a close view showing the weight-bearing axis point passing medial to the medial tibial eminence (**b**)

Imaging

Imaging is an important diagnostic tool to augment the assessment of posterolateral knee injury. Plain radiography is used to rule out the presence of avulsions and tibial plateau fractures. In chronic cases, long-leg radiographs should be obtained to assess for the presence of a varus mechanical axis deformity (Fig. 3.10). Varus stress radiographs at 0 and 20° offer an objective and retrievable assessment of lateral compartment gapping. The mean side-to-side difference in lateral compartment gapping in isolated grade III FCL injuries is 2.1 and 2.7 mm at 0 and 20°, respectively (Fig. 3.11) [12]. The side-to-side difference in lateral compartment increases to 3.4 and 4.0 mm in knees with a complete grade III PLC injury. In addition, intra- and interobserver reliability is high, indicating that varus stress radiography is a reliable tool in the diagnostic armamentarium [12, 25].

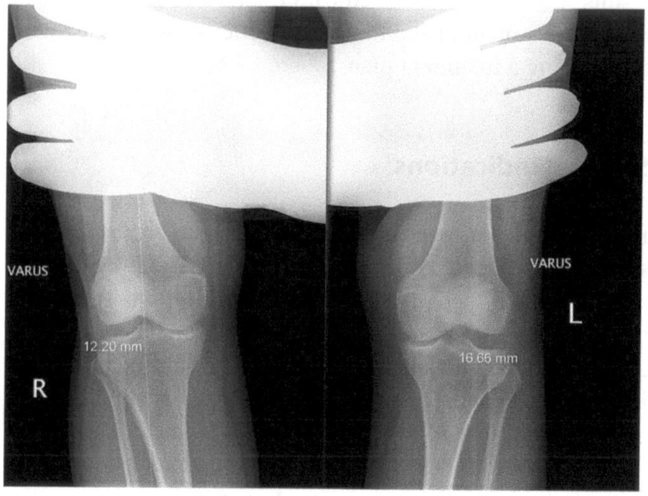

Fig. 3.11 Varus stress radiographs are an objective and a retrievable method of assessing lateral compartment stability

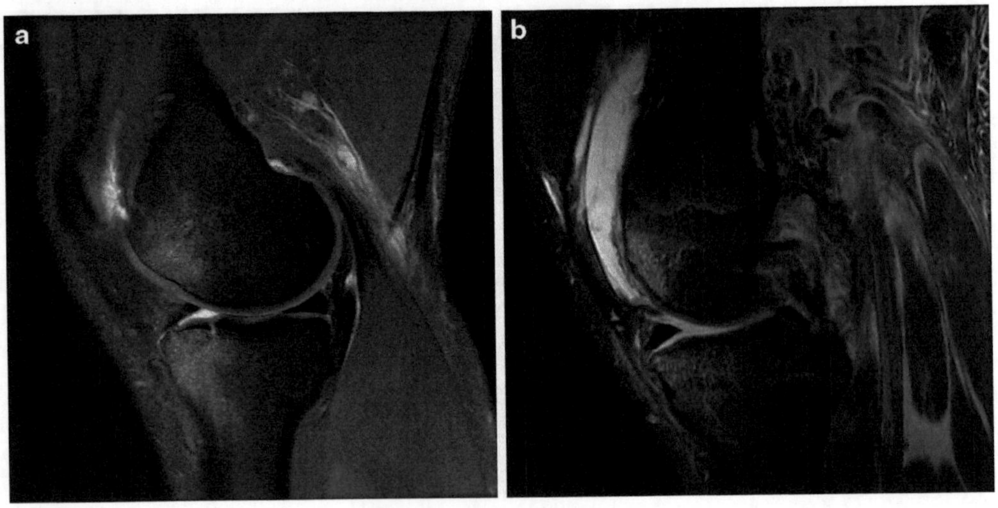

Fig. 3.12 Magnetic resonance images demonstrating bone bruising on the anteromedial femoral condyle (**a**) and bone bruising on the anteromedial femoral condyle plus a fracture on the anteromedial tibial plateau (**b**)

Magnetic resonance imaging (MRI) is essential to further assess PLC structural integrity in the FCL, PFL, PLT, cruciate ligaments, and medial and lateral menisci. High sensitivities have been reported for the detection of injury to the FCL and PLT femoral attachment (94.4 and 93.3 %, respectively); however, the sensitivity of the PFL has been reported to be much lower (68.8 %). In addition, while the FCL has been reported to have a specificity of 100 %, the femoral attachments of the PLT and PFL have been reported to have lower specificity values (80 and 66.7 %, respectively) [26]. It is also important to assess for the presence of bone bruise patterns on MRI, which often present as a secondary sign of a PLC injury (Fig. 3.12). In a prospective series of 102 acute PLC injuries, 55 % of patients had a bone bruise on the anterior aspect of the medial femoral condyle [4]. Together, imaging results should be synthesized with findings on physical exam to identify structural and functional deficits and to assist with formulating a treatment plan.

Surgical Indications

In acute injuries, primary repair of the PLT or FCL avulsions may be performed within the first 2–3 weeks after injury. Primary repair is contraindicated for midsubstance tears, with reconstruction yielding superior outcomes [27, 28]. Nonoperative management should be considered for the initial management of grade I and II injuries, focusing on edema management, range of motion, and quadriceps muscle exercises [11]. However, many patients with low-grade injury may not always present for treatment.

Patients with combined acute or chronic PLC and cruciate ligament injury should undergo posterolateral reconstruction to avoid recurrent instability and the risk of cruciate ligament graft failure [18, 19]. Therefore, PLC reconstruction functions in two major ways: (1) to eliminate symptomatic lateral knee instability that leads to increased stress on the medial compartment of the knee [4] and (2) to protect concurrent cruciate ligament reconstructions by limiting the strain on reconstruction grafts [18, 19].

While primary reconstruction is indicated in patients with acute grade III injuries [11, 29], limb alignment must be assessed first in patients with chronic posterolateral knee injuries. In chronically injured knees, limb alignment must be assessed during surgical planning. Failure to correct underlying varus alignment places the soft tissue posterolateral reconstruction grafts at a high risk of failure. When varus alignment is detected, a proximal tibial opening wedge osteotomy can be used, which resolved posterolateral instability without reconstruction in 38 % of patients in one case series [30].

Surgical Techniques

Grade III injuries to the FCL, PFL, and PLT almost always require repair or reconstruction. Numerous techniques have been described that can be divided into nonanatomic procedures, including the "arcuate complex" advancement [31], biceps femoris tenodesis [32], anterior or posterior tibialis allograft reconstruction [28], single femoral tunnel reconstruction [33], and anatomic procedures utilizing two femoral tunnels with or without popliteus bypass and PFL reconstruction [3, 34–36]. The authors prefer an anatomic reconstruction utilizing a split Achilles tendon allograft to reconstruct the FCL, PFL, and PLT, which has been validated to improve clinical outcomes after surgery [3, 5, 15].

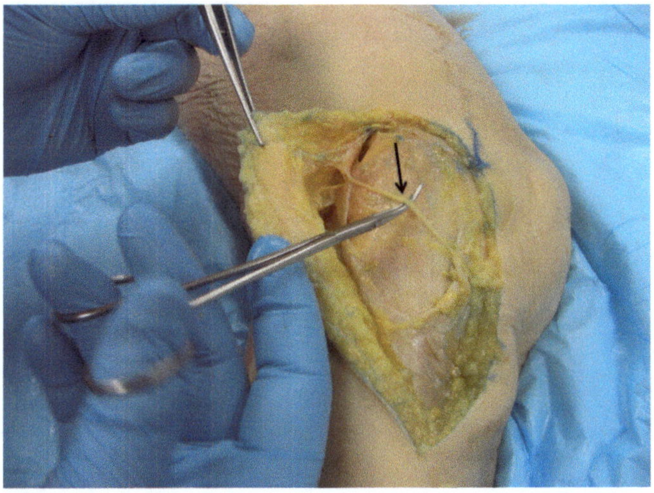

Fig. 3.13 The saphenous nerve courses across the medial aspect of the knee and may be at risk of iatrogenic injury during medial knee surgery (*arrow*)

Posteromedial Corner Anatomy

Introduction

The posteromedial corner (PMC) of the knee is a very commonly injured area of the knee. The most clinically relevant structures of the PMC are the superficial medial collateral ligament (sMCL), the deep medial collateral ligament (dMCL), and the posterior oblique ligament (POL) [37]. In addition, the saphenous nerve courses through the medial aspect of the knee and must be avoided during medial knee surgery (Fig. 3.13). The understanding of the anatomy of each of these ligamentous structures as well as relevant bony landmarks of the medial knee has continued to evolve, which has resulted in a more refined approach to repairing and reconstructing these ligaments.

Medial Femoral Bony Landmarks

The qualitative and quantitative anatomy of the prominent femoral bony landmarks of the medial epicondyle, adductor tubercle, and gastrocnemius tubercle has helped to allay the confusion in the literature regarding the attachment sites of the PMC ligaments [38–41]. LaPrade et al. examined the relationship of all three bony landmarks and reported the qualitative and quantitative relationships among these structures [40]. The medial epicondyle is the most anterior and distal of the three medial bony landmarks (Fig. 3.14). The adductor tubercle is at the distal edge of the medial supracondylar line on the distal aspect of the femur, located 12.6 mm proximal and 8.3 mm posterior to the medial epicondyle. The newly described gastrocnemius tubercle can be referenced off either the medial epicondyle or the adductor tubercle. This structure is 9.4 mm distal and 8.7 mm posterior to the adductor tubercle and adjacent to a depression where the medial gastrocnemius tendon attaches. In addition, it can be located 6.0 mm proximal and 13.7 mm posterior to the medial epicondyle.

Superficial Medial Collateral Ligament

The anatomy of the sMCL was first reported by Brantigan and Voshell, which they termed the tibial collateral ligament [42]. The authors reported that the sMCL attached to the femur at the medial epicondyle and split into two separate attachments on the tibia. Later reports clarified that the sMCL has one femoral attachment and two tibial attachments (Fig. 3.15) [40]. The femoral attachment is located in a depression 3.2 mm proximal and 4.8 mm posterior to the medial epicondyle and 26.8 mm proximal to the femoral joint line (Fig. 3.16). The authors reported that there was no functional attachment between the sMCL and dMCL or any bursae between the two structures. In addition, Wijdicks et al. reported the sMCL attachments in relation to radiographic reference points [43]. The femoral attachment of the sMCL was reported to be 30.5 mm distal to the femoral

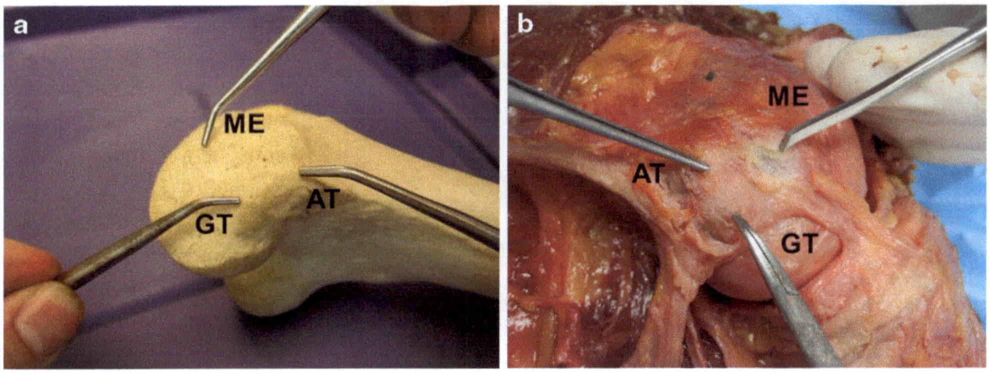

Fig. 3.14 Bony medial knee landmarks (**a–b**) can be readily identified during a medial knee dissection. *AT* adductor tubercle, *GT* gastrocnemius tubercle, *ME* medial epicondyle

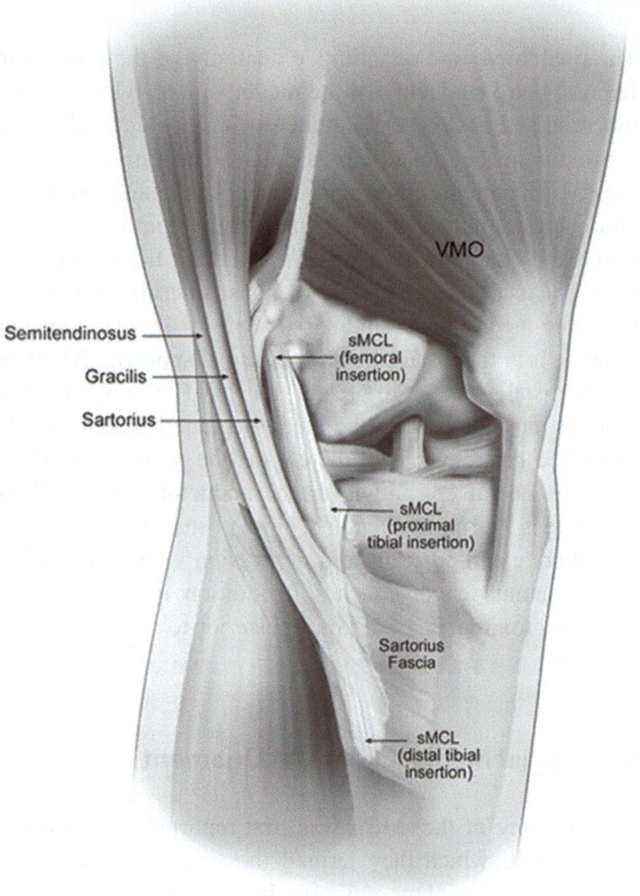

Fig. 3.15 An illustration of the anatomic orientation of the superficial medial collateral ligament, sartorius, gracilis, semitendinosus, and VMO. *sMCL* superficial medial collateral ligament, *VMO* vastus medialis obliquus

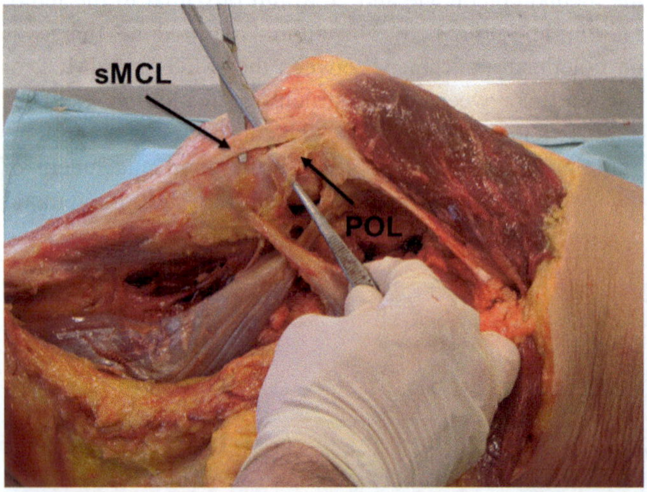

Fig. 3.16 The sMCL consists of one femoral and two tibial attachments; femoral attachments of other ligamentous and tendinous attachments in relation to the sMCL. *MGT* medial gastrocnemius tendon, *MPFL* medial patellofemoral ligament, *sMCL* superficial medial collateral ligament, *VMO* vastus medialis obliquus

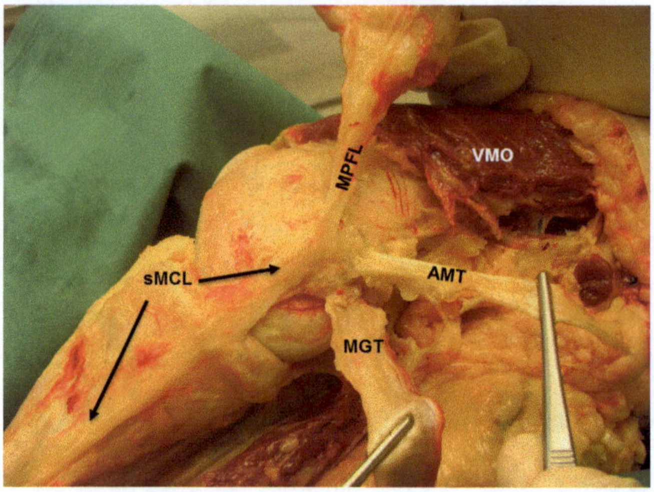

Fig. 3.17 The deep medial collateral ligament consists of a proximal meniscofemoral division and a distal meniscotibial division. *MF* meniscofemoral division, *MFC* medial femoral condyle, *MM* medial meniscus, *MT* meniscotibial division, *sMCL* superficial medial collateral ligament

condylar line on anteroposterior views and 6.0 mm from the medial epicondyle on lateral views.

The tibial attachments of the sMCL are separated from the tibia by the inferior medial genicular artery and vein, fascia, and adipose tissue [41]. The proximal attachment of the sMCL attaches primarily to the deep soft tissue, which was reported to mostly consist of the anterior arm of the semimembranosus tendon. LaPrade et al. reported that the proximal tibial attachment was 12.2 mm distal to the tibial joint line [40], and a similar distance of 11.2 mm distal to the tibial joint line was found on anteroposterior radiographic views [43]. The distal tibial attachment of the sMCL inserts anterior to the posteromedial crest of the tibia within the pes anserine bursa. This attachment was located 61.2 mm distal to the tibial joint line in one study. Wijdicks et al. reported that on anteroposterior radiographic view, the distal attachment was 60.1 mm distal to the tibial joint line [43].

Deep Medial Collateral Ligament

The dMCL is a distinct thickening of the medial joint capsule [40]. This thickening is most distinct along the anterior aspect of the joint capsule, which parallels the fibers of the anterior sMCL. LaPrade et al. reported that the dMCL is consisted of meniscofemoral and meniscotibial ligament components (Fig. 3.17). The meniscofemoral attachment of the dMCL is longer than the meniscotibial attachment and located, an average of 15.7 mm, proximal to the femoral joint line. The meniscotibial attachment, which was reported to be shorter and thicker, attaches only 3.2 mm distal to the tibial joint line.

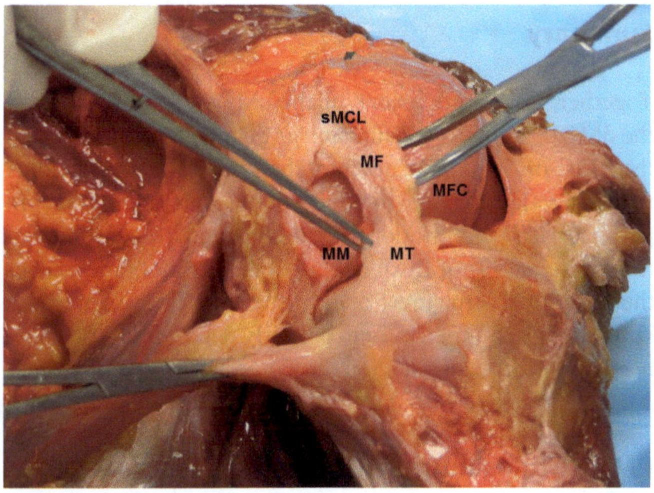

Fig. 3.18 The POL is located posterior to the sMCL and attaches adjacent to the gastrocnemius tendon. *POL* posterior oblique ligament, *sMCL* superficial medial collateral ligament

Posterior Oblique Ligament

The POL was originally considered to be confluent with and the posterior aspect of the sMCL [37, 38, 42, 44]. However, later reports by Hughston et al. defined the POL as a thickening of the capsular ligament that attaches proximally to the adductor tubercle and posterodistally to the tibia, which is anatomically and functionally distinct from the sMCL (Fig. 3.18) [39]. This study also differentiated the POL into three different arms: (1) the central arm that attaches adjacent to the articular cartilage of the posterior tibial plateau, (2) the superior or capsular arm that is continuous with the posterior capsule and the proximal oblique popliteal ligament, and (3) the inferior or superficial arm that attaches both distally to the soft tissue covering the semimembranosus tendon and distally to the semimembranosus tendon insertion. Current literature has quantitatively assessed the relationships of the POL to the main clinically relevant bony landmarks of the medial femur. The POL was found to be much closer to the newly defined gastrocnemius tendon than the adductor tubercle [40]. LaPrade et al. reported that the femoral POL attachment is 1.4 mm distal and 2.9 mm anterior to the gastrocnemius tubercle, and 7.7 mm distal and 6.4 mm posterior to the adductor tubercle. These findings were later confirmed radiographically [43].

The central arm is the largest and thickest portion of the POL [41], and it courses from the distal semimembranosus tendon to provide reinforcement to the posteromedial capsule and medial meniscus. The central arm may be differentiated from the sMCL due to the posterior orientation of its fibers, in comparison to the sMCL fibers that run anteriorly. Distally, the central arm is reported to attach to the posteromedial medial meniscus, meniscotibial dMCL, and posteromedial tibia without a direct bony attachment site.

The capsular arm and superficial arms of the POL are both much thinner than the central arm [37, 41]. The capsular arm is a thin fascial expansion off the anterior and distal semimembranosus tendon, which runs posterolateral to the meniscofemoral dMCL. The capsular arm has no osseous attachment and instead attaches to the soft tissue over the medial gastrocnemius tendon, adductor magnus tendon femoral attachment, and adductor magnus tendon expansion to the medial gastrocnemius. Lastly, the superficial arm of the POL is a thin fascial expansion that runs medially to the anterior arm of the semimembranosus. Proximally, the superficial arm courses into the central arm, while distally the superficial arm follows the posterior border of the sMCL until it blends into the distal tibial attachment of the semimembranosus tendon.

Summary

The sMCL, dMCL, and POL, all have a unique anatomy that in many cases, have only recently been clarified through quantitative studies. The authors believe that the three bony landmarks on the femur—the adductor tubercle, medial epicondyle, and the recently defined gastrocnemius tubercle—are essential for understanding the native anatomy of these structures. As with almost all structures in the knee, the knowledge of this anatomy is essential for developing repair and reconstruction techniques for after injury.

PMC Biomechanics

Introduction

An appreciation for the biomechanics of the posteromedial knee structures is critical for understanding which injured structures need repair or reconstruction. In addition, this understanding will allow for accurate intraoperative and postoperative assessment of the function of reconstructed structures. This section highlights the static and dynamic forces that the sCML, dMCL, and POL have on native knee function.

Superficial Medial Collateral Ligament

The sMCL is the largest medial knee structure, and is composed of proximal and distal divisions. These divisions are conjoined, but function as distinct structures [45, 46]. Sequential sectioning studies and force generation studies have demonstrated that the proximal division not only acts as a primary static stabilizer to valgus motion in all knee flexion angles, but also contributes to internal and external rotation restraint. The proximal division acts as a secondary restraint to external rotation at 90° of knee flexion, and a secondary internal rotation restraint at 0, 30, and 90°. The distal division of the sMCL is a primary stabilizer of internal rotation at all knee flexion angles, a primary stabilizer of external rotation at 30° flexion, and a secondary stabilizer of external rotation at 0, 20, and 60° of knee flexion [45]. In load response testing, the proximal division of the sMCL demonstrated force against valgus stress at all knee flexion angles [46]. However, the distal division of the sMCL varied its force depending on the knee flexion angle, with its highest valgus restraint force at 60° of knee flexion. Therefore, the two divisions of the sMCL function independently and share load depending on knee flexion angle and stress directions. Due to the separate functions of the two divisions of the sMCL, these structures must be treated as distinct ligaments in order to properly restore native knee function in injured ligaments.

Deep Medial Collateral Ligament

The dMCL also has two distinct divisions separated by the attachment to the medial meniscus [45, 46]. The meniscofemoral division of the dMCL functions as a primary restraint to internal rotation at 20, 60, and 90° of knee flexion; a secondary internal rotation restraint at 0 and 30° of flexion; a secondary valgus stabilizer at all knee flexion angles; and a secondary external rotation restraint at 30 and 90° of knee flexion. The meniscotibial division of the dMCL is a secondary valgus stabilizer at 60° of knee flexion, and a secondary internal rotation restraint at 0, 30, and 90° of knee flexion. Therefore, these divisions both have several roles in knee stabilization, but the only primary function is internal rotation restraint by the meniscofemoral division of the dMCL.

Posterior Oblique Ligament

The POL is a thickening of the joint capsule posterior to the MCL, which courses from anterosuperior to posterodistal. The main function of the POL is as a primary stabilizer of internal rotation at all knee flexion angles [45, 47]. It also serves as a secondary external rotation restraint at 30° of knee flexion, a secondary valgus stabilizer at 0 and 30°, and a restraint to posterior tibial translation in extension [37, 47]. Force studies have shown that the POL and sMCL have a shared load response at all knee flexion angles, with significant force generation in internal rotation, external rotation, and valgus stress [46, 48, 49]. This dynamic relationship displays the importance of both the sMCL and the POL in native knee mechanics.

Summary

Together, the two divisions of the sMCL, two divisions of the dMCL, and the POL function as distinct structures within the PMC of the knee. These are the primary knee structures to limit valgus laxity, internal rotation, external rotation, posterior tibial translation in extension, and anterior tibial translation at 90° of flexion. Due to the distinct functions of the individual structures, one must carefully evaluate each structure in an injured knee to properly determine which may need repair or reconstruction.

PMC Surgical Implications

Introduction

The PMC of the knee is a complex arrangement with several distinct structures and functions. Injuries to the medial knee are the most common ligamentous knee injury, and often occur with concomitant cruciate or PLC injury. One study showed that 22 of 23 (96%) patients with combined ACL and sMCL injuries also tore their POL. In addition, 8 out of 23 (35%) had complete PMC injury to the sMCL, dMCL, and POL [50]. Untreated laxity of the medial and posteromedial knee can result in subjective instability, higher stress on native or allograft ACLs and PCLs, and contribute to late cruciate ligament graft failure [47]. The sMCL is widely known to have an abundant vascular supply with strong healing potential [37, 47]. However, it remains unclear whether other structures of the PMC of the knee share this trait or are at higher risk of persistent laxity. Therefore, careful examination and imaging must be considered before a treatment plan is developed for medial knee injury.

Physical Exam

A comprehensive physical exam should be conducted to assess for osseous injury and to determine the integrity of all ligamentous structures of the knee. Initial inspection and palpation may reveal ecchymosis on the medial knee and tenderness to palpation over the superficial MCL or POL. Patients with medial-sided knee injury will have increased laxity with valgus stress. Specifically, the widest opening will be present at 30°, but can also be appreciated at full extension. Joint space opening on valgus stress testing with the knee at full extension indicates injury to the capsule, POL, or both [47]. Valgus opening at 30°, but not at 0°, makes POL injury less likely. A widely accepted grading system for medial knee injury is the American Medical Association Standard

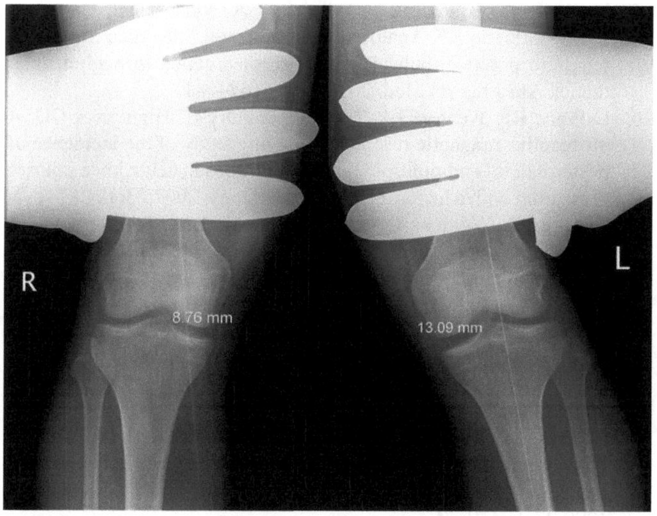

Fig. 3.19 Valgus stress radiographs offer an objective means to quantify medial compartment gapping and correlate with medial knee injury

Nomenclature of Athletic Injuries Scale [51]. In this system, grade I injury shows tenderness to palpation over the medial knee, but no laxity on valgus stress. Grade II injury displays partial tears of the medial knee and laxity with a firm endpoint, while grade III injury displays complete ligamentous disruption and subjective gapping to valgus stress. In addition, medial knee injury is qualitatively described by the grade 1+, 2+, and 3+ system. Grade 1+ has a subjective increase of 3–5 mm of valgus opening, 2+ has an increase of 6–10 mm, and grade 3+ has greater than 10 mm of medial opening with valgus stress compared to the contralateral side [51]. However, it is important to recognize that the American Medical Association (AMA) grading system is based upon subjective data and does not represent the true objective amount of medial compartment gapping with a medial knee injury which is most objectively documented with the use of valgus stress radiographs. The dial test, anteromedial drawer test, Lachman maneuver, posterior drawer test, and varus stress test should also be performed. The synergistic result of these maneuvers will display the likely pattern of injury and involved structures.

Imaging

Simple and advanced imaging modalities are important in the assessment of medial and PMC knee injury. Valgus stress radiographs at 0 and 20° are essential to objectively quantify valgus laxity. An isolated grade III sMCL injury has been reported to result in 1.7 and 3.2 mm of increased gapping with valgus stress at 0 and 20° compared to the contralateral side, respectively. With complete tear to both structures of the MCL and POL injury, valgus opening increases to 6.5 and 9.8 mm at 0 and 20°, respectively (Fig. 3.19) [52]. In addition, plain anteroposterior and lateral radiographs can rule out associated osseous injury, heterotopic ossification (Pellegrini-Stieda disease), tibial plateau fracture, or avulsion. In chronic cases, long-leg radiographs should be obtained to assess for the presence of a valgus mechanical axis deformity. MRI is critical to directly assess for medial-sided ligamentous integrity and to evaluate for concomitant ACL, PCL, and lateral-sided knee injury. Studies have reported that MRI can reliably predict MCL injury in 87 % of patients [53]. These results will confirm physical exam findings and aid in the development of a treatment plan.

Surgical Indications

Acute, isolated medial knee injuries have been clinically proven to have strong healing potential due to the robust vasculature of the sCML [54–56]. Numerous natural history studies have also reported a strong healing potential of the MCL when the other ligaments in the knee are uninjured [57–59]. Therefore, there is a general consensus that acute, isolated grade I, II, or III medial knee injuries should initially be treated nonoperatively with protected range of motion and an acute rehabilitation program. Combined ACL or PCL injury with grade I or II medial knee injury should first be treated conservatively to allow the medial and PMC to heal prior to surgical reconstruction of the cruciate ligaments.

Combined acute grade III injury to the medial knee with grade III gapping in full extension with an ACL or a PCL tear is often an indication for repair or reconstruction of the medial knee. Medial knee laxity may increase the risk of cruciate graft failure if untreated [37, 47]. Therefore, the medial knee must be repaired or reconstructed not only to correct symptomatic valgus instability but also to reduce the strains placed upon cruciate reconstruction grafts.

Chronic medial knee injury with symptomatic valgus laxity or severe, acute medial and posteromedial knee injury are also indications for surgical repair or reconstruction [37, 47]. In chronically injured knees, nonoperative management is unlikely to result in spontaneous healing and reconstruction is generally necessitated. In severe, acutely injured knees including disruption of the POL, nonoperative management is less likely to result in a return to native knee mechanics. Therefore, surgery may be considered depending on the characteristics of the patient and risk factors for surgery.

Surgical Techniques

In a PMC injury where the sMCL, dMCL, and POL are disrupted, repair or reconstruction is often necessary. Several techniques have been developed to reconstruct these ligaments including direct repair [39], primary repair with augmentation [60], pes anserine transfer [39, 61], and autograft or allograft reconstruction [62, 63]. If the POL is deemed repairable, the authors prefer acute repair of the POL with possible augmentation at full extension. If unrepairable, two allografts for reconstruction of both the sMCL and POL are performed [63]. The POL should be fixed at full extension and the sMCL at 30° of flexion according to previous biomechanical studies [44, 47, 63].

References

1. LaPrade RF, Ly TV, Wentorf FA, Engebretsen L. The posterolateral attachments of the knee: a qualitative and quantitative morphologic analysis of the fibular collateral ligament, popliteus tendon, popliteofibular ligament, and lateral gastrocnemius tendon. Am J Sports Med. 2003;31(6):854–60.
2. LaPrade RF, Tso A, Wentorf FA. Force measurements on the fibular collateral ligament, popliteofibular ligament, and popliteus tendon to applied loads. Am J Sports Med. 2004;32(7):1695–701.
3. LaPrade RF, Johansen S, Wentorf FA, Engebretsen L, Esterberg JL, Tso A. An analysis of an anatomical posterolateral knee reconstruction: an in vitro biomechanical study and development of a surgical technique. Am J Sports Med. 2004;32(6):1405–14.
4. Geeslin AG, LaPrade RF. Location of bone bruises and other osseous injuries associated with acute grade III isolated and combined posterolateral knee injuries. Am J Sports Med. 2010;38(12):2502–8.
5. LaPrade RF, Johansen S, Agel J, Risberg MA, Moksnes H, Engebretsen L. Outcomes of an anatomic posterolateral knee reconstruction. J Bone Joint Surg Am. 2010;92(1):16–22.
6. LaPrade RF, Spiridonov SI, Coobs BR, Ruckert PR, Griffith CJ. Fibular collateral ligament anatomical reconstructions: a prospective outcomes study. Am J Sports Med. 2010;38(10):2005–11.
7. LaPrade RF, Wozniczka JK, Stellmaker MP, Wijdicks CA. Analysis of the static function of the popliteus tendon and evaluation of an anatomic reconstruction: the "fifth ligament" of the knee. Am J Sports Med. 2010;38(3):543–9.
8. Pietrini SD, LaPrade RF, Griffith CJ, Wijdicks CA, Ziegler CG. Radiographic identification of the primary posterolateral knee structures. Am J Sports Med. 2009;37(3):542–7.
9. Gollehon DL, Torzilli PA, Warren RF. The role of the posterolateral and cruciate ligament in the stability of the human knee. A biomechanical study. J Bone Joint Surg Am. 1987;69:233–42.
10. Grood ES, Stowers SF, Noyes FR. Limits of movement in the human knee. Effect of sectioning the posterior cruciate ligament and posterolateral structures. J Bone Joint Surg Am. 1988;70:88–97.
11. Lunden JB1, Bzdusek PJ, Monson JK, Malcomson KW, LaPrade RF. Current concepts in the recognition and treatment of posterolateral corner injuries of the knee. J Orthop Sports Phys Ther. 2010;40(8):502–16.
12. LaPrade RF, Heikes C, Bakker AJ, Jakobsen RB. The reproducibility and repeatability of varus stress radiographs in the assessment of isolated fibular collateral ligament and grade-III posterolateral knee injuries. An in vitro biomechanical study. J Bone Joint Surg Am. 2008;90(10):2069–76.
13. Coobs BR, LaPrade RF, Griffith CJ, Nelson BJ. Biomechanical analysis of an isolated fibular (lateral) collateral ligament reconstruction using an autogenous semitendinosus graft. Am J Sports Med. 2007;35(9):1521–7.
14. Maynard MJ, Deng X, Wickiewicz TL, Warren RF. The popliteofibular ligament: rediscovery of a key element in posterolateral stability. Am J Sports Med. 1996;24:311–6.
15. McCarthy M, Camarda L, Wijdicks CA, Johansen S, Engebretsen L, LaPrade RF. Anatomic posterolateral knee reconstructions require a popliteofibular ligament reconstruction through a tibial tunnel. Am J Sports Med. 2010;38(8):1674–81.
16. LaPrade RF, Wentorf FA, Fritts H, Gundry C, Hightower CD. A prospective magnetic resonance imaging study of the incidence of posterolateral and multiple ligament injuries in acute knee injuries presenting with a hemarthrosis. Arthroscopy. 2007;23(12):1341–7.
17. Griffith CJ, Wijdicks CA, Goerke U, Michaeli S, Ellermann J, LaPrade RF. Outcomes of untreated posterolateral knee injuries: an in vivo canine model. Knee Surg Sports Traumatol Arthrosc. 2011;19(7):1192–7.
18. LaPrade RF, Muench C, Wentorf F, Lewis JL. The effect of injury to the posterolateral structures of the knee on force in a posterior cruciate ligament graft: a biomechanical study. Am J Sports Med. 2002;30(2):233–8.
19. LaPrade RF, Resig S, Wentorf F, Lewis JL. The effects of grade III posterolateral knee complex injuries on anterior cruciate ligament graft force. A biomechanical analysis. Am J Sports Med. 1999;27(4):469–75.
20. Hughston JC, Norwood LA Jr. The posterolateral drawer test and external rotational recurvatum test for posterolateral rotatory instability of the knee. Clin Orthop Relat Res. 1980 Mar-Apr;147:82–87.
21. LaPrade RF, Ly TV, Griffith C. The external rotation recurvatum test revisited: reevaluation of the sagittal plane tibiofemoral relationship. Am J Sports Med. 2008;36(4):709–12.
22. LaPrade RF, Terry GC. Injuries to the posterolateral aspect of the knee. Association of anatomic injury patterns with clinical instability. Am J Sports Med. 1997;25(4):433–8.
23. Fanelli GC, Feldmann D. Management of combined anterior cruciate ligament/posterior cruciate ligament/posterolateral complex injuries of the knee. Oper Tech Sports Med. 1999;7:143–9.
24. Hughston JC, Andrews JR, Cross MJ, Moschi A. Classification of knee ligament instabilities. Part II. The lateral compartment. J Bone Joint Surg Am. 1976;58(2):173–9.
25. Gwathmey FW Jr, Tompkins MA, Gaskin CM, Miller MD. Can stress radiography of the knee help characterize posterolateral corner injury? Clin Orthop Relat Res. 2012;470(3):768–73.
26. LaPrade RF, Gilbert TJ, Bollom TS, Wentorf F, Chaljub G. The magnetic resonance imaging appearance of individual structures of the posterolateral knee. A prospective study of normal knees and knees with surgically verified grade III injuries. Am J Sports Med. 2000;28(2):191–9.
27. Levy BA, Dajani KA, Morgan JA, Shah JP, Dahm DL, Stuart MJ. Repair versus reconstruction of the fibular collateral ligament and posterolateral corner in the multiligament-injured knee. Am J Sports Med. 2010;38(4):804–9.
28. Stannard JP, Brown SL, Farris RC, McGwin G Jr, Volgas DA. The posterolateral corner of the knee: repair versus reconstruction. Am J Sports Med. 2005;33(6):881–8.
29. Geeslin AG1, LaPrade RF. Outcomes of treatment of acute grade-III isolated and combined posterolateral knee injuries: a prospective case series and surgical technique. J Bone Joint Surg Am. 2011;93(18):1672–83.
30. Arthur A, LaPrade RF, Agel J. Proximal tibial opening wedge osteotomy as the initial treatment for chronic posterolateral corner deficiency in the varus knee: a prospective clinical study. Am J Sports Med. 2007;35(11):1844–50.
31. Hughston JC, Jacobson KE. Chronic posterolateral rotatory instability of the knee. J Bone Joint Surg Am. 1985;67(3):351–9.
32. Wascher DC, Grauer JD, Markoff KL. Biceps tendon tenodesis for posterolateral instability of the knee. An in vitro study. Am J Sports Med. 1993;21(3):400–6.
33. Larson RV, Sidles JA, Beals CT. Isometry of lateral collateral and popliteofibular ligaments and a technique for reconstruction. University of Washington research report, 1996. pp. 42–4.

34. Bicos J, Arciero RA. Novel approach for reconstruction of the posterolateral corner using a free tendon graft technique. Sports Med Arthrosc Rev. 2006;14:28–36.
35. Noyes FR, Barber-Westin SD. Surgical reconstruction of severe posterolateral corner injuries of the knee using allograft tissues. Am J Sports Med. 1995;23:2–12.
36. Sekiya JK, Kurtz CA. Posterolateral corner reconstruction of the knee: surgical technique utilizing a bifid Achilles tendon allograft and a double femoral tunnel. Arthroscopy. 2005;21:1400.
37. Wijdicks CA, Griffith CJ, Johansen S, Engebretsen L, LaPrade RF. Injuries to the medial collateral ligament and associated medial structures of the knee. J Bone Joint Surg Am. 2010;92(5):1266–80.
38. Fischer RA, Arms SW, Johnson RJ, Pope MH. The functional relationship of the posterior oblique ligament to the medial collateral ligament of the human knee. Am J Sports Med. 1985;13(6):390–7.
39. Hughston JC, Eilers AF. The role of the posterior oblique ligament in repairs of acute medial (collateral) ligament tears of the knee. J Bone Joint Surg Am. 1973;55:923–40.
40. LaPrade RF, Engebretsen AH, Ly TV, Johansen S, Wentorf FA, Engebretsen L. The anatomy of the medial part of the knee. J Bone Joint Surg Am. 2007;89(9):2000–10.
41. Loredo R, Hodler J, Pedowitz R, Yeh LR, Trudell D, Resnick D. Posteromedial corner of the knee: MR imaging with gross anatomic correlation. Skeletal Radiol. 1999;28(6):305–11.
42. Brantigan OC, Voshell AF. The tibial collateral ligament: its function, its bursae, and its relation to the medial meniscus. J Bone Joint Surg Am. 1943;25(1):121–31.
43. Wijdicks CA, Griffith CJ, LaPrade RF, Johansen S, Sunderland A, Arendt EA, Engebretsen L. Radiographic identification of the primary medial knee structures. J Bone Joint Surg Am. 2009;91(3):521–9.
44. Slocum DB, Larson RL. Rotatory instability of the knee. Its pathogenesis and a clinical test to determine its presence. J Bone Joint Surg Am. 1968;50(2):211–5.
45. Griffith CJ, LaPrade RF, Johansen S, Armitage B, Wijdicks C, Engebretsen L. Medial knee injury: Part 1, static function of the individual components of the main medial knee structures. Am J Sports Med. 2009;37(9):1762–70.
46. Griffith CJ, Wijdicks CA, LaPrade RF, Armitage BM, Johansen S, Engebretsen L. Force measurements on the posterior oblique ligament and superficial medial collateral ligament proximal and distal divisions to applied loads. Am J Sports Med. 2009;37(1):140–8.
47. Tibor LM, Marchant MH Jr, Taylor DC, Hardaker WT Jr, Garrett WE Jr, Sekiya JK. Management of medial-sided knee injuries, part 2: posteromedial corner. Am J Sports Med. 2011;39(6):1332–40.
48. Wijdicks CA, Ewart DT, Nuckley DJ, Johansen S, Engebretsen L, LaPrade RF. Structural properties of the primary medial knee ligaments. Am J Sports Med. 2010;38(8):1638–46.
49. Wijdicks CA, Griffith CJ, LaPrade RF, Spiridonov SI, Johansen S, Armitage BM, Engebretsen L. Medial knee injury: part 2, load sharing between the posterior oblique ligament and superficial medial collateral ligament. Am J Sports Med. 2009;37:1771–6.
50. Halinen J, Lindahl J, Hirvensalo E, Santavirta S. Operative and nonoperative treatments of medial collateral ligament rupture with early anterior cruciate ligament reconstruction: a prospective randomized study. Am J Sports Med. 2006;34:1134–40.
51. American Medical Association. Committee on the Medical Aspects of Sports. Standard nomenclature of athletic injuries. Chicago: American Medical Association; 1966. pp. 99–100.
52. LaPrade RF, Bernhardson AS, Griffith CJ, Macalena JA, Wijdicks CA. Correlation of valgus stress radiographs with medial knee ligament injuries: an in vitro biomechanical study. Am J Sports Med. 2010;38(2):330–8.
53. Yao L, Dungan D, Seeger LL. MR imaging of tibial collateral ligament injury: comparison with clinical examination. Skeletal Radiol. 1994;23:521–4.
54. Ellsasser JC, Reynolds FC, Omohundro JR. The non-operative treatment of collateral ligament injuries of the knee in professional football players. An analysis of seventy-four injuries treated nonoperatively and twenty-four injuries treated surgically. J Bone Joint Surg Am. 1974;56(6):1185–90.
55. Indelicato PA. Non-operative treatment of complete tears of the medial collateral ligament of the knee. J Bone Joint Surg Am. 1983;65:323–9.
56. Indelicato PA, Hermansdorfer J, Huegel M. Nonoperative management of complete tears of the medial collateral ligament of the knee in intercollegiate football players. Clin Orthop Relat Res. 1990;256:174–7.
57. Inoue M, McGurk-Burleson E, Hollis JM, Woo SL. Treatment of the medial collateral ligament injury. I: the importance of anterior cruciate ligament on the varus-valgus knee laxity. Am J Sports Med. 1987;15(1):15–21.
58. Weiss JA, Woo SL, Ohland KJ, Horibe S, Newton PO. Evaluation of a new injury model to study medial collateral ligament healing: primary healing versus nonoperative treatment. J Orthop Res. 1991;9(4):516–28.
59. Woo SL, Young EP, Ohland KJ, Marcin JP, Horibe S, Lin HC. The effects of transection of the anterior cruciate ligament on healing of the medial collateral ligament. A biomechanical study of the knee in dogs. J Bone Joint Surg Am. 1990;72(3):382–92.
60. Gorin S, Paul DD, Wilkinson EJ. An anterior cruciate ligament and medial collateral ligament tear in a skeletally immature patient: a new technique to augment primary repair of the medial collateral ligament and an allograft reconstruction of the anterior cruciate ligament. Arthroscopy. 2003;19:E21–6.
61. Nicholas JA. The five-one reconstruction for anteromedial instability of the knee. Indications, technique, and the results in fifty-two patients. J Bone Joint Surg Am. 1973;55:899–922.
62. Yoshiya S, Kuroda R, Mizuno K, Yamamoto T, Kurosaka M. Medial collateral ligament reconstruction using autogenous hamstring tendons: technique and results in initial cases. Am J Sports Med. 2005;33:1380–5.
63. Coobs BR, Wijdicks CA, Armitage BM, Spiridonov SI, Westerhaus BD, Johansen S, Engebretsen L, LaPrade RF. An in vitro analysis of an anatomical medial knee reconstruction. Am J Sports Med. 2010;38(2):339–47.

Part III

Diagnosis and Evaluation

Clinical and Arthroscopic Evaluation of the Posterior-Cruciate-Ligament-Injured Knee

4

Brian M. Devitt and Daniel B. Whelan

Introduction

Although the posterior cruciate ligament (PCL) is the strongest ligament of the knee, it is rarely reconstructed in isolation [1, 2]. It has generally been accepted that multi-ligamentous knee injuries involving the PCL require operative intervention [1]. Yet, the treatment of PCL injuries in isolation is less clearly defined and remains somewhat controversial.

Isolated tears of the PCL have traditionally been treated nonoperatively with relative success [3–5]. As such, the requirement for operative intervention for isolated PCL injured knees has been reported to be as low as 3 % [5]. Indeed, there are numerous examples of high-level athletes, who have sustained PCL injuries and have returned to pre-injury levels without surgical intervention in the short to intermediate term [6]. Nonetheless, long-term clinical studies have reported that non-operative treatment frequently leads to early-onset osteoarthritis of the patellofemoral and medial compartments and an overall deterioration in knee function [7–11]. Therefore, it is becoming clear that whereas some patients may cope reasonably well with a deficient PCL, others have significantly reduced knee function and require operative intervention to regain knee stability [12, 13].

A key element in assessing a patient with an injured PCL, whether in isolation or part of a multi-ligamentous injured knee, is to determine the extent of knee instability and the functional limitations this places on the patient. The acuteness of the injury also needs to be considered as part of this process. The assessment not only encompasses a thorough history and physical examination but also requires advanced imaging. This chapter provides a comprehensive review of the steps required to provide a clinical and arthroscopic evaluation of a patient with a PCL injured knee.

D. B. Whelan (✉)
Division of Orthopaedic Surgery, St. Michael's Hospital, 800-55 Queen Street East, Toronto, ON M5C 1Rl, Canada
e-mail: wheland@smh.ca

B. M. Devitt
Orthopaedic Surgery, Sports Surgery Clinic, Santry Demense, Dublin 9, Ireland

History

"We all pay lip service to a careful history, but how many of us are patient enough to elicit one?" Alan Graham Apley [14]

A good history provides the first clue in solving the mystery of the multi-ligamentous injured knee. A majority of mechanical disorders almost diagnose themselves to the attentive listener. Let the patient tell his/her own story. It is often helpful in taking a history to differentiate between an acute and chronic injury by asking the following open-ended questions:

Acute injury—Tell me what happened to your knee?
Chronic injury—Tell me about your knee?

The 'history' like all good stories should have a beginning, middle and an end. Start with the index trauma, which is of critical importance. By exploring the mechanism of injury, one can often ascertain the structures at risk; e.g. PCL injuries typically occur by direct impact to the anterior aspect of the tibia with a flexed knee or by hyperextension, hyperflexion, or rotational injuries with associated varus or valgus stress [15]. Particular attention should be given to the energy or velocity imparted to the knee during the injury; was the injury a result of a motor vehicle accident, a sporting injury, or an ultralow velocity mechanism [16]?

Following the initial injury, the examiner needs to discover what happened next: Did the knee swell up immediately? Could the patient bear weight? Did the knee feel unstable? Or worse, was the knee dislocated and needed to be reduced? Was there any concern about the blood supply to the foot? Enquire as to what treatment was initiated acutely and which investigations were performed.

In concluding the history, explore with the patients the current symptoms they are suffering, including pain, stiffness

G. C. Fanelli (ed.), *Posterior Cruciate Ligament Injuries*,
DOI 10.1007/978-3-319-12072-0_4, © Springer International Publishing Switzerland 2015

and instability. Pain alone is incredibly important and may be the overwhelming symptom in patients with chronic injury. Interrogating the patient as to the nature of pain is very beneficial in directing treatment. Enquiry should also hone in on the functional limitations the patient endures; what can you not do today that you were able to do prior to the injury? Do you trust your knee?

Physical Examination

A well-performed, systematic and clearly documented physical examination is a key component to diagnosing and treating a multi-ligamentous injured knee.

Physical examination represents a quick, sensitive and reproducible method to establish an anatomical diagnosis, provide a realistic prognosis and direct further investigations. It should be considered as the primary investigation in the evaluation of an injured patient, preceding other radiological investigations.

Life, Limb, Joint

Given the high incidence of vascular and neurological injury associated with multi-ligamentous knee injuries, assessment of the neurovascular status takes primacy in terms of the initial assessment of the limb [17]. Based on the clinical suspicion ascertained from the history, the specific ligamentous injury is identified primarily by comparing the excursion of the tibia on the femur in the affected and unaffected knee. To this end, nature has been considerate by providing a normal side for comparison. Assessing for the presence of pathology to the knee involves imparting stress to the knee through a range of motion.

The concept of 'look, feel, move' provides a useful and simplistic framework for the systematic assessment of the injured limb, ensuring that relevant findings are not overlooked.

Look

The entire limb should be inspected, paying particular attention for the presence of skin changes, abrasions, ecchymosis, or old scars. In the acute setting, one should rule out any evidence of active bleeding, gross mal-alignment or open injury.

The 'dimple sign' over the medial aspect of the knee is indicative of a knee dislocation that may require open reduction, and may occur as a result of buttonholing of the medial femoral condyle through the anteromedial joint capsule or entrapment of the adductor magnus tendon (Fig. 4.1) [18, 19].

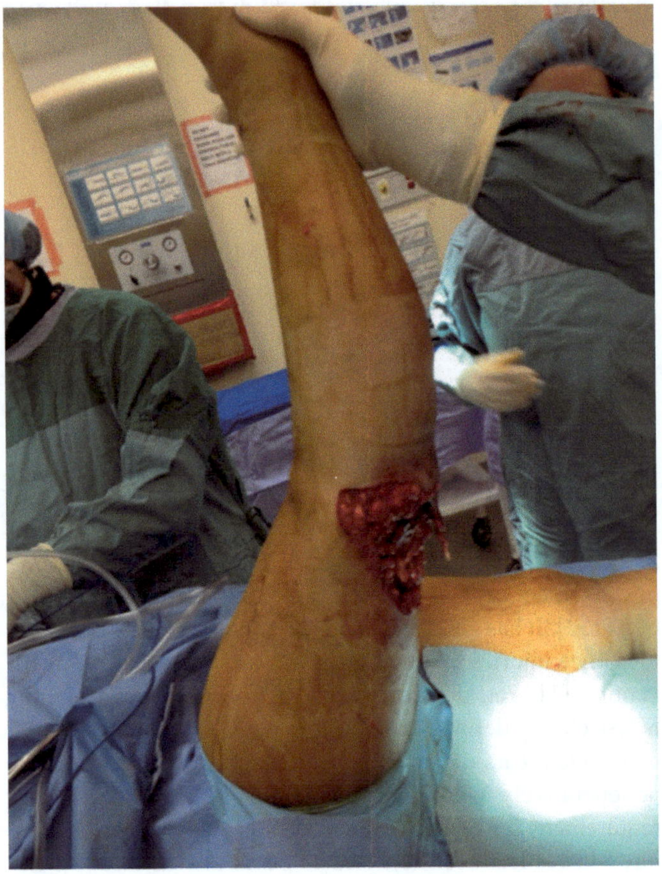

Fig. 4.1 An intra-operative clinical photograph revealing extensive soft-tissue injury on the posterior aspect of the knee with an associated recurvatum deformity

The state of the skin is also quite revealing as to the direction, force and mechanism of injury. Pay particular attention to observe the anterior aspect of the tibia for the presence of bruising; this is a common site for a haematoma in the setting of a PCL injury as a result of direct impact to the anterior aspect of the tibia following a fall on the flexed knee. In addition, be mindful to inspect the posterior aspect of the knee, which is also instructive as to the extent of the injury (Fig. 4.2). The shape of the joint and upper and lower limb segments, their general alignment and any atrophy or swelling (localized or diffuse) should be noted; all of this preceding the 'laying on of hands'.

Feel

Vascular Assessment

The physical examination continues with an evaluation of the vascular status of the lower extremity. Be observant for signs of vascular injury (Table 4.1). Examine the temperature of the distal extremity. Palpate for both the dorsalis pedis and posterior tibial pulses. Hard signs should alert the

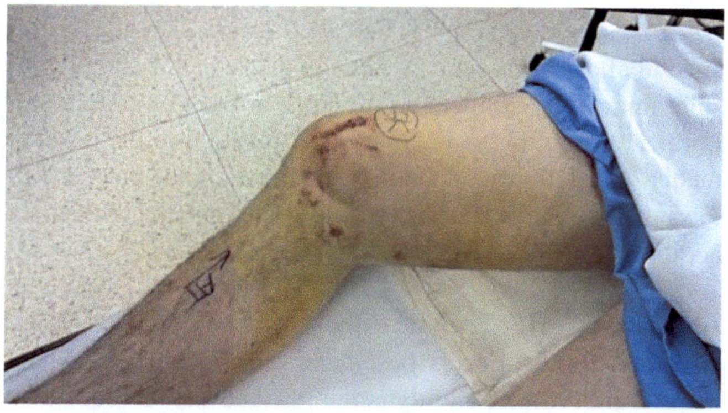

Fig. 4.2 Ecchymosis on the medial aspect of the knee with a positive 'dimple' sign (*white arrow*), indicative of an irreducibly dislocated knee with soft-tissue interposition between the femur and tibia

Table 4.1 Signs of vascular injury

Hard signs	Active haemorrhage
	Distal ischemia
	Expanding haematoma
Soft signs	Limb colour
	Capillary refill

treating surgeon to the need for emergent vascular imaging and involvement of a vascular surgeon. Soft signs, on the other hand, are less reliable; however, at the very least they should heighten the clinical suspicion and prompt the use of further vascular studies.

Neurological Assessment

Assessment of neurological function in the setting of knee dislocation can be challenging. In the context of a multisystem injury, the compliance of the patient may be compromised by a head injury or intoxication. The peroneal nerve is the most commonly injured nerve, due to its proximity, with less frequent injury to the tibial nerve [20]. Both the sensory and motor function of these nerves must be evaluated and documented, particularly before and after any manoeuvres or intervention.

The Form of the Knee

Palpation of the knee requires a subtle gradient of force application. The examiner should commence with the normal side with sufficient pressure to feel the subtleties of the knee's form. The process complements the visual inspection.

Increasing pressure may be applied to distinguish induration—the hardness of the different tissue planes. Induration provides insight into the severity and site of the injury. It is often helpful to bend the knee during this process to localize the source of the injury, and identify specific anatomical structures.

The skin, soft tissues and bones should be palpated methodically in an orderly manner to distinguish between normal and altered anatomy. The precise relationship of tender points to the joint line and ligamentous attachments is instructive in identifying the site of the lesion.

The final palpation is conducted with slightly more force to identify tenderness and/or gaps in the underlying soft tissue. It is critical that the patient is aware that you will be probing with increased vigour and can expect a certain degree of discomfort. It is important not to neglect the extensor mechanism of the knee, in particular the inferior pole of the patella, which, if tender, may indicate a concomitant injury to the PCL, which may have resulted from an anteriorly applied force; e.g. a dashboard injury.

Move

Examination of the knee should consist of active and passive motion. It is helpful to ask the patient to move the well leg within the range of motion that is comfortable and possible, which provides the standard for comparison. In an acutely injured knee, this portion of the examination may be painful. The examiner should be confident and decisive and try to avoid excessive force, which can induce pain and cause guarding or even further injury.

Ask the patient to move the injured leg within the limits of comfort. This process is important in demonstrating the range of motion available to position the leg for the ligamentous examination. Passive movement of the joint may be carried out gently to assess any resistance to full extension or further flexion. Focus on the effect of passive movement by looking at the patient's face.

Limits of Motion

An initial assessment of the limits of motion is very important. First, start by asking the patient to fully extend the knee. An inability to fully extend the knee may indicate meniscal pathology, hamstring spasm or a comprised extensor mechanism. This assessment is very beneficial also in ascertaining the need for acute surgical intervention or the requirement for preoperative physical therapy to improve the range of motion.

Flexion, both active and passive, is tested next. Note the limits of motion with each test and try to identify the location of any discomfort. Knee flexion of at least 90° is required to be able to carry out a conclusive examination of the PCL. If this angle cannot be achieved initially, the patient should be re-examined sequentially following physical therapy until it is reached. Ice may be helpful in reducing swelling and pain and facilitate an improved physical examination. Failing this, an examination under anaesthetic (EUA) may be warranted. Joint line tenderness on maximal flexion may indicate meniscal pathology, which should not be overlooked.

Special Tests

There are a myriad of special tests, which may be carried out to assess the knee. The key factor is to choose a series of tests, which are comprehensive enough to assess the entirety of the knee and are also reproducible to the examiner. Listed below are preferred tests of the authors.

Varus/Valgus Stability

If the patient can reach hyperextension, it is the ideal position to start. Stability in this position infers that the medial and lateral capsuloligamentous structures and the PCL are intact. This finding alone is extremely informative. However, laxity in this position to either varus or valgus angulation is a worrying sign, indicating disruption of key ligamentous structures. If in hyperextension the knee is lax to varus angulation, then the posterolateral corner and the PCL are probably disrupted (Fig. 4.3). Likewise, if in hyperextension the joint is lax to valgus angulation, the medial capsuloligamentous structures and the PCL are probably disturbed (Fig. 4.4).

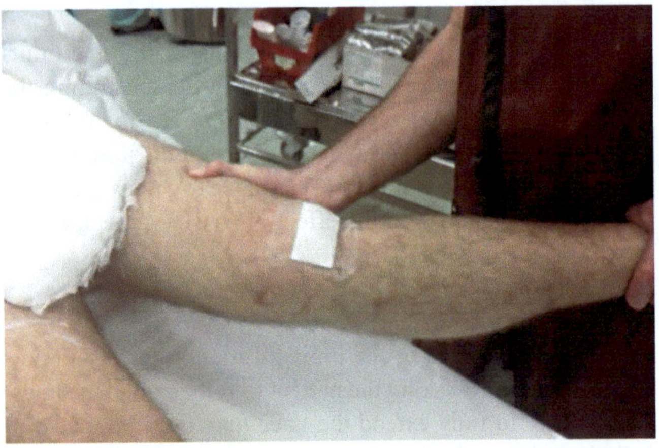

Fig. 4.3 Valgus instability in hyperextension: Valgus opening in full extension with no end point. This finding is indicative of injury to not only the medial structures but also the posteromedial capsule and likely the posterior cruciate ligament

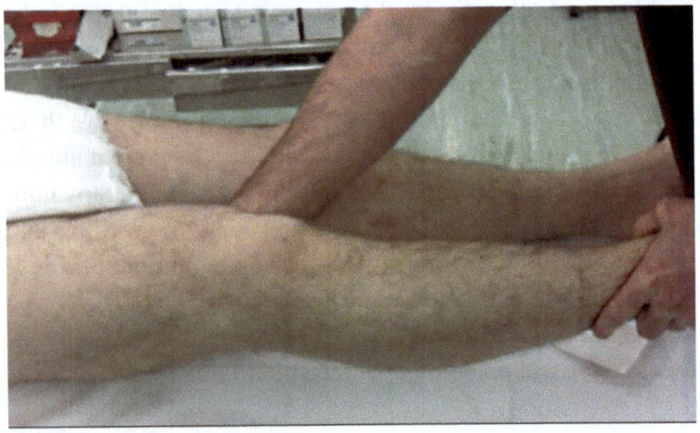

Fig. 4.4 Testing of varus stability in full extension: The knee is tested in full extension to assess if there is lateral and posterolateral corner instability

At 0° flexion, the ACL and PCL are sufficiently slackened to allow diagnostic evaluation of medial or lateral capsular injuries by application of varus and valgus angulation. Further flexion to 30° facilitates examination of the isolated medial and lateral collateral ligaments (LCLs) because, in this position, the posterolateral and posteromedial corners, in addition to the cruciate ligaments, are relaxed.

Anteroposterior Translation

Anteroposterior glide is best determined with the fingers. Prior to performing any dynamic manoeuvres, be confident that you can palpate both the medial and lateral joint line. As the examination of both posterior and anterior drawers is conventionally performed in the same position, one must be able to distinguish between subtle changes in anteroposterior translation.

> An anterior drawer is only present when one has proved that the posterior drawer is absent. Werner Müller [21]

The first component to these series of tests is to assess the relationship of the tibial plateau to the femur in the sagittal plane. Position the patient supine with the hips flexed to 45° and the knee at 90° of flexion. Prior to performing any tests, keen surveillance is essential. Flex both knees together, and inspect the silhouette of the knee in the sagittal plane, from each side (Fig. 4.5). Begin with the uninjured side. The key structures to observe are the anterior tibial tubercle and the association with the patellar tendon and the anterior aspect of the patella. In the presence of a disrupted PCL, and more often than not a concomitant posteromedial or posterolateral lesion, the tibial plateau will be translated posteriorly with respect to the femur, which is termed 'posterior sag'.

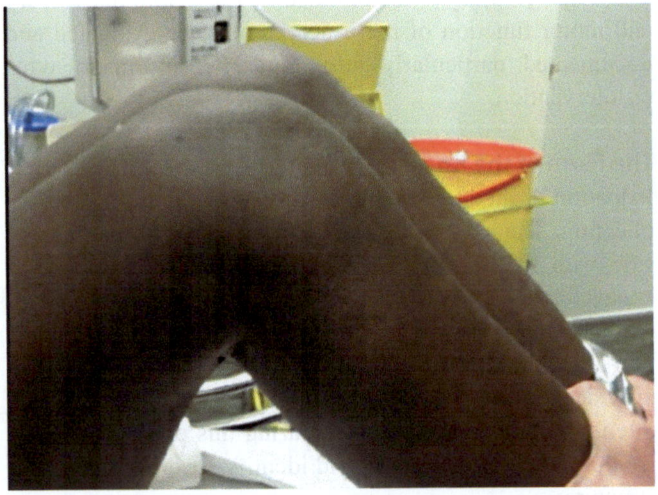

Fig. 4.5 Inspection of relative tibial translation: The patient is placed supine on the table with hips flexed to 45° and knees to 90°. Observe the silhouette of the knees. Note the loss of the contour of the joint line and prominence of the tibial tuberosity on the right knee compared to the opposite side, suggesting posterior subluxation of the tibia

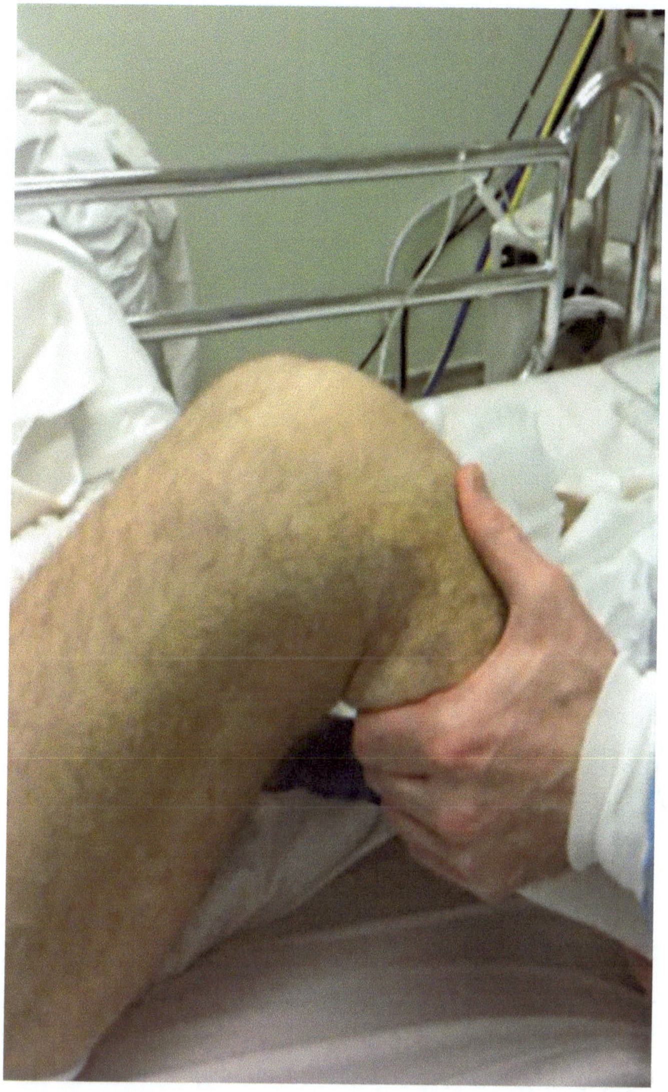

Fig. 4.6 Posterior drawer testing in neutral rotation. The patient is supine with the knees flexed to 90°. A posterior force is exerted anteriorly on the proximal tibia. Translation at the joint line can be appreciated with the thumbs

Müller also describes a test where the patient is asked to actively extend the knee from the flexed position [21]. The force of the quadriceps will translate the tibia anteriorly to allow the knee to straighten, which is visible from the sagittal position. This test is also known as the 'quadriceps active' test. A modification of this test is performed by holding the foot and asking the patient to contract his/her quadriceps against resistance.

Pure posterior glide involves symmetrical posterior translation of both tibial plateaus with neither internal nor external rotation. This is a rare situation. Posterior drawer alone without any peripheral lesions is due to an isolated PCL lesion, which is not a common finding. Peripheral structures compensate for the absence of a PCL and give rise to a hard end point at the extreme of posterior translation [22]. The accuracy of the interpretation can, therefore, be uncertain.

Table 4.2 IKDC—Grading of joint translation

Normal	Nearly normal	Abnormal	Sev. abnormal
0–2 mm	3–5 mm	6–10 mm	>10 mm

Associated posteromedial or posterolateral lesions also influence the response to posterior translation. A soft end point is typically present in this circumstance. Failure to discriminate between this finding and an anterior drawer is not unusual, as injury to the anterior cruciate ligament (ACL) is a more common finding.

The Posterior and Anterior Drawer Test

The foot is fixed firmly in a neutral position with the knee flexed to 90°. The posterior aspect of the proximal tibia is held with both hands, placing the fingers into the popliteal fossa (Fig. 4.6). The movement for posterior drawer first requires the joint to be reduced to a neutral position. It is, therefore, advisable to place the thumbs of each hand on either side of the patellar tendon so that one can palpate any posterior subluxation and to confirm that the joint is in neutral alignment. Feel the tightness of the hamstrings with the index and middle fingers and ask the patient to relax. The tibia is then pulled forward in order to feel the anterior shift of the tibial plateau. The tibia is then pushed backwards by applying a force with the thumbs on the tibial tuberosity. This manoeuvre is gently repeated, as required. It is important to be conscious of the end point in the anterior and posterior direction. Observe for a change in shape of the joint with each sequential movement. It is possible to increase the force of the anterior pull by placing the thumbs against the femoral condyle and levering the tibia forward. The parallel orientation of the thumbs on either side of the patellar tendon also facilitates detection of any rotatory movement, which may occur in addition to anteroposterior glide. The extent of translation can be quantified according to the International Knee Documentation Committee (IKDC) values (Table 4.2) or based on grading of the step-off (Fig. 4.7) [23].

Rotatory Stability

The appreciation of increased rotatory excursion requires careful attention to detail and can be subtle. Failure to diagnose and rotatory instability may result in failed surgical treatment and a poor prognosis. The pathophysiology of injuries to the posteromedial and posterolateral corners can be difficult to interpret with physical examination, and, therefore, it is advisable to spend some time teasing out abnormalities that are detected.

The Anteromedial Rotatory Drawer

The patient is supine with the hip flexed to 45°, the knee flexed at 90° and the foot fixed on the examining table in 15° of external rotation. In this position, the ACL and collateral ligaments are lax, which permits anterior and lateral

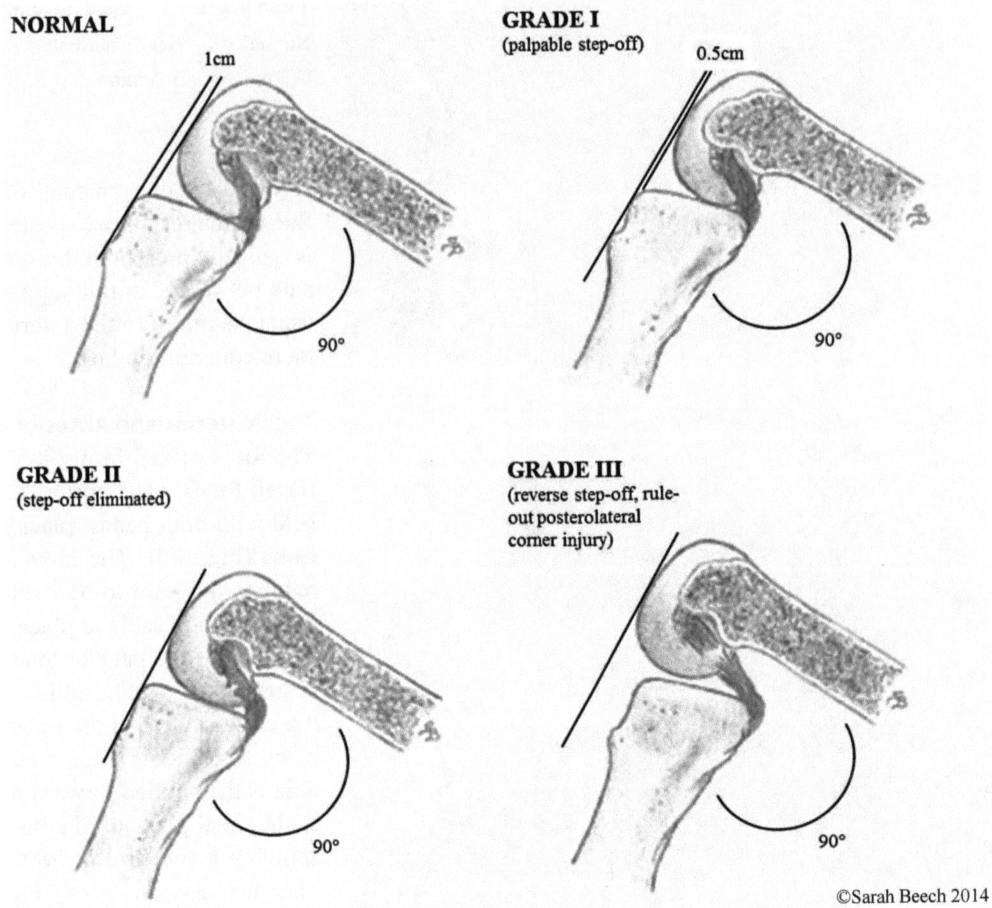

Fig. 4.7 Assessment of step-off in the PCL-deficient knee as classified by Petrie and Harner [23]. *PCL* posterior cruciate ligament. (Figure courtesy of Sarah Beech)

displacement of the medial tibial plateau. An anteriorly direct force is applied to pull the tibia directly forward. Depending on the severity of injury to the medial capsule, the medial collateral ligament (MCL) and the ACL, there will be a progressive increase in the pathological external rotation of the tibia with respect to the femur. The medial tibial plateau glides forward while the lateral plateau hardly moves at all. The axis of rotation occurs around the PCL on the lateral wall of the medial femoral condyle. If the ACL is intact, this drawer is purely rotational. Slocum, who was the first to describe this test in 1968, stated that greater than 30° external rotation should be considered pathological [24]. Accordingly, it is very important to rule out the presence of hypermobility of the contralateral limb to avoid false positive results. The quantification of this test, as proposed by Slocum, falls outside the IKDC classification, and is listed in Table 4.3.

Table 4.3 Slocum classification of rotatory instability

1+	Half a thumb—13 mm
2+	Between half and three quarters of a thumb—13–19 mm
3+	Greater than three quarters of a thumb—> 19 mm

The Anterolateral Rotatory Drawer

This test is performed in the same position with the foot internally rotated. A positive drawer in this position is indicative of a deficient ACL, which according to Noyes is the first restraint to anterior shift in internal rotation. This manoeuvre also examines the integrity of the anterolateral femoral tibial ligament [25]. Anterolateral rotation is only possible if these fibres are deficient.

Posterior Rotatory Stability

The addition of rotation to the posterior drawer is used as a further test to assess the integrity of the PCL and posterior corners of the knee. The key determinant in drawing conclusion from these tests is quantifying the ratio of translation to rotation that occurs, which should be compared to posterior drawer in neutral rotation. In internal rotation, the PCL tightens and apposes the surface of the tibia to the femur, preventing any posterior sliding of the medial tibial plateau. If the PCL is ruptured the axis of rotation shifts from a central position to a lateral position, provided the posterolateral structures are intact. This results in the medial tibial plateau translating posteriorly to a greater extent than the lateral tibial plateau. Translation predominates over rotation.

This is defined, therefore, as a posteromedial translatory rotatory laxity.

The Posterolateral Rotatory Drawer

The patient is in the same position as for all other drawer tests. The foot is fixed in slight external rotation and posterior directed force is applied to the anterior tibial tuberosity [26]. In this position, the PCL relaxes so that there can be rotatory and translatory posterolateral laxity. The ratio of translation to rotation should be compared to that observed when the posterior drawer is in the neutral position. Pure rotatory laxity occurs with an isolated posterolateral corner injury. There is an increase in external rotation, but posterior translation will not increase with external rotation of the foot, as the PCL is intact. The result is a decrease in the ratio of translation to external rotation. In the case of a PCL rupture without injury to the posterolateral corner, application of a posterior drawer in this position will result in increase in the ratio of posterior translation to external rotation as the centre of rotation is displaced peripherally.

The Posteromedial Translatory Rotatory Drawer

Internally rotating the foot tightens the PCL at 90° of knee flexion, resulting in coaptation of the femur and tibia, which prevents posterior sliding of the medial tibial plateau. Application of a posteriorly directed force to the anterior tibia, in this setting, will result in a hard end point, thereby confirming the presence of an intact PCL. However, if the PCL is deficient, coaptation does not occur and the axis of rotation shift laterally, provided the posterolateral structures are intact, which will result in a greater degree of medial-to-lateral tibial subluxation. In the absence of a PCL and a disrupted posterolateral corner, the axis of rotation is more centrally located, allowing posterior translation of the lateral tibial plateau along with the medial tibial plateau [27]. It is, therefore, necessary to assess the magnitude of the relative translation between the lateral tibial plateau and the medial tibial plateau. The more this ratio increases, the more posterior laxity become global.

The Lachman Test

The Lachman test is one of the most sensitive tests to assess ACL integrity when performed by experienced hands [28]. This test does require practice to master and relies upon having a relaxed and compliant patient. The advantage this test has over the anterior drawer relates to the fact that it is not always possible to flex the patient's knee to 90° in an acutely injured knee, in the setting of an effusion or haemarthrosis, whereas flexion to 30° is normally attainable. The reflex contraction of the hamstrings can be strong, particularly in an athletic population, and has a greater effect on preventing anterior translation at higher degrees of flexion. Finally, the bony osteology of the medial compartment and the addition of the secondary restraints, provided by the medial meniscus and posterior oblique ligament (POL), are more effective in resisting anterior translation at 90° than 30°.

The examination is performed with the patient supine and the examiner on the side of the knee to be examined. With the patient relaxed, the knee is placed in 30° of flexion. While stabilizing the femur with one hand, place the other hand on the posterior aspect of the upper tibia and apply an anterior force to draw the tibia forward on the femur (Fig. 4.8). When the test is positive, there is an anterior shift of the tibia with respect to the femur with a soft end point. This is in contrast to a hard end point when the ACL is still intact. A soft end point, which occurs with increased anterior excursion, denotes that the ACL is ruptured without doubt. However, a hard end point is more difficult to interpret as it may not indicate that the ACL is intact for two reasons—the ACL may be simply attenuated and stretched and tighten at a greater degree of tibial excursion, or the secondary peripheral structures are compensating to produce the hard end point. In this test, as in any test, it is very important to compare with opposite side to rule out any congenital laxity and quantify the side-to-side difference in translation.

The Recurvatum Test

Testing in full extension may also reveal a recurvatum deformity, which points to a posterolateral lateral injury or

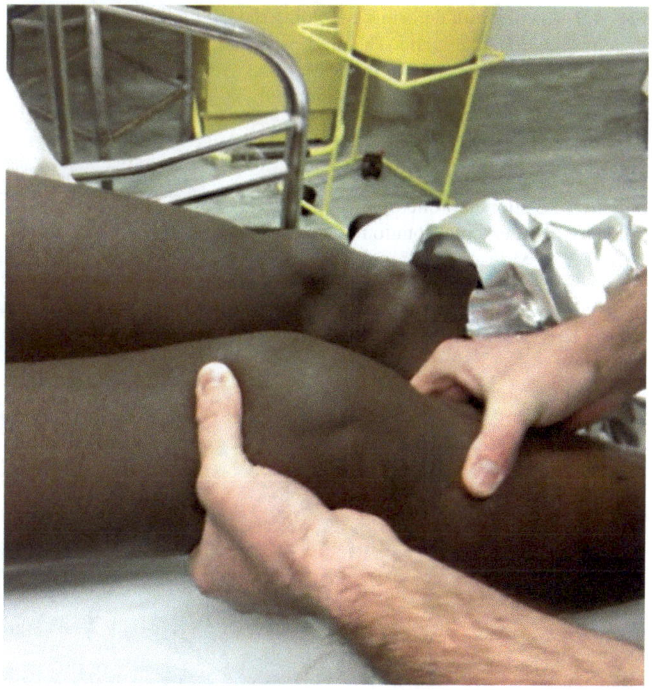

Fig. 4.8 The Lachman test: The knee is flexed to 30°. The proximal tibia is pulled anteriorly with one hand while the femur is held steady with the opposite hand

possibly even a posteromedial injury. Classically, the description of this test involves the examiner lifting the patient's great toe and observing the relative amount of genu recurvatum present [29]. The amount of relative knee hyperextension present should be compared to the contralateral normal knee and may be measured by a goniometer or heel-height differences. In addition to the hyperextension seen, the tibia commonly rotates into external rotation and a varus alignment is often noted at the knee (Fig. 4.9). A positive finding of this test should alert the examiner to the possibility of a posterolateral corner injury, which is typically with an associated cruciate ligament injury [30, 31].

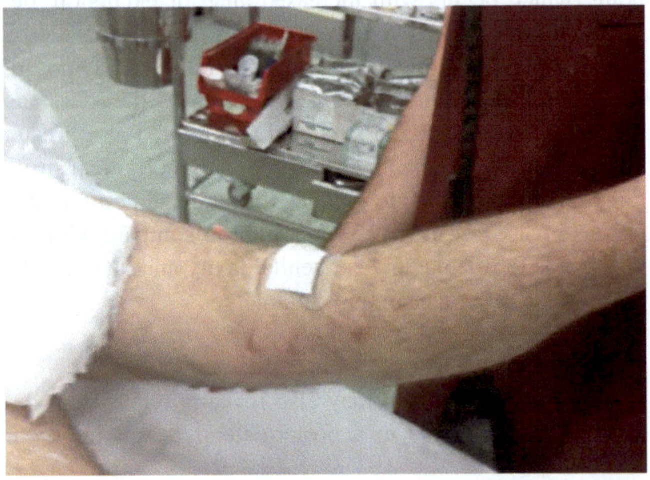

Fig. 4.9 Recurvatum deformity: Holding the leg by the foot or toe, the knee is seen to hyperextend. This finding is indicative of a PCL rupture and suggestive of an injury to the posterolateral corner of posteromedial structures. *PCL* posterior cruciate ligament

Prone Examination of Knee

The prone examination affords the opportunity of assessing the posterior aspect of the knee. Initial observation is carried out to identify the presence of any scars, swellings, atrophy or bruising on the posterior aspect of the lower leg. Extra-articular bruising is often easier to appreciate posteriorly, as it typically accumulates here, as the lower limb is usually in a supine, dependent position following injury. This position also facilitates further testing of rotational stability through the dial tests.

The Dial Test

The dial test is performed to determine the amount of external rotation of the tibia, which occurs on the femur. Conventionally, it is used to differentiate between isolated posterolateral corner injury and a combined PCL and posterolateral corner injury. The test is performed by flexing both knees to 30° and maximally externally rotating both feet (Fig. 4.10). Compare the uninjured side to the affected side and assess for any increase in rotation. The test is repeated at 90° of flexion. An isolated posterolateral corner is diagnosed if there is a positive dial test at 30° with a normal dial test at 90°. A positive dial test at 90° usually indicates a combined posterolateral corner and cruciate ligament injury, but it may also indicate a severe medial knee injury, which can be isolated or combined with a PCL disruption.

Functional Tests

Of particular importance, is the use of functional and dynamic examinations, which require the assumption of different

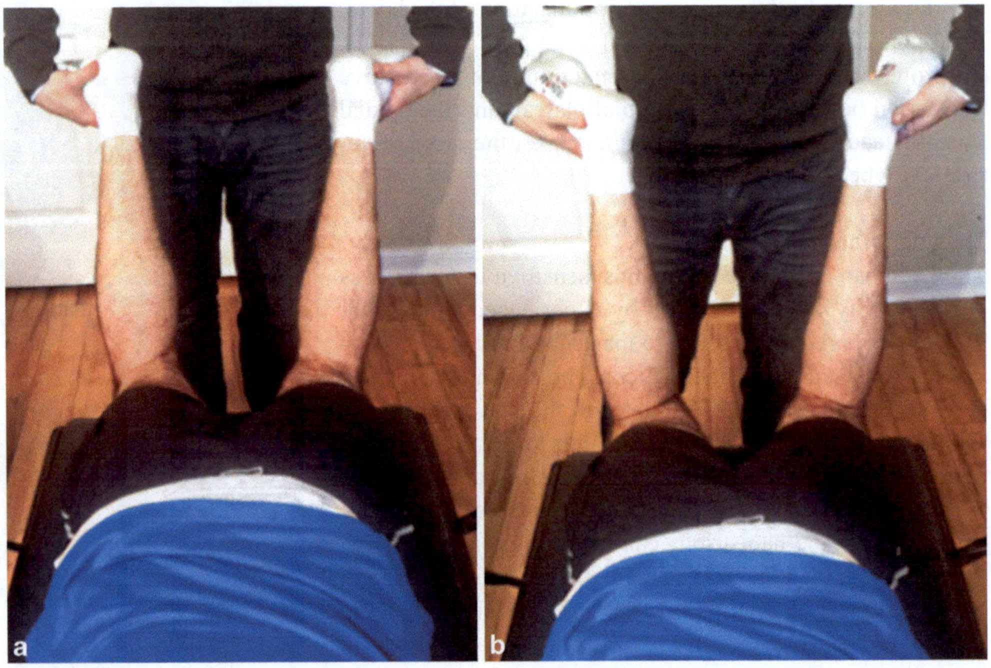

Fig. 4.10 The dial test: The patient is positioned prone. A comparison of external rotation of both feet is made at (**a**) 30° and (**b**) 90° of flexion

positions; standing, walking, or running gives the examiner a keener appreciation of the limitation of function of the joint and the patient. It is vital to recognize mechanical mal-alignment, which may have a significant influence on the outcome of a soft tissue reconstruction and may point to the requirement for bony correction. Pay particular attention to a thrust when the patient is walking. Adequate exposure to appreciate subtle compensatory movement of the lower limb when ambulating is very important. In complex instabilities, it is often beneficial to film functional activities and to examine them in slow motion. A comparison can be made postoperatively to assess any changes with treatment.

Diagnostic Studies

Vascular Studies

Aside from physical examination, additional vascular studies may be warranted in the context of an acute knee dislocation or multi-ligamentous injury. Many surgeons advocate that an ankle-brachial index (ABI) be performed in all patients suspected of having a knee dislocation [32]; however, this is not universal practice. The ABI is a fast and reliable test with relatively no associated morbidity to the patient. The ABI is recorded by means of a Doppler ultrasound probe by measuring the systolic pressure in the affected leg at a level just proximal to the ankle and dividing this value by the systolic pressure in the ipsilateral arm. A value of >0.9 has been found to be a reliable marker of normal arterial patency. Further investigation by arteriography or imaging with vascular reconstructions is indicated in the presence of abnormal physical findings and an ABI <0.9.

In a systematic review of patients who sustained vascular injury following a knee dislocation, Medina et al. identified that selective angiography was the most frequently used diagnostic modality (61 %, 14 of 23), followed by nonselective angiography and duplex ultrasonography (22 %, 5 of 23), ABI (17 %, 4 of 23) and magnetic resonance (MR) angiography (9 %, 2 of 23) [17]. As is evident from this review, considerable debate still exists regarding the optimal diagnostic method for detecting vascular injury. Historically, conventional angiography has been regarded as the gold standard for diagnosis and was routinely ordered following knee dislocation. More recently, many authors now advocate the use of selective angiography, suggesting only those patients with abnormal pulses or ABI undergo angiography [33–36]. Supporters of the routine angiography would argue that the grave clinical consequences of a missed vascular injury diagnosis, while those of the latter cite the accuracy of non-invasive screening exams as well as the costs and risks associated with angiography [17].

Imaging Studies

Plane Radiography

A standard knee series, including bilateral standing anteroposterior (AP), AP flexion 45° weight bearing, lateral and Merchant patellar radiographs, should be evaluated for any evidence of avulsion fractures, tibial subluxation and associated knee injuries (Fig. 4.11). In the event of having access to plain radiographs performed prior to reduction, these should be scrutinized closely to assess the direction of the dislocation.

If there is any suggestion of mal-alignment in the setting of chronic multi-ligamentous instability, long-leg standing radiographs should be performed to assess the mechanical axis and plan for corrective osteotomies should they be required (Fig. 4.12).

Stress Radiography

Stress radiography has been gaining popularity for the diagnosis of multi-ligamentous knee injuries. It involves the application of a standardized force to the knee to produce abnormal joint displacement. It has been demonstrated to reliable measure posterior laxity in patients with PCL injuries, in addition to being a good predictor of concomitant posterolateral corner injuries [37, 38].

In their study, LaPrade et al. concluded that clinicians should be suspicious of an isolated fibular collateral ligament injury if opening on clinician-applied varus stress radiographs increases by approximately 2.7 mm and a grade-III posterolateral corner injury if values increase by approxi-

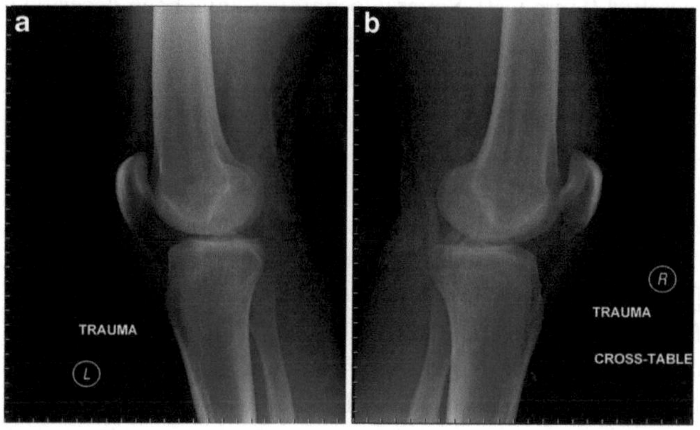

Fig. 4.11 **a** Lateral radiograph of the left (*unaffected*) knee. Note the position of the tibia with respect to the femur. **b** Lateral radiograph of the PCL injured knee. There is an avulsion fracture of the tibia insertion of the PCL (*large white arrow*) with posterior subluxation of the tibia (*black arrow*). Also, note the fracture to the inferior pole of the patella (*small white arrow*). *PCL* posterior cruciate ligament

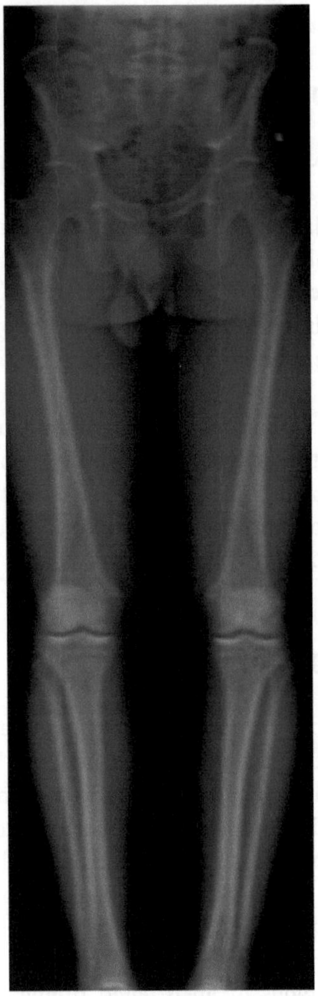

Fig. 4.12 Long-leg film of bilateral limbs. Used to assess the mechanical axis of both lower limbs to determine the requirement of osteotomies in the treatment of multi-ligamentous knee injuries

mately 4.0 mm [37]. Several techniques have been described to deliver a posteriorly directed force during stress radiography to assess the integrity of the PCL [39–43]. These methods have included hamstring contraction, gravity assisted, the Telos device (Austin and Associates, Fallston, Maryland), and single-leg kneeling [41, 44–46]. The Telos device and kneeling have been shown to be superior to other methods for reproducibly demonstrating posterior knee instability [40]. Schulz et al. have reported that subjects with isolated PCL injuries demonstrated 5–12 mm of increased posterior displacement compared with the uninjured extremity. Subjects with combined posterior knee injuries to the PCL, posterolateral corner and/or posteromedial corner had increased posterior displacement measuring >12 mm compared with the contralateral side [47].

In a further study using stress radiographs to diagnose medial-sided injuries, LaPrade et al. concluded that a grade-III medial collateral ligament injury should be suspected with greater than 3.2 mm of medial compartment gapping compared to the contralateral knee at 20° of flexion, and this injury will also result in gapping in full extension [48].

Magnetic Resonance Imaging

Magnetic resonance imaging (MRI) has become the gold standard imaging modality for assessing the multi-ligamentous injured knee. The ability of MRI to identify associate tendon, ligament and meniscal injury is unparalleled with other imaging modalities. Furthermore, the specific site of ligamentous injury, proximal, distal or mid-substance, can be clearly defined (Fig. 4.13). The information garnered from MRI scans is invaluable for preoperative planning. In addition, MRI is extremely useful in offering clues as to the mechanism of injury, particularly with the location of bone bruising patterns (Fig. 4.14). Finally, the state of the cartilage may also be ascertained which may be helpful as a prognostic indicator. However, one must interpret MRIs with a degree of caution, particularly in the setting of chronic PCL injuries. Tewes et al. reported that MRI scans are unreliable to assess for chronic PCL tears and should not be used to infer functional status in cases with chronic injuries [49].

While MRIs are extremely useful, they only provide static images, and are incapable of determining the limits of motion or the function of the affected knee. Therefore, history and physical examination should always precede MR imaging and guide the interpretation of findings. A systematic approach should to be adopted during the interpretation

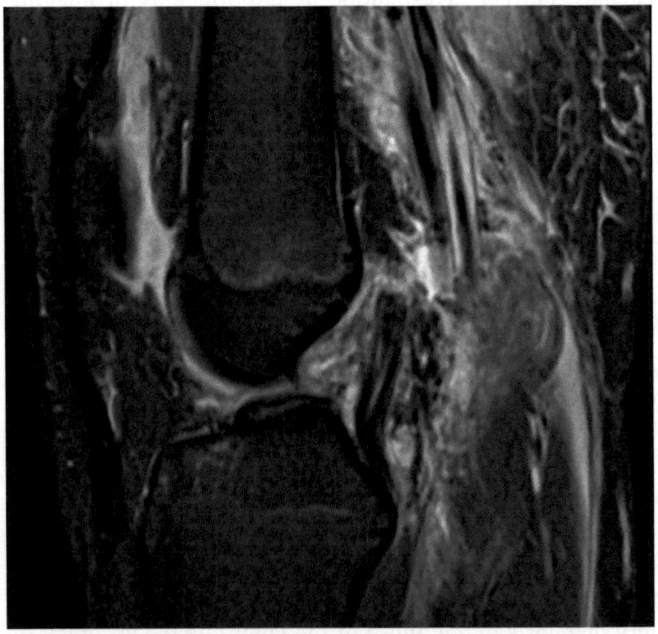

Fig. 4.13 T2 Sagittal MRI of the right knee, demonstrating an acutely injured PCL. The femoral origin of the PCL has been torn off (*white arrow*), and there is evidence of increased signal in the substance of the ligament (*yellow arrow*). *PCL* posterior cruciate ligament

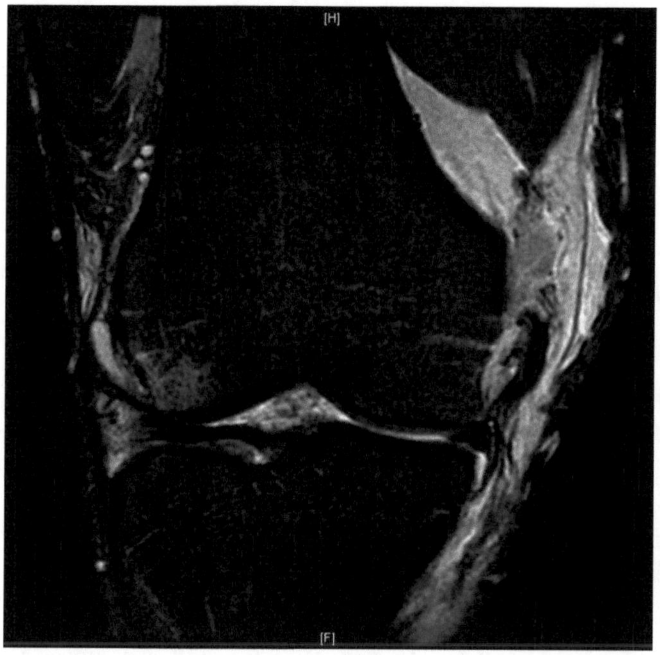

Fig. 4.14 3-Tesla T2 Coronal view of the right knee, demonstrating an acute tear of the proximal medial collateral ligament with lateral-sided bone bruising to the lateral femoral condyle. The injury sustained was a traumatic valgus load

of scans to avoid missing significant injuries. It should be noted, that MRI is less reliable and accurate in diagnosing chronic multi-ligamentous injuries, as a previously torn ligament, which has healed with scar, may appear morphologically intact although physiologically incompetent.

Characterization of PCL injury by MRI requires three planes of view—axial, coronal and sagittal. Dedicated coils improve signal-to-noise ratio and a small field of view helps with spatial resolution and a small field of view (10–14 cm) helps to improve spatial resolution [50]. Higher magnet strength has also resulted in improved image quality.

The PCL is best visualised in the sagittal oblique plane. PCL tears may be categorized into intra-substance, partial, complete or avulsion. Intra-substance tears are characterized by oedema and haemorrhage within the ligament. Partial tears demonstrate an interruption of a portion of one of the margins of the ligament and may present with a circumferential ring of haemorrhage. Complete tears show a loss of continuity of the tendon and may include increased signal at the margins of the tear. Avulsions are usually found at the tibial insertion and the PCL will be retracted along with its bony fragment (Fig. 4.15).

On the medial side of the knee, the key structures that should be visualized are the superficial MCL, the deep MCL and the medial meniscus. Observe for the presence and location of signal change, which is indicative of oedema and haemorrhage. The continuity of the medial structures, the MCL, POL, the menisco-femoral and meniscotibial

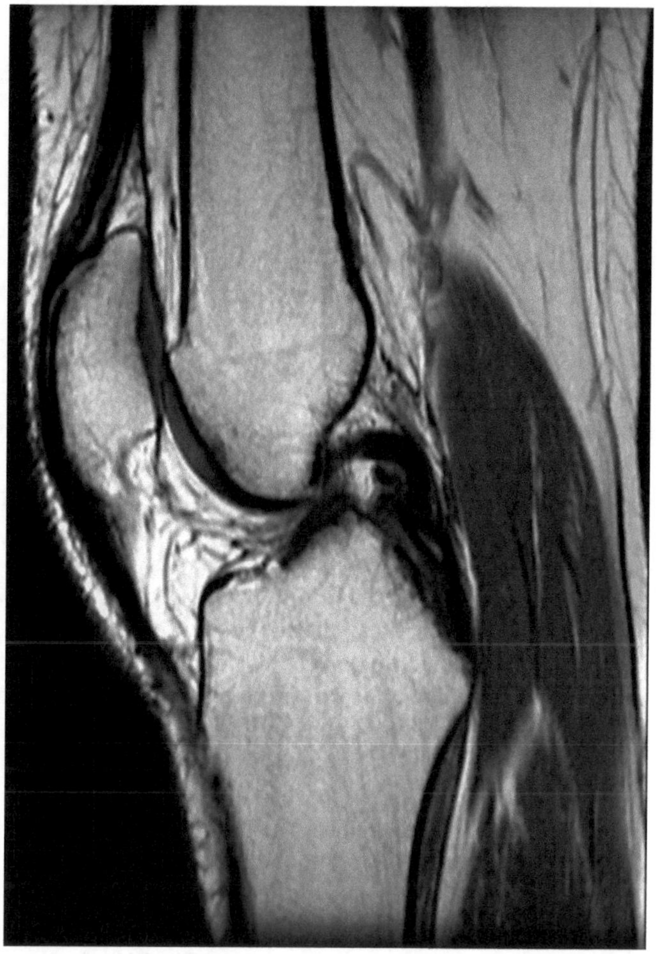

Fig. 4.15 T1 Sagittal image of the right knee. The *white arrow* marks the avulsed fragment of bone along with the PCL from the tibial insertion

ligaments should be ascertained. Although it is possible to grade injuries based on MRI, this should always be correlated with clinical examination.

The structures that need to be identified on the lateral and posterolateral side of the knee on MRI are the iliotibial band (ITB), LCL, biceps femoris, popliteus complex and capsular structures. Injury may occur to all or a variety of these structures. It is critical, however, to recognize injury to the key stabilizers, such as the LCL, the conjoined tendon of the biceps femoris and the popliteofibular ligament.

The ITB, the terminal extension of the tensor fascia lata, inserts distally onto Gerdy's tubercle. It is uncommon to injure the ITB, but discontinuity or significant injury to this structure represents a very high energy injury.

Meniscal injuries are important to recognize in the context of multi-ligamentous knee injuries [51]. The high energy involved in this injury pattern frequently results in meniscal damage, including root avulsions [52]. The presence of a displaced meniscal tear may dictate that early intervention is warranted. Meniscal root avulsions may also be overlooked, given the complexity of the injury; however, failure to recognize these and address them at the time of surgery may have a negative effect on the outcome.

Computerized Tomography

Computerized tomography (CT) scans continue to play a role in the assessment of PCL injuries [53]. Their value is probably greatest in the assessment of ligamentous injury with associated fractures or avulsions (Fig. 4.16). In addition, in the setting of revision surgery, CT scans, and in particular 3D reconstruction, can accurately identify the location and size of the tunnels.

Examination Under Anaesthesia

The examination under anaesthesia (EUA) should always be a concomitant of the arthroscopic examination. Subtle laxities may become much more apparent with complete muscle relaxation. As usual, examination with the good leg should be performed initially. A comparison should be made between the EUA findings and those in the office to constantly try to improve one's technique and diagnostic accuracy. In addition, it is often useful to film the examination for further scrutiny and to compare and contrast the effect of surgical reconstruction. Ideally, the same systematic approach should be used and recorded contemporaneously. The EUA findings are an important addition to the operative noted.

The EUA is particularly useful when examining a patient who had a decreased range of motion (flexion <90°) at initial presentation. The PCL can only be truly assessed with certainty at this angle. It is not uncommon to discover a PCL injury at EUA, which had previously gone undiagnosed. This obviously has significant implications for surgical planning, particularly in relation to the requirement for allograft, and may perhaps delay surgery. Therefore, it is important to always keep an open mind to the possibility of a PCL injury, particularly in a seriously injured knee with reduced range of motion.

Arthroscopic Evaluation

A thorough diagnostic arthroscopic evaluation should be carried out as part of any ligament reconstruction procedure. It is important to employ a methodical approach to avoid overlooking subtle injuries to the posterolateral and posteromedial corners, the menisci and all articular surfaces. Ensure that all compartments of the knee are adequately scrutinized and, if necessary, probed.

A key factor in successful diagnosis in the multi-ligamentous injured knee is getting adequate visualization of the entire knee. A standard 4-mm 30° arthroscopy is used initially. However, surgeons embarking on this surgery should be familiar using a 70° arthroscope and adept at gaining access to the posteromedial and posterolateral aspect of the knee. In addition, one should be prepared to make accessory portals posteromedially and posterolaterally, as necessary.

The patient is placed supine on the operating table. Prior to using a tourniquet, it is vital to be aware of the vascular status of the patient and whether any emergent revascularization procedure was carried out. If there are no vascular issues, a tourniquet should be placed high on the thigh. The knee should be held in the position the surgeon is most familiar and comfortable with, ensuring that adequate flexion can be achieved, and there is sufficient space proximally for making accessory portals.

The authors use an outflow portal routinely on the lateral aspect of the suprapatellar pouch, which is particularly useful for venting the knee and improving visibility in the acutely injured knee. A standard anterolateral parapatellar portal is used for the arthroscope and an anteromedial parapatellar portal for the instruments. A systematic approach is used to explore the patellofemoral joint, the femoral notch

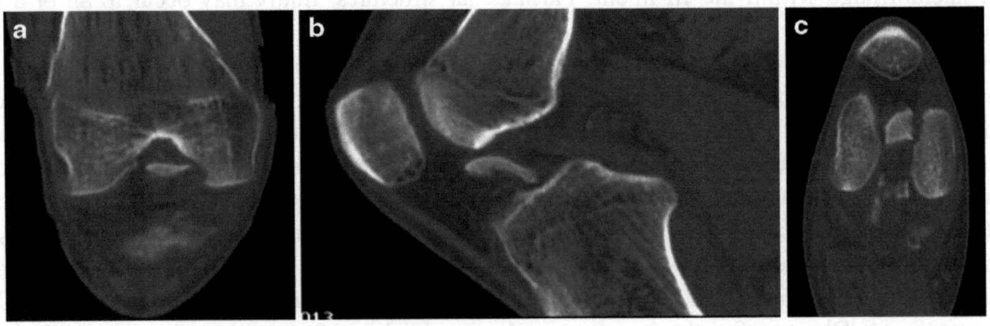

Fig. 4.16 **a** CT scan—coronal image of a right knee, demonstrating a femoral side PCL avulsion fragment from the medial wall of the lateral wall of the medial femoral condyle. **b** CT scan—sagittal image of right knee, demonstrating an avulsed fragment of bone within the femoral notch. **c** CT scan—axial image of the right knee, showing a comminuted avulsion fracture of the lateral wall of the medial femoral condyle at the origin of the PCL. *CT* computerized tomography, *PCL* posterior cruciate ligament

and medial and lateral compartments. A list of the specific structures in each compartment is provided in Table 4.4. Discussed below are some of the specific findings related to PCL injuries and other discoveries suggestive of associated knee pathology.

Table 4.4 Checklist for arthroscopic assessment of the PCL injured knee

Patellofemoral joint	Haemarthrosis/haemosiderin deposition
	Arthrofibrosis
	Patella chondrosis
	Medial patellofemoral ligament injury
	Trochlear chondrosis
Lateral gutter	Lateral gutter drive through
	Popliteal tendon avulsion
	Loose bodies
	Meniscal extrusion
Medial gutter	Deep MCL avulsion
	Meniscal extrusion
	Loose bodies
Femoral notch	ACL injury—torn, empty wall sign, injection
	Pseudo-laxity ACL
	PCL injury—torn, injection, loss of tension
	Posteromedial drive through sign
Lateral compartment	Lateral drive through sign
	Meniscotibial (coronary) ligament of lateral meniscus
	Popliteal meniscal fascicle (Posterosuperior and inferior)
	Popliteus tendon
	Horns of lateral meniscus (posterior and anterior)
	Meniscofemoral ligaments (Wrisberg and Humphreys)
	Articular cartilage (femoral condyle and tibial plateau)
Medial compartment	Medial drive-through sign
	Meniscotibial ligament of medial meniscus Meniscocapsular ligament (femoral)
	Horns of medial meniscus (posterior and anterior)
	Articular cartilage (femoral condyle and tibial plateau)

MCL medial cruciate ligament, *ACL* anterior cruciate ligament, *PCL* posterior cruciate ligament

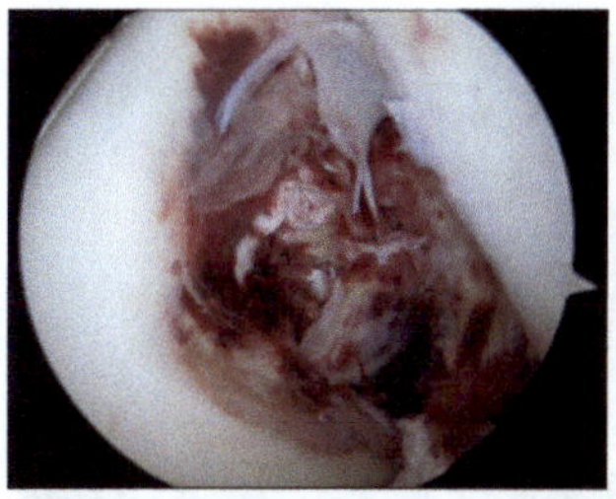

Fig. 4.17 Arthroscopic image from anterolateral portal of an acutely torn PCL. *PCL* posterior cruciate ligament

A number of arthroscopic findings, specifically related to the multi-ligamentous injured knee, have been described. Immediately upon introduction of the arthroscope into the suprapatellar pouch, one gets an impression of the general state of the knee. The presence of a haemarthrosis is indicative of an acute injury; whereas haemosiderin staining and a scarred, thickened synovium herald a more chronic process. The patellofemoral articulation is important to explore initially to assess the presence of associated articular lesions, which may be acute from the initial trauma or chronic as a result of altered biomechanics in a PCL-deficient knee.

On examination of the femoral notch, one should observe for injection of the femoral footprint of the PCL or the presence of haematoma around a frankly torn PCL (Fig. 4.17). In a chronic injury, there may be an abundance of amorphous scar tissue in the notch, which should be removed with care to delineate the bundles of the PCL. Examine the ACL for concomitant injury and also for the presence of the pseudo-laxity (Fig. 4.18); this phenomenon occurs as a result of posterior subluxation of the tibia and an apparent redundancy of the ACL. It is not uncommon for this to be mistaken as a torn ligament. By applying an anterior translation under visualization, the normal contour of the ligament is restored.

The drive-through sign was first described in the posterolateral knee ligament injuries as the ability to pass the arthroscope easily between the lateral femoral condyle and the tibial plateau due to excessive opening of the lateral

Fig 4.18 **a** Arthroscopic image of the ACL, demonstrating 'pseudo-laxity' due to the posterior subluxation of the tibia in the setting of a chronically injured PCL. **b** A normal appearance of the ACL following the application of an anterior translation force to reduce the tibia. *ACL* anterior cruciate ligament, *PCL* posterior cruciate ligament

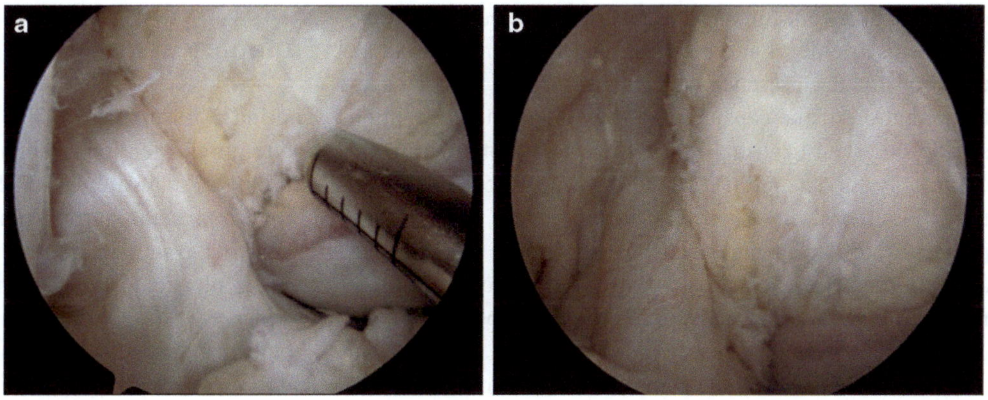

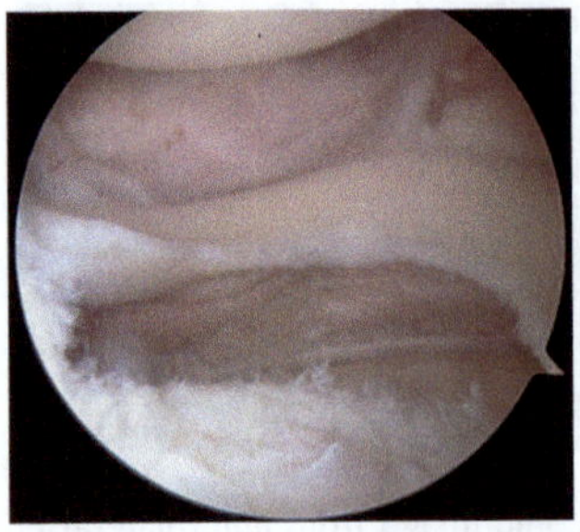

Fig. 4.19 An arthroscopic image of the lateral drive-through sign of a left knee with a combined PCL and PLC injury. *PCL* posterior cruciate ligament, *PLC* posterolateral corner

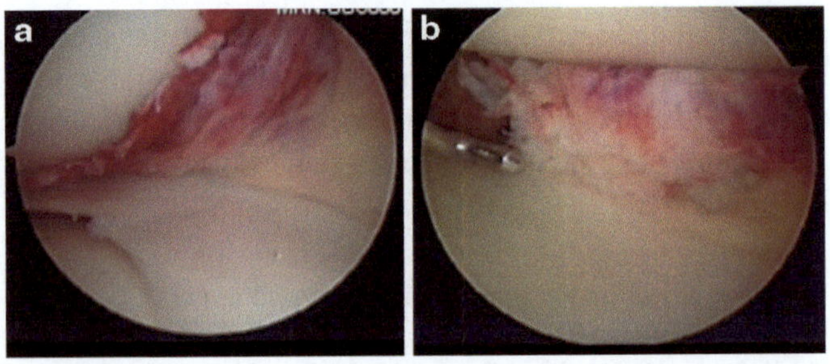

Fig. 4.20 **a** Arthroscope image of the medial compartment of the knee, demonstrating a tear the medial capsule with invagination of the capsule into the joint superior to the medial meniscus. **b** Arthroscopic image of the lateral compartment in a posterolateral corner injury. Note the presence of a torn lateral capsule

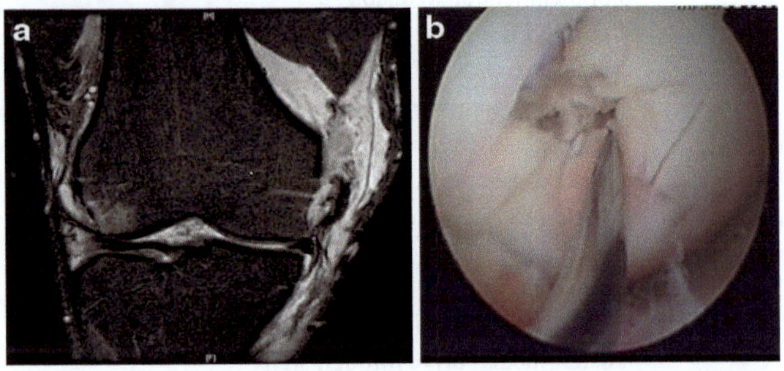

Fig. 4.21 **a** T2 coronal MRI of right knee—observe the increased signal on the lateral femoral condyle which is suggestive of impaction of the lateral compartment following a valgus injury. **b** Arthroscopic image of the lateral femoral condyle in the same patient. Note the devastating cartilage injury as a result of impaction. *MRI* magnetic resonance imaging

compartment [54] (Fig. 4.19). Feng et al. have also described a lateral gutter drive-through sign in the arthroscopic knee surgery as the entry of the arthroscope into the posterolateral compartment through the interval between the popliteal tendon and the lateral femoral condyle to indicate the presence of posterolateral corner peel-off lesions [55, 56].

In addition, a posteromedial drive-through sign has also been reported, demonstrating a very high positive predictive value (91.7 %) for the diagnosis of PCL injury, in particular grade-III ruptures [57]. The posteromedial compartment can be viewed either through a posteromedial portal or through the intercondylar notch from the anterolateral or anteromedial portal. When the posteromedial compartment is viewed through an anterolateral portal via the intercondylar notch, the arthroscope passes the space between the medial femoral condyle and the PCL. In the majority of patients with an intact PCL, this passage of the arthroscopy typically necessitates a slight degree of knee flexion and valgus stress due to the limited space between the medial femoral condyle and the PCL. However, when there is PCL insufficiency, the arthroscope passes easily between the medial femoral condyle and the PCL as a result of an enlarged space; valgus stress or manipulation with a trocar at 80–90° of knee flexion is not required. A number of authors have documented this occurrence in patients with partial or complete PCL deficiency [58–60].

It is also extremely important to assess the lateral and medial compartments for the presence of meniscal pathology. The meniscofemoral and meniscotibial ligaments should be explored for the presence of tears or in more severe cases incarceration of the capsule (Fig. 4.20). Particular attention should be given to visualize the meniscus roots, which are commonly torn in multi-ligamentous injury [51, 52]. Sonnery-Cottet et al. have recently claimed that a lesion to the posterior horn of medial meniscus often goes undiagnosed and report on the value of assessing the posterior horn of the medial meniscus by visualization through the posteromedial portal to improve the accuracy of the diagnosis [61]. To gain access to the posteromedial compartment, the arthroscope is introduced through the anterolateral portal deeply into the notch and underneath the PCL; it may be necessary to use a blunt trocar.

At all times, be aware of the integrity of the articular cartilage in all compartments. Seek to correlate any suspicious lesions on MRI with direct visualization and probing. Cartilage lesions may vary from minor scuffing to osteochondral fractures to degenerative changes in a chronic situation (Fig. 4.21).

Summary

The initial assessment of PCL injured knees is challenging and requires attention to detail to avoid missing concomitant pathology. An awareness of the mechanism of injury is vital and an important starting point in the quest to discover the extent of the injury and provide appropriate treatment. The treating physician needs patience, vigilance and a variety of diagnostic tools to reach a precise diagnosis. Each injury should be approached in a methodical and systematic manner to ensure an accurate initial assessment and ultimately improve outcomes.

References

1. Arøen A., Verdonk P. Posterior cruciate ligament, exploring the unknown. Knee Surg Sports Traumatol Arthrosc. 2013;21:996–7.
2. Race A, Amis AA. PCL reconstruction. In vitro biomechanical comparison of 'isometric' versus single and double-bundled 'anatomic' grafts. J Bone Joint Surg Br. 1998;80(1):173–9.
3. Fowler PJ, Messieh SS. Isolated posterior cruciate ligament injuries in athletes. Am J Sports Med. 1987;15(6):553–7.
4. Parolie JM, Bergfeld JA. Long-term results of nonoperative treatment of isolated posterior cruciate ligament injuries in the athlete. Am J Sports Med. 1986;14(1):35–8.
5. Shelbourne KD, Clark M, Gray T. Minimum 10-year follow-up of patients after an acute, isolated posterior cruciate ligament injury treated nonoperatively. Am J Sports Med. 2013;41(7):1526–33.
6. Toritsuka Y, Horibe S, Hiro-Oka A, Mitsuoka T, Nakamura N. Conservative treatment for rugby football players with an acute isolated posterior cruciate ligament injury. Knee Surg Sports Traumatol Arthrosc. 2004;12(2):110–14.
7. Allen CR, Kaplan LD, Fluhme DJ, Harner CD. Posterior cruciate ligament injuries. Curr Opin Rheumatol. 2002;14(2):142–9.
8. Boynton MD, Tietjens BR. Long-term followup of the untreated isolated posterior cruciate ligament-deficient knee. Am J Sports Med. 1996;24(3):306–10.
9. Covey CD, Sapega AA. Injuries of the posterior cruciate ligament. J Bone Joint Surg Am. 1993;75(9):1376–86.
10. Dejour H, Walch G, Peyrot J, Eberhard P. The natural history of rupture of the posterior cruciate ligament. Rev Chir Orthop Reparatrice Appar Mot. 1988;74(1):35–43.
11. Keller PM, Shelbourne KD, McCarroll JR, Rettig AC. Nonoperatively treated isolated posterior cruciate ligament injuries. Am J Sports Med. 1993;21(1):132–6.
12. Ahn JH, Lee YS, Choi SH, Chang MJ, Lee DK. Singlebundle transtibial posterior cruciate ligament reconstruction using a bioabsorbable cross-pin tibial back side fixation. Knee Surg Sports Traumatol Arthrosc. 2013;21(5):1023–8.
13. Aroen A, Sivertsen EA, Owesen C, Engebretsen L, Granan LP. An isolated rupture of the posterior cruciate ligament results in reduced preoperative knee function in comparison with an anterior cruciate ligament injury. Knee Surg Sports Traumatol Arthrosc. 2013;21(5):1017–22.
14. Apley AG. Intelligent kneemanship. Postgrad Med J. 1964;40: 519–20.
15. Kannus P, Bergfeld J, Järvinen M, Johnson RJ, Pope M, Renström P, Yasuda K. Injuries to the posterior cruciate ligament of the knee. Sports Med. 1991;12(2):110–31.
16. Werner BC, Gwathmey FW Jr, Higgins ST, Hart JM, Miller MD. Ultra-low velocity knee dislocations: patient characteristics, complications, and outcomes. Am J Sports Med. 2014;42(2):358–63.
17. Medina O, Arom GA, Yeranosian MG, Petrigliano FA, McAllister DR. Vascular and Nerve Injury After Knee Dislocation: A Systematic Review. Clin Orthop Relat Res. 2014 Feb 20. [Epub ahead of print].
18. Silverberg DA, Acus R. Irreducible posterolateral knee dislocation associated with interposition of the vastus medialis. Am J Sports Med. 2004;32(5):1313–6.
19. Braun DT, Muffly MT, Altman GT. Irreducible posterolateral knee dislocation with entrapment of the adductor magnus tendon and medial skin dimpling. J Knee Surg. 2009;22(4):366–9.
20. Niall DM, Nutton RW, Keating JF. Palsy of the common peroneal nerve after traumatic dislocation of the knee. J Bone Joint Surg Br. 2005;87(5):664–7.
21. Müller, PD Dr Werner. The knee: form, function, and ligament reconstruction. Berlin: Springer; 1982.
22. Zehms CT, Whiddon DR, Miller MD, Quinby JS, Montgomery SL, Campbell RB, Sekiya JK. Comparison of a double bundle arthroscopic inlay and open inlay posterior cruciate ligament reconstruction using clinically relevant tools: a cadaveric study. Arthroscopy. 2008;24(4):472–80.
23. Petrie RS, Harner CD. Evaluation and management of the posterior cruciate injured knee. Oper Tech Sports Med. 1999;7(3): 93–103.
24. Slocum DB, Larson RL. Rotatory instability of the knee: its pathogenesis and a clinical test to demonstrate its presence. 1968. Clin Orthop Relat Res. 2007 Jan;454:5–13; discussion 3–4.
25. Claes S, Vereecke E, Maes M, Victor J, Verdonk P, Bellemans J. Anatomy of the anterolateral ligament of the knee. J Anat. 2013;223(4):321–8.
26. Hughston JC, Andrews JR, Cross MJ, Moschi A. Classification of knee ligament instabilities. Part II. The lateral compartment. J Bone Joint Surg Am. 1976;58(2):173–9.
27. Hughston JC, Andrews JR, Cross MJ, Moschi A. Classification of knee ligament instabilities. Part I. The medial compartment and cruciate ligaments. J Bone Joint Surg Am. 1976;58(2): 159–72.
28. Peeler J, Leiter J, MacDonald P. Accuracy and reliability of anterior cruciate ligament clinical examination in a multidisciplinary sports medicine setting. Clin J Sport Med. 2010;20(2):80–5.
29. Hughston JC, Norwood LA. The posterolateral drawer test and external rotation recurvatum test for posterolateral rotatory instability of the knee. Clin Orthop Rel Res. 1980;147:82–7.
30. LaPrade RF, Ly TV, Griffith C. The external rotation recurvatum test revisited: reevaluation of the sagittal plane tibiofemoral relationship. Am J Sports Med. 2008;36(4):709–12.
31. Thaunat M, Pioger C, Chatellard R, Conteduca J, Khaleel A, Sonnery-Cottet B. The arcuate ligament revisited: role of the posterolateral structures in providing static stability in the knee joint. Knee Surg Sports Traumatol Arthrosc. 2013 Aug 31.
32. Nicandri GT, Dunbar RP, Wahl CJ. Are evidence-based protocols which identify vascular injury associated with knee dislocation underutilized? Knee Surg Sports Traumatol Arthrosc. 2010;18(8):1005–12.
33. Mills WJ, Barei DP, McNair P. The value of the ankle-brachial index for diagnosing arterial injury after knee dislocation: a prospective study. J Trauma. 2004;56(6):1261–5.
34. Hollis JD, Daley BJ. 10-year review of knee dislocations: is arteriography always necessary? J. Trauma. 2005;59:672–5; discussion 675–6.
35. Klineberg EO, Crites BM, Flinn WR, Archibald JD, Moorman CT 3rd. The role of arteriography in assessing popliteal artery injury in knee dislocations. J. Trauma. 2004;56:786–90.
36. Nicandri GT, Chamberlain AM, Wahl CJ. Practical management of knee dislocations: a selective angiography protocol to detect limb-threatening vascular injuries. Clin. J. Sport Med. Off. J. Can. Acad. Sport Med. 2009;19:125–9.
37. LaPrade RF, Heikes C, Bakker AJ, Jakobsen RB. The reproducibility and repeatability of varus stress radiographs in the assessment of isolated fibular collateral ligament and grade-III posterolateral knee injuries. An in vitro biomechanical study. J Bone Joint Surg Am. 2008;90(10):2069–76.
38. Jackman T, LaPrade RF, Pontinen T, Lender PA. Intraobserver and interobserver reliability of the kneeling technique of stress radiography for the evaluation of posterior knee laxity. Am J Sports Med. 2008;36(8):1571–6.
39. Jacobsen K. Stress radiographical measurements of post-traumatic knee instability: a clinical study. Acta Orthop Scand. 1977;48:301–10.
40. Jung T, Reinhardt C, Scheffler S, Weiler A. Stress radiography to measure posterior cruciate ligament insufficiency: a comparison of five different techniques. Knee Surg Sports Traumatol Arthrosc. 2006;14:1116–21.
41. Louisia S, Siebold R, Canty J, Bartlett RJ. Assessment of posterior stability in total knee replacement by stress radiographs:

prospective comparison of two different types of mobile bearing implants. Knee Surg Sports Traumatol Arthrosc. 2005;13:476–82.
42. Margheritini F, Mancini L, Mauro CS, Mariani PP. Stress radiography for quantifying posterior cruciate ligament deficiency. Arthroscopy. 2003;19:706–11.
43. Puddu G, Gianni E, Chambat P, De Paulis F. The axial view in evaluating tibial translation in cases of insufficiency of the posterior cruciate ligament. Arthroscopy. 2000;16:217–20.
44. Chassaing VDF, Touzard R, Ceccaldi JP, Miremad C. Etude radiologique du L.C.P.: a 90° de flexion. Rev Chir Orthop. 1995;81(Suppl):35–8.
45. Stäubli HU, Noesberger B, Jakob RP. Stress radiography of the knee: cruciate ligament function studied in 138 patients. Acta Orthop Scand Suppl. 1992;249:1–27.
46. Schulz MS, Russe K, Lampakis G, Strobel MJ. Reliability of stress radiography for evaluation of posterior knee laxity. Am J Sports Med. 2005;33:502–6.
47. Schulz MS, Russe K, Weiler A, Eichhorn HJ, Strobel MJ. Epidemiology of posterior cruciate ligament injuries. Arch Orthop Trauma Surg. 2003;123:186–91.
48. Laprade RF, Bernhardson AS, Griffith CJ, Macalena JA, Wijdicks CA. Correlation of valgus stress radiographs with medial knee ligament injuries: an in vitro biomechanical study. Am J Sports Med. 2010;38(2):330–8.
49. Tewes DP, Fritts HM, Fields RD, Quick DC, Buss DD. Chronically injured posterior cruciate ligament: magnetic resonance imaging. Clin Orthop Relat Res. 1997;335:224–32.
50. Grover JS, Bassett LW, Gross ML, et al. Posterior cruciate ligament: MRI imaging. Radiology. 1990;174:527–30.
51. Beasley L, Robertson D, Armfield D, et al. Medial meniscus root tears: an unsolved problem—demographic, radiographic, and arthroscopic findings. Pittsburgh Orthop J. 2005;16:155.
52. Koenig JH, Ranawat AS, Umans HR, et al. Meniscal root tears: diagnosis and treatment. Arthroscopy. 2009;25:1025–32.
53. Griffith JF, Antonio GE, Tong CW, Ming CK. Cruciate ligament avulsion fractures. Arthroscopy. 2004;20(8):803–12.
54. LaPrade RF. Arthroscopic evaluation of the lateral compartment of knees with grade 3 posterolateral knee complex injuries. Am J Sports Med 1997. 25(5):596–602.
55. Feng H, Zhang H, Hong L, Wang XS, Zhang J. The "lateral gutter drive-through" sign: an arthroscopic indicator of acute femoral avulsion of the popliteus tendon in knee joints. Arthroscopy 2009. 25(12):1496–9.
56. Shen J, Zhang H, Lv Y, Hong L, Wang X, Zhang J, Feng H. Validity of a novel arthroscopic test to diagnose posterolateral rotational instability of the knee joint: the lateral gutter drive-through test. Arthroscopy 2013. 29(4):695–700.
57. Nha KW, Bae JH, Kwon JH, Kim JG, Jo DY, Lim HC. Arthroscopic posteromedial drive-through test in posterior cruciate ligament insufficiency: a new diagnostic test. Knee Surg Sports Traumatol Arthrosc. 2014 Feb 15. [Epub ahead of print]
58. Ahn JH, Nha KW, Kim YC, Lim HC, Nam HW, Wang JH. Arthroscopic femoral tensioning and posterior cruciate ligament reconstruction in chronic posterior cruciate ligament injury. Arthroscopy 2006. 22(3):e341–4.
59. Yang JH, Yoon JR, Jeong HI, Hwang DH, Woo SJ, Kwon JH, Nha KW. Second-look arthroscopic assessment of arthroscopic single-bundle posterior cruciate ligament reconstruction: comparison of mixed graft versus achilles tendon allograft. Am J Sports Med. 2012. 40(9):2052–60
60. Lim HC, Bae JH, Wang JH, Yang JH, Seok CW, Kim HJ, Kim SJ. Double-bundle PCL reconstruction using tibial double cross-pin fixation. Knee Surg Sports Traumatol Arthrosc. 2010;18(1):117–22.
61. Sonnery-Cottet B, Conteduca J, Thaunat M, Gunepin FX, Seil R. Hidden lesions of the posterior horn of the medial meniscus: a systematic arthroscopic exploration of the concealed portion of the knee. Am J Sports Med. 2014. [Epub ahead of print]

Instrumented Measurement of the Multiple-Ligament-Injured Knee: Arthrometry, Stress Radiography, Rotationometry, and Computer Navigation

5

Sasha Carsen, Robert Timothy Deakon and Don Johnson

Introduction

The multiple-ligament-injured knee presents a variety of unique challenges. Among the many significant challenges are the accurate clinical diagnosis and classification of the ligamentous and soft-tissue injuries. The history (i.e., mechanism) and clinical exam are the most important elements of assessment of the knee. Instrumented ligament laxity measurement is an important adjunctive diagnostic tool available to the clinician.

The most important application of instrumented examination in the dislocated knee is for confirmation of the clinical diagnosis determined from history and physical examination. This quantitative information used in conjunction with appropriate diagnostic imaging can lead to a more accurate diagnosis of the anatomical structures affected and, in turn, more effective and safer treatment of the patient's knee injury. Any application of physical stress to the knee joint, however, should take place only after the patient has been deemed to be in stable condition and a possible vascular lesion has been ruled out. In addition, appropriate analgesia is of paramount importance, as many of the instrumented measurements require some level of stress on the joint and therefore can lead to significant pain. Muscular "guarding" by the patient due to discomfort can lead to erroneous measurements being obtained.

S. Carsen (✉)
Division of Orthopaedic Surgery, University of Ottawa, Children's Hospital of Eastern Ontario, 401 Smyth Road, Ottawa, ON K1H 8L1, Canada
e-mail: scarsen@hotmail.com

R. T. Deakon
Halton Healthcare Services, Oakville Trafalgar Site, Orthopaedic Surgery, 250 Wyecroft Rd., Unite 18, Oakville, ON L6K3T7, Canada

D. Johnson
Department of Orthopaedics, The Ottawa Hospital, Ottawa, ON, Canada

Indications and Reasons for Instrumented Measurement

While not essential for diagnosis, there are a number of advantages to using instrumented measurements of knee ligament laxity to enhance the standard physical examination. Objective measurements are helpful to the clinician when documenting the extent of injury and are essential to the researcher. They can also be helpful when communicating with the extended health care team in certain cases, including the primary care sports medicine physician, physiatrist, physiotherapist, or athletic trainer.

Diagnosis

Accurate diagnosis of the multiple-ligament-injured knee is crucial, as it ultimately defines the type and extent of surgical intervention necessary to restore function. X-ray and magnetic resonance imaging (MRI) form an indispensable part of the clinical workup but MRI, in particular, should not be relied upon in isolation to determine the correct medical treatment. For instance, the difference between a partial and a complete ligamentous rupture may be difficult or impossible to determine using MRI imaging alone, but that difference could have a profound effect on surgical planning.

Instrumented testing can provide a more objective and dependable measure of laxity, and, therefore, assist with differentiation of complete versus partial ligament injuries, leading to a safer and more effective treatment.

Although advanced soft-tissue imaging is now relatively standard, there are cases and situations where these evaluations may not be diagnostically helpful. Patients may have significant artifact secondary to previous injury or surgery rendering the examinations uninterpretable.

Some patients will have a contraindication for MRI, such as indwelling ferrous metallic material, pacemaker, or defibrillator. Another growing problem is the difficulty encountered in imaging patients who are morbidly obese, a patient

G. C. Fanelli (ed.), *Posterior Cruciate Ligament Injuries,*
DOI 10.1007/978-3-319-12072-0_5, © Springer International Publishing Switzerland 2015

group that also happens to be at greater risk for multiligament knee injury.

Postop

By comparing instrumented measures pre- and postoperatively, one can quantify the clinical effect of the surgical intervention. A direct comparison with the same measurement tool using the same technique can provide immediate postoperative information to the surgeon on the effect of the repair or reconstruction.

Follow-Up/Rehab

In follow-up, either post-injury or postoperatively, repeated instrumented measurement can provide insight into the integrity of the repair or reconstruction, or reveal residual clinical instability. This can be especially beneficial after a reinjury, as postoperative changes may make imaging-based diagnosis more challenging. Having an objective measurement to compare against can lead to a clearer clinical picture.

Methods of Measurement

Stress Radiography

Posterior Stress

Stress radiographs are most indicated and most helpful in defining the posterior displacement of the tibia relative to the femur [1]. The degree of that displacement reflects the integrity of the posterior cruciate ligament (PCL) and the posterolateral or posteromedial corners (PMCs) of the knee. There are numerous described techniques for stressing the posterior structures, and the four most common are presented below.

Hamstring Contraction

The active resisted hamstring contraction radiograph is performed by having the patient assume the lateral decubitus position with the index knee dependent, and flexed 90°over an X-ray cassette to obtain a true lateral view. The patient is then asked to actively contract their hamstrings against resistance at the heel, while knee flexion is maintained at 90° (Fig. 5.1). The resultant lateral radiograph of the knee can then be measured, assessing the posterior tibial displacement. In one comparative study, the hamstring contraction stress view showed similar results to the Telos stress device, and far greater accuracy than the axial stress view [2].

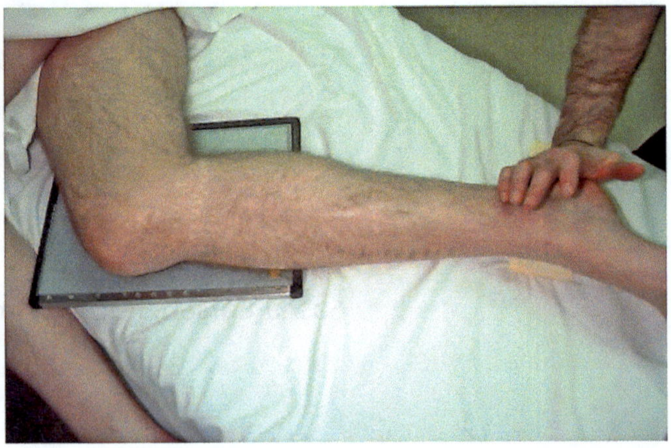

Fig. 5.1 The active resisted hamstring contraction stress X-ray. The patient is performing an active maximal hamstring contraction against resistance in the lateral position. The X-ray is done during the maximal contraction. (From Carsen and Johnson 2013 [36]. Reprinted with permission)

Axial View

A modified axial patellofemoral radiograph has been described as a quick and easy form of stress view to assess the integrity of the posterior structures of the knee. The patient is positioned supine with the knees flexed to 70°, feet flat on the table in moderate plantar flexion, and the tibia in neutral rotation. The X-ray beam is then directed from distal to proximal and parallel to the longitudinal axis of the patella, at an upward angle of 10° to the X-ray table. Early results of the technique were promising [3]. However, more recent multi-technique comparisons have shown it to be a less reliable technique compared to the alternative stress views [2, 4].

Posterior Sag/Gravity View

The patient is positioned supine on the X-ray table, and both the hip and knee are flexed to 90°. The tibia is held in place in neutral rotation. A true lateral radiograph of the knee is then obtained. The method is quick and easy, but has not compared favorably to other stress views [4].

Kneeling Stress View

The stress view yielding the best and most reliable results thus far is the kneeling stress view. The patient kneels on a bench or similar structure with the knee over the edge of the bench (i.e., the femoral condyles are past the bench, while the tibial tubercle is supported by it). The knee is maintained at 90° of flexion. A true lateral radiograph of the knee is then taken. Measurement of displacement is then performed using the posterior cortex of the tibia and posterior cortex of the

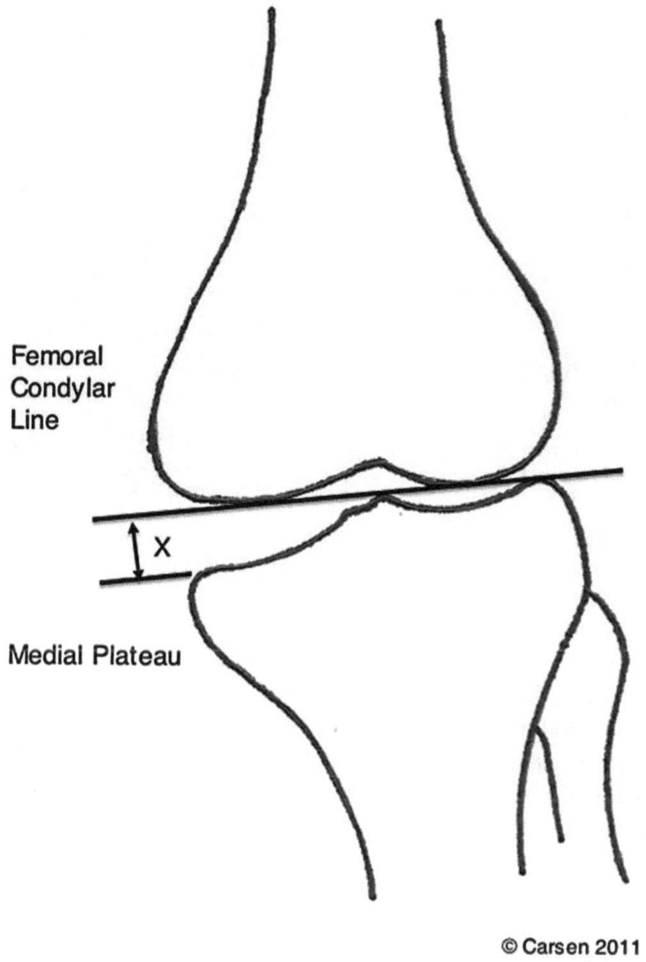

Fig. 5.2 The opening of the medial joint space is measured in millimeters. (From Carsen and Johnson 2013 [36]. Reprinted with permission)

distal femur. The kneeling stress view was found to have very high inter- and intra-observer reliability [5], and to be reliable evaluation of posterior laxity [6].

Of note, however, a recent study comparing Telos stress views to kneeling stress views showed significantly different displacement measurements—both pre- and post-reconstructive surgery [7]. This has been hypothesized to likely be due to the difference in force placed on the anterior tibia with the two techniques. Further study will therefore be required to better define normative displacement measurements for the kneeling exam. Moreover, a larger comparative study to other available methods is necessary to determine the value of the kneeling stress view in quantitating the posterior instability.

Valgus Stress

A valgus force applied to the knee will put stress on the medial collateral ligament (MCL) opening the medial compartment and allow for grading of MCL injury. The patient is positioned supine on a radiolucent table, and their knees bound together. The examiner is then able to apply valgus stress to both knees by attempting to separate the patient's feet from the foot of the bed. The knees should be maintained in approximately 10–15° of flexion, and the feet slightly externally rotated while performing the stress. An anteroposterior (AP) radiograph is then taken of the knee at the endpoint of displacement. Displacement is measured from the medial plateau to the femoral condylar line [8] and the uninjured knee is used as the control (normal) value (Fig. 5.2).

Varus Stress

Varus stress radiography has been found to correlate well with MRI findings and be helpful in determining which lateral/posterolateral corner injuries should be surgically repaired or reconstructed [9]. Gawthmey et al. found that a lateral joint opening averaging 18.6 mm (range 10.0–36.5 mm) was associated with a complete posterolateral corner (PLC) disruption on MRI while an opening of 12.8 mm (range 7.5–17.0 mm) was reflective of a partial tear. Opening in operative cases that underwent PLC stabilization was, on average, 16.5 mm (11.0–36.5 mm) versus 11.0 mm (range 7.5–13.5 mm) in those that were treated nonoperatively [9].

Advantages

- Cost-effective
- Some protocols have very good reliability and effectiveness

Disadvantages

- Training for clinicians and radiation technologists
- Standardization of protocols is necessary to obtain comparable data

Instrumented Stress Radiography

Telos Stress Radiography

The Telos Stress Device (Austin and Associates Inc. Fallson MD) is a commercially available system that allows for the application of consistent and reproducible stress forces to the index knee joint, while radiographs are obtained (Fig. 5.3). Measurement of displacement on the radiograph can then be performed. Depending on the patient's position and device's orientation, it can be used to stress the tibiofemoral joint

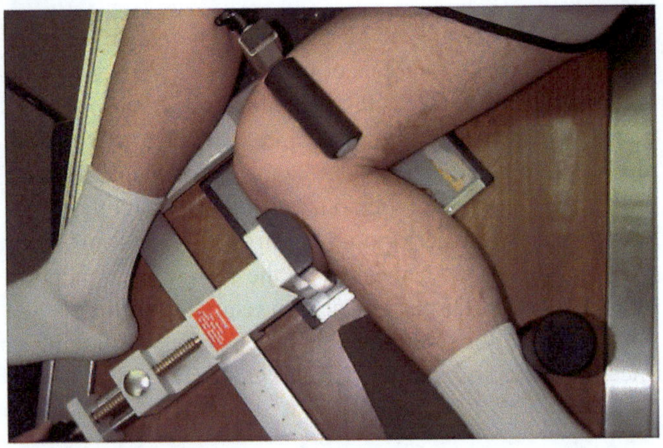

Fig. 5.3 The stress X-ray examination of the PCL-deficient knee with the Telos device. (From Carsen and Johnson 2013 [36]. Reprinted with permission). *PCL* posterior cruciate ligament

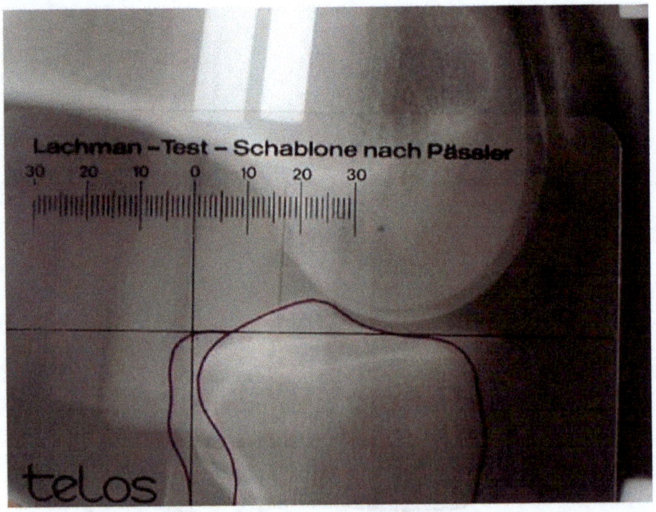

Fig. 5.4 The Telos stress X-ray with the measuring template. (From Carsen and Johnson 2013 [36]. Reprinted with permission)

anteriorly, posteriorly, medially, or laterally, thereby assessing the ACL, PCL/PLC/posteromedial corner (PMC), MCL, and lateral collateral ligament (LCL), respectively.

Posterior Stress

To perform a posterior stress X-ray utilizing the Telos device, the patient is positioned in the lateral decubitus position, index knee dependent on the radiolucent table. The knee is positioned at 90° of flexion inside the Telos device (Fig. 5.3). The knee must be in neutral rotation. A 15-kPa force is exerted on the anterior tibial tubercle, and a lateral X-ray is performed. The knee must be positioned in a true lateral position, which should be confirmed by superimposition of the lateral and medial femoral condyles on the radiograph.

Measurement of displacement is performed by using the Telos template, aligning the inferior horizontal line parallel to and overlying the tibial plateau. The perpendicular "zero" line is then lined up with the posterior border of the tibial plateau. The measurement of posterior displacement is then made in millimeters between the posterior border of the tibial plateau and the posterior border of femoral condyles.

The degree of posterior displacement is measured with a template on the lateral stress X-ray (Fig. 5.4). In this example, the posterior displacement is 17 mm.

The difficulties with this method are:

- It is essential to have a true lateral X-ray with the femoral condyles overlapping as shown in Fig. 5.4.
- The template must be accurately positioned to ensure reproducible measurements.

One of the most significant challenges with the Telos system is ensuring standardized measurement. Following a standardized protocol when performing the radiographs produces reliable and reproducible measurements [10].

A recently published study conducted over 12 years using the Telos device for the evaluation of knee instability in more than 1000 patients found it to be reliable and effective at diagnosing posterior laxity [11]. They found that a measurement of greater than 8 mm of posterior displacement was diagnostic for complete PCL rupture, while a measurement of greater than 12 mm was indicative of injury to secondary supporting structures as well (PLC and/or PMC).

Anterior Stress

The Telos system has not been as helpful in assessing the magnitude of anterior laxity of the knee. Rijk et al. found that an anterior displacement of more than 7 mm was abnormal, with a false-negative rate of 12% [12]. The patient and device positioning for anterior stress testing is essentially identical to the posterior stress exam, with the position reversed.

Recently, Dejour et al. demonstrated that the Telos device in conjunction with clinical examination (pivot shift test) was helpful in differentiating partial from complete ACL ruptures [13].

Advantages

- Accurate measurement of the posterior displacement with a template.

Disadvantages

- The use of X-rays/radiation.
- The radiological technician must be trained in the correct use of the device.
- Expense of the Telos device.

Knee Ligament Arthrometers

KT-1000/2000

The KT-1000 and KT-2000 (the KT-2000 is essentially the same as the KT-1000 but with an added graphic plotting interface) are arthrometers that measure anterior–posterior tibiofemoral translation (i.e., translation in the sagittal plane only).

Anterior

The KT-1000 knee ligament arthrometer (MEDMetric Corp., San Diego, CA), developed by Dale Daniel and Larry Malcolm [14], has become the standard for the measurement of ACL laxity. Starting from its introduction in the early 1980s, it has continued to be found to be accurate and reliable in the measurement of anterior translation of the tibia on the femur [15]. It has proven to have strong reliability, with good inter- and intra-rater performance [16]. It has recently performed equally compared with intra-operative computer-assisted surgery/navigation [17]. The device is used with the patient supine and a support platform placed under both thighs to maintain approximately 25–35° flexion of both knees. The feet are supported on the lateral aspects by a second platform to ensure the same relative rotation of both lower legs. This position is ideal for the performance of an instrumented Lachman test on both knees. The arthrometer is placed secured with Velcro straps on the knee and lower leg such that the force pad is located over the tibial tubercle, and the patellar pad is resting on the anterior surface of the patella. The patella pad is gently stabilized while the force handle is pushed and pulled to achieve tibiofemoral translation readings (Fig. 5.5). The maximum manual test has been found to have the highest diagnostic value for the determination of ACL laxity and is performed by using a hand behind the calf to produce a maximal anterior translation force [18].

The best results with the KT-1000 are obtained when comparing side-to-side difference within the same patient, and when the same examiner performs the repetitive exams. Though the KT-1000 arthrometer is simple to use, there is still an association of increased accuracy and reproducibility with the experienced user.

Posterior

The KT-1000 has not, however, achieved the same level of acceptance for the quantitative measurement of posterior instability. Daniel [19] described the method of measuring posterior laxity by first determining the quadriceps neutral point.

The principle of the measurement as described by Daniel is to determine the four levels of anterior-to-posterior motion:

- Anterior
- Quadriceps neutral
- Posterior sag
- Posterior displacement

Initially, the patient contracts the quadriceps muscle sufficiently to bring the tibial forward to the "quadriceps neutral" position.

The posterior motion from this point is then recorded as the posterior sag, and then the posterior displacement with 20 pounds of posterior force is measured and noted as the posterior displacement (Fig. 5.6). The total amount of posterior motion is determined when these two later values are added.

In our experience, it is often difficult to get the patient to contract their quadriceps sufficiently to bring the tibia fully forward to the neutral position. This amount of forward displacement is often underestimated. Johnson presented a study to the PCL study group in 1995, comparing the KT value against the stress X-ray [20]. The results were:

When the millimeters of displacement of the KT is expressed as a percentage of the Telos:

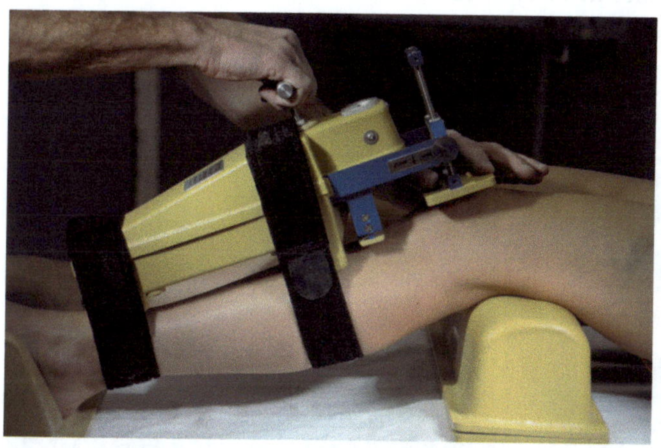

Fig. 5.5 This photo shows the KT-1000 device used to measure the anterior tibial displacement

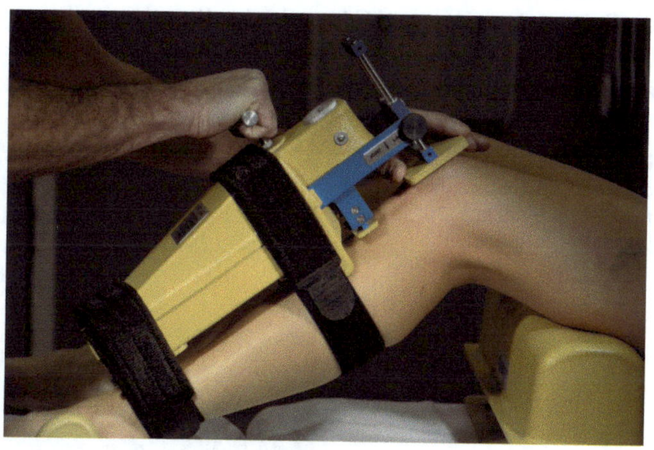

Fig. 5.6 This photo demonstrates the KT-1000 device positioned to measure posterior tibial translation

>10 mm of posterior displacement—the KT is 65% of the Telos
<10 mm of posterior displacement—The KT is 72% of the Telos

The KT-1000 measurement underestimates the degree of posterior instability when compared with the Telos stress X-ray, and this difference is more pronounced when the posterior displacement is greater than 10 mm. The PCL-deficient knee is, therefore, best quantitatively evaluated with stress X-rays.

This underestimation of displacement by the KT-1000 was also confirmed by Noyes et al. [21], who found that stress radiography was superior to both arthrometer and clinical posterior drawer testing. His group determined that 8 mm of posterior displacement was the cutoff for complete PCL rupture [21].

This study confirms that the measurement of the posterior displacement is more accurate with the stress X-ray, especially in cases where the posterior displacement is greater than 10 mm.

Another study by Harner et al. [22] compared a novice and an experienced user of the KT-1000 device and found that the device was a moderately reliable tool to evaluate PCL laxity. This was a small group of patients, most having less than 10 mm of posterior laxity.

Advantages

- Widely used and accepted method of measurement of anterior displacement in the ACL-deficient knee
- Widely available

Disadvantages

- Underestimates the degree of posterior instability, especially when more than 10 mm of posterior displacement is present.

Knee Laxity Tester

The use of the knee laxity tester (KLT) arthrometer (Orthopedic Systems Inc., Hayward CA) or Stryker Knee Laxity Tester (Stryker Inc., Kalamazoo, MI) likely hit its peak in the 1990s, and though the arthrometer is no longer available, it is still used by some and was highly tested. Like the KT-1000, the KLT measures tibiofemoral translation in the sagittal plane.

Anterior

The technique is similar to the KT-1000, and has produced similar results [23].

Posterior

The measurement of posterior laxity has been described by Cannon [24]. The patient is positioned sitting with the knee flexed to 90° over the end of a table. The patient actively contracts the quadriceps. At this quads' neutral point, the instrument is set to 0. The tibia is then displaced posteriorly with a 20- and 40-pound force. The displacements are recorded. The authors [25] found that the arthrometric measurements correlated well with the clinical examination. The arthrometer was also able to detect subtle grade 1 injuries.

Advantages

- The knee is held in the 90° position and it may be easier for the patient to perform the quads active test

Disadvantages

- The instrument is not widely available
- The 71° position was determined by Daniel to be the optimum position to measure the quads active position.

Rotationometer/Laxiometer

The ligament augmentation and reconstruction system (LARS) rotational laxiometer (LARS, Dijon France) was developed specifically to measure the degree of rotation of the tibia relative to the femur. It is a simple device, which can be strapped externally to the subjects' tibia and measures rotation in a noninvasive manner. Objective measurement of external and internal rotation of the tibia at 30 and 90° of knee flexion provides an indication of clinical PLC and PMC laxity (Fig. 5.7).

This device has been validated by measuring the normal variation of tibial rotation [26]. Baseline values of the degree

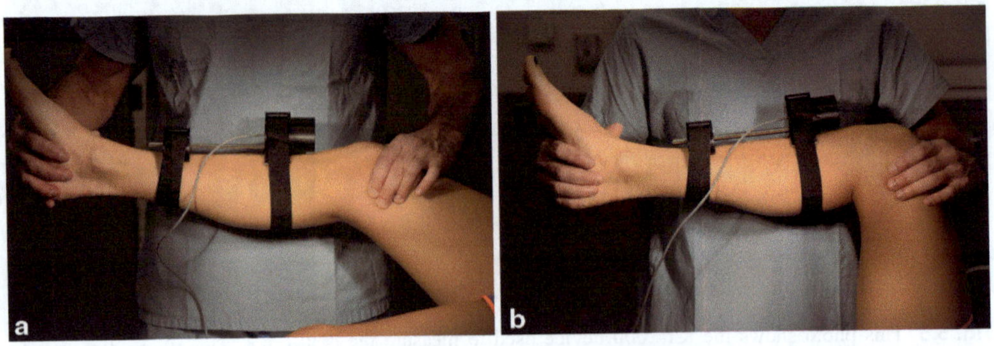

Fig. 5.7 The rotational laxiometer used to measure the external rotation of the tibia at 30° (**a**) and 90° (**b**) of knee flexion

of normal external rotation of the tibia at 30 and 90° have also been established. Three authors each examined 30 asymptomatic patients to determine the side-to-side difference. At 90°, the side-to-side difference was 4.4° (range 3.7–5.1) and at 30° the difference was 5.5° (range 4.7–6.3) [26].

It can be extrapolated that any measurement above these numbers is abnormal and indicative of pathological posterolateral corner laxity. The LARS rotational laxiometer is also a useful device to assess the rotational stability of reconstructed knees postoperatively. One caveat to the use of the rotational laxiometer, as pointed out by the validating authors [26], is that the device is not able to measure the moment applied by the observer during testing or to cancel out the coupled motion of the femur. It is also important to note that when using this device in the presence of PCL deficiency, it is necessary to correct for the posterior sag of the tibia by first performing a quadriceps contraction neutralization prior to evaluating tibial rotation.

Advantages

- Measures external/internal tibial rotation

Disadvantages

- The device requires two people to operate properly when posterior sag is present.
- The device is expensive and not widely available

Computer-Assisted Navigation

Recently, there has been significant progress in the area of computer-assisted surgery (CAS). The role of computer navigation in soft-tissue knee reconstruction surgery has largely focused on accurate tunnel and fixation positioning. However, with increasingly accurate mapping and navigation technology, many of the CAS systems, such as the OrthoPilot system (Aesculap Implant Systems, Center Valley, PA), are now able to intraoperatively measure knee kinematics in multiple planes.

With growing interest in CAS, there have been a number of groups studying the accuracy of various systems in accurately mapping and plotting the kinematics of the knee. Results thus far have been promising, with accuracy measured within 1 mm or 1–2° [27–29]. A recent study comparing computer navigation to the KT-1000 in determining the degree of ACL deficiency found the two approaches to yield comparable results [17]. The keys to obtaining accurate measurements with CAS are familiarity with program (each system has its own learning curve), accurate placement of bony navigation markers, and proper system calibration.

The future of CAS holds great promise, and it should allow for improved accuracy and reproducibility in the measurement of laxity of the knee in all planes and, in particular, in complex multiplanar movements. It is likely to be of value in assessing immediate pre- and post-reconstruction kinematic alterations in complex multiligament reconstructions. However, there are still a number of hurdles for computer navigation to overcome. The systems are still very costly, and most centers will not have access to them. They require appropriate training and support. Computer navigation is an important tool for instrumented measurement, but will not negate the need for other instrumented measures, as it currently is only used in the operative setting. CAS has also not been shown to be of clinical benefit over traditional surgical approaches in the performance of ACL reconstruction [30]. Given these limitations, at this time, computer navigation does not have a significant role to play in preoperative diagnosis or in follow-up.

Advantages

- Accuracy
- Immediate post-reconstruction measurement

Disadvantages

- Costly
- Facility availability
- Only currently used in the operating room (OR) setting

Future Directions

The use of instrumented measurements of ligament laxity in the multiple-ligament-injured knee is currently undergoing somewhat of a renaissance. The development of arthrometers and measurement tools to quantitate knee instability became prevalent in the early 1980s when a number of devices were designed and produced. Among these, the KT-1000 arthrometer has been proven to be the device of choice in evaluating anterior tibiofemoral translation and has now been utilized in well over 500 published peer-reviewed studies. As our ability to restore knee function through surgical stabilization has improved, our interest has increased in obtaining more accurate preoperative and postoperative knee laxity measurements. A better understanding of the soft-tissue anatomy and kinematics of the knee, the advent of anatomic ligament reconstruction including multiple-bundle reconstructions, and the wider introduction and adoption of computer navigation have all led to an increased interest and need for accurate and reproducible objective measures. Recent general reviews have highlighted the current state of instrumented measurement, the most recent outcomes and evidence for their use, and also experience with new techniques and devices [31, 32].

One of the remaining challenges is the accurate determination of rotational laxity. Rotational instability has proven itself to be more difficult to reliably assess than linear translation and displacement, and its clinical importance over the long term is still to be fully appreciated. There are several tools that have been recently developed by respected research groups attempting to better characterize and define ligamentous laxity [32–35]. Most of these systems incorporate electromagnetic markers that are placed on surface landmarks on the lower extremity as well as some form of standardized force applied in rotation and translation. While these systems will be unlikely to play a role in the average clinician's practice, they will help to continue to shed light on the complex kinematics of the knee and lead us to better understand the various soft-tissue deficiencies that must be addressed in the multiple-ligament-injured knee, and their relative importance.

Conclusion

The cornerstone of assessment of the multiple-ligament-injured knee is obtaining a thorough history and performing a detailed clinical exam. History and physical exam along with advanced soft-tissue imaging provide much of the information necessary for initial assessment and management. Instrumented measurement can provide a useful adjunct, and allows for more objective clinical testing and more reliable measurements that can be used to analyze outcomes of a single patient or groups of patients. Familiarity and experience with the instrumented measure being used is essential to gathering accurate reproducible measurements.

The choice of instrumented measurement systems should be based on both the ligaments being tested and the resources available.

In the setting of computer-assisted surgery, very accurate measurements can be taken intraoperatively both pre- and post-reconstruction. Unfortunately, these systems are still not widely available, are expensive to purchase, and do not create measurements that are interchangeable with other instrumented means. The use of computer navigation for the purpose of instrumented measurement is still in its infancy.

The KT-1000 arthrometer is widely available and has proven itself reliable and accurate in the measurement of anterior tibial translation, but is not nearly as effective at gauging posterior laxity. The KT-1000 is the tool of choice for objectively assessing the ACL. The posterior structures, the PCL and PLC, are best assessed using the Telos Stress Radiography system. However, the system's cost and limited clinical adoption make it an unlikely option for many clinicians. The LARS rotational laxiometer can be an objective adjunct to a clinical exam of tibiofemoral rotation, and is of benefit in assessing and following PCL injuries. Recent renewed interest in stress radiography has produced a number of comparison trials of stress radiography, and thus far it appears that kneeling stress radiographs show great promise as a reliable measure of posterior laxity.

References

1. Chassaing V, Deltour F, Touzard R, Ceccaldi JP, Miremad C. Etude radiologique du L.C.P. Ã 90 de flexion. Rev Chir Orthop Reparatrice Appar. 1995;81:35–8.
2. Margheritini F, Mancini L, Mauro CS, Mariani PP. Stress radiography for quantifying posterior cruciate ligament deficiency. Arthrosc: J Arthrosc Rela Surg. 2003;19(7):706–11.
3. Puddu G, Giannì E, Chambat P, De Paulis F. The axial view in evaluating tibial translation in cases of insufficiency of the posterior cruciate ligament. Arthroscopy. 2000;16(2):217–20.
4. Jung TM, Reinhardt C, Scheffler SU, Weiler A. Stress radiography to measure posterior cruciate ligament insufficiency: a comparison of five different techniques. Knee Surg Sports Traumatol Arthrosc. 2006;14(11):1116–21.
5. Jackman T, LaPrade RF, Pontinen T, Lender PA. Intraobserver and interobserver reliability of the kneeling technique of stress radiography for the evaluation of posterior knee laxity. Am J Sports Med. 2008;36(8):1571–6.
6. Osti L, Papalia R, Rinaldi P, Denaro V, Bartlett J, Maffulli N. The kneeling view: evaluation of the forces involved and side-to-side difference. Knee. 2009;16(6):463–5.
7. Garofalo R, Fanelli GC, Cikesb A, N'Deleb D, Kombotb C, Marianid PP, Mouhsine E. Stress radiography and posterior pathological laxity of knee: comparison between two different techniques. Knee. 2009;16(4):251–5.
8. Sawant M, Murty AN, Ireland J. Valgus knee injuries: evaluation and documentation using a simple technique of stress radiography. Knee. 2004;11(1):25–8.
9. Gwathmey FW Jr, Tompkins MA, Cree MG, Miller MD. Can stress radiography of the knee help characterize posterolateral corner inury? Clin Orthop Relat Res. 2012;470(3):768–73.
10. Schulz MS, Russe K, Lampakis G, Strobel MJ. Reliability of stress radiography for evaluation of posterior knee laxity. Am J Sports Med. 2005;33(4):502–6.
11. Schulz MS, Steenlage ES, Russe K, MJ Strobel. Distribution of posterior tibial displacement in knees with posterior cruciate ligament tears. J Bone Joint Surg Am. 2007;89:332–8.
12. Rijke AM, Goitz HT, McCue FC 3rd, Delp JL, Lam D, Port SE. Graded stress radiography of injured anterior cruciate ligaments. Invest Radiol. 1991;26:926–33.
13. Dejour D, Ntagiopoulos PG, Saggin PR, Panisset JC. The diagnostic value of clincal tests, magnetic resonance imaging, and instrumented laxity in the differentiation of complete versus partial anterior cruciate ligament tears. Arthroscopy. 2013;29(3):491–9.
14. Daniel D, Malcolm LL, Stone ML, Sachs R, Burks R. Instrumented measurement of anterior laxity of the knee. J Bone Joint Surg (Am) 1985;67:720–6.
15. Malcolm LL, Daniel DM, Stone ML, Sachs R. The measurement of anterior knee laxity after ACL reconstructive surgery. Clin Orthop Rela Res. 1985;196:35–41.

16. Hanten WP, Pace MB. Reliability of measuring anterior laxity of the knee joint using a knee ligament arthrometer. Phys Ther. 1987;67:357–9.
17. Monaco E, Labianca L, Maestri B, De Carli A, Conteduca F, A Ferretti. Instrumented measurements of knee laxity: KT-1000 versus navigation. Knee Surg Sports Traumatol Arthrosc. 2009;17(6):617–21.
18. Bach BR Jr, Warren RF, Flynn WM, Kroll, M, Wickiewiecz TL. Arthrometric evaluation of knees that have a torn anterior cruciate ligament. J Bone Joint Surg Am. 1990;72:204–8.
19. Daniel DM, Stone ML, Barnett P, et al. Use of the quadriceps active test to diagnose posterior cruciate ligament disruption and measure posterior laxity of the knee. J Bone Joint Surg. 1988;70(A):386–91.
20. Johnson DH. Personal communication, PCL Study Group, 1995.
21. Hewett TE, Noyes FR, Lee MD. Diagnosis of complete and partial posterior cruciate ligament ruptures: stress radiography compared with KT1000 arthrometer and posterior drawer testing. Am J Sports Med. 1997;25(5):648–55.
22. Huber FE, Irragang JJ, Harner C, Lephart S. Intratester and intertester reliability of the KT-1000 arthrometer in the assessment of posterior laxity of the knee. Am J Sports Med. 1997;25(4):479–85.
23. Anderson AF, Snyder RB, Federspiel CF, Lipscomb AB. Instrumented evaluation of knee laxity: a comparison of five arthrometers. Am J Sports Med. 1992;20(2):135–40.
24. Cannon WD, Vittori JM. The use of instrumented testing to measure knee displacement. In: Aichroth P, Cannon WD, editors. Knee surgery: current practice. London: Martin Dunitz Ltd; 1992. pp. 206–216.
25. Eakin CL, Cannon WD. Arthrometric evaluation of posterior cruciate ligament injuries. Am J Sports Med. 1998:26(1);96–102.
26. Bleday RM, Fanelli GC, Giannotti BF, Edson CJ, Barrett TA. instrumented measurement of the posterolateral corner. Arthroscopy. 1998;14(5):489.
27. Colombet P, Robinson J, Christel P, Franceschi JP, Djian P. Using navigation to measure rotation kinematics during ACL reconstruction. Clin Orthop Rela Res. 2007;454:59–65.
28. Seon JK, Song EK, Park SJ, Cho SG, Cho SB, Yoon TR. Measurement of anteroposterior and rotational stability of knee using navigation system. Proceedings of British Society For computer aided orthopaedic surgery, Feb 2008. J Bone Joint Surg Br. 2009;91(SUPP III):395.
29. Yamamoto Y, Ishibashi Y, Tsuda E, Tsukada H, Maeda S, Toh S. Comparison between clinical grading and navigation data of knee laxity in ACL-deficient knees. Sports Med Arthrosc Rehab Ther Technol. 2010;2:27.
30. Young SW, Safran MR, Clatworthy M. Applications of computer navigation in surgey: an evidence-based review. Curr Rev Musculoskelet Med. 2013;6:150–7.
31. Pugh L, Mascarenhas R, Arneja S, Chin PYK, Leith JM. Current concepts in instrumented knee-laxity testing. Am J Sports Med. 2009;37(1):199–210.
32. Branch TP, Mayr HO, Browne JE, Campbell JC, Stoehr S, Jacobs CA. Instrumented examination of anterior cruciate ligament injuries: minimizing flaws of the manual clinical examination. Arthrosc: J Arthrosc Rela Surg. 2010;26(7):997–1004.
33. Musahl V, Bell KM, Tsai AG, Costic RS, Allaire R, Zantop T, Irrgang JJ, Fu FH. Development of a simple device for measurement of rotational knee laxity. Knee Surg Sports Traumatol Arthrosc. 2007;15(8):1009–12.
34. Tsai AG, Musahl V, Steckel H, Bell KM, Zantop T, Irrgang JJ, Fu FH. Rotational knee laxity: reliability of a simple measurement device in vivo. BMC Musculoskelet Disord. 2008;9:35.
35. Lorbach O, Wilmes P, Maas S, Zerbe T, Busch L, Kohn D, Seil R. A non-invasive device to objectively measure tibial rotation: verification of the device. Knee Surg Sports Traumatol Arthrosc. 2009;17(7):756–62.
36. Carsen S, Johnson D. Instrumented measurement of the multiple ligament injured knee: arthrometry, stress radiography, rotationometry, and computer navigation in Fanelli GC: The mulitple ligament injured knee: a practical guide to management. 2nd ed. New York: Springer; 2013.

MRI of PCL, Posteromedial, and Posterolateral Corner Injuries of the Knee

6

W. James Malone, Satre Stuelke, Robert R. Snowden and Joel S. Salesky

Introduction

Imaging is complementary to the history and physical examination in confirming suspected injuries. Imaging is especially valuable when the clinical examination is limited by large body habitus, guarding, and in the setting of complex injuries. Imaging, furthermore, decreases the chance of unsuspected and thus undiagnosed injuries, which if untreated may result in instability, repair failure, and early osteoarthritis [1]. Radiographic imaging provides evaluation of osseous injuries, both large and small. Radiographs should be scrutinized for small avulsion fractures not only because they are often unapparent on magnetic resonance imaging (MRI) but also that they alert us to other more substantial injuries. MRI evaluates directly for ligamentous injury and evaluates for coexistent injuries of the articular cartilage and menisci. MRI evaluation of the posterior cruciate ligament (PCL) as well as the medial and lateral stabilizers is the focus of this chapter.

Initial Radiographic Evaluation

Imaging protocols vary depending on preference, but at our institution this typically includes standing anteroposterior (AP) views of both knees, a tunnel view, 30° flexion lateral view, and sunrise view of the patella. Radiographs may demonstrate indirect and direct signs of PCL tear, for example, radiographic posterior drawer and PCL avulsion fracture [2] (Figs. 6.1 and 6.12b respectively). The "reverse Segond" fracture is a subtle avulsion fracture on X-ray, and is associated with PCL tear [3] (Fig. 6.2). The "arcuate sign" is an osseous avulsion of the fibular head involving some combination of the arcuate complex (arcuate ligament, fabellofibular, popliteofibular ligaments) and/or the conjoined insertion of fibular collateral ligament (FCL)/biceps femoris. Both injuries have a high association with PCL tears [4–6] (Fig. 6.3).

MRI

When evaluating the dynamic and static knee stabilizers, the obtained MRI should be of high resolution. Optimally, imaging should be on a 1.5-Tesla magnet or higher, with small field-of-view (FOV) images of the knee, and should be tailored to evaluate ligaments, tendons, and cartilage. That is to say, large FOV images that cover from the mid femur through the mid tibia result in lower-resolution images, and potentially missed pathology. A high-quality exam is important to accurately evaluate the large stabilizers, but it is even more important to evaluate the complex, blending medial and lateral capsular stabilizers, subtle coexistent meniscal tears, and articular cartilage defects. MRI should be performed in the acute setting, because as normal healing progresses and edema resolves, injuries may become less conspicuous.

PCL

The knee is typically imaged in extension, where the anterior cruciate ligament (ACL) is taut and straight, and the PCL is lax and curved. This position is comfortable for the patient, and allows for the technologist to utilize a knee coil for high-resolution MR images. Unlike the ACL, the normal PCL is homogeneously low signal on both T2 and proton density

W. J. Malone (✉)
Department of Radiology, MC 20-07, Geisinger Medical Center, 100 North Academy Avenue, Danville, PA 17822, USA
e-mail: wjmalone@geisinger.edu

S. Stuelke · R. R. Snowden
Department of Radiology, Geisinger Medical Center, Danville, PA, USA
e-mail: satre.md.mfa@gmail.com

J. S. Salesky
Department of Radiology, Geisinger Wyoming Valley Medical Center, Wilkes-Barre, PA 18711, USA
e-mail: jsalesky@geisinger.edu

G. C. Fanelli (ed.), *Posterior Cruciate Ligament Injuries*,
DOI 10.1007/978-3-319-12072-0_6, © Springer International Publishing Switzerland 2015

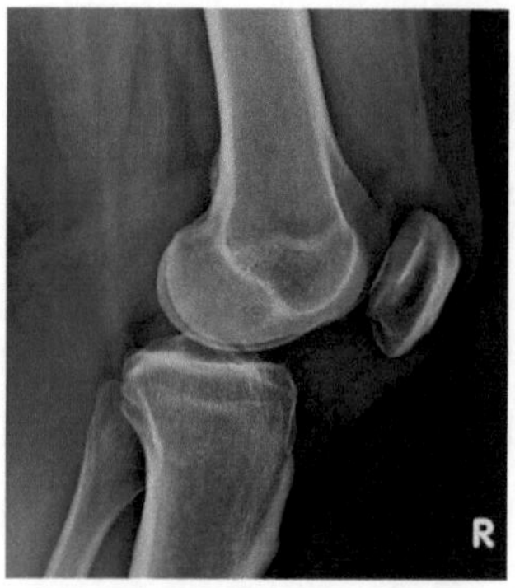

Fig. 6.1 X-ray showing posterior displacement of the tibia on the femur. The radiographic posterior drawer is indicative of PCL tear. *PCL* posterior cruciate ligament

(PD) weighted sequences, lacking internal striations that may be seen in the normal ACL [7, 8] (Fig. 6.4). The knee is not typically imaged in flexion, because a knee coil cannot be utilized, resulting in lower resolution images. However, when imaged in flexion, the PCL appears taut and remains homogeneously low in signal (Fig. 6.5). The normal PCL should measure 6 mm or less, when measured from anterior to posterior in the sagittal plane [9]. Like the ACL, the PCL has two functional bundles, the posteromedial bundle (PMB) and anterolateral bundle (ALB), named according to

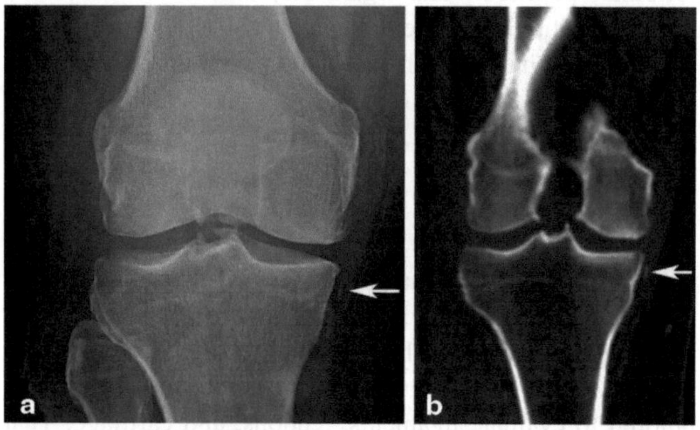

Fig. 6.2 **a** and **b** X-ray and CT respectively showing reverse segond fracture, which is osseous avulsion of meniscotibial ligament. *CT* computerized tomography

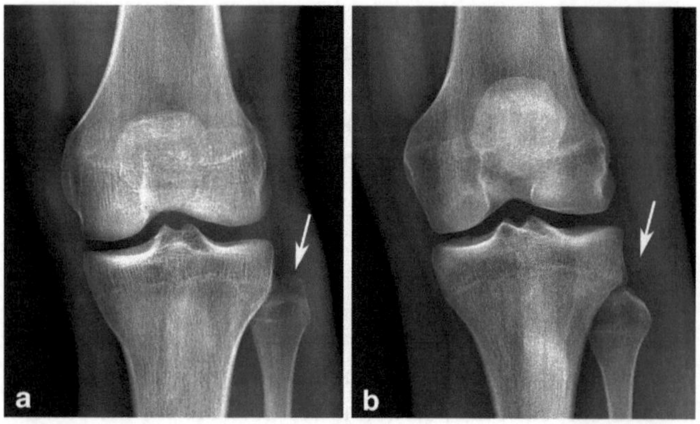

Fig. 6.3 Two different patients with X-rays demonstrating the "arcuate sign." **a** Nondisplaced avulsion fracture of fibular head. **b** Mildly displaced avulsion fracture of the fibular head

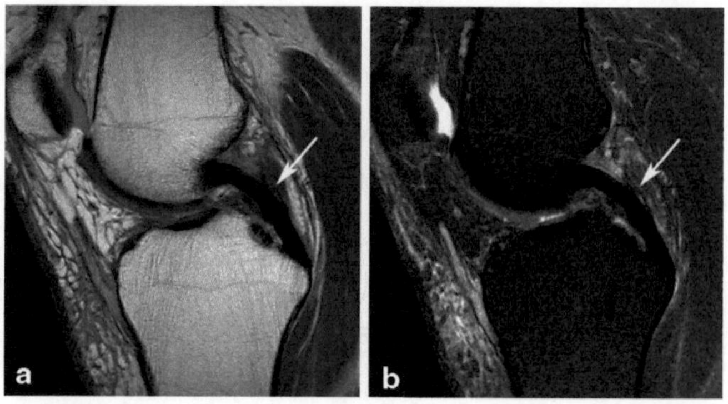

Fig. 6.4 **a** and **b** Normal PCL. Sagittal PD nonfat-suppressed image and sagittal T2 fat-suppressed image demonstrate normal appearance of PCL. The PCL is not taut like ACL when imaged in extension and thus has curved rather than straight morphology. The normal PCL is hypointense on PD and T2 weighted images. *PCL* posterior cruciate ligament, *PD* proton density, *ACL* anterior cruciate ligament

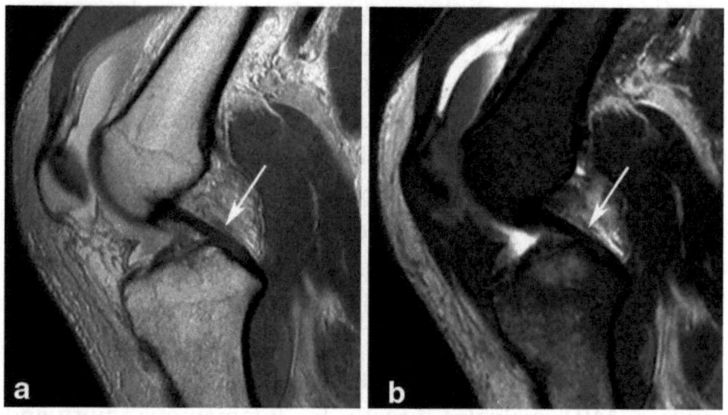

Fig. 6.5 **a** and **b** Normal PCL in flexion. Coronal PD nonfat-suppressed and T2 fat-suppressed image shows knee imaged in mild flexion without a knee coil. PCL is taut in flexion rather than usual curved appearance in extension. Note lower quality images due to imaging without a knee coil. *PCL* posterior cruciate ligament, *PD* proton density

their femoral attachments [10]. In the axial plane, the separate bundles can often be distinguished from one another (Fig. 6.6). The meniscofemoral ligaments can often be seen coursing adjacent to the PCL, with the posterior meniscofemoral ligament (Wrisberg) being more common than the anterior meniscofemoral ligament (Humphey). Not uncommonly both meniscofemoral ligaments are present [11].

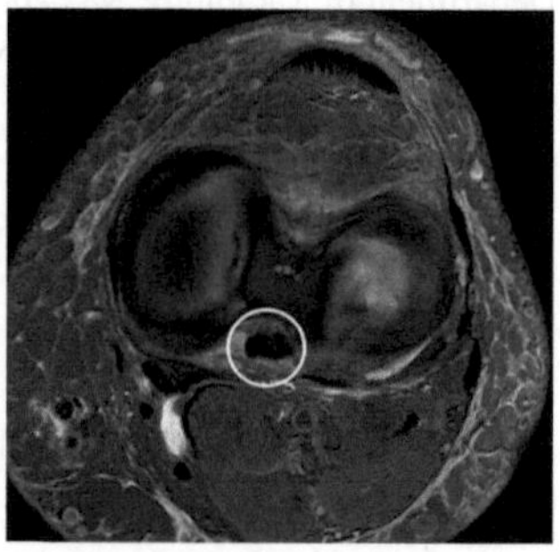

Fig. 6.6 Normal PCL. Axial T2 fat-suppressed image shows normal PCL, which is homogeneously low in signal. Anterolateral and posteromedial bundles are intact, but blend imperceptibly with one another. *PCL* posterior cruciate ligament

MRI is the radiologic study of choice in diagnosing acute PCL tears [7]. The sagittal MRI sequences quickly screen for PCL injury and determine the site of failure at the femoral attachment, midsubstance, or tibial attachment. MRI readily demonstrates acute high-grade injuries to the PCL (Figs. 6.7, 6.8, 6.9). However, unlike ACL tears, PCL tears are more commonly partial rather than complete [7]. In the sagittal plane, partially torn PCL tears often demonstrate a "stretched" appearance with thickening greater than 6 mm and intrasubstance signal changes, the latter of which may be seen only on PD sequence but not on T2 weighted sequences [9]. There are two potential pitfalls if one relies only on the sagittal plane when evaluating PCL tears. First, partial tears may be interpreted as complete tears. Second, mucoid degeneration may mimic a PCL tear in the setting of a functionally stable ligament. In this regard, we have found that the axial plane is complementary to the sagittal plane and can safeguard against the aforementioned pitfalls.

In the axial plane, the anterolateral and PMBs are often apparent and side by side, so we can better determine if the tear is partial or complete, depending on if one or both bundles are torn (compare Figs. 6.7 and 6.10 respectively). Mucoid degeneration of the ACL has been described as a pitfall resulting in false positive ACL tears on MRI [12]. More recently, mucoid degeneration of the PCL was described [13]. Both mucoid degeneration and partial PCL tears may demonstrate thickening and intrasubstance signal changes in the sagittal plane. The axial images help us to distinguish mucoid degeneration from PCL tear, because the former demonstrates the "tram-track" sign. The tram-track sign is defined as a single, linear striation in the PCL that does not surface, so is surrounded by low signal in all planes [13] (Fig. 6.11). In contradistinction, incomplete PCL tears demonstrate multiple heterogeneous internal striations that extend to the outer surface somewhere along the course of the ligament in the sagittal and/or axial planes (compare Figs. 6.10 and 6.11).

Although chronic PCL injuries may be apparent on MRI (Figs. 6.12 and 6.13), MRI is not as sensitive in diagnosing chronic compared to acute PCL tears [14, 15]. Furthermore, MRI may appear normal as soon as 3 months following low-

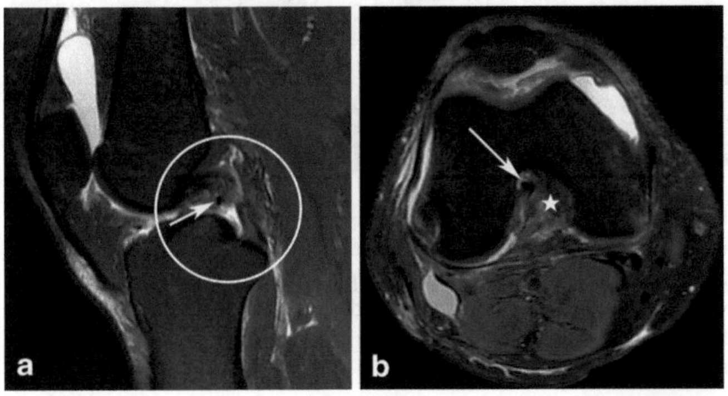

Fig. 6.7 Complete PCL tear. **a** Complete midsubstance disruption with intact femoral and tibial attachments intact. Note subjacent Humphries ligament (*arrow*). **b** Axial image shows empty notch (*star*) other than ACL (*arrow*), consistent with complete PCL tear involving PM and AL bundles. *PCL* posterior cruciate ligament, *ACL* anterior cruciate ligament, *PM* posteromedial, *AL* Anterolateral

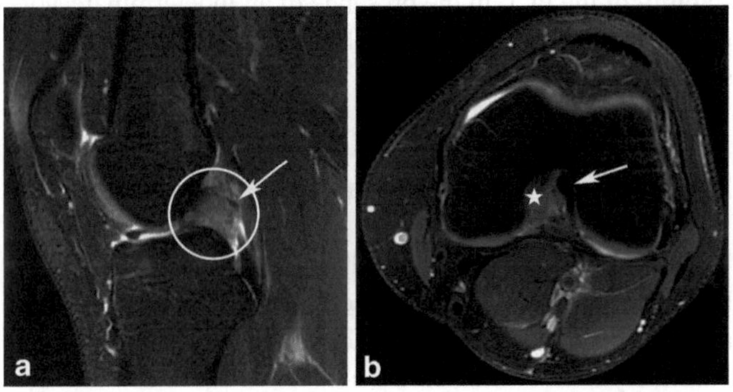

Fig. 6.8 Complete PCL tear. **a** Fat-suppressed T2 sagittal demonstrates complete proximal disruption of PCL. Note overlying Wrisburg ligament (*arrow*). **b** Axial image shows empty notch (*star*) other than ACL (*arrow*), consistent with complete tear involving PM and AL bundles. *PCL* posterior cruciate ligament, *ACL* anterior cruciate ligament, *PM* posteromedial, *AL* anterolateral

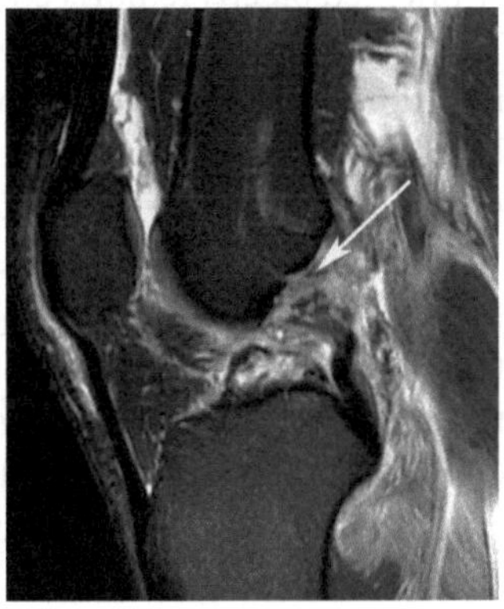

Fig. 6.9 Femoral avulsion PCL. Sagittal T2 fat-suppressed image demonstrating femoral avulsion of PCL (*arrow*). Axial image at femoral attachment showed complete tear (not shown). *PCL* posterior cruciate ligament

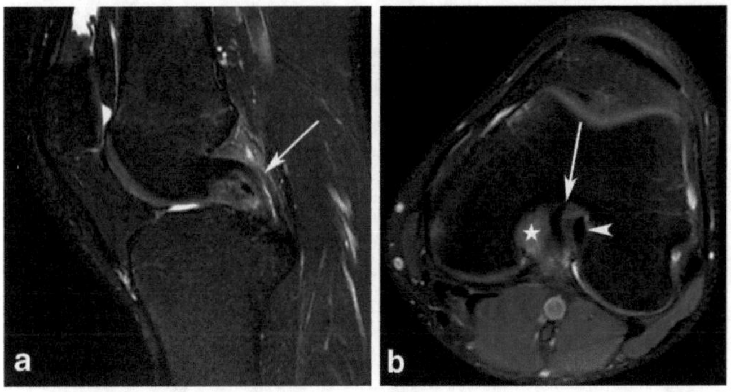

Fig. 6.10 Partial PCL tear. **a** Sagittal and axial T2 fat-suppressed images showing moderate grade midsubstance PCL injury. Intrasubstance striated signal changes with no visualization of tibial attachment. **b** *Arrowhead* shows normal ACL. PCL is dimutive with intact AL bundle (*arrow*) and fluid signal at expected location of torn PM bundle (*star*). *PCL* posterior cruciate ligament, *ACL* anterior cruciate ligament, *AL* anterolateral, *PM* posteromedial

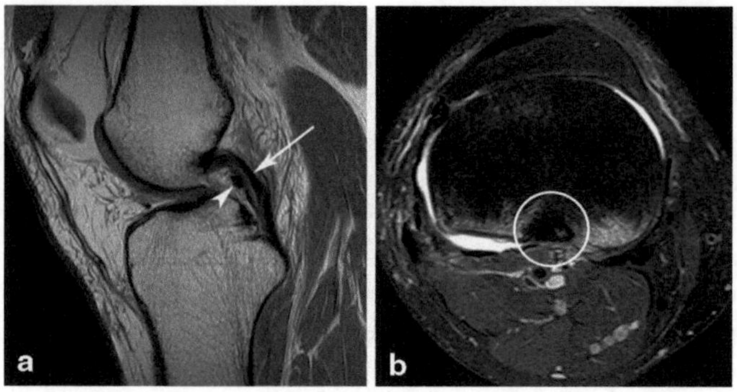

Fig. 6.11 PCL mucoid degeneration. **a** Nonfat-suppressed proton density (*PD*) image demonstrates mild linear intrasubstance fluid bright signal changes. **b** Axial T2 fat-suppressed image midsubstance of PCL. Signal changes do not reach the surface of the ligament on sagittal or axial sequences. Femoral and tibial attachments are intact. Note Humphries ligament (*arrowhead*). *PCL* posterior cruciate ligament

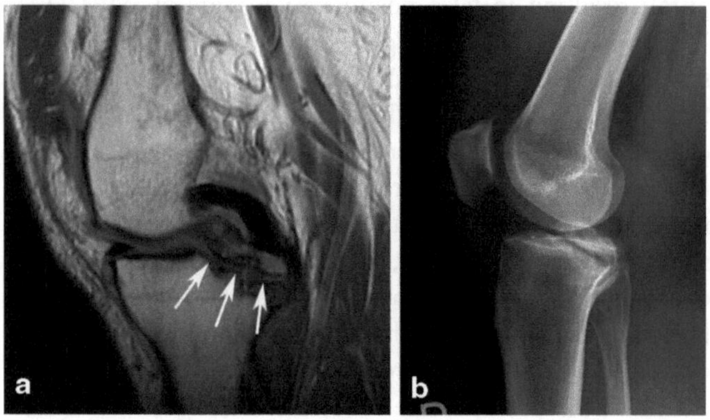

Fig. 6.12 Osseous avulsion of PCL. **a** Nonfat-suppressed PD images show intact PCL with osseous avulsion of PCL at tibial attachment (*arrows*). **b** Corresponding X-ray shows osseous avulsion as well. Note hypointense fracture margins on MRI and sclerotic fracture margins on X-ray, consistent with chronic rather than acute injury. *PCL* posterior cruciate ligament, *PD* proton density, *MRI* magnetic resonance imaging

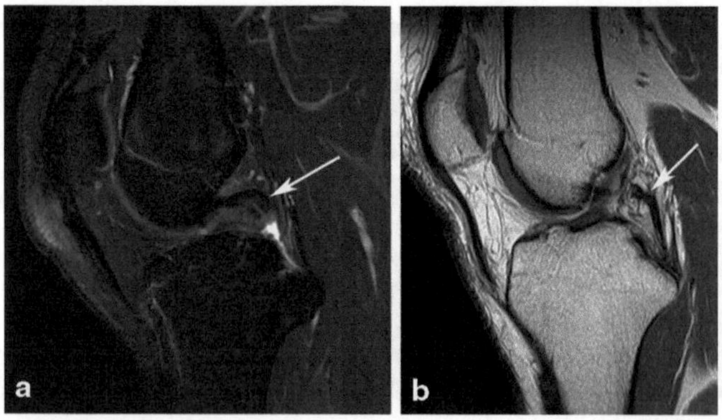

Fig. 6.13 Two patients with high-grade chronic tears. **a** T2 fat-suppressed image shows remote, complete nonosseous avulsion of PCL at tibial attachment with proximal retraction. **b** PD nonfat-suppressed images show marked attenuation of PCL with nonvisualization of femoral attachment, consistent with chronic tear. *PCL* posterior cruciate ligament, *PD* proton density

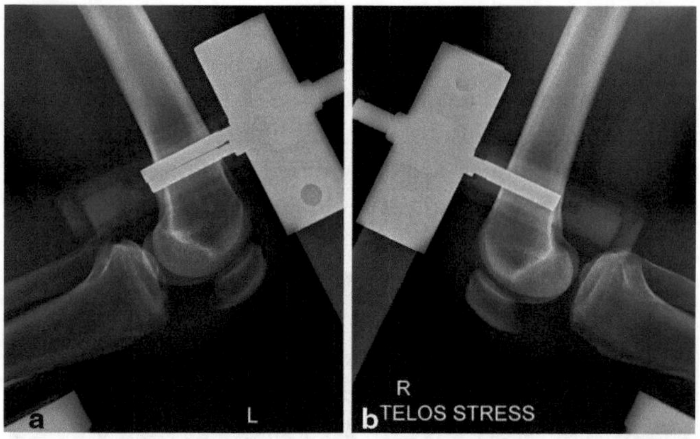

Fig. 6.14 **a** and **b** Stress radiographs of both knees with history of remote injury and only mildly thickened PCL on MRI (MRI not shown). Note posterior displacement of the right tibia on the femur in right knee with stress, with ~10-mm corrected side: side differential compared to normal left knee. *PCL* posterior cruciate ligament, *MRI* magnetic resonance imaging

to moderate-grade PCL injuries [16]. Stress radiographs, such as the Telos system, are accurate in their ability to evaluate for functional instability of the PCL [17, 18]. Given the above challenges in diagnosing chronic partial PCL tears on MRI, stress radiographs are useful to evaluate functional stability of the PCL in the presence of an indeterminate MRI that demonstrates mild PCL thickening and/or mild PCL signal changes (Fig. 6.14).

Lateral and Posterolateral Corner Stabilizers

The large lateral stabilizers such as the iliotibial band (ITB), FCL, biceps tendon, and the conjoined insertion of biceps and FCL are well seen on MRI, and hence injuries are accurately characterized. MRI evaluation of the smaller ligamentous and capsular structures, such as the popliteofibular ligament and capsular ligaments, are challenging due to their diminutive size, oblique course relative to traditional imaging planes, and anatomic variation [1].

The FCL courses obliquely from anterior to posterior in the lateral and posterolateral aspect of the knee. The obliquely oriented biceps femoris courses from posterior to anterior. These two structures converge to form a "conjoined tendon insertion" as they insert onto the lateral aspect of the fibular head [19, 20]. Both structures are homogeneously low in signal on all pulse sequences, with the exception of their conjoined insertion, which we note often demonstrates faint, thin striations (Fig. 6.15). Injuries to the biceps, FCL, and their conjoined insertion are relatively straightforward due to the size of these structures. Figures 6.16, 6.17, and 6.18 demonstrate various injuries to the FCL.

The popliteus tendon and popliteofibular ligament are strong stabilizers of the PLC of the knee. The origin of the

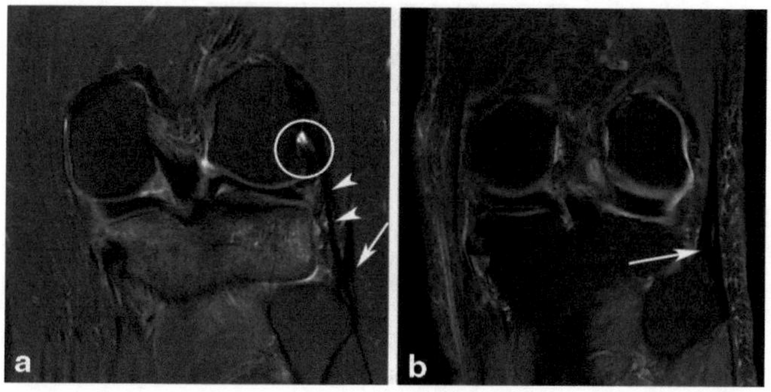

Fig. 6.15 Normal FCL, biceps, and popliteus origin on coronal T2 fat-suppressed images. **a** Normal FCL (*arrowheads*) and partially imaged biceps tendon at their conjoined insertion (*arrow*). Note popliteus origin as well (*circle*). **b** Normal biceps tendon insertion is striated (*arrow*), which does not indicate pathology. *FCL* fibular collateral ligament

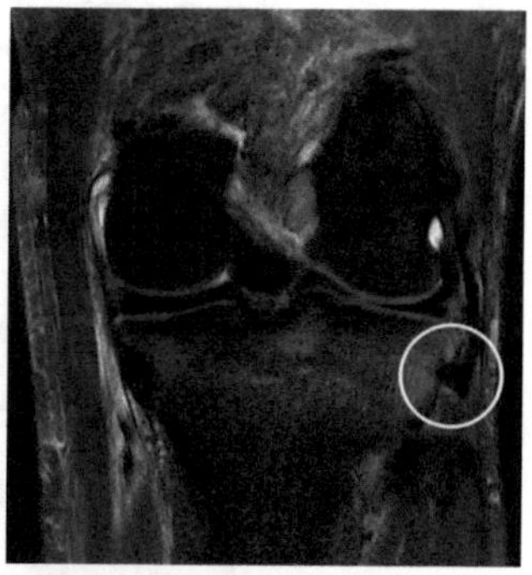

Fig. 6.18 Avulsion of conjoined tendon insertion. Coronal T2 fat-suppressed image showing avulsion of FCL at the fibular attachment with proximal retraction of ~ 1 cm (*circle*). More posteriorly located biceps tendon insertion was intact (not shown). *FCL* fibular collateral ligament

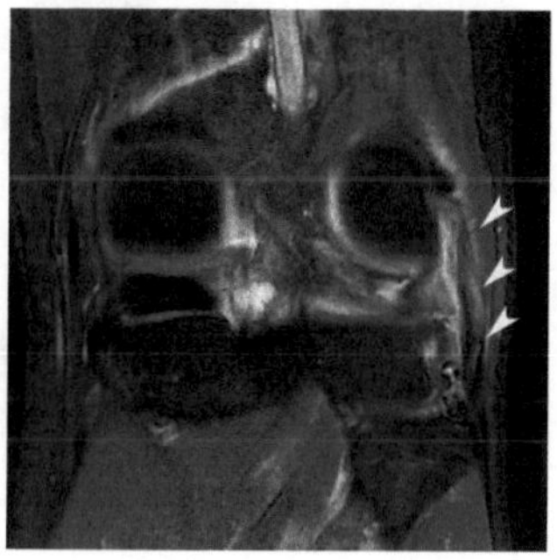

Fig. 6.16 Moderate- to high-grade FCL tear. Coronal T2 fat-suppressed image showing moderate- to high-grade injury to FCL, as denoted by intrasubstance and periligamentous edema (*arrowheads*). *FCL* fibular collateral ligament

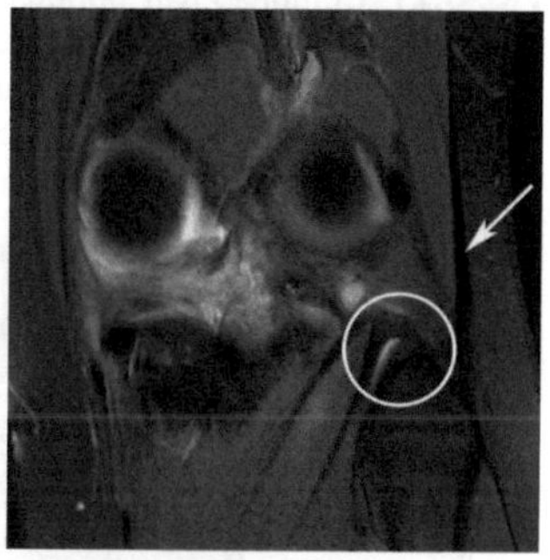

Fig. 6.19 Normal popliteofibular ligament coming off popliteus tendon. Coronal T2 fat-suppressed image sequence showing normal appearance of popliteofibular ligament (*circle*). Note normal biceps tendon (*arrow*)

popliteus tendon is intra-articular from a sulcus on the lateral femoral condyle, inferior and anterior to the proximal attachment of the FCL [19, 20]. As the popliteus tendon wraps posteromedially, it become extra-articular at the meniscal hiatus and gives off a branch that acts as a pulley; this popliteofibular ligament courses laterally and inserts on the medial aspect of the fibular styloid process, medial to the attachment of the fabellofibular ligament and arcuate ligament [19–21].

The popliteus origin is consistently seen on MRI (Fig. 6.15a). Although it is generally a low signal on all pulse sequences, we often see mild signal changes and striations in the absence of injury. The normal popliteofibular ligament is consistently present [22], but can be difficult to visualize on MRI [19, 23]. The popliteofibular ligament courses on average approximately 40° to the horizontal plane [24] and is best seen on coronal sequences (Fig. 6.19). At times, fat surrounding the ligament makes it more conspicuous on traditional nonfat-suppressed PD or T2 weighted sequences (Fig. 6.20). Complicating the evaluation of this ligament is that there is known anatomic variation, whereas at times the popliteofibular ligament may have a more vertical course, and multiple bands have been described [17, 19, 20, 25].

Injury to the popliteus complex may occur throughout its course (Figs. 6.21, 6.22, 6.23, 6.24, 6.25, 6.26). An empty popliteus notch is indicative of tear (Fig. 6.21). An injury may occur in isolation, but multiligament involvement is

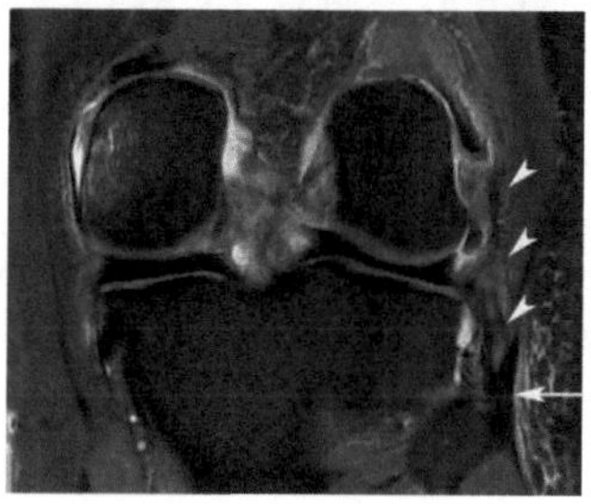

Fig. 6.17 Complete disruption of FCL. Coronal T2 fat-suppressed image with nonvisualization of FCL (*arrowheads*) with the exception of edematous distal fibers at conjoined insertion, consistent with high-grade injury. Partially imaged biceps insertion was intact (*arrow*). Popliteus origin and popliteofibular ligament were intact (not shown). *FCL* fibular collateral ligament

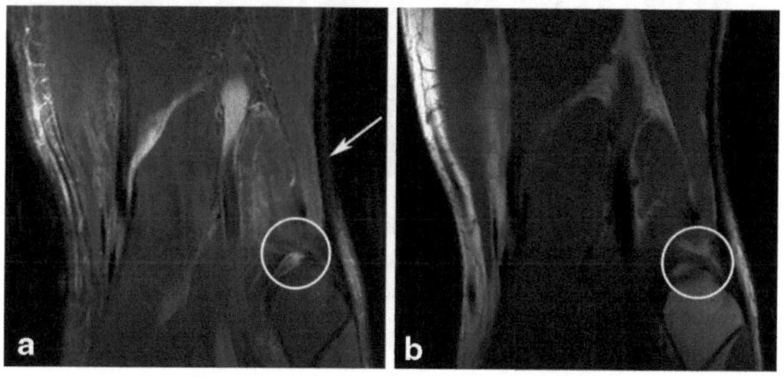

Fig. 6.20 Normal popliteofibular ligament. **a** Popliteofibular ligament not as well seen on coronal T2 fat-suppressed image. **b** Popliteofibular ligament better seen on coronal T1 nonfat-suppressed image (*circle*) with fat serving as contrast against ligament. Note normal biceps tendon (*arrow*)

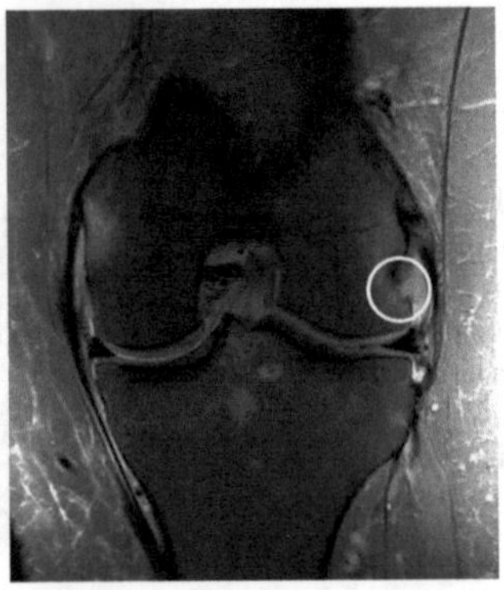

Fig. 6.21 Complete tear popliteus origin. Coronal T2 fat-suppressed image showing empty groove at expected popliteus origin (*circle*) immediately subjacent to FCL attachment, consistent with complete avulsion. *FCL* fibular collateral ligament

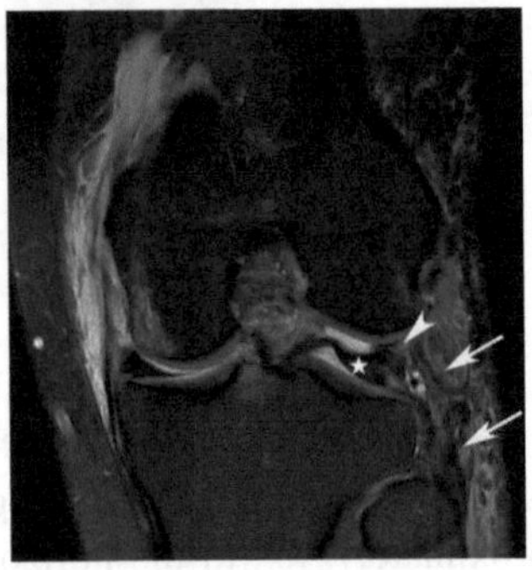

Fig. 6.22 High-grade posterolateral corner injury. Coronal T2 fat-suppressed image showing popliteus avulsion from the femoral attachment, displaced into the lateral joint (*arrowhead*), partially obscured by the superimposed lateral meniscus (*star*). Nonvisualized FCL and conjoined insertion, completely torn at femoral attachment (*arrows*). *FCL* fibular collateral ligament

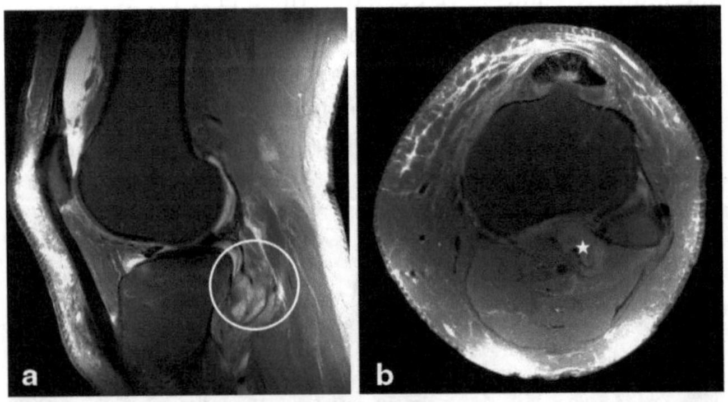

Fig. 6.23 **a** and **b** Moderate- to high-grade popliteus strain. Sagittal and axial T2 fat-suppressed images showing strain popliteus myotendinous junction (*circle* and *star* respectively)

common. A torn tendon may be retracted far proximally and become entrapped in the joint (Fig. 6.22). Despite the difficulties in visualizing the noninjured popliteofibular ligament, injury to the popliteofibular ligament is often

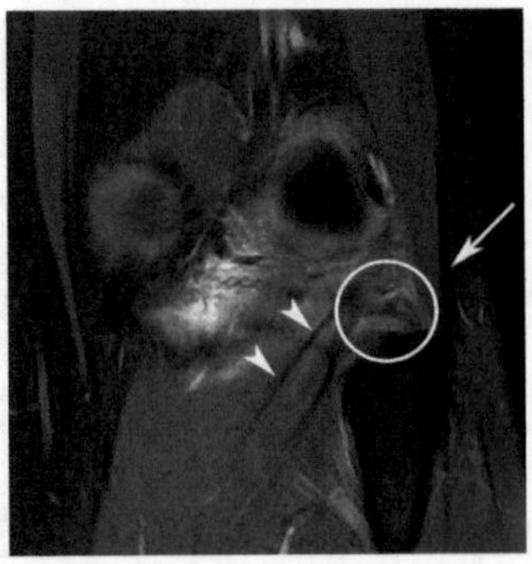

Fig. 6.24 Moderate-grade popliteofibular ligament injury. Coronal T2 fat-suppressed image showing mild intrasubstance and surrounding periligamentous edema, consistent with moderate sprain (*circle*). Normal biceps (*arrow*) and popliteus tendon (*arrowheads*)

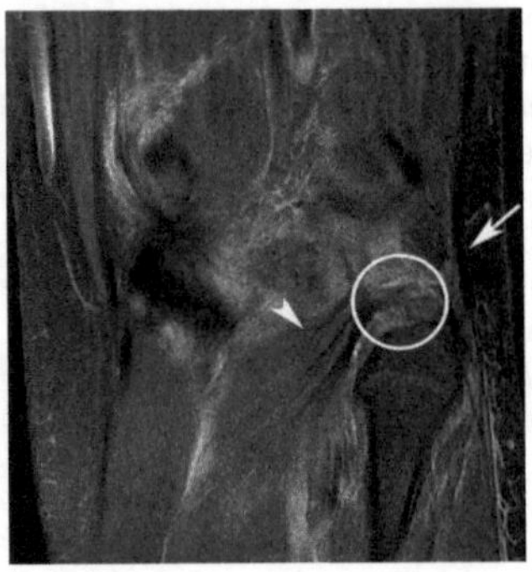

Fig. 6.25 Moderate- to high-grade popliteofibular ligament injury. Coronal T2 fat-suppressed image showing disorganization of fibers of the popliteofibular ligament with intrasubstance and surrounding edema (*circle*). Normal popliteus tendon (*arrowhead*) and biceps (*arrow*)

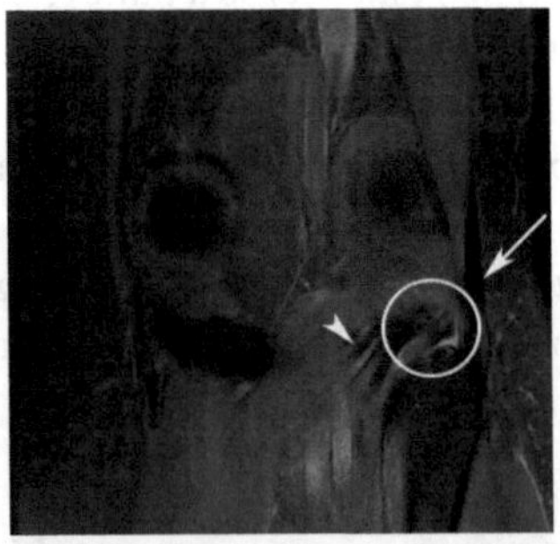

Fig. 6.26 Complete popliteofibular ligament tear. Coronal T2 fat-suppressed image showing linear fluid gap at popliteofibular ligament insertion (*circle*), consistent with complete disruption. This is likely a chronic injury given no surrounding edema. Normal biceps (*arrow*) and popliteus tendon (*arrowhead*)

apparent because the surrounding edema makes the ligament more conspicuous. Injuries run the gamut from low-grade sprains with mild surrounding edema to complete avulsion (Figs. 6.24, 6.25, 6.26). If no edema is present posterolaterally, acute injury to the popliteus and posterior capsule (discussed below) is unlikely, despite nonvisualization of these structures on MRI.

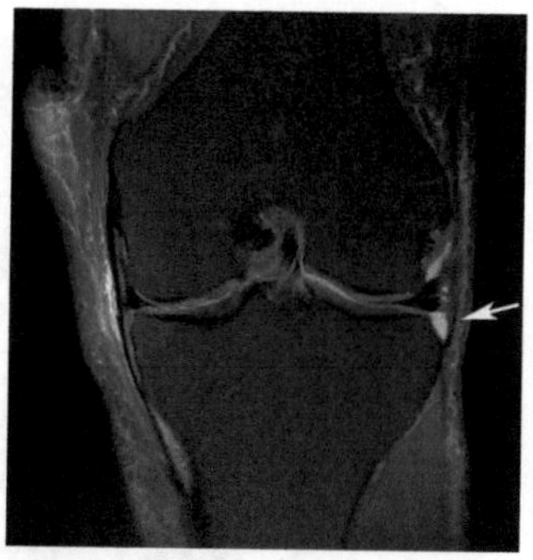

Fig. 6.27 Normal mid-lateral capsule. Coronal T2 fat-suppressed image showing normal mid-lateral capsule at the interval between ITB insertion and FCL (*arrow*). *FCL* fibular collateral ligament, *ITB* iliotibial band

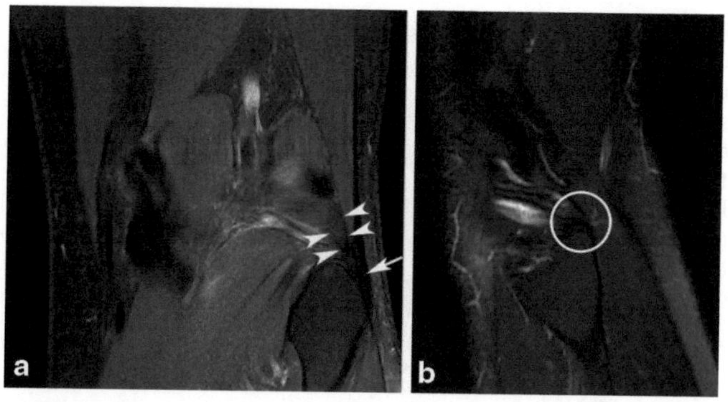

Fig. 6.30 Lateral capsule on coronal and sagittal T2 fat-suppressed images respectively. **a** Edema surrounding and thus highlighting thin V shape of medial and lateral limbs of arcuate ligament complex (*arrowheads*). Note adjacent biceps (*arrow*). **b** Edema does not track posterior to popliteofibular ligament insertion to fibular styloid process on lateral view (*circle*), so post capsule is intact

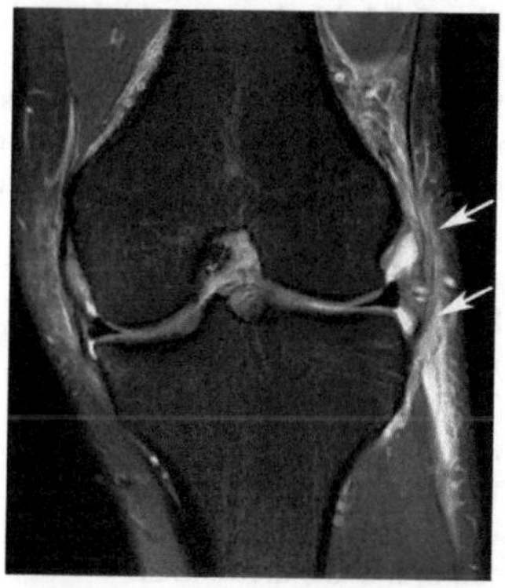

Fig. 6.28 Moderate-grade mid-lateral capsule injury without complete disruption. Coronal T2 fat-suppressed image with diffusely attenuated and edematous AOB (*arrows*). *AOB* anterior oblique band

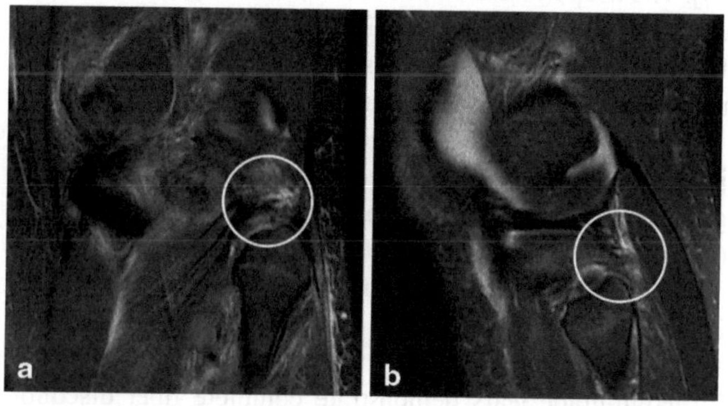

Fig. 6.31 Moderate- to-high-grade injury to the popliteofibular ligament on coronal and sagittal T2 fat-suppressed images, respectively. **a** Note disorganization of fibers of the posterior capsule on coronal image (circle). **b** There is fluid signal posterior to the fibular head on sagittal image (*circle*), consistent with high-grade posterolateral capsule injury

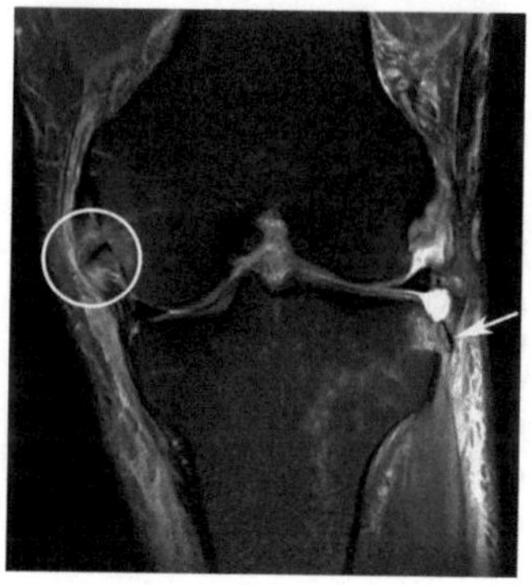

Fig. 6.29 Segond fracture. Coronal T2 fat-suppressed image showing Segond fracture, which is osseous avulsion of the AOB at its tibial attachment (*arrow*). Also, note injury to superficial and deep MCL (*circle*) with osseous avulsion at meniscofemoral ligament attachment. *AOB* anterior oblique band, *MCL* medial collateral ligament

The mid-lateral capsule is specifically the anterior oblique band (AOB), which is formed by contributions from the ITB and FCL [26]. The normal mid-lateral capsule is located in the interval between the ITB and FCL, and is low signal and relatively thin (Fig. 6.27). Figure 6.28 demonstrates injury to the mid-lateral capsule. Avulsion fracture at the tibial attachment of the AOB is termed the Segond fracture [26] (Fig. 6.29).

The posterolateral capsule is formed by a number of structures, most notably the fabellofibular and arcuate ligaments, with contributions from the popliteus and lateral gastrocnemius. These smaller capsular structures are not consistently present in dissection, vary in size and thickness, and can be present alone or in combination [20, 22, 27–30]. An injury to the posterolateral capsule is challenging to characterize due to the anatomic variation in this region, the small size of these structures, and location that is not well evaluated with traditional imaging planes [1]. Knowledge of the insertional geometry of the popliteofibular ligament and arcuate complex onto the fibular head is instrumental to accurate diagnosis [31]. In the setting of PLC injury, marrow edema may be present in the fibular head, and the surrounding soft tissue edema is helpful in highlighting the normal anatomy (Fig. 6.30). Soft tissue edema, disorganization of fibers, and fluid tracking posterior to the popliteus tendon are indicative of moderate to high-grade injury of the posterolateral capsule [27] (Fig. 6.31).

Medial and Posteromedial Stabilizers

Warren initially described three layers stabilizing the medial knee, which includes the sartorius fascia, superficial medial collateral ligament (MCL), and deep MCL [32]. The prominent superficial component of the MCL in the middle third of the knee is traditionally referred to as the MCL, which, due to its size, is well seen in all planes and on all sequences. The more superficial sartorius fascia is thin, so is best seen

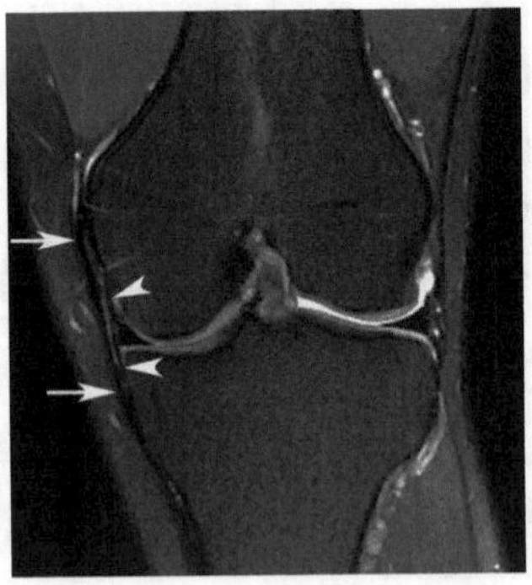

Fig. 6.32 Normal MCL. Coronal T2 fat-suppressed image showing normal superficial MCL (*arrows*) and underlying menisco-femoral and meniscotibial ligaments of the deep MCL (*arrowheads*). *MCL* Medial collateral ligament

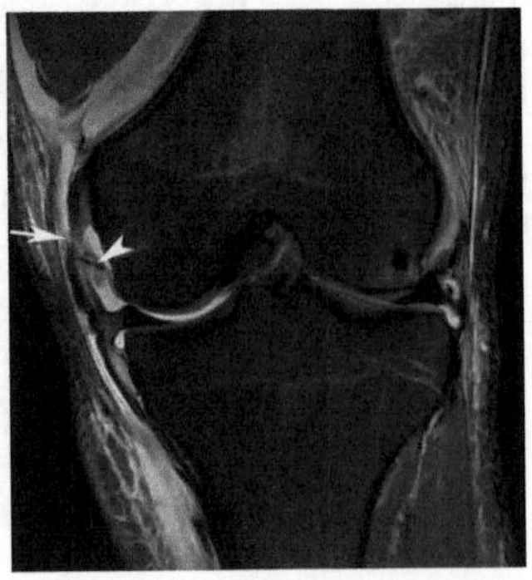

Fig. 6.34 Moderate to high-grade MCL injury. Coronal T2 fat-suppressed image showing focal disruption of superficial MCL near the femoral attachment (*arrow*) and osseous avulsion of MF ligament (*arrowhead*). Tibial attachment of superficial MCL and meniscotibial ligament are both intact. *MF* meniscofibular, *MCL* medial cruciate ligament

without fat suppression, and may be inconspicuous on T2 fat-suppressed sequence. The deep MCL is likewise thin, but is located just deep to the MCL. The deep MCL forms the capsule in the middle third of the knee, and is made up of the meniscotibial (MT) and meniscofibular (MF) ligaments [32, 33]. The deep MCL is best seen when fluid signal or fat is interposed between the superficial and deep MCL (Fig. 6.32). If the deep MCL is flush against the larger overlying MCL, it may be hard to distinguish (Fig. 6.33).

The imaging criteria utilized for all other ligamentous injuries are also used for the medial stabilizers [34, 35]. Low-grade injuries demonstrate periligamentous signal changes (edema and/or hemorrhage) without internal signal changes or fiber discontinuity. Moderate-grade injuries demonstrate intrasubstance signal changes in addition to periligamentous signal changes, sometimes with areas of partial discontinuity. High-grade tears demonstrate complete fiber discontinuity, often exemplified by a wavy ligament. Care should be taken as to which layers of the MCL are torn, as well as describing the location of injury (i.e., at the femoral attachment, tibial attachment, or midsubstance). Figures 6.34, 6.35, 6.36, 6.37, and 6.38 demonstrate various MCL injuries and descriptions of these injuries. Of note, atraumatic edema from osteoarthritis and/or meniscal tear may mimic low-grade MCL tear [36, 37].

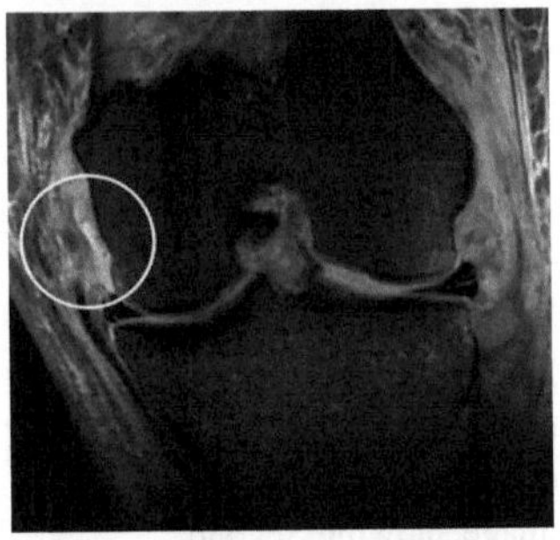

Fig. 6.35 Complete proximal MCL tear. Coronal T2 fat-suppressed image showing complete disruption of superficial and deep components of MCL at femoral attachment. *MCL* medial cruciate ligament

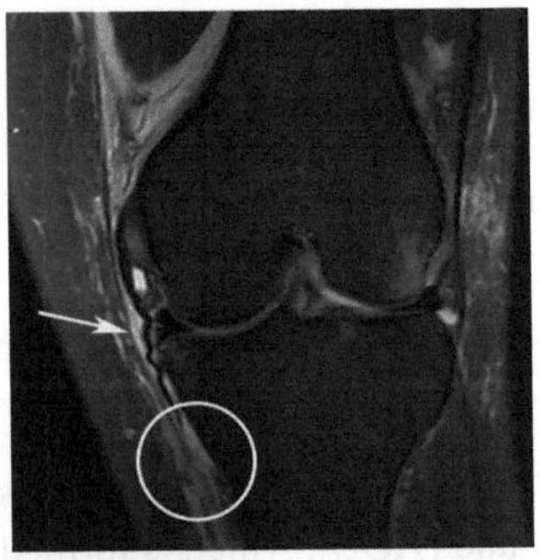

Fig. 6.36 T2 fat-suppressed image showing distal avulsion of MCL (*circle*) with resultant retraction and "wavy" appearance to MCL (*arrow*). *MCL* medial cruciate ligament

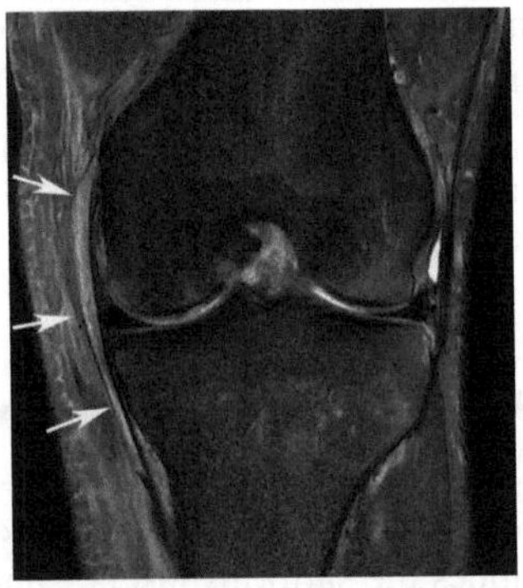

Fig. 6.33 Low-grade MCL sprain. Coronal T2 fat-suppressed image showing fluid/edema superficial to MCL displaces the overlying sartorius fascia (*arrows*). As is often the case, the meniscofemoral and meniscotibial ligaments are taut against and therefore blend with and are indistinguishable from overlying superficial MCL. *MCL* Medial collateral ligament

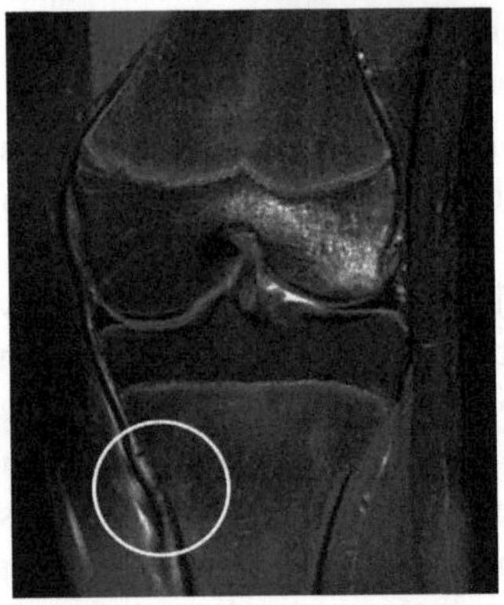

Fig. 6.37 Complete distal MCL tear. Coronal T2 fat-suppressed image showing more subtle MCL tear with distal attachment of MCL (*circle*), which is peeled off tibia but only minimally displaced. Note the bone contusion from "clip" injury medially. *MCL* medial cruciate ligament

When one moves from the middle third to the posterior third of the knee, the deep MCL blends with the posterior oblique ligament (POL) and capsule. The posteromedial capsule is further reinforced by contributions from fibers of the medial gastrocnemius as well as the semimembranosus [27, 32, 33, 38]. The POL is well visualized on MRI and, like the deep MCL, has MF and MT components (Fig. 6.39). Injury to the POL is graded similar to the MCL, and may be diffuse (Fig. 6.40), may occur to the meniscofemoral or meniscotibial components (Fig. 6.41), may strip off the meniscus (meniscocapsular separation; Fig. 6.42), or may pull off the periphery of the meniscus in the form of a longitudinal vertical tear (Fig. 6.43). The POL serves as a bridge between the meniscus and the semimbranosus tendon, and this coupling of the meniscus to the semimembranosus provides motor function to the meniscus via its capsular attachments, resulting in meniscal retraction during knee flexion [39, 40]. Tear in any of the above locations has the potential to decouple the meniscus and semimembranosus tendon, increasing risk of meniscal tear.

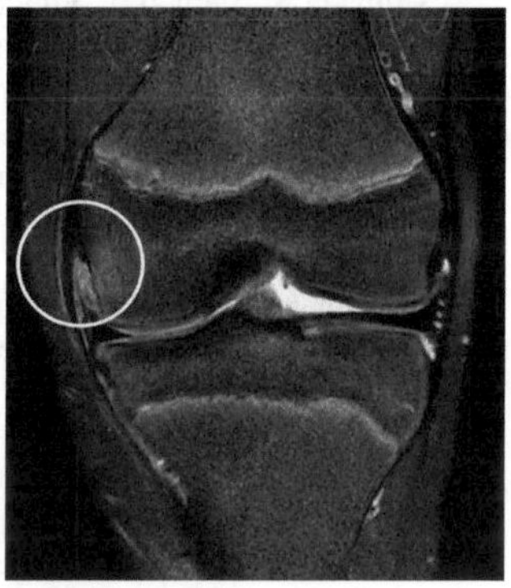

Fig. 6.38 Deep MCL sprain. Coronal T2 fat-suppressed image showing MCL sprain with edema surrounding deep > superficial MCL. Meniscofemoral ligament present but is torn off at femoral attachment (*circle*). Meniscotibial ligament intact. *MCL* medial cruciate ligament

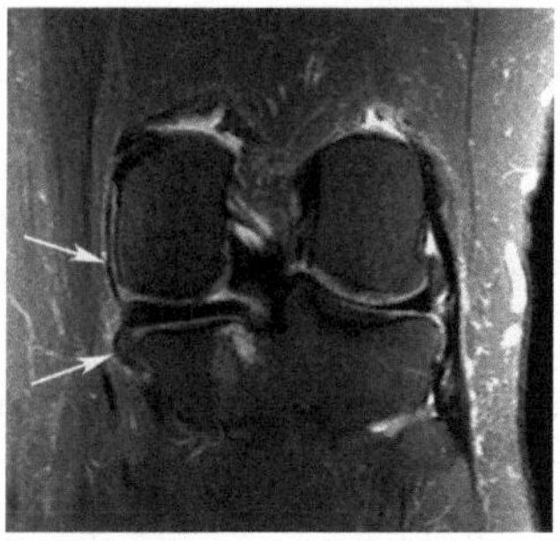

Fig. 6.39 Normal POL ligament. Coronal T2 fat-suppressed image showing normal POL stabilizing the medial meniscus (*arrows*). The appearance is similar to MF and MT ligaments seen in middle 1/3 of knee, but is located posteriorly, and there is no overlying MCL. *MF* meniscofemoral, *MT* meniscotibial, *POL* posterior oblique ligament, *MCL* medial collateral ligament

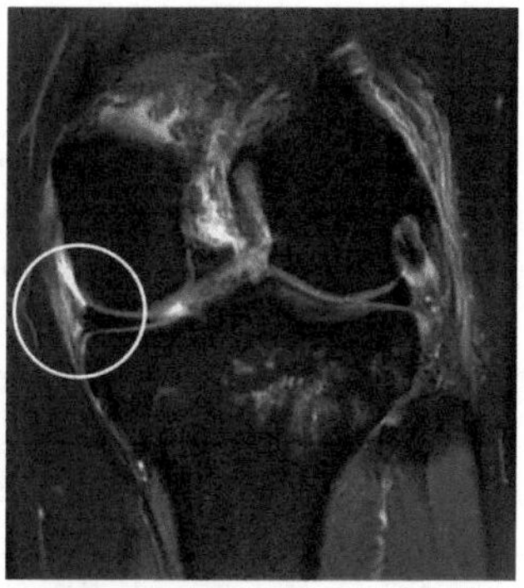

Fig. 6.40 Moderate-grade POL injury. Coronal T2 fat-suppressed image showing attenuated and edematous MF > MT portions of POL without complete disruption. *MF* meniscofemoral, *MT* meniscotibial, *POL* posterior oblique ligament

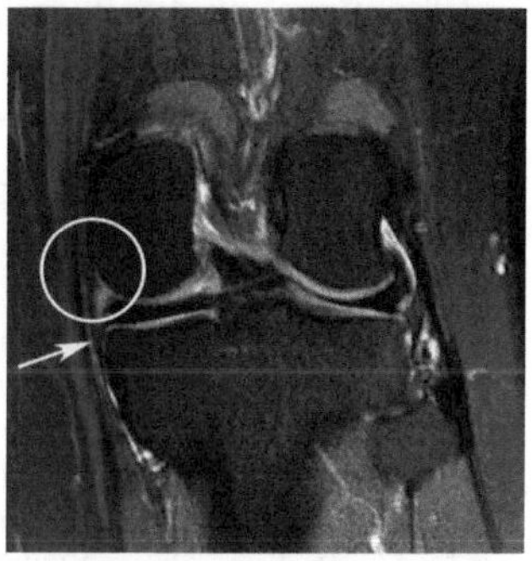

Fig. 6.41 High-grade POL injury. Coronal T2 fat-suppressed image showing disruption of MF portion of POL (*circle*). Meniscotibial portion is intact (*arrow*). *MF* meniscofemoral, *POL* posterior oblique ligament

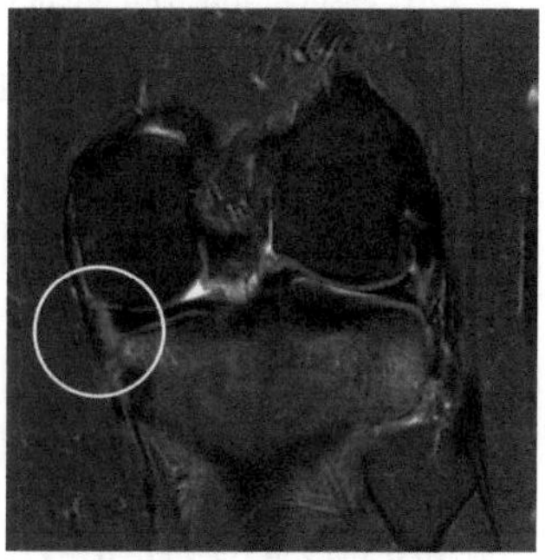

Fig. 6.42 Meniscocapsular separation. Coronal T2 fat-suppressed image showing fluid gap between MF and MT portions of POL and medial meniscus (*circle*). *MF* meniscofemoral, *MT* meniscotibial, *POL* posterior oblique ligament

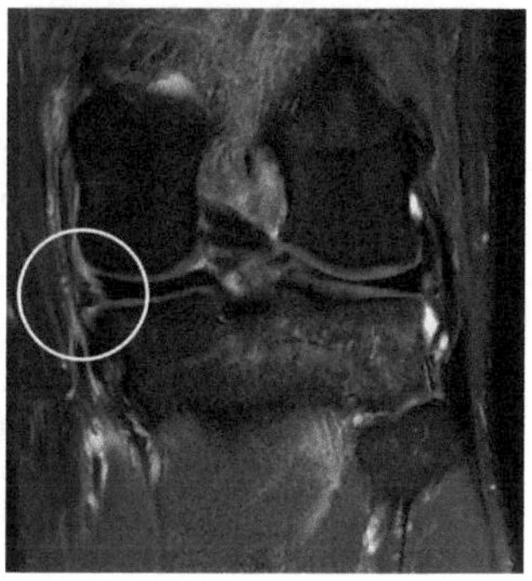

Fig. 6.43 Peripheral meniscal tear. Coronal T2 fat-suppressed image showing moderate diffuse sprain of POL without detachment from the meniscus. However, note peripheral longitudinal vertical meniscal tear, decoupling the POL and the meniscus. *POL* posterior oblique ligament

Conclusion

High-quality radiographs and MRI accurately evaluate the normal anatomy and acute injuries of the PCL, medial knee, and lateral knee. X-rays complement MRI by evaluating for fractures, gross ligamentous injury, and can pick up tiny avulsion fractures that may be subtle or missed on MRI. MRI not only confirms clinically suspected injuries but helps to diagnose unsuspected injuries as well. MRI is complementary, but less accurate in the evaluation of chronic injuries, and may be supplemented with functional imaging in this setting. Imaging studies combined with history and clinical exam and functional studies together provide a precise diagnosis to plan the complex ligamentous repair and reconstruction.

References

1. Malone WJ, Verde F, Weiss D, Fanelli GC. MR imaging of knee instability. Magn Reson Imaging Clin N Am. 2009 vi–vii;17(4):697–724.
2. Gottsegen CJ, Eyer BA, White EA, Learch TJ, Forrester D. Avulsion fractures of the knee: imaging findings and clinical significance. Radiographics. 2008;28(6):1755–70.
3. Escobedo EM, Mills WJ, Hunter JC. The "reverse Segond" fracture: association with a tear of the posterior cruciate ligament and medial meniscus. AJR Am J Roentgenol. 2002;178(4):979–83.
4. Huang GS, Yu JS, Munshi M, Chan WP, Lee CH, Chen CY, et al. Avulsion fracture of the head of the fibula (the "arcuate" sign): MR imaging findings predictive of injuries to the posterolateral ligaments and posterior cruciate ligament. AJR Am J Roentgenol. 2003;180(2):381–87.
5. Juhng SK, Lee JK, Choi SS, Yoon KH, Roh BS, Won JJ. MR evaluation of the "arcuate" sign of posterolateral knee instability. AJR Am J Roentgenol. 2002;178(3):583–8.
6. Shindell R, Walsh WM, Connolly JF. Avulsion fracture of the fibula: the 'arcuate sign' of posterolateral knee instability. Nebr Med J. 1984;69(11):369–71.
7. Sonin AH, Fitzgerald SW, Hoff FL, Friedman H, Bresler ME. MR imaging of the posterior cruciate ligament: normal, abnormal, and associated injury patterns. Radiogr : Rev Publ Radiolog Soc N Am Inc. 1995;15(3):551.
8. Roberts CC, Towers JD, Spangehl MJ, Carrino JA, Morrison WB. Advanced MR imaging of the cruciate ligaments. Magn Reson Imaging Clin N Am. 2007;15(1):73–86.
9. Rodriguez W, Jr, Vinson EN, Helms CA, Toth AP. MRI Appearance of Posterior Cruciate Ligament Tears. Am J Roentgenol. 2008;191(4):W155–9.
10. Amis AA, Gupte CM, Bull AMJ, Edwards A. Anatomy of the posterior cruciate ligament and the meniscofemoral ligaments. Knee Surg Sports Traumatol Arthrosc Off J ESSKA. 2006;14(3):257–63.
11. Bintoudi A, Natsis K, Tsitouridis I. Anterior and posterior meniscofemoral ligaments: MRI evaluation. Anat Res Int 2012;2012:839724–5.
12. Bergin D, Morrison WB, Carrino JA, Nallamshetty SN, Bartolozzi AR. Anterior cruciate ligament ganglia and mucoid degeneration: coexistence and clinical correlation. AJR Am J Roentgenol. 2004;182(5):1283–7.
13. Vinson EN, Helms CA. Imaging for evaluation of posterolateral corner injury. J Knee Surg. 2005;18(2):151–6.
14. Tewes DP, Fritts HM, Fields RD, Quick DC, Buss DD. Chronically injured posterior cruciate ligament: magnetic resonance imaging. Clin Orthop Relat Res. 1997;335:224–32.
15. Christopher TJS, James PR, Neil PT. The accuracy of magnetic resonance imaging in diagnosing chronic posterior cruciate ligament injury. The Knee. 2004;11(4):265–70.
16. Shelbourne KD, Jennings RW, Vahey TN. Magnetic resonance imaging of posterior cruciate ligament injuries: assessment of healing. Am J Knee Surg. 1999;12(4):209–13.
17. Stäubli HU, Birrer S. The popliteus tendon and its fascicles at the popliteal hiatus: gross anatomy and functional arthroscopic evaluation with and without anterior cruciate ligament deficiency. Arthroscopy. 1990;6(3):209–20.
18. Schulz MS, Steenlage ES, Russe K, Strobel MJ. Distribution of posterior tibial displacement in knees with posterior cruciate ligament tears. J Bone Joint Surg Am. 2007;89(2):332–8.
19. Munshi M, Pretterklieber ML, Kwak S, Antonio GE, Trudell DJ, Resnick D. MR imaging, MR arthrography, and specimen correlation of the posterolateral corner of the knee: an anatomic study. AJR Am J Roentgenol. 2003;180(4):1095–101.
20. Diamantopoulos A, Tokis A, Tzurbakis M, Patsopoulos I, Georgoulis A. The posterolateral corner of the knee: evaluation under microsurgical dissection. Arthroscopy. 2005;21(7):826–33.
21. Brinkman JM, Schwering PJ, Blankevoort L, Kooloos JG, Luites J, Wymenga AB. The insertion geometry of the posterolateral corner of the knee. J Bone Joint Surg Br. 2005;87(10):1364–8.
22. Watanabe Y, Moriya H, Takahashi K, Yamagata M, Sonoda M, Shimada Y, Tamaki T. Functional anatomy of the posterolateral structures of the knee. Arthroscopy. 1993;9(1):57–62.
23. De Maeseneer M, Shahabpour M, Vanderdood K, De Ridder F, Van Roy F, Osteaux M. Posterolateral supporting structures of the knee: findings on anatomic dissection, anatomic slices and MR images. Eur Radiol. 2001;11(11):2170–7.
24. LaPrade RF, Ly TV, Wentorf FA, Engebretsen L. The posterolateral attachments of the knee: a qualitative and quantitative morphologic analysis of the fibular collateral ligament, popliteus tendon, popliteofibular ligament, and lateral gastrocnemius tendon. Am J Sports Med. 2003;31(6):854–60.
25. Ullrich K, Krudwig WK, Witzel U. Posterolateral aspect and stability of the knee joint. I. Anatomy and function of the popliteus muscle-tendon unit: an anatomical and biomechanical study. Knee Surg Sports Traumatol Arthrosc. 2002;10(2):86–90.
26. Campos JC, Chung CB, Lektrakul N, Pedowitz R, Trudell D, Yu J, Resnick D. Pathogenesis of the Segond fracture: anatomic and MR imaging evidence of an iliotibial tract or anterior oblique band avulsion. Radiology. 2001;219(2):381–6.
27. De Maeseneer M, Van Roy P, Shahabpour M, Gosselin R, De Ridder F, Osteaux M. Normal anatomy and pathology of the posterior capsular area of the knee: findings in cadaveric specimens and in patients. AJR Am J Roentgenol. 2004;182(4):955–62.
28. Seebacher JR, Inglis AE, Marshall JL, Warren RF. The structure of the posterolateral aspect of the knee. J Bone Joint Surg Am. 1982;64(4):536–41.
29. Maynard MJ, Deng X, Wickiewicz TL, Warren RF. The popliteofibular ligament. Rediscovery of a key element in posterolateral stability. Am J Sports Med. 1996;24(3):311–6.
30. Sudasna S, Harnsiriwattanagit K. The ligamentous structures of the posterolateral aspect of the knee. Bull Hosp Jt Dis Orthop Inst. 1990;50(1):35–40.
31. Lee J, Papakonstantinou O, Brookenthal KR, Trudell D, Resnick DL. Arcuate sign of posterolateral knee injuries: anatomic, radiographic, and MR imaging data related to patterns of injury. Skeletal Radiol. 2003;32(11):619–27.
32. Warren LF, Marshall JL. The supporting structures and layers on the medial side of the knee: an anatomical analysis. J Bone Joint Surg Am. 1979;61(1):56–62.

33. LaPrade RF, Engebretsen AH, Ly TV, Johansen S, Wentorf FA, Engebretsen L. The anatomy of the medial part of the knee. J Bone Joint Surg Am. 2007;89(9):2000–10.
34. Schweitzer ME, Tran D, Deely DM, Hume EL. Medial collateral ligament injuries: evaluation of multiple signs, prevalence and location of associated bone bruises, and assessment with MR imaging. Radiology. 1995;194(3):825–9.
35. Stoller DW. Magnetic resonance imaging in orthopaedics and sports medicine. 3rd ed. Baltimore: Lippincott Williams & Wilkins; 2007. pp. 553–4.
36. Bergin D, Keogh C, O'Connell M, Rowe D, Shah B, Zoga A, et al. Atraumatic medial collateral ligament oedema in medial compartment knee osteoarthritis. Skeletal Radiol. 2002;31(1):14–8.
37. Bergin D, Hochberg H, Zoga AC, Qazi N, Parker L, Morrison WB. Indirect soft-tissue and osseous signs on knee MRI of surgically proven meniscal tears. AJR Am J Roentgenol. 2008;191(1):86–92.
38. Hughston JC, Eilers AF. The role of the posterior oblique ligament in repairs of acute medial (collateral) ligament tears of the knee. J Bone Joint Surg Am. 1973;55(5):923–40.
39. Hughston JC. Knee ligaments:injury and repair. St. Louis: Mosby Year-Book; 1993.
40. Sims WF, Jacobson KE. The posteromedial corner of the knee: medial-sided injury patterns revisited. Am J Sports Med. 2004;32(2):337–45.

Part IV
Non-Surgical Treatment

Nonoperative Treatment and Natural History of Posterior Cruciate Ligament Injuries

7

K. Donald Shelbourne

Introduction

Posterior cruciate ligament (PCL) injuries are uncommon and only a few of these injuries may be seen each year in a general orthopedist's practice. PCL injuries can occur with athletic activity and activities in daily life but are more commonly seen with trauma, where the PCL can be torn along with other ligamentous structures. Although one can detect a PCL injury, if trained properly, the injury can be missed unless the physician suspects it based on the patient history. Even when the diagnosis is made, it can be difficult to develop a treatment protocol for patients with PCL injuries because of the varying degrees of the injury and the lack of consensus among orthopedic surgeons as to the best treatment approach.

Orthopedic surgeons are trained to focus on surgical solutions to musculoskeletal injuries, always striving to restore perfect anatomy. Through the years, PCL reconstruction surgery has been developed and improvements in techniques have been made. But it is still unclear as to whether surgical treatment will provide better results than nonoperative management.

The nonoperative treatment approach to PCL injuries found in this chapter is in contrast to most opinions. This approach is based on more than 30 years of an orthopedic practice that has been devoted to knee injuries only. The practice began in 1982 at a time when PCL reconstructions were infrequently done, mostly because the PCL injury was not recognized and, when it was, the surgical procedures available could not reliably restore the native anatomy or stability. In 1983, a true natural history study of PCL injuries was begun at my institution. Only a few natural history studies have been conducted of PCL injuries, as most reports of nonoperative treatment include patients who sought treatment for chronic PCL instability [1–4].

K. D. Shelbourne (✉)
Shelbourne Knee Center, 1815 N. Capitol Ave.,
Indianapolis, IN 46202, USA
e-mail: tgray@fixknee.com

This chapter reviews the findings of natural history studies of PCL injuries and other studies from investigators seeking to find answers to the treatment of PCL injuries. The mechanism of injury, patient history, and clinical diagnosis will be outlined. The nonoperative treatment with both isolated PCL injuries and PCL injury in combination with other ligamentous instability will be described. Finally, results of nonoperative treatment will be compared and contrasted with current outcomes of PCL reconstruction.

Mechanism of Injury

Understanding the common mechanisms of PCL injuries is essential to clinically suspect and diagnose PCL tears. PCL injuries can occur in isolation or with other ligamentous injuries, and they can occur from low- or high-velocity impact or force. High-velocity PCL injuries can occur from trauma such as automobile accidents, where the front of the tibia comes in contact with the dashboard and is forced backwards. This same mechanism of impact on the front of the tibia occurs in athletics and everyday life when a person falls with the foot in plantar flexion. A blow to the proximal tibia is probably the most common mechanism of injury for isolated PCL injuries.

Hyperflexion of the knee is another method of isolated PCL injury, with the PCL usually tearing near its tibial attachment or at midsubstance [5, 6]. With hyperflexion, the anterolateral portion is damaged but the posteromedial portion remains intact [7, 8]. Another mechanism for an isolated PCL injury is an external rotation force on a weightbearing leg with the knee in near full extension (Fig. 7.1) [9].

PCL injuries are more commonly found in conjunction with other ligamentous injuries. Shelbourne et al. identified a combined PCL-medial collateral injury (MCL) in patients who had sustained a valgus external rotation force to a flexed knee with a planted but nonweightbearing foot (Fig. 7.2) [10]. This injury typically occurs when the foot gets stuck on a surface or in a hole, the weight is on the other leg, there is

G. C. Fanelli (ed.), *Posterior Cruciate Ligament Injuries,*
DOI 10.1007/978-3-319-12072-0_7, © Springer International Publishing Switzerland 2015

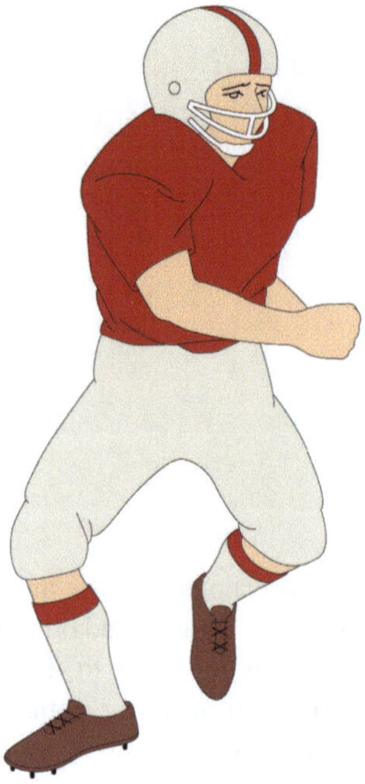

Fig 7.1 The *right foot* is fixed but becomes unloaded as the athlete shifts his weight and forward momentum to his *left leg*. The *right knee* is minimally flexed and sustains a relative external rotation twist while the *body* and the *right femur* are anteriorly translating and internally rotating

valgus stress on the knee, and the tibia is externally rotated. The injured MCL is easily recognized but the PCL can be slight and often missed on physical examination.

PCL injuries in conjunction with a dislocated knee, either medial or lateral, can have varying degrees of injury and subsequent laxity and have implications for treatment. When the injury occurs as a result of major trauma, as in the case with automobile accidents, the more serious injuries to the rest of the body take precedence in emergency care. The injury to the PCL may not be recognized or addressed until the patient later has symptoms affecting function. Given that the PCL injury is frequently overlooked, the incidence of the injury with major trauma may never be known.

Therefore, an understanding of the mechanisms of injury for PCL injuries, whether isolated or combined with other knee structures, will raise suspicion for the injury and proper examination techniques will lead to an accurate diagnosis and appropriate management.

Clinical Diagnosis/Physical Examination

As previous stated, being suspect of PCL injury by understanding the mechanisms of injury is very important for diagnosing a PCL injury. With an isolated injury to the PCL, the patient usually feels the injury was significant but perhaps not debilitating. The patient can usually bear weight but may walk with a slightly flexed knee, avoiding terminal extension and external rotation. In contrast to anterior cruciate ligament (ACL) tears, the patient usually denies hearing or feeling a "pop" and the presence of an effusion may be minimal. Most isolated PCL injuries seen acutely after the injury are accompanied by posterior knee pain, a mild hemarthrosis and difficulty squatting. The patient will often report that "something is not right" in the injured knee, but cannot elaborate on what feels wrong.

If the knee injury includes a PCL injury with other ligaments injured, the swelling is usually much greater. Patients with PCL/MCL injuries have the symptoms of an isolated MCL injury, with pain and tenderness on the medial side of the knee and a feeling of medial instability in the knee. The patient may have localized swelling along the ligament. If the PCL injury is part of a knee dislocation with ACL and either medial or lateral collateral ligament (LCL) injuries, the patient will have a significant hemarthrosis. If there has been a significant capsular injury, swelling may dissect into the subcutaneous tissues resulting in the development of edema and ecchymosis in the leg below the knee. The main concern with multiple ligament dislocations is the possibility of neurovascular injury. Careful assessment must be made of the vascular and neurologic status of the limb, and consultation with a vascular surgeon may be required. Patients with ACL, PCL, and lateral-side knee injuries have an almost 30 % incidence of peroneal nerve injury [11].

If not seen acutely after a PCL injury, many of the patient's symptoms will resolve and activities can be resumed without the patient knowing of the injury. Patients usually will not seek treatment unless they develop chronic knee symptoms, with pain being the most common complaint [1, 12]. Instability is usually a secondary complaint in about 20–45 % of patients with chronic PCL-deficient knees [1, 12].

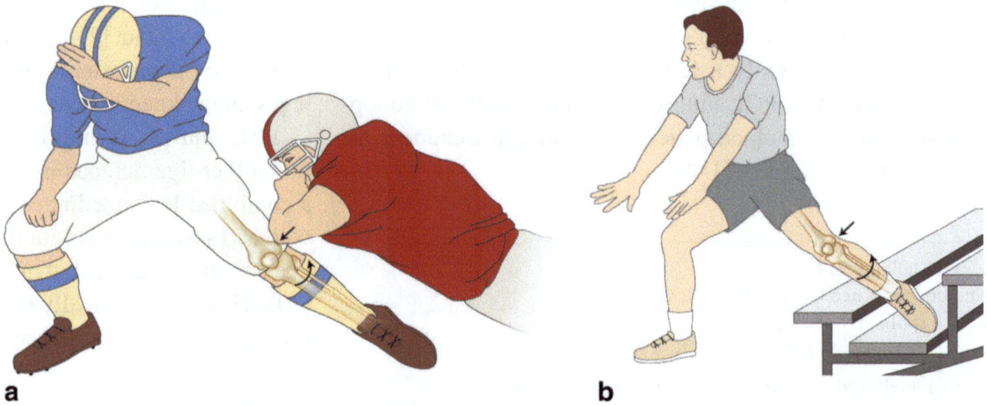

Fig. 7.2 Combined PCL–MCL injuries can occur when the *foot* is planted or fixed, but not weight bearing, and the *leg* is either struck on the lateral side (**a**) or the *foot* being stuck causes a valgus stress with external rotation of the tibia (**b**). PCL posterior cruciate ligament, MCL medial collateral injury

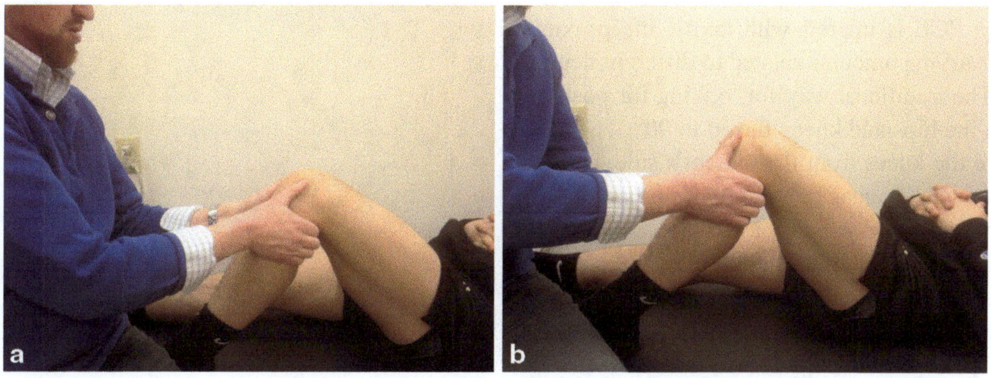

Fig. 7.3 Posterior drawer test: The patient is supine and has the *hip* and *knee* flexed to about 90°. The examiner sits at the edge of the patient's *foot* so the *foot* cannot slide on the exam table. This allows the patient to relax his/her *leg* completely. The examiner places his/her *hands* so that the *thumbs* can feel for the normal prominence of the tibia in relation to the femoral condyles (**a**). The *index fingers* can be used to feel for relaxation of the hamstring muscles. The examiner pushes directly posterior on the tibia and feels for translation of the tibia and the loss of normal prominence of the tibia. When the tibia is completely flush with the femoral condyles upon posterior force, the patient has 2+ posterior laxity (**b**)

Table 7.1 Grade of posterior cruciate ligament laxity as evaluated with posterior drawer examination

Grade	Difference on posterior drawer (mm)	Anatomical landmarks
1	3–5	Tibial plateau prominence remains anterior to femoral condyles
1.5	6–8	Tibial plateau prominence not quite flush with the femoral condyles
2	9–10	Tibial plateau and femoral condyles lie flush
2.5	11–13	Anterior tibial plateau is slightly posterior to the femoral condyles
3	>13	Anterior tibial plateau is grossly posterior to the femoral condyles

Physical Examination

Physical examination serves to confirm the diagnosis suspected from the patient's history. Physical examination of the acutely injured knee can be difficult due to pain, swelling, muscle spasm, limited range of motion (ROM), and patient apprehension. The normal, uninjured knee should be examined first so that a normal baseline for the patient can be determined by the examiner for all parameters, including knee stability. An examination of the normal knee allows the patient to know what to expect when the clinician examines the injured knee and may instill some confidence in the patient, allowing them to relax somewhat, thus making the examination a little easier.

The best physical examination test for diagnosing PCL injuries has been found to be the posterior drawer test, which was found to be 96 % accurate, 90 % sensitive and 99 % specific with an interobserver agreement for the grade of injury of 81 % [13]. The posterior drawer examination is performed with the knee bent at 90° of flexion. The examiner places his leg over the patient's toes so the patient can relax the leg and the foot is stabilized on the examination table. The examiner places both hands on the front of the tibia with the thumbs over the femoral condyles. Force is applied and directed posteriorly to evaluate posterior excursion (Fig. 7.3). Posterior laxity is graded as described in Table 7.1, with grade 2 laxity indicating that the tibia is flush with the femoral condyles. Translation greater than 13 mm is classified as a grade 3 injury, which usually indicates that other knee ligamentous injuries are present.

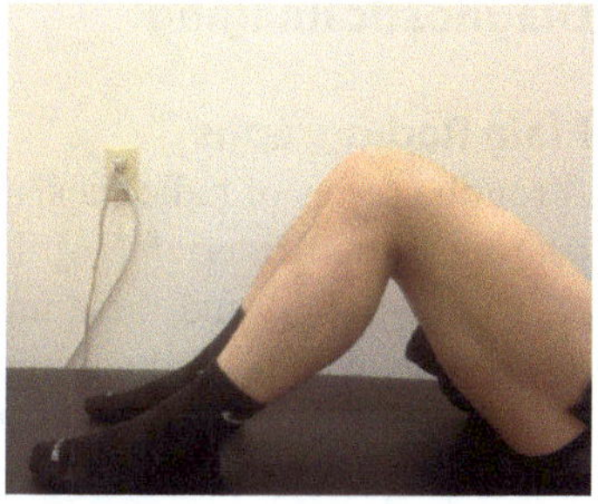

Fig. 7.4 Posterior sag: The *knee* in the foreground shows posterior sag of the tibia compared with the normal *knee* that can be seen with PCL injury.PCL posterior cruciate ligament

The accuracy of the posterior drawer exam comes with experience. If the posterior drawer exam becomes a part of the regular routine of a thorough knee examination for any patient with a knee injury, the clinician gains experience for feeling differences in PCL laxity and the feel of an endpoint of stability. If the patient's knee cannot be bent to 90° due to significant injury or swelling, one can reexamine the patient a few days later to give time for the initial pain and swelling to subside.

With both knees bent to 90° for the posterior drawer exam, the clinician can also observe for posterior sag of the tibia in the involved knee compared with the normal knee (Fig. 7.4). With an intact PCL, the anteromedial proximal tibia will be about 1 cm anterior to the distal femoral condyles. When the PCL is injured with laxity, the proximal tibia will sag to varying amounts related to different degrees of PCL injury. The traditional way for looking for posterior sag is with both the hips and knees flexed to 90°. The clinician can observe the knees from the patient's side, and this method has the added advantage of gravity for producing sag of the tibia. However, this method may cause more pain for a patient with an acute PCL injury and may not be possible. Other tests to assess clinical integrity of the PCL include the reverse Lachman test, the dynamic posterior shift test [14], and the quadriceps active drawer test [15].

When a multiple ligament injury is suspected, further ligamentous testing should be performed. The medial and LCL can be examined by applying valgus and varus stresses respectively at 30° of knee flexion. Repeating these tests at 0° of flexion will also assess the capsular and cruciate components to valgus and varus stability. Repeating the posterior drawer test with the tibia placed in internal rotation will assess the medial structures. If the posterior drawer decreases with internal tibial rotation, the medial structures are most likely intact. In combined ligament injuries (PCL/MCL or PCL/ACL/MCL), the usual tightening observed when the posterior drawer is performed with the patient's tibia in internal rotation is lost.

Diagnostic Imaging

Plain Radiographs

A routine series of radiographs include a 45° flexed weight-bearing posteroanterior [16], lateral, and Merchant's view [17] radiographs, and these images should be obtained for all patients with acute knee injuries. The radiographs, however, are not diagnostic for a PCL injury. Occasionally, an avulsion fracture of the tibial PCL insertion may be seen, but these are fairly uncommon [18]. A modified axial view has been described that allows for measuring of the amount of posterior tibial translation, which is compared to the uninjured side [19].

Magnetic Resonance Imaging

In the acute setting, magnetic resonance imaging (MRI) of the PCL-injured knee has been reported to be 99–100 % sensitive and specific [20, 21]. We do not recommend routine MRI examinations for patients with PCL tears because the severity of damage to the PCL as seen on the MRI does not correlate with function or laxity. In my opinion, MRI diagnosis of PCL injuries with knee dislocations has led to unnecessary surgical treatment of the PCL. This overtreatment stems from a lack of knowledge that the PCL can heal [22, 23], even when a "complete tear" is diagnosed from the MRI scan [22].

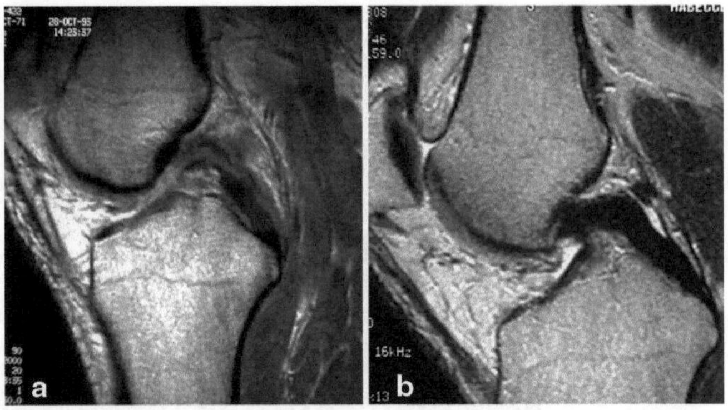

Fig. 7.5 The MRI scan (**a**) of an acute PCL injury determined to be a complete PCL tear. A follow-up scan (**b**) at 8 months after injury shows the PCL to be in continuity. PCL posterior cruciate ligament, MRI magnetic resonance imaging

Tewes et al. [23] obtained follow-up MRI scans at an average of 20 months after injury for 13 patients with high-grade PCL tears. The results showed that the PCLs of 10 of 13 patients (77 %) had regained continuity, although with an abnormal appearance. Clinical or functional status did not correlate with the degree of posterior laxity.

In a similar study, Shelbourne et al. [22] obtained MRI scans acutely after injury and then again at a mean of 3.2 years after injury on 27 patients with isolated acute PCL tears and 17 patients with acute PCL injuries in combination with other ligamentous injuries. The investigators assessed the healing potential of partial and complete tears as graded on the MRI scans. The results showed that all partial and most complete (19 of 22) PCL tears regained continuity on MRI scans and that location, severity, and associated ligament injury were not factors. The healed PCL did demonstrate abnormal morphology in 25 of the 37 continuous PCLs at follow-up.

Ahn et al. [24] evaluated PCL laxity in 49 patients who were treated with casting and bracing after acute PCL injury to determine if there would be a change in laxity with treatment. The grade of laxity at initial evaluation was grade 1 in 13 patients and grade 2 in 25 patients. At a mean of 24 months after injury, the grades of PCL instability improved grade 0 in 3 patients, grade 1 in 21 patients, and grade 2 in 14 patients.

The time to obtain PCL healing after acute injury is as yet unknown. However, Shelbourne et al. [25] described the development of a firm endpoint and painless posterior drawer at follow-up examination of acute PCL injured knees at about 2 weeks after injury.

Given the findings of these studies showing a "normal" PCL in the chronic setting, MRI evaluation of the PCL for patients who suffer chronic instability may not be helpful (Fig. 7.5). Therefore, treatment decisions should not be based on MRIs, but on clinical examination.

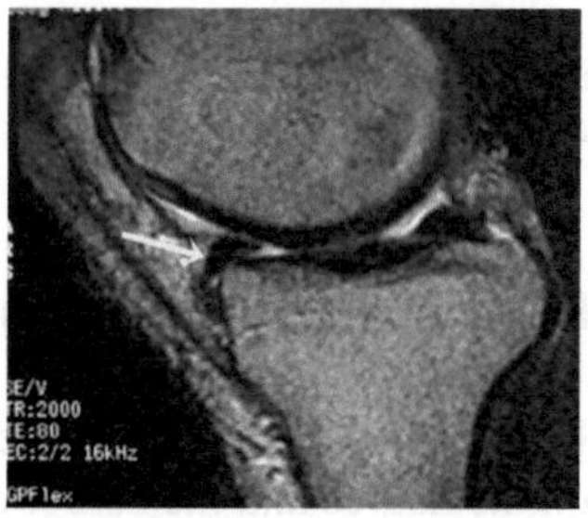

Fig. 7.6 MRI scanning in PCL lax knees often shows the posterior medical meniscus (*white arrow*) to be behind the femur and out of contact with the femoral condyle. PCL posterior cruciate ligament, MRI magnetic resonance imaging

With PCL laxity, the MRI scan will often show the posterior medial meniscus to be behind the femur and out of contact with the femoral condyle. If this is seen on a scan with the PCL in continuity, it may serve as an adjunctive sign of a previous PCL tear that has healed with PCL laxity (Fig. 7.6).

Natural History Studies

Most published studies of PCL injuries treated nonoperatively were conducted retrospectively and included patients who sought treatment because of chronic PCL laxity and painful symptoms or include patients with multiple knee ligament injuries [1–4]. These studies do not give a true picture of the natural history of isolated PCL injuries and may represent a worse outcome than what would be found from evaluating a population of patients prospectively after acute isolated PCL injury.

Only a few PCL studies report long-term subjective or objective results for isolated, PCL injuries in patients followed prospectively after an acute injury [25–27].

Patel et al. [26] evaluated 57 patients (58 knees) who were seen acutely for isolated PCL injuries and were treated nonoperatively with rehabilitation to restore the knee ROM and strength. Patients were evaluated again at a mean of 6.9 years after the injury and they were not being seen because they were having troubling symptoms. No correlation was found between subjective scores and length of follow-up or between subjective scores and grade of PCL laxity. The mean Lysholm score was 85.2 ± 10 points. Radiograph showed medial compartment degenerative changes in ten knees (seven mild grade 1; three knees moderate grade 2) and four knees had mild grade 1 patellofemoral changes.

In a subjective follow-up study of 215 patients at a mean of 7.8 years after acute, isolated PCL injury, a similar lack of correlation was found between subjective scores and grade of PCL laxity [27]. The subjective results were lower than scores of normative data of patients with no history of injury to the knee, but the scores did not decrease significantly with time.

Shelbourne et al. [25] reported the natural history of 133 patients after acute, isolated PCL injury. Sixty-eight of the patients returned for objective follow-up at a mean of 5.4 years after the injury and the other 65 returned subjective surveys. There was no statistically significant difference in subjective survey scores between patients who returned for both objective and subjective follow-up and patients who were able to return surveys only. No change in laxity was found from initial exam to final follow-up, and patients with greater laxity did not have worse subjective or objective scores. No correlation was found between radiographic joint space narrowing and grade of laxity. Ten of 67 patients (1 patient refused radiographs) had evidence of arthrosis in the injured knee alone, and 15 patients had arthrosis in the both the injured and noninjured knees. Regardless of PCL laxity, one half of the patients returned to the same sport at the same level, one third of the patients returned to the same sport at a lower level, and one sixth of patients were not able to return to the same sport.

In a longer-term follow-up study of the same population, Shelbourne et al. [28] obtained objective and subjective follow-up for 44 of the original 68 patients who were evaluated objectively in the original study [25]. These evaluations were performed at a mean of 14.3 years after injury (range, 10–21 years) and subjective follow-up was obtained from all 68 patients at a mean of 17.6 years after injury. PCL laxity did not increase with time.

The mean knee ROM for the PCL injured knee was from 4° of hyperextension to 138° of flexion compared with 4° of hyperextension and 137° of flexion in the noninjured knee. Eight patients (18 %) had trace effusion in one or both knees and one patient had a mild effusion in both knees. There was no difference in mean quadriceps muscle strength based on PCL laxity and the mean for all patients was 97.2 % of the noninjured knee.

The overall grade of radiographs were rated as normal in 26 patients (59 %), nearly normal in 13 patients (30 %), abnormal in 4 patients (9 %), and severely abnormal in 1 patient (2 %). The grade of osteoarthritis (OA) on radiographs was not different in any knee compartment based on PCL laxity grade. Five patients (11 %) had medial joint space narrowing greater than 2 mm. When comparing radiographic ratings of the same patients in the original follow-up study [25], seven patients (16 %) had increased degenerative changes in at least one compartment of the knee; five of the seven patients had grade 2 PCL laxity. However, the same five patients had similar degenerative changes in the noninjured knee as well.

Mean International Knee Documentation Committee (IKDC) and modified Cincinnati Knee Rating System (CKRS) subjective scores at a mean of 17 years after injury were 73.4 ± 21.7 and 81.3 ± 17.4 points, respectively; there was no difference in subjective scores between PCL laxity grades. There was no difference in subjective scores between patients who completed a minimum 10-year objective follow-up and patients who completed surveys only. Forty patients had completed at least four CKRS surveys through time, and an evaluation of consistency of scores revealed that the scores were consistent for less than half of the patients. Nine patients had consistently improving scores through time, 5 patients had consistently declining scores through time, and 12 (30 %) were inconsistent.

An activity-level survey revealed that 20 patients (45 %) were still participating in jumping/pivoting sports at a mean of 17 years after their injury. Seventeen patients were still participating in recreational sports such as tennis and golf. Only seven patients (16 %) reported that they were limited to activities of daily living.

The incidence of meniscus tears associated with isolated PCL injury has been reported to be between 5 and 28 %, with common tears being in the lateral meniscus [7, 25, 29–31]. Although meniscus tears are not that common with PCL injuries, the medial meniscus does not function normally because the meniscus is posterior to the femur with posterior laxity. I believe this is what may cause osteoarthritic changes in the medial compartment to occur in some patients with PCL laxity.

Patellofemoral arthritis is thought to be common with PCL injuries, but the data from true natural history studies do not confirm this thought. The incidence of patellofemoral arthrosis has been reported to be between 7 and 16 % with follow-up between 6 and 14 years [12, 25, 26, 32]. Anterior knee pain can be seen in patients with PCL laxity, but the pain may be caused from the posterior translation of the tibia on the femur and anterior impingement of the meniscus with knee extension versus arthrosis of the patellofemoral joint as has been proposed.

Nonoperative Rehabilitation

Isolated PCL Injury

The patient's symptoms and physical examination may vary greatly depending on the severity of the PCL injury. With mild injuries, the patient may have only minimal swelling and ill-defined symptoms. Other patients may have had an injury that stopped them from the activity or sport in which they were participating. Regardless of the degree of injury or symptoms, the goals of rehabilitation are the same: Minimize effusion, restore knee extension and flexion, and then restore any loss of strength or function to return the patient to his or her activities.

Cold/compression with elevation is used to reduce the effusion. Exercises to restore normal knee extension, such as towel stretch and heel prop exercises, are performed. Full flexion can be obtained with the use of heel slide exercises. Strengthening exercises include single-leg extension, leg press, and squats. The use of a stationary bicycle or stair-climbing machine can be used to increase endurance. The patient then progresses through functional activities before returning to sports.

PCL with Multiple Ligament Knee Injuries

Different treatment approaches are recommended depending on the degree and the combination of each injured structure. The initial treatment approach is based on recognizing that the PCL and MCL can heal without surgery, and the ACL and lateral structures generally do not. Thus, most ligament injuries do not require acute surgery and, in most cases, immediate surgery is not desirable because of the increased incidence of arthrofibrosis and long-term loss of knee ROM.

An understanding of the healing response of individual structures provides an explanation for potential postoperative stiffness associated with acute surgery. The long-term goal of treatment is for the patient to obtain a functionally stable knee with full ROM. In observing a young, athletically active population, I have found that patients who have a stable but stiff knee have disability and would much rather prefer a knee that has full ROM that would allow a functional activity level. Once an accurate diagnosis has been made and associated injuries have been evaluated, the treatment plan for the knee is formalized.

Combined ACL, PCL, MCL Injury, or PCL/MCL Injury

Our goal with an ACL, PCL, and MCL injury is to allow the PCL and MCL to heal and then address ACL instability as needed for the individual patient. The patient's leg is initially placed in a cylinder cast with 20° of flexion and encouraged to weight-bear. The goal is to prevent valgus stress, allow healing of the MCL and PCL. We recommend using a cast instead of a splint or brace because a cast provides more rigid weightbearing support, allows for more comfortable weightbearing, and mandates compliance. In addition, because residual medial laxity in combination with cruciate ligament injuries can be problematic, a cast is preferred to assure healing of the MCL with minimal laxity. The cast is changed weekly so that ligament healing can be evaluated and because a decrease in swelling typically makes the cast loose. Gentle valgus stress testing is performed to check for an endpoint. Once stability is achieved in the MCL with a stable endpoint and the patient is pain free and can comfortably bear weight, the cast is discontinued. Typically, a firm endpoint can be felt upon physical examination at about 2 weeks after injury for a proximal MCL injury and at 4–5 weeks after injury with a distal MCL injury.

Once MCL healing is confirmed clinically, knee rehabilitation for ROM and strength can begin. Once full ROM has been established, knee stability can be reevaluated. Casting usually allows the PCL to heal with a good endpoint on posterior drawer examination. This treatment approach usually results in no medial laxity, acceptable posterior laxity, and ACL deficiency. Depending on the patient's activity level and athletic goals, an ACL reconstruction may be warranted. In some patients, this approach also allows for healing of the ACL, which may provide enough stability to allow patients to do well functionally without having the ACL reconstructed.

Combined ACL, PCL, and Lateral-Side Knee Injury

A lateral-side knee dislocation requires semi-urgent attention. Our philosophy is to balance obtaining ROM and decreased swelling with the ability to repair the lateral structures. While medial structures tear interstitially and can heal, lateral-side structures almost always tear distally to the knee joint and retract proximally above the joint. Consequently, injured lateral-side structures will not heal properly without surgical repair. I recommend semi-acute surgery for lateral-side repair, allow the PCL to heal, and perform ACL reconstruction according to the patient's need.

The initial goals and program for rehabilitation are again to decrease swelling and restore normal ROM without causing further injury to the lateral compartment. Because of lateral instability, the patient most likely will need to have a splint and use crutches for ambulation for protection.

The patient is typically prescribed an antiembolism stocking, a cold/compression device, and a continuous passive motion (CPM) machine. The patient also attends several preoperative physical therapy sessions with the goal of decreasing swelling, improving leg control, and achieving satisfactory ROM. Our goal is to have knee extension equal to that of the opposite knee and about 130° of knee flexion before surgery.

Repair of the lateral complex in less than 2 weeks from injury usually is reliable in reestablishing lateral stability; results of surgical repair more than 3 weeks from injury are less predictable. If the initial injury is unrecognized, patients can have significant disability. An ACL reconstruction may be needed but I still recommend that the PCL be left to heal.

Treatment Outcomes: Nonoperative Versus PCL Reconstruction

It could probably be said that there is a consensus for treating isolated PCL injuries that are grade 2 or less in laxity, with grade 2 laxity being defined as the femoral condyles being flush with the tibia on posterior drawer exam. Most would agree that patients with grade 2 or less PCL laxity should be treated nonoperatively with rehabilitation for the acute injury so the patient can return to his or her daily and sporting activities [31]. It is when PCL laxity is greater than grade 2 or when the PCL is torn in combination with other ligamentous injuries that surgery is commonly recommended, although I believe PCL reconstruction is recommended unnecessarily in many cases.

Given that the PCL can heal, even when other ligaments are damaged, my recommendation would be to allow the PCL to heal and treat other ligamentous injuries as is needed for the individual patient. With an acute knee dislocation, the PCL injury can appear as "complete" on the MRI, and physicians may rely on the diagnosis from the MRI because physical examination of PCL laxity can be difficult to detect with acute knee dislocations. PCL reconstruction is more commonly performed in combination with ACL reconstruction in patients who suffer with knee dislocations. I believe, however, that the PCL can be left to heal, and ACL laxity and other medial or lateral ligamentous laxity can be addressed nonoperatively or surgically as indicated for the patient.

The only knee ligamentous injury that requires semi-acute surgery is a lateral-side knee dislocation, which occurs only rarely. Most knee dislocations are medial-side injuries, and these injuries are known to cause extreme stiffness, especially when surgery is performed acutely after the injury. There are many advantages in waiting for the knee swelling to resolve, restoring normal ROM, and waiting to reevaluate ligamentous laxity and function before determining whether any surgery is needed for the patient.

One of the main complications with PCL reconstruction for knee dislocations is knee ROM problems after surgery, with the rate of ROM deficits being reported to be from 7 to 30 % [33–39]. Knee ROM loss has been found to be related to the presence of OA after ACL reconstruction [40, 41] and we would expect that ROM deficits after PCL reconstruction would also be related to development of OA.

The purpose of PCL reconstruction would be to restore normal laxity, with the hope of preventing the development of osteoarthritic changes in the joint. It is unclear, however, whether PCL reconstruction can restore normal PCL stability. In studies that reported both initial laxity and laxity after PCL reconstruction, the rate of achieving grade 0 or normal PCL stability ranged from 0 to 90 %, with most reporting less than 50 % success [33–38, 42–44]. Several investigators concluded that PCL reconstruction can improve PCL stability but may not be able to normalize it [43–47].

Long-term follow-up of more than 10 years after nonoperative management or PCL reconstruction that also include radiographic evaluation for OA is limited to only a few studies. The long-term outcome of nonoperative treatment shows an incidence of OA to range from 17 to 53 % as compared with a range of 36–59 % with PCL reconstruction. At a mean of 7 years after PCL injury, Patel et al. [26] found that 10 of 58 knees (17%) had evidence of OA. Parolie et al. [12] found arthritis in 36% of their patients at a mean of 8.4 years after PCL injury. Boynton and Tietjens [32] reported articular degeneration in the medial tibiofemoral compartment in 53% of their patients at a mean time of 13.2 years after PCL injury. Finally, at a mean of 14 years after injury, Shelbourne et al. [28] found evidence of some OA in 41% of patients overall, but moderate to severe OA was found in only 11% of patients.

These results of nonoperative treatment compare favorably with long-term outcome of PCL reconstruction for isolated PCL injuries. With a mean of 9 years after PCL reconstruction, Hermans et al. [45] found medial joint line narrowing in 59% of their patients and the IKDC ratings of radiographs were normal for 9 of 22 patients (41%), nearly normal for 10 (45%), and abnormal for 3 (9%). Jackson et al. [34] found evidence of OA in 8 of 22 patients at 10 years after PCL reconstruction; 4 patients had osteophytes but normal joint space width, and 4 (18%) had moderate degenerative changes. If PCL reconstruction is being done to prevent OA in the future, it appears that, thus far, this goal has not been met.

Long-term subjective evaluations of patients after nonoperative treatment and PCL reconstruction are strikingly similar. At a mean of 17 years after nonoperative treatment, Shelbourne et al. [28] found that patients had a mean IKDC score of 73 points, which compares to IKDC scores of 75 and 87 found by studies of operative treatment that had much less follow-up times of 9–10 years [45].

Given that objective and subjective results found in the long-term after nonoperative treatment of isolated PCL injuries is so similar to treatment with PCL reconstruction, I question recommendations for surgical approach to these injuries, especially when considering the expense and potential morbidity PCL reconstruction can cause.

Summary

The trend for treatment of PCL injuries is toward performing more PCL reconstructions. However, the natural history of PCL shows that the injured PCLs can heal without treatment, even in the presence of other ligamentous injuries. Ten-year follow-up shows that PCL laxity does not change with time from injury and patients with lesser PCL laxity do not have better subjective survey scores or less radiographic evidence of OA than patients with greater PCL laxity. Radiographic evaluation showed the prevalence rate of OA being abnormal or severely abnormal was 11% at a mean of 14 years after injury. The mean IKDC subjective survey score was 73 points at a mean of 17 years after injury. Both objective and subjective results of nonoperative treatment of PCL injuries compare favorably with long-term outcome of PCL reconstruction.

References

1. Dandy DJ, Pusey RJ. Long term results of unrepaired tears of the posterior cruciate ligament. J Bone Joint Surg Br. 1982;64:92–4.
2. Dejour H, Walch G, Peyrot J, et al. The natural history of rupture of the posterior cruciate ligament. French J Ortho Surg. 1988;2:112–20.
3. Keller PM, Shelbourne KD, McCarroll JD, et al. Nonoperatively treated isolated posterior cruciate ligament injuries. Am J Sports Med. 1993;21:132–6.
4. Torg JS, Barton TM, Pavlov H, et al. Natural history of posterior cruciate ligament—deficient knee. Clin Orthop Relat Res. 1989;246:208–16.
5. Kennedy JC, Hawkins RJ, Willis RB, et al. Tension studies of human knee ligaments. Yield point, ultimate failure and disruption of the cruciate and tibial collateral ligaments. J Bone Joint Surg Am. 1976;58:350–5.
6. Trickey EL. Rupture of the posterior cruciate ligament of the knee. J Bone Joint Surg Br. 1968;50:334–41.
7. Fowler PJ, Messieh SS. Isolated posterior cruciate ligament injuries in athletes. Am J Sports Med. 1987;15:553–7.
8. Harner CD, Xerogeanes JW, Livesay, GA, et al. The human posterior cruciate ligament complex: an interdisciplinary study. Ligament morphology and biomechanical evaluation. Am J Sports Med. 1995;23:736–45.
9. Shelbourne KD, Rubinstein RA Jr. Isolated posterior cruciate ligament rupture: an unusual mechanism of injury. A report of 3 cases. Am J Knee Surg. 1993;6:84–6.
10. Shelbourne KD, Mesko JW, McCarroll JR, Rettig AC. Combined medial collateral ligament—posterior cruciate rupture. Mechanism of injury. Am J Knee Surg. 1990;3:41–4.
11. DeLee JC, Riley MB, Rockwood CA. Acute straight lateral instability of the knee. Am J Sports Med. 1983;11:404–11.
12. Parolie JM, Bergfield JA. Long term results of non operative treatment of isolated posterior cruciate ligament injury in the athlete. Am J Sports Med. 1986;14:35–8.
13. Rubinstein RA Jr, Shelbourne KD, McCarroll JR, VanMeter CD, Rettig AC. The accuracy of clinical examination in the setting of posterior cruciate ligament injury. Am J Sports Med. 1994; 22:550–7.
14. Shelbourne KD, Benedict F, McCarroll JR, et al. Dynamic posterior shift test. An adjuvant in evaluation of posterior tibial subluxation. Am J Sports Med. 1989;17:275–7.
15. Daniel DM, Stone ML, Barnett P, Sachs R. Use of the quadriceps active test to diagnose posterior cruciate ligament disruption and measure posterior laxity of the knee. J Bone Joint Surg Am. 1988;70:386–91.
16. Rosenberg TD, Paulos LE, Parker RD, et al. The forty-five-degree posteroanterior flexion weight-bearing radiograph of the knee. J Bone Joint Surg Am. 1988;70:1479–83.
17. Merchant AC, Mercer RL, Jocobsen RH, et al. Roentgenographic analysis of patellofemoral congruence. J Bone Joint Surg Am. 1974;56:1391–6.
18. Strand T, Molster AO, Engesaeter LB, et al. Primary repairs in posterior cruciate ligament injuries. Acta Ortho Scand. 1984;55: 545–7.
19. Paddu G, Gianni E, Chambat PD, De Paulis F. The axial view in evaluating tibial translation in cases of in sufficiency of the posterior cruciate ligament. Arthroscopy. 2000;2:217–20.
20. Fischer SP, Fox JM, Del Pizzo W, et al. Accuracy of diagnoses from magnetic resonance imaging of the knee. A multicenter analysis of 1014 patients. J Bone Joint Surg Am. 1991;73:2–10.
21. Polly DW Jr, Callaghan JJ, Sikes RA, et al. The accuracy of selective magnetic resonance imaging compared with the findings of arthroscopy of the knee. J Bone Joint Surg Am. 1988;70A:192–8.

22. Shelbourne KD, Jennings RW, Vahey TN. Magnetic resonance imaging of posterior cruciate ligament injuries: assessment of healing. Am J Knee Surg. 1999;12:209–3.
23. Tewes DP, Fritts HM, Fields RD, et al. Chronically injured posterior cruciate ligament. Magnetic resonance imaging. Clin Orth Relat Res. 1997;335:224–32.
24. Ahn JH, Lee SH, Choi SH, Wang JH, Jang SW. Evaluation of clinical and magnetic resonance imaging results after treatment with casting and bracing for the acutely injured posterior cruciate ligament. Arthroscopy. 2011;27:1679–87.
25. Shelbourne KD, Davis TJ, Patel DV. The natural history of acute isolated non-operatively treated posterior cruciate ligament injuries. A prospective study. Am J Sports Med. 1999;27:276–83.
26. Patel DV, Allen AA, Warren RF, Wickiewicz TG, Simonian PT. The nonoperative treatment of acute, isolated (partial or complete) posterior cruciate ligament-deficient knees: an intermediate-term follow-up study. HSS J. 2007;3:137–46.
27. Shelbourne KD, Muthukaruppan Y. Subjective results of nonoperatively treated, acute, isolated posterior cruciate ligament injuries. Arthroscopy. 2005;21:457–61.
28. Shelbourne KD, Clark M, Gray T. Minimum 10-year follow-up of patients after an acute, isolated posterior cruciate ligament injury treated nonoperatively. Am J Sports Med. 2013;41;1526–33.
29. Geissler WB, Whipple TL. Intra-articular abnormalities in association with posterior cruciate ligament injuries. Am J Sports Med. 1993;21:846–9.
30. Hamada M, Shino K, Mitsuoka T, et al. Chondral injury associated with acute isolated posterior cruciate ligament injury. Arthroscopy. 2000;16:59–63.
31. Wind WM, Bergfeld JA, Parker RD. Evaluation and treatment of posterior cruciate ligament injuries. Revisited. Am J Sports Med. 2004;32:1765–75.
32. Boynton MD, Tietjens BR. Long term follow-up of the untreated isolated posterior cruciate ligament deficient knee. Am J Sports Med. 1996;24:306–10.
33. Chan YS, Yang SC, Chung CH, Chen AC, Yuan LJ, Hsu KY, Wang CJ. Arthroscopic reconstruction of the posterior cruciate ligament with use of a quadruple hamstring tendon graft with 3- to 5-year follow-up. Arthroscopy. 2006;22:762–70.
34. Jackson WFM, van der Tempel WM, Salmon LJ, Williams HA, Pinczewski LA. Endoscopically-assisted single-bundle posterior cruciate ligament reconstruction: results at minimum ten-year follow-up. J Bone Joint Surg Br. 2008;90:1328–33.
35. Jenner JT, van der Hart CP, Willems WJ. Mid-term results of arthroscopic reconstruction in chronic posterior cruciate ligament instability. Knee Surg Sports Traumatol Arthrosc. 2006;14: 848–53.
36. Shon OJ, Lee DC, Park CH, Kim WH, Jung KA. A comparison of arthroscopically assisted single and double bundle tibial inlay reconstruction for isolated posterior cruciate ligament injury. Clin Orthop Surg. 2010;2:76–84.
37. Wu CH, Chen ACY, Yuan LJ, Chang CH, Chan YS, Hsu KY, Wang CJ, Chen WJ. Arthroscopic reconstruction of the posterior cruciate ligament by using a quadriceps tendon autograft: a minimum 5-year follow-up. Arthroscopy. 2007;23:420–7.
38. Zhao J, Huangfu X. Arthroscopic single-bundle posterior cruciate ligament reconstruction: retrospective review of 4- versus 7-strand hamstring tendon graft. Knee. 2007;14:301–5.
39. Zhao J, Xiaoqiao H, He Y, Yang X, Liu C, Lu Z. Sandwich-style posterior cruciate ligament reconstruction. Arthroscopy. 2008;24: 650–9.
40. Shelbourne KD, Gray T. Minimum 10-year results after anterior cruciate ligament reconstruction: how the loss of normal knee motion compounds other factors related to the development of osteoarthritis after surgery. Am J Sports Med. 2009;37:471–80.
41. Shelbourne, KD, Urch SE, Gray T, Freeman H. Loss of normal knee motion after anterior cruciate ligament reconstruction is associated with radiographic arthritic changes after surgery. Am J Sports Med. 2012;40:108–13.
42. Chen B, Gao S. Double-Bundle posterior cruciate ligament reconstruction using a non-hardware suspension fixation technique and 8 strands of autogenous hamstring tendons. Arthroscopy. 2009;25:777–82.
43. Garofalo R, Jolles BM, Moretti B, Siegrist O. Double-bundle transtibial posterior cruciate ligament reconstruction with a tendon-patellar bone-semitendinosus tendon autograft: clinical results with a minimum of 2 years' follow-up. Arthroscopy. 2006;12:1331–8.
44. Wajsfisz A, Christel P, Djian P. Does reconstruction of isolated chronic posterior cruciate ligament injuries restore normal knee function? Orthop Traumatol Surg Res. 2010;96:388–93.
45. Hermans S, Corten K, Bellemans J. Long-term results of isolated anterolateral bundle reconstructions of the posterior cruciate ligament: A 6- to 12- year follow-up study. Am J Sports Med. 2009;37:1499–507.
46. Lien, OA, Aas EJ, Johansen S, Ludvigsen TC, Figved W, Engebretsen L. Clinical outcome after reconstruction for isolated posterior cruciate ligament injury. Knee. 2010;18:1568–72.
47. MacGillivray JD, Stein BE, Park M, Allen AA, Wickiewicz TL, Warren RF. Comparison of tibial inlay versus transtibial techniques for isolated posterior cruciate ligament reconstruction: minimum 2-year follow-up. Arthroscopy. 2006;22:320–8.

Part V

Surgical Treatment

Graft Selection in Posterior Cruciate Ligament Surgery

8

Natalie L. Leong, Nima Kabir and David R. McAllister

Introduction

There are many factors to take into account when assessing patients with PCL injuries. Here, we present a brief overview of some of the issues influencing management of PCL rupture. The type of graft selected by a surgeon can have a significant impact on the clinical management and outcome of these patients. Thus, it is necessary for surgeons to have a broad understanding of the variety of graft options available. Unfortunately, for multiple reasons, many surgeons do not have much specific knowledge surrounding the tissue grafts that are commercially available to them at individual hospitals and surgery centers [1]. There exists wide variation among allograft distributors with regard to the donor pool from which the grafts are obtained, the screening process of donors, and possible sterilization processes. In addition, there are multiple different allograft tissue types that can be selected for PCL reconstruction. In this chapter, we will present the medically relevant differences among the many graft options currently utilized in PCL reconstruction including a discussion of their biomechanical properties and biological differences.

Patient Factors

Several patient-related factors including patient age, activity level, acuity of injury, surgical history, and medical comorbidities are important to consider. The age of the patient is a key factor in developing an appropriate treatment plan specific to a given patient. In skeletally immature patients, the surgeon may consider employing surgical techniques and specific grafts to minimize the risk of physeal arrest and the risk of resultant angular deformities. Allografts may be particularly beneficial in middle-aged and older patients who are hoping to avoid donor-site morbidity associated with the use of autografts, to minimize postoperative pain, and to reduce time away from work. In addition, a patient's desired activity level, the types of activities in which they participate, and their profession can also influence management and graft selection.

The acuity of the PCL injury and presence of concomitant injuries can also influence the reconstructive approach. With an isolated tear, the PCL has a greater likelihood of spontaneous healing than the anterior cruciate ligament (ACL) in the subacute or acute stages [2]. However, residual laxity or PCL rupture associated with other injuries, such as those causing posterolateral rotary instability, may necessitate surgical intervention [3]. In high-energy PCL injuries, which generally involve multiple ligaments, compromise of vascular structures, compartment syndrome, or the presence of an open or irreducible joint can necessitate an urgent surgical intervention consisting of revascularization, surgical reduction, or compartment release; however, most surgeons prefer to delay ligament reconstruction for a few weeks in an attempt to decrease swelling of the soft tissue envelope. In general, definitive ligament repairs and/or reconstructions performed within 2–3 weeks from the time of injury have been associated with better outcomes [4–7]. Chronic injuries may necessitate ligament reconstructions be performed in conjunction with osteotomies either concurrently or in a staged one [8, 9].

Prior surgical procedures can present challenges as a result of retained hardware, prior autograft tissue harvest, prior tunnel placement, tunnel osteolysis, and geography of prior skin incisions. Additionally, medical comorbidities, psychological impairment, and concomitant central nervous system (CNS) injury all can influence surgical recommendations.

N. L. Leong (✉)
Department of Orthopedic Surgery, University of California Los Angeles, Los Angeles, CA, USA
e-mail: nleong@mednet.ucla.edu

N. Kabir · D. R. McAllister
Department of Orthopedic Surgery, David Geffen School of Medicine at UCLA, Los Angeles, CA, USA

G. C. Fanelli (ed.), *Posterior Cruciate Ligament Injuries*,
DOI 10.1007/978-3-319-12072-0_8,

Graft Factors

The goal of surgical intervention is to obtain an anatomic repair, when possible, or reconstruction of any associated ligamentous and capsular injuries. Several options exist regarding the material used to perform PCL reconstruction with the mainstays of treatment consisting of either allograft or autograft. Each option has a multitude of advantages and disadvantages, which will be further discussed. It is essential that treating surgeons have an understanding of the particular grafts that are available for implantation in their individual surgical practice because the recruitment of donors, harvesting, screening, possible sterilization, and assaying of grafts can vary among graft distributors. The use of allograft versus autograft tissue for ligamentous reconstruction is still debated in the literature with some authors advocating autograft as the gold standard and yet others have been demonstrating decreased pain and stiffness with equivalent objective and subjective outcomes with allograft compared to autograft [10–16]. Some authors recommend use of different autografts for specific surgical techniques, such as a hamstring tendon autograft for transtibial tunnel PCL reconstruction and use of quadriceps tendon autograft for femoral inlay [17, 18]. Others suggest use of Achilles tendon allograft for single-bundle reconstruction with a tibialis anterior allograft for the second graft in a double-bundle procedure [19]. Despite the controversy, the efficacy of all of these graft options has been demonstrated and, thus, both appear to be good choices [13, 20–29].

Availability of Graft

Limited supply of both autograft and allograft tendons can restrict the availability of grafts for clinical use. Autograft is particularly limited in the case of multiligamentous injuries that require multiple grafts, and harvesting can cause donor-site morbidity. For these reasons, many authors have advocated the use of allograft tissues for PCL reconstruction. However, allograft also has limited availability, and this availability can vary greatly by geographic region. Allograft distributors acquire specimens from a limited donor pool, as the preferred grafts arise from uninjured, young, appropriately screened donors who have themselves or by proxy of their family members voluntarily agreed to donate their tissues [1]. Although the grafts are tested for infectious diseases including hepatitis B virus (HBV), hepatitis C virus (HCV), and HIV, it is still possible that these illnesses or others could be transmitted.

Although unavailable in the USA, an alternative to autograft and allograft ligaments in other countries is synthetic grafts. Synthetic grafts theoretically would have the advantages of availability, consistency, and appropriate mechanical strength, while eliminating concerns regarding autograft morbidity as well as the risk of disease transmission associated with allograft. Carbon fiber, Dacron, bundled polytetrafluoroethylene (GORE-TEX™), ABC carbon, polyester, and ligament augmentation devices have all been investigated either in animal models or even implanted clinically in the past. Some of these implants exhibited promising initial results; however, longer term follow-up demonstrated recurrent instability and chronic effusions as a result of catastrophic failures, chronic inflammatory reactions, particulate debris, or poor biologic scaffolding properties [30–39]. As a result, the use of synthetic ligaments for PCL reconstruction is not currently recommended, and none of these are unconditionally approved by the Food and Drug Administration (FDA) for clinical use in the USA.

Bioengineered ligament grafts are also not currently approved for implantation in the USA. However, clinical applications of this technology are actively being pursued and have demonstrated considerable promise. Hopefully, bioengineered ligaments will be available in the future as their use could potentially eliminate the risks currently associated with the use of both autografts and allografts [40–46].

Autograft

Several autograft tissue options are available for harvest either in the ipsilateral or contralateral extremity among patients with a posterior cruciate ligament injury, including bone–patellar tendon–bone (B-PT-B), hamstring (semitendinosus and/or gracilis), and quadriceps tendon–patellar bone (QTB). A meta-analysis of 12 studies of autograft used in isolated PCL reconstruction found that hamstring tendon was used in 72% of patients, followed by B-PT-B in 16%, and QTB in 12% [13]. The extensor mechanism acts synergistically with the PCL to prevent posterior tibial translation; thus, weakening the quadriceps is a theoretical concern when using it as an autograft [47]. For this and other reasons, QTB is less popular than other graft options [48, 49]. However, good short- and long-term results have been reported for PCL reconstruction with quadriceps tendon [50, 51], hamstring [52–59], and B-PT-B autografts [52, 57, 60], with no significant difference found in direct comparisons of QTB with hamstrings [51] or B-PT-B with hamstring grafts [52, 60]. Thus, there is no uniformly ideal autograft choice. Each graft has its own strengths and weaknesses with regard to biomechanical properties, ease of harvest, morbidity, biology of healing, and fixation strength.

Autograft does enjoy several advantages over the use of allograft for ligamentous reconstructions. Autograft tissues have no risk of transmission of an infectious disease; they exhibit faster incorporation with adjacent tissues, and have no risk of immune-mediated tissue rejection. Additionally, autograft tissues are not exposed to sterilization or other sterilization modalities, which could have a negative impact on both the biomechanical and biological properties of the graft.

However, donor-site morbidity is associated with autograft tissue harvest, potentially representing a distinct disadvantage. Autograft hamstring harvest has been associated with symptomatic neuroma, numbness, arthrosis, symptomatic hardware requiring removal, posterior knee pain tunnel osteolysis, and terminal flexion hamstring weakness [1–66]. B-PT-B harvest is associated with patella fracture, patellar tendon rupture, infrapatellar contracture, loss of range of motion, arthrosis, patellar tendonitis, quadriceps weakness, and, most significantly, an increased incidence of anterior knee pain [29, 49, 62, 67–75]. QTP has a similar constellation of associated complications to B-PT-B, albeit to a lesser degree, consisting of a low incidence of decreased range of motion, anterior knee numbness, and anterior knee pain [76, 77]. Moreover, the larger skin and soft tissue incisions as well as bony cuts that are associated with autograft harvest expose an already injured body region to further trauma. Although some authors propose that hamstring tendons can regenerate after harvesting and that anterior knee pain is not exclusively observed in autograft B-PT-B grafted patients, there is no doubt that the risk of morbidity associated with autograft tissue harvest is significant and necessitates appropriate surgeon consideration and preoperative patient counseling [47, 78, 79]. This is of particular importance in patients with multiple ligament injuries in which multiple grafts will be required for surgical reconstruction. Also, there can be a limited quantity of available autografts. For these reasons, most surgeons prefer allograft, when available, for most PCL reconstructions.

Surgical Technique

Harvesting of autograft tissue can be performed via multiple approaches with regard to separate skin incisions and desired dimensions of the harvested graft; however, the basic techniques described below are quite similar. A brief surgical description of specific autograft harvesting techniques is discussed below.

Patellar Tendon

An infrapatellar midline incision is performed, slightly medial to the midline. Dissection is carried out down to the subcutaneous tissue and the paratenon is identified. The paratenon is sharply incised and reflected, thus exposing the patellar tendon. A central section of the tendon is excised measuring 9–11 mm wide throughout its length. Bone plugs of 20–30 mm in length on both the tibia and the patella are created with an oscillating saw and osteotomies [61].

Hamstrings

The hamstring tendons insert 2 cm distal and 2 cm medial to the tibial tubercle. The sartorius fascia is identified and incised. The semitendinosus and gracilis tendons are located directly beneath the Sartorius fascia with the interval between them being more easily distinguishable proximally. Careful blunt and sharp dissection can be used to further isolate the tendons and to free them from the surrounding tissues. A tendon stripper is passed up the tendons proximally to release them from the muscle [20].

Quadriceps Tendon

Quadriceps tendon autograft is harvested through a longitudinal midline incision extending from the superior pole of the patella. After dissecting through subcutaneous tissues, the prepatellar retinaculum is isolated and preserved. The quadriceps tendon and its junction with the vastus medialis obliquus and vastus lateralis obliquus are identified proximally (Fig. 8.1). An incision is carried out through some or all layers of the quadriceps tendon. The graft may be harvested with or without a bone plug from the superior patella [80, 81].

Allograft

The American Orthopaedic Society for Sports Medicine (AOSSM) has estimated that approximately 60,000 allografts were used in knee reconstruction procedures alone in 2005 [82]. Because of potential graft necrosis and the relatively large size of the native PCL, larger graft options are preferred for allograft PCL reconstruction. The Achilles tendon (Figs. 8.2 and 8.3), with its large cross-sectional area, is currently the most frequently used graft for acute (43 %) and chronic (50 %) PCL reconstructions [78] due to its large size. Double-stranded anterior and posterior tibial tendons (Figs. 8.4 and 8.5) are also commonly used allografts. Other allograft options include B-PT-B (Fig. 8.6), hamstrings (Fig. 8.7), and QTB (Figs. 8.1 and 8.8).

Surgeons are attracted to allograft ligament reconstructions because they eliminate donor-site morbidity as well as the additional risks associated with autograft tissue harvest. Furthermore, allografts provide multiple graft size options, shorter operative and tourniquet times, as well as fewer incisions as a result of not needing to harvest autograft tissue

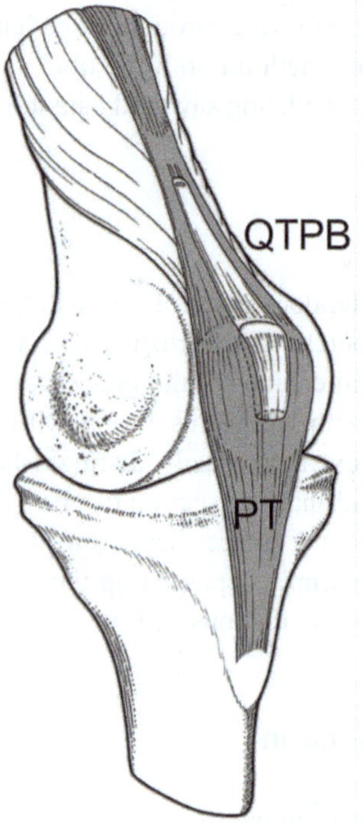

Fig. 8.1 Diagram of quadriceps tendon-patella bone (QTPB) harvesting. PT denotes patellar tendon [119]

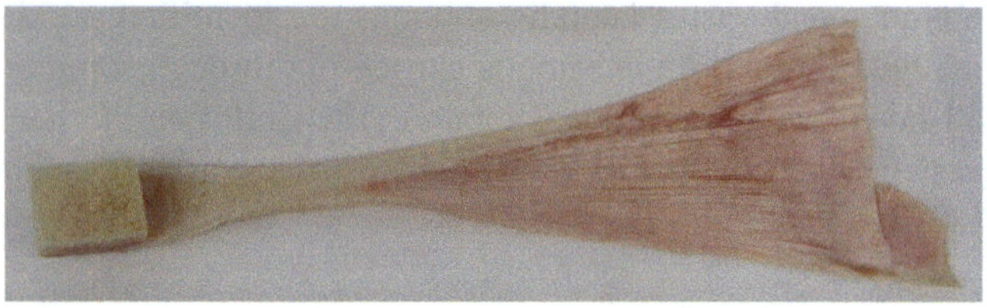

Fig. 8.2 Achilles tendon–bone allograft removed from package. Image kindly provided by Musculoskeletal Transplant Foundation (MTF) [120]

[22, 27, 83, 84]. Unfortunately, the use of allograft tissues is also associated with its own set of complications, such as small risk of infectious disease transmission, slower incorporation of graft tissue, and the potential for immunologic rejection [1, 21, 34, 85–91].

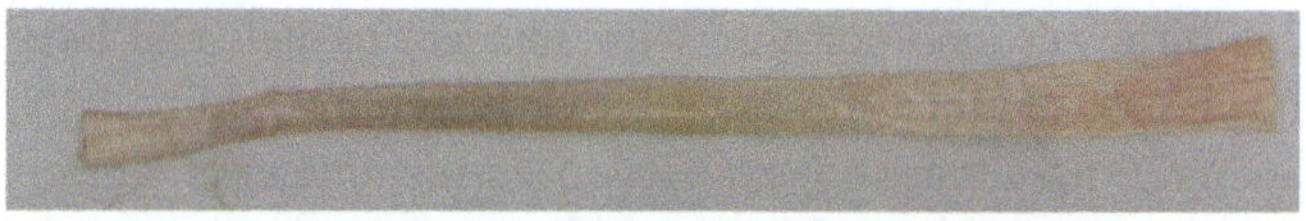

Fig. 8.4 Tibialis anterior allograft. Image kindly provided by Musculoskeletal Transplant Foundation (MTF) [120]

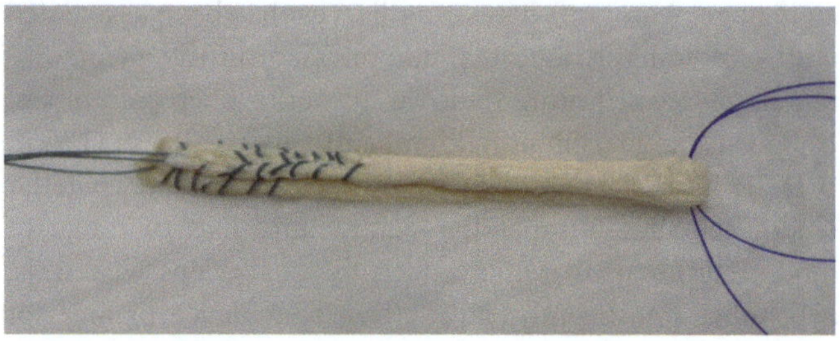

Fig. 8.5 Tibialis anterior allograft ready for implantation. Image kindly provided by Musculoskeletal Transplant Foundation (MTF) [120]

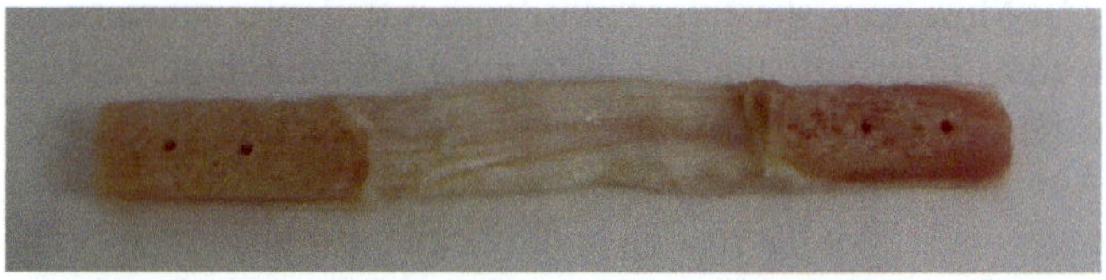

Fig. 8.6 Bone–patellar tendon–bone allograft ready for implantation. Image kindly provided by Musculoskeletal Transplant Foundation (MTF) [120]

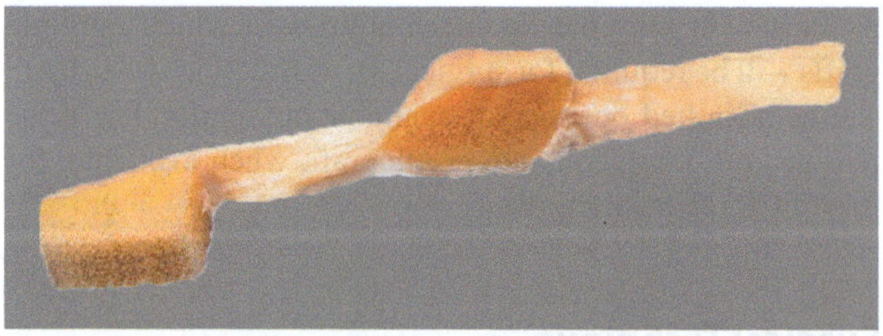

Fig. 8.7 Quadriceps tendon–patellar bone–patellar tendon–tibial bone allograft after removal of packaging [120]

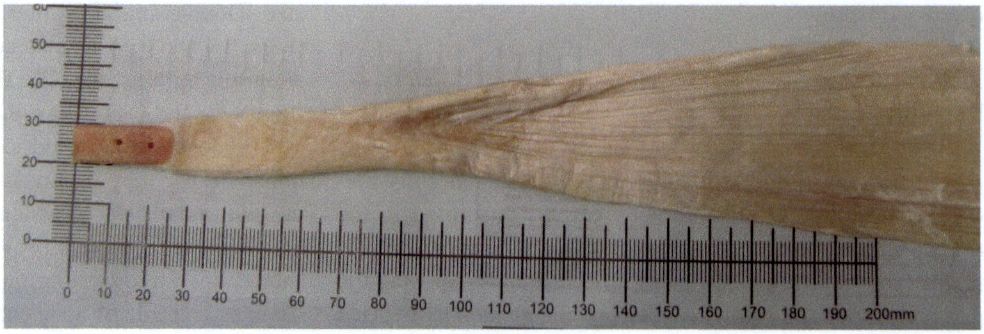

Fig. 8.3 Achilles tendon–bone allograft being prepared for implantation. Image kindly provided by Musculoskeletal Transplant Foundation (MTF) [120]

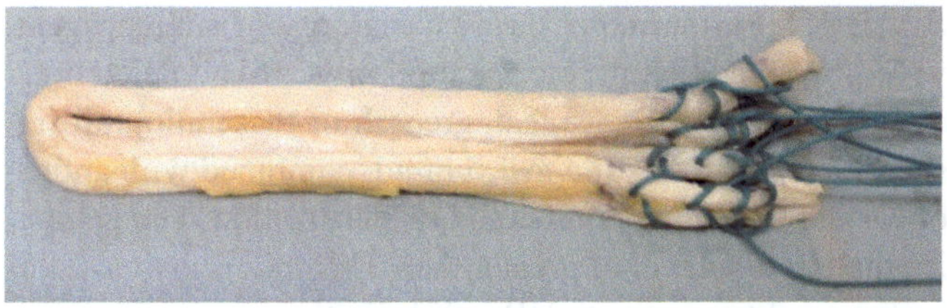

Fig. 8.8 Quadrupled hamstrings allograft

Risk of Infectious Disease Transmission

Infectious disease transmission, albeit exceedingly rare, is a distinct possibility when implanting allograft musculoskeletal tissues and there have been multiple documented cases of disease transmission in this manner, some of which have resulted in the death of the patient [1]. It is possible to transmit human immunodeficiency (HIV) virus type 1 and type 2, HBV, HCV, bacteria, such as clostridia or treponema pallidum, fungi, parasites, West Nile virus (WNV), and human transmissible spongiform encephalopathies.

The risk of HIV transmission in a properly screened donor ranges between 1 in 173,000 and 1 in 1 million and the corresponding risk of HCV is 1 in 421,000 for unprocessed tissue [1]. The most concerning incident regarding HIV transmission in the setting of allograft ligament implantation was in 1986 when a fresh-frozen B-PT-B allograft, which was not secondarily sterilized and was derived from a young male donor with no known risk factors for HIV whom tested negative for HIV-1 antibodies, was implanted into a patient [86]. Three weeks following surgery the recipient was treated with supportive therapy for flu-like illness and lymphopenia was noted. The patient was not diagnosed with HIV until several years later after an investigation was carried out to identify the cause of seroconversion in a woman whose only risk factor for HIV was the receipt of bone allograft from the same donor. Other non-musculoskeletal allografts from the same donor also resulted in disease transmission. At the time of this incident, HIV testing of donors was performed via detecting the presence of anti-HIV antibodies, which may take several months to become detectable in the peripheral blood of recently infected individuals [86]. Currently, nucleic acid testing (NAT) is now required by American Association of Tissue Banks (AATB). HIV, although it is a retrovirus, synthesizes DNA that is detectable within the leukocytes it infects and NAT can be carried out effectively within 48 h of a donor's death. In addition to this case of HIV transmission, there have been at least two separate documented reports of hepatitis C transmission as a result of receiving patellar ligament allografts from infected donors [92, 93]. Again, these incidents occurred as a result of harvesting tissue from an anti-HCV antibody negative donor where NAT was not performed. Although the pool of allograft donors who fall into the category of anti-HCV antibody negative yet HCV-RNA positive is unknown, in 2003 this serology pattern was present in approximately four out of every one million blood transfusion donors [92]. Although sterilization of allografts will be discussed later, it should be noted that studies have demonstrated that although freeze-drying and radiation may decrease the already low risk of HIV transmission it does not eliminate this risk completely [86, 94, 95].

In addition to viral transmissions, several bacterial infections have resulted from musculoskeletal allograft implantation [1, 96]. Allograft tissues distributed by vendors operating with questionable standards that occurred between 2001 and 2005 prompted the FDA to require more stringent surveillance of organizations procuring allograft tissue. As a result, all tissue banks are now required to register with the FDA and follow Current Good Tissue Practice requirements designed to minimize risk to allograft recipients [1, 96]. These examples bring three points to light: (1) there is a definite time lag between a donor contracting a virus and our current ability to detect its presence (approximately 7–10 days with NAT testing), (2) secondary processing and sterilization processes have the potential to effectively decrease the risk of viral disease transmission yet, and (3) there will always be a finite risk to patients when implanting musculoskeletal allografts [1, 97].

As mentioned previously, the risk of HIV and HCV is exceedingly low and the authors are unaware of any documented transmissions in the setting of appropriately screened donors and modern NAT. Additionally, an investigation by Greenberg et al. in a large series of patients failed to demonstrate an increased risk of bacterial disease transmission associated with implantation of allograft tissues [98]. Again, this underscores the importance of the surgeon becoming knowledgeable about the procurement practices of their allograft provider so that the surgeon can help patients make informed decisions about their care.

Delayed Incorporation of Allograft

Healing of a ligament graft occurs in three phases: inflammatory, proliferative, and remodeling. Within the inflammatory phase, neutrophils and other inflammatory cells arise and the water content of the graft increases ultimately leading to decreased biomechanical properties of the tendon itself. Graft necrosis then occurs, which is believed to be the cause of the permanent strength loss observed in reconstructed ligaments, when compared to their biomechanical strength at the time of implantation [87]. Next is the proliferative phase in which fibroblasts and synovial cells infiltrate the graft from the bone tunnels and vascular granulation tissue engrafts into the ligament matrix. Finally, the disorganized fibroblast and extracellular matrix mass is reorganized into a more highly cellular tissue with tensile-strength properties. This process is termed "ligamentization." Although a similar pattern of revascularization and incorporation of the graft with host tissue occurs among both autograft and allograft tissues, it has been well documented that autograft tissues incorporate faster than allograft tissues [87–90, 99]. It may take up to one and a half times longer for allograft to completely remodel and gain comparable strength to autograft [100]. ACL retrieval studies at autopsy suggest that allograft incorporation continues for more than 2 years [101]. Despite the slower rate of incorporation, the eventual healing is almost identical to the healing of autograft [102, 103]. Inherent to this delayed incorporation is the potential for graft rejection. Although this has been reported in musculoskeletal allograft, it rarely impacts the clinical course of the patient [104, 105].

Procurement of Allograft Donor Tissue

The screening of acceptable donors is quite rigorous as this is the first barrier to preventing disease transmission. Prospective donors or their relevant family begin by completing a questionnaire detailing their medical, social, and sexual history. An inquiry is made regarding drug use, neurologic diseases, autoimmune diseases such as rheumatoid arthritis, metabolic disease, collagen disorders, and exposure to hepatitis, HIV, or Creutzfeld–Jacob disease, or unprotected anal sex. Any positive response disqualifies them as a donor. Next, a thorough physical exam is performed, evaluating for signs of infectious diseases such as sexually transmitted diseases, hepatosplenomegaly, lymphadenopathy, thrush, and skin lesions. Again, any positive findings disqualify the donor. Next, a blood sample is obtained. The FDA requires that recovered tissue must be negative for HIV-1 NAT, HCV NAT, and hepatitis B core antibody. American Association of Tissue Banks (AATB)-accredited banks require additional testing for HIV type 1 and type 2 antibody, hepatitis B surface antigen, total antibody to hepatitis B core antigen (IgG and IgM), HTLV-I/HTLV-II antibody, HCV antibody, a syphilis assay, as well as NAT for HCV and HIV-1. Tissues are then harvested using sterile techniques within 15 h of asystole for an unrefrigerated donor or within 24 h of asystole for refrigerated donors. Specimens are contained in wet ice for transport with a maximum of 72 h on wet ice before transfer to colder environment is required [1, 96, 97].

Sterilization of Allografts

In 2006, a survey of 365 members of the AOSSM indicated that 86 % of them utilized allografts, yet 21 % were not aware of whether their allograft source was accredited by the AATB [1]. Furthermore, the vast majority of surgeons surveyed believed that the sterilization process had deleterious effects on the biomechanical strength of these allograft tissues. Gamma irradiation to 1.5 mrad, combined with antibiotic soaks, is a common method of sterilization. Yet, gamma irradiation to a level of greater than 3.5 mrad is estimated to be required to eliminate HIV [95]. Furthermore, gamma irradiation above 3 mrad has been shown to decrease allograft maximum failure force by up to 27 % and strain energy to maximum force by up to 40 % and, as a result, doses below 2.5 mrad are currently recommended to prevent damage to graft biomechanical properties [97, 106]. In response to this, research involving the use of free radical scavengers in conjunction with radiation is currently underway in order to balance adequate prevention of infectious disease with the preservation of biomechanical properties [107].

Ethylene oxide (EtO) was formerly a commonly implemented sterilization technique. However, after an association of a resultant chronic inflammatory reactions (effusions) and increased graft failures with its use was demonstrated, it was eliminated from AATB approved tissue banks [108, 109].

There are many other proprietary sterilization techniques involving serial soaks alternating tissue-culture-grade water with denatured 70 % ethanol, biologic detergents, dimehtylsulfoxide, antibiotics, or hydrogen peroxide. Additional treatments may consist of ultrasound, centrifugation, and repeated irradiation cycles [96]. Some tissue banks with proprietary sterilization techniques claim that tissue integrity is not damaged by the sterilization processes [110]. However, sterilized grafts have been associated with poor clinical outcomes in several investigations [111–113].

Storage of Allograft

Cryopreservation is a process of slowly cooling a graft while extracting the intracellular water using various chemical soaks such as dimethylsulfoxide or glycerol. Following the chemical soaks, a controlled rate of progressive freezing to −135 °C is carried out, with the graft ultimately being stored at −196 °C for up to 10 years. This controlled freezing in cryoprotectant solution inhibits the formation of ice crystals and thus preserves collagen integrity. It was theorized that this would also preserve cellular integrity and thus be associated with an increased risk of graft rejection. However, a minimal histological inflammatory response at the allograft ligament as well as normal, rather than accelerated, rejection of corresponding allograft full-thickness skin graft was demonstrated. This, as well as a complete absence of donor DNA by 4 weeks post-transplantation, indicated that there was minimal cell survival among these cryopreserved allografts [113].

Fresh-frozen treatment of allografts is the most commonly utilized storage modality and consists of rapid freezing of the graft to −80 °C or −100 °C without additional sterilization processing. It has been shown to eliminate cellular components that lead to immunologic rejection of allograft tissue [88]. Freeze-dried samples are created by removing the marrow and blood from the specimen and freezing the tissue for a quarantine period. After quarantine, the tissues are thawed, treated with antibiotic soaks, and exposed to serial alcohol rinses in order to dehydrate the specimens. They are subsequently lyophilized and packaged. The resultant graft can be stored for up to 5 years. There is very little immunogenic response when implanted. However, unlike freeze-dried bone, the biomechanical properties of freeze-dried tendons have been demonstrated to be inferior to fresh-frozen specimens and the potential for viral disease transmission is not completely eliminated [94, 114, 115].

Author's Recommendation

It is clear that allograft tissue plays a substantial role in PCL reconstruction. Any surgeon utilizing banked tissue should become familiar with the practices, protocols, and proven results of whichever allograft vendor is to be utilized. Some organizations providing allograft tissues surpass the requirements of the AATB and US Food and Drug Administration (US FDA). It is our recommendation that surgeons, at the very least, utilize allograft tissues from organizations whose processing and distribution comply with all of the required AATB and US FDA criteria for current good manufacturing practices. Furthermore, surgeons should be familiar with any sterilization processes used for grafts which will be implanted. Because of the potential deleterious effects of the sterilization processes on both the biomechanical and biological properties of allografts, the authors currently utilize only fresh-frozen nonirradiated allografts from an AATB member tissue bank. Routine culturing of allograft tissue in the operating room immediately prior to implantation is not currently recommended because there is little correlation with swab culture results and future allograft-associated infection [1, 116].

Conclusion

Graft selection in PCL reconstruction remains controversial, as there is a relative paucity of research on graft options for PCL reconstruction as compared to ACL reconstruction. While much of the knowledge of graft selection is based upon the experience with ACL grafts, the PCL is biomechanically different from the ACL [117, 118], and thus the results of specific graft use in PCL reconstruction may vary from those of the ACL [13]. To date, the literature has not shown significant differences in clinical outcomes with the use of autograft versus allograft or among the different types of each graft. Thus, the patient's specific characteristics and goals should be considered to help the patient make an informed decision.

References

1. McAllister DR, Joyce MJ, Mann BJ, Vangsness CT. Allograft update: the current status of tissue regulation, procurement, processing, and sterilization. Am J Sports Med. 2007;35(12):2148–58.
2. Lee YS, Jung YB. Posterior cruciate ligament: focus on conflicting issues. Clin Orthop Surg. 2013;5(4):256–62.
3. Jung YB, Jung HJ, Kim SJ, Park SJ, Song KS, Lee YS, et al. Posterolateral corner reconstruction for posterolateral rotatory instability combined with posterior cruciate ligament injuries: comparison between fibular tunnel and tibial tunnel techniques. Knee Surg Sports Traumatol Arthrosc. 2008;16(3):239–48.
4. Levy BA, Dajani KA, Whelan DB, Stannard JP, Fanelli GC, Stuart MJ, et al. Decision making in the multiligament-injured knee: an evidence-based systematic review. Arthroscopy. 2009;25(4):430–8.
5. Tzurbakis M, Diamantopoulos A, Xenakis T, Georgoulis A. Surgical treatment of multiple knee ligament injuries in 44 patients: 2–8 years follow-up results. Knee Surg Sports Traumatol Arthrosc. 2006;14(8):739–49.
6. Harner CD, Waltrip RL, Bennett CH, Francis KA, Cole B, Irrgang JJ. Surgical management of knee dislocations. J Bone Joint Surg Am. 2004;86-A(2):262–73.
7. Fanelli GC, Orcutt DR, Edson CJ. The multiple-ligament injured knee: evaluation, treatment, and results. Arthroscopy. 2005;21(4):471–86.
8. Ranawat A, Baker CL, Henry S, Harner CD. Posterolateral corner injury of the knee: evaluation and management. J Am Acad Orthop Surg. 2008;16(9):506–18.
9. LaPrade RF, Johansen S, Agel J, Risberg MA, Moksnes H, Engebretsen L. Outcomes of an anatomic posterolateral knee reconstruction. J Bone Joint Surg Am. 2010;92(1):16–22.
10. Montgomery SR, Johnson JS, McAllister DR, Petrigliano FA. Surgical management of PCL injuries: indications, techniques, and outcomes. Curr Rev Musculoskelet Med. 2013;6(2):115–23.
11. Nancoo TJ, Lord B, Yasen SK, Smith JO, Risebury MJ, Wilson AJ. Transmedial all-inside posterior cruciate ligament reconstruction using a reinforced tibial inlay graft. Arthrosc Tech. 2013;2(4):e381–8.
12. Höher J, Scheffler S, Weiler A. Graft choice and graft fixation in PCL reconstruction. Knee Surg Sports Traumatol Arthrosc. 2003;11(5):297–306.
13. Hudgens JL, Gillette BP, Krych AJ, Stuart MJ, May JH, Levy BA. Allograft versus autograft in posterior cruciate ligament reconstruction: an evidence-based systematic review. J Knee Surg. 2013;26(2):109–15.
14. Olson EJ, Harner CD, Fu FH, Silbey MB. Clinical use of fresh, frozen soft tissue allografts. Orthopedics. 1992;15(10):1225–32.
15. Wang CJ, Chan YS, Weng LH, Yuan LJ, Chen HS. Comparison of autogenous and allogenous posterior cruciate ligament reconstructions of the knee. Injury. 2004;35(12):1279–85.
16. Ahn JH, Yoo JC, Wang JH. Posterior cruciate ligament reconstruction: double-loop hamstring tendon autograft versus Achilles tendon allograft–clinical results of a minimum 2-year follow-up. Arthroscopy. 2005;21(8):965–9.

17. Lin YC, Chen SK, Liu TH, Cheng YM, Chou PP. Arthroscopic transtibial single-bundle posterior cruciate ligament reconstruction using patellar tendon graft compared with hamstring tendon graft. Arch Orthop Trauma Surg. 2013;133(4):523–30.
18. Margheritini F, Frascari Diotallevi F, Mariani PP. Posterior cruciate ligament reconstruction using an arthroscopic femoral inlay technique. Knee Surg Sports Traumatol Arthrosc. 2011;19(12):2033–5.
19. Fanelli GC, Edson CJ. Surgical treatment of combined PCL-ACL medial and lateral side injuries (global laxity): surgical technique and 2- to 18-year results. J Knee Surg. 2012;25(4):307–16.
20. Rihn JA, Groff YJ, Harner CD, Cha PS. The acutely dislocated knee: evaluation and management. J Am Acad Orthop Surg. 2004;12(5):334–46.
21. Harner CD, Olson E, Irrgang JJ, Silverstein S, Fu FH, Silbey M. Allograft versus autograft anterior cruciate ligament reconstruction: 3- to 5-year outcome. Clin Orthop Relat Res. 1996;(324):134–44.
22. Wascher DC, Becker JR, Dexter JG, Blevins FT. Reconstruction of the anterior and posterior cruciate ligaments after knee dislocation. Results using fresh-frozen nonirradiated allografts. Am J Sports Med. 1999;27(2):189–96.
23. Fanelli GC, Giannotti BF, Edson CJ. Arthroscopically assisted combined posterior cruciate ligament/posterior lateral complex reconstruction. Arthroscopy. 1996;12(5):521–30.
24. Fanelli GC, Tomaszewski DJ. Allograft use in the treatment of the multiple ligament injured knee. Sports Med Arthrosc. 2007;15(3):139–48.
25. Noyes FR, Barber-Westin SD. Reconstruction of the anterior and posterior cruciate ligaments after knee dislocation. Use of early protected postoperative motion to decrease arthrofibrosis. Am J Sports Med. 1997;25(6):769–78.
26. Noyes FR, Barber-Westin SD. The treatment of acute combined ruptures of the anterior cruciate and medial ligaments of the knee. Am J Sports Med. 1995;23(4):380–9.
27. Shapiro MS, Freedman EL. Allograft reconstruction of the anterior and posterior cruciate ligaments after traumatic knee dislocation. Am J Sports Med. 1995;23(5):580–7.
28. Shelton WR, Treacy SH, Dukes AD, Bomboy AL. Use of allografts in knee reconstruction: I. Basic science aspects and current status. J Am Acad Orthop Surg. 1998;6(3):165–8.
29. Buss DD, Warren RF, Wickiewicz TL, Galinat BJ, Panariello R. Arthroscopically assisted reconstruction of the anterior cruciate ligament with use of autogenous patellar-ligament grafts. Results after twenty-four to forty-two months. J Bone Joint Surg Am. 1993;75(9):1346–55.
30. Rushton N, Dandy DJ, Naylor CP. The clinical, arthroscopic and histological findings after replacement of the anterior cruciate ligament with carbon-fibre. J Bone Joint Surg Br. 1983;65(3):308–9.
31. Jenkins DH, McKibbin B. The role of flexible carbon-fibre implants as tendon and ligament substitutes in clinical practice. A preliminary report. J Bone Joint Surg Br. 1980;62-B(4):497–9.
32. Weiss AB, Blazina ME, Goldstein AR, Alexander H. Ligament replacement with an absorbable copolymer carbon fiber scaffold–early clinical experience. Clin Orthop Relat Res. 1985;(196):77–85.
33. Mäkisalo S, Skutnabb K, Holmström T, Grönblad M, Paavolainen P. Reconstruction of anterior cruciate ligament with carbon fiber. An experimental study on pigs. Am J Sports Med. 1988;16(6):589–93.
34. Arnoczky SP, Warren RF, Minei JP. Replacement of the anterior cruciate ligament using a synthetic prosthesis. An evaluation of graft biology in the dog. Am J Sports Med. 1986;14(1):1–6.
35. Glousman R, Shields C, Kerlan R, Jobe F, Lombardo S, Yocum L, et al. Gore-Tex prosthetic ligament in anterior cruciate deficient knees. Am J Sports Med. 1988;16(4):321–6.
36. Indelicato PA, Pascale MS, Huegel MO. Early experience with the GORE-TEX polytetrafluoroethylene anterior cruciate ligament prosthesis. Am J Sports Med. 1989;17(1):55–2.
37. Guidoin MF, Marois Y, Bejui J, Poddevin N, King MW, Guidoin R. Analysis of retrieved polymer fiber based replacements for the ACL. Biomaterials. 2000;21(23):2461–74.
38. Mody BS, Howard L, Harding ML, Parmar HV, Learmonth DJ. The ABC carbon and polyester prosthetic ligament for ACL-deficient knees. Early results in 31 cases. J Bone Joint Surg Br. 1993;75(5):818–21.
39. Kumar K, Maffulli N. The ligament augmentation device: an historical perspective. Arthroscopy. 1999;15(4):422–32.
40. Tovar N, Bourke S, Jaffe M, Murthy NS, Kohn J, Gatt C, et al. A comparison of degradable synthetic polymer fibers for anterior cruciate ligament reconstruction. J Biomed Mater Res A. 2010;93(2):738–47.
41. Farng E, Urdaneta AR, Barba D, Esmende S, McAllister DR. The effects of GDF-5 and uniaxial strain on mesenchymal stem cells in 3-D culture. Clin Orthop Relat Res. 2008;466(8):1930–7.
42. Petrigliano FA, McAllister DR, Wu BM. Tissue engineering for anterior cruciate ligament reconstruction: a review of current strategies. Arthroscopy. 2006;22(4):441–51.
43. Koski JA, Ibarra C, Rodeo SA. Tissue-engineered ligament: cells, matrix, and growth factors. Orthop Clin North Am. 2000;31(3):437–52.
44. Wolfman NM, Hattersley G, Cox K, Celeste AJ, Nelson R, Yamaji N, et al. Ectopic induction of tendon and ligament in rats by growth and differentiation factors 5, 6, and 7, members of the TGF-beta gene family. J Clin Invest. 1997;100(2):321–30.
45. Altman GH, Horan RL, Martin I, Farhadi J, Stark PR, Volloch V, et al. Cell differentiation by mechanical stress. FASEB J. 2002;16(2):270–2.
46. Leong NL, Petrigliano FA, McAllister DR. Current tissue engineering strategies in anterior cruciate ligament reconstruction. J Biomed Mater Res A. 2014;102(5):1614–24.
47. Cross MJ, Roger G, Kujawa P, Anderson IF. Regeneration of the semitendinosus and gracilis tendons following their transection for repair of the anterior cruciate ligament. Am J Sports Med. 1992;20(2):221–3.
48. Squires N, West R, Harner C. Anterior cruciate ligament reconstruction: general considerations. In: ElAttrache N, Harner C, Mirzayan R, Sekiya J, editors. Philadelphia: Lippincott, Williams and Wilkins; 2007.
49. West RV, Harner CD. Graft selection in anterior cruciate ligament reconstruction. J Am Acad Orthop Surg. 2005;13(3):197–207.
50. Wu CH, Chen AC, Yuan LJ, Chang CH, Chan YS, Hsu KY, et al. Arthroscopic reconstruction of the posterior cruciate ligament by using a quadriceps tendon autograft: a minimum 5-year follow-up. Arthroscopy. 2007;23(4):420–7.
51. Chen CH, Chen WJ, Shih CH. Arthroscopic reconstruction of the posterior cruciate ligament: a comparison of quadriceps tendon autograft and quadruple hamstring tendon graft. Arthroscopy. 2002;18(6):603–12.
52. Lien OA, Aas EJ, Johansen S, Ludvigsen TC, Figved W, Engebretsen L. Clinical outcome after reconstruction for isolated posterior cruciate ligament injury. Knee Surg Sports Traumatol Arthrosc. 2010;18(11):1568–72.
53. Wong T, Wang CJ, Weng LH, Hsu SL, Chou WY, Chen JM, et al. Functional outcomes of arthroscopic posterior cruciate ligament reconstruction: comparison of anteromedial and anterolateral trans-tibia approach. Arch Orthop Trauma Surg. 2009;129(3):315–21.
54. Chen B, Gao S. Double-bundle posterior cruciate ligament reconstruction using a non-hardware suspension fixation technique and 8 strands of autogenous hamstring tendons. Arthroscopy. 2009;25(7):777–82.
55. Zhao J, Xiaoqiao H, He Y, Yang X, Liu C, Lu Z. Sandwich-style posterior cruciate ligament reconstruction. Arthroscopy. 2008;24(6):650–9.

56. Zhao J, Huangfu X. Arthroscopic single-bundle posterior cruciate ligament reconstruction: retrospective review of 4- versus 7-strand hamstring tendon graft. Knee. 2007;14(4):301–5.
57. Seon JK, Song EK. Reconstruction of isolated posterior cruciate ligament injuries: a clinical comparison of the transtibial and tibial inlay techniques. Arthroscopy. 2006;22(1):27–32.
58. Chan YS, Yang SC, Chang CH, Chen AC, Yuan LJ, Hsu KY, et al. Arthroscopic reconstruction of the posterior cruciate ligament with use of a quadruple hamstring tendon graft with 3- to 5-year follow-up. Arthroscopy. 2006;22(7):762–70.
59. Houe T, Jørgensen U. Arthroscopic posterior cruciate ligament reconstruction: one- vs. two-tunnel technique. Scand J Med Sci Sports. 2004;14(2):107–11.
60. Jung YB, Tae SK, Jung HJ, Lee KH. Replacement of the torn posterior cruciate ligament with a mid-third patellar tendon graft with use of a modified tibial inlay method. J Bone Joint Surg Am. 2004;86-A(9):1878–83.
61. Miller SL, Gladstone JN. Graft selection in anterior cruciate ligament reconstruction. Orthop Clin North Am. 2002;33(4):675–83.
62. Freedman KB, D'Amato MJ, Nedeff DD, Kaz A, Bach BR. Arthroscopic anterior cruciate ligament reconstruction: a meta-analysis comparing patellar tendon and hamstring tendon autografts. Am J Sports Med. 2003;31(1):2–11.
63. L'Insalata JC, Klatt B, Fu FH, Harner CD. Tunnel expansion following anterior cruciate ligament reconstruction: a comparison of hamstring and patellar tendon autografts. Knee Surg Sports Traumatol Arthrosc. 1997;5(4):234–8.
64. Yasuda K, Tsujino J, Ohkoshi Y, Tanabe Y, Kaneda K. Graft site morbidity with autogenous semitendinosus and gracilis tendons. Am J Sports Med. 1995;23(6):706–14.
65. Tashiro T, Kurosawa H, Kawakami A, Hikita A, Fukui N. Influence of medial hamstring tendon harvest on knee flexor strength after anterior cruciate ligament reconstruction. A detailed evaluation with comparison of single- and double-tendon harvest. Am J Sports Med. 2003;31(4):522–9.
66. Nakamura N, Horibe S, Sasaki S, Kitaguchi T, Tagami M, Mitsuoka T, et al. Evaluation of active knee flexion and hamstring strength after anterior cruciate ligament reconstruction using hamstring tendons. Arthroscopy. 2002;18(6):598–602.
67. McCarroll JR. Fracture of the patella during a golf swing following reconstruction of the anterior cruciate ligament. A case report. Am J Sports Med. 1983;11(1):26–7.
68. Shaw DR, Chen JT, Lester RG. X-ray appearance and clinical significance of left atrial wall calcification. Invest Radiol. 1976;11(6):501–7.
69. Marumoto JM, Mitsunaga MM, Richardson AB, Medoff RJ, Mayfield GW. Late patellar tendon ruptures after removal of the central third for anterior cruciate ligament reconstruction. A report of two cases. Am J Sports Med. 1996;24(5):698–701.
70. Langan P, Fontanetta AP. Rupture of the patellar tendon after use of its central third. Orthop Rev. 1987;16(5):317–21.
71. Paulos LE, Rosenberg TD, Drawbert J, Manning J, Abbott P. Infrapatellar contracture syndrome. An unrecognized cause of knee stiffness with patella entrapment and patella infera. Am J Sports Med. 1987;15(4):331–41.
72. Järvelä T, Paakkala T, Kannus P, Toivanen J, Järvinen M. Ultrasonographic and power Doppler evaluation of the patellar tendon ten years after harvesting its central third for reconstruction of the anterior cruciate ligament: comparison of patients without or with anterior knee pain. Am J Sports Med. 2004;32(1):39–46.
73. Rosenberg TD, Franklin JL, Baldwin GN, Nelson KA. Extensor mechanism function after patellar tendon graft harvest for anterior cruciate ligament reconstruction. Am J Sports Med. 1992;20(5):519–25; discussion 25–6.
74. Bach BR, Levy ME, Bojchuk J, Tradonsky S, Bush-Joseph CA, Khan NH. Single-incision endoscopic anterior cruciate ligament reconstruction using patellar tendon autograft. Minimum two-year follow-up evaluation. Am J Sports Med. 1998;26(1):30–40.
75. Ritchie JR, Parker RD. Graft selection in anterior cruciate ligament revision surgery. Clin Orthop Relat Res. 1996;(325):65–77.
76. Han HS, Seong SC, Lee S, Lee MC. Anterior cruciate ligament reconstruction: quadriceps versus patellar autograft. Clin Orthop Relat Res. 2008;466(1):198–204.
77. Geib TM, Shelton WR, Phelps RA, Clark L. Anterior cruciate ligament reconstruction using quadriceps tendon autograft: intermediate-term outcome. Arthroscopy. 2009;25(12):1408–14.
78. Rispoli DM, Sanders TG, Miller MD, Morrison WB. Magnetic resonance imaging at different time periods following hamstring harvest for anterior cruciate ligament reconstruction. Arthroscopy. 2001;17(1):2–8.
79. Shelton WR, Papendick L, Dukes AD. Autograft versus allograft anterior cruciate ligament reconstruction. Arthroscopy. 1997;13(4):446–9.
80. Noyes FR, Barber-Westin SD. Anterior cruciate ligament revision reconstruction: results using a quadriceps tendon-patellar bone autograft. Am J Sports Med. 2006;34(4):553–64.
81. Fulkerson JP, Langeland R. An alternative cruciate reconstruction graft: the central quadriceps tendon. Arthroscopy. 1995;11(2):252–4.
82. Eagan MJ, McAllister DR. Biology of allograft incorporation. Clin Sports Med. 2009;28(2):203–14, vii.
83. Indelicato PA, Linton RC, Huegel M. The results of fresh-frozen patellar tendon allografts for chronic anterior cruciate ligament deficiency of the knee. Am J Sports Med. 1992;20(2):118–21.
84. Noyes FR, Barber-Westin SD. Reconstruction of the anterior cruciate ligament with human allograft. Comparison of early and later results. J Bone Joint Surg Am. 1996;78(4):524–37.
85. Fu FH, Bennett CH, Lattermann C, Ma CB. Current trends in anterior cruciate ligament reconstruction. Part 1: Biology and biomechanics of reconstruction. Am J Sports Med. 1999;27(6):821–30.
86. Simonds RJ, Holmberg SD, Hurwitz RL, Coleman TR, Bottenfield S, Conley LJ, et al. Transmission of human immunodeficiency virus type 1 from a seronegative organ and tissue donor. N Engl J Med. 1992;326(11):726–32.
87. Arnoczky SP, Tarvin GB, Marshall JL. Anterior cruciate ligament replacement using patellar tendon. An evaluation of graft revascularization in the dog. J Bone Joint Surg Am. 1982;64(2):217–24.
88. Arnoczky SP, Warren RF, Ashlock MA. Replacement of the anterior cruciate ligament using a patellar tendon allograft. An experimental study. J Bone Joint Surg Am. 1986;68(3):376–85.
89. Jackson DW, Grood ES, Goldstein JD, Rosen MA, Kurzweil PR, Cummings JF, et al. A comparison of patellar tendon autograft and allograft used for anterior cruciate ligament reconstruction in the goat model. Am J Sports Med. 1993;21(2):176–85.
90. Jackson DW, Corsetti J, Simon TM. Biologic incorporation of allograft anterior cruciate ligament replacements. Clin Orthop Relat Res. 1996;(324):126–33.
91. Amiel D, Kleiner JB, Roux RD, Harwood FL, Akeson WH. The phenomenon of "ligamentization": anterior cruciate ligament reconstruction with autogenous patellar tendon. J Orthop Res. 1986;4(2):162–72.
92. Centers for Disease Control and Prevention. Hepatitis C virus transmission from an antibody-negative organ and tissue donor–United States, 2000-2002. MMWR Morb Mortal Wkly Rep. 2003;52(13):273–4, 6.
93. Conrad EU, Gretch DR, Obermeyer KR, Moogk MS, Sayers M, Wilson JJ, et al. Transmission of the hepatitis-C virus by tissue transplantation. J Bone Joint Surg Am. 1995;77(2):214–24.

94. Buck BE, Resnick L, Shah SM, Malinin TI. Human immunodeficiency virus cultured from bone. Implications for transplantation. Clin Orthop Relat Res. 1990;(251):249–53.
95. Conway B, Tomford W, Mankin HJ, Hirsch MS, Schooley RT. Radiosensitivity of HIV-1–potential application to sterilization of bone allografts. AIDS. 1991;5(5):608–9.
96. Vangsness CT, Wagner PP, Moore TM, Roberts MR. Overview of safety issues concerning the preparation and processing of soft-tissue allografts. Arthroscopy. 2006;22(12):1351–8.
97. Barnam B, Johnson DL. Surgical Principles: allograft tissues. In: Delee J, Drez D, Miller M, Editors. Philadelphia: Saunders Elsevier; 2009.
98. Greenberg DD, Robertson M, Vallurupalli S, White RA, Allen WC. Allograft compared with autograft infection rates in primary anterior cruciate ligament reconstruction. J Bone Joint Surg Am. 2010;92(14):2402–8.
99. Hohbach C, Meissner HP, Schmidt H, Seeliger H. Morphological and electrophysiological studies of islets of Langerhans in diabetic mice. Verh Dtsch Ges Pathol. 1978;62:367.
100. Cordrey LJ. A comparative study of fresh autogenous and preserved homogenous tendon grafts in rabbits. J Bone Joint Surg Br. 1963;45-B:182–95.
101. Vollmann J, Winau R. History of informed medical consent. Lancet. 1996;347(8998):410.
102. Shino K, Kawasaki T, Hirose H, Gotoh I, Inoue M, Ono K. Replacement of the anterior cruciate ligament by an allogeneic tendon graft. An experimental study in the dog. J Bone Joint Surg Br. 1984;66(5):672–81.
103. Nikolaou PK, Seaber AV, Glisson RR, Ribbeck BM, Bassett FH. Anterior cruciate ligament allograft transplantation. Long-term function, histology, revascularization, and operative technique. Am J Sports Med. 1986;14(5):348–60.
104. Shino K, Inoue M, Horibe S, Hamada M, Ono K. Reconstruction of the anterior cruciate ligament using allogeneic tendon. Long-term followup. Am J Sports Med. 1990;18(5):457–65.
105. Rodeo SA, Seneviratne A, Suzuki K, Felker K, Wickiewicz TL, Warren RF. Histological analysis of human meniscal allografts. A preliminary report. J Bone Joint Surg Am. 2000;82-A(8):1071–82.
106. Gibbons MJ, Butler DL, Grood ES, Bylski-Austrow DI, Levy MS, Noyes FR. Effects of gamma irradiation on the initial mechanical and material properties of goat bone-patellar tendon-bone allografts. J Orthop Res. 1991;9(2):209–18.
107. Seto A, Gatt CJ, Dunn MG. Improved tendon radioprotection by combined cross-linking and free radical scavenging. Clin Orthop Relat Res. 2009;467(11):2994–3001.
108. Jackson DW, Windler GE, Simon TM. Intraarticular reaction associated with the use of freeze-dried, ethylene oxide-sterilized bone-patella tendon-bone allografts in the reconstruction of the anterior cruciate ligament. Am J Sports Med. 1990;18(1):1–10; discussion 10–1.
109. Rihn JA, Harner CD. The use of musculoskeletal allograft tissue in knee surgery. Arthroscopy. 2003;19(Suppl 1):51–66.
110. Jones DB, Huddleston PM, Zobitz ME, Stuart MJ. Mechanical properties of patellar tendon allografts subjected to chemical sterilization. Arthroscopy. 2007;23(4):400–4.
111. Borchers JR, Pedroza A, Kaeding C. Activity level and graft type as risk factors for anterior cruciate ligament graft failure: a case-control study. Am J Sports Med. 2009;37(12):2362–7.
112. Rappé M, Horodyski M, Meister K, Indelicato PA. Nonirradiated versus irradiated Achilles allograft: in vivo failure comparison. Am J Sports Med. 2007;35(10):1653–8.
113. Jackson DW, Simon TM, Kurzweil PR, Rosen MA. Survival of cells after intra-articular transplantation of fresh allografts of the patellar and anterior cruciate ligaments. DNA-probe analysis in a goat model. J Bone Joint Surg Am. 1992;74(1):112–8.
114. Indelicato PA, Bittar ES, Prevot TJ, Woods GA, Branch TP, Huegel M. Clinical comparison of freeze-dried and fresh frozen patellar tendon allografts for anterior cruciate ligament reconstruction of the knee. Am J Sports Med. 1990;18(4):335–42.
115. Jackson DW, Grood ES, Arnoczky SP, Butler DL, Simon TM. Freeze dried anterior cruciate ligament allografts. Preliminary studies in a goat model. Am J Sports Med. 1987;15(4):295–303.
116. Veen MR, Bloem RM, Petit PL. Sensitivity and negative predictive value of swab cultures in musculoskeletal allograft procurement. Clin Orthop Relat Res. 1994;(300):259–63.
117. Kennedy JC, Hawkins RJ, Willis RB, Danylchuck KD. Tension studies of human knee ligaments. Yield point, ultimate failure, and disruption of the cruciate and tibial collateral ligaments. J Bone Joint Surg Am. 1976;58(3):350–5.
118. Race A, Amis AA. The mechanical properties of the two bundles of the human posterior cruciate ligament. J Biomech. 1994;27(1):13–24.
119. Dargel J, et al. Biomechanical testing of quadriceps tendon-patellar bone grafts: an alternative graft source for press-fit anterior cruciate ligament reconstruction? Arch Ortho Trauma Surg 2006;126:265–70. (Reprinted with permission from Springer).
120. Kremen T, McAllister DR. Graft selection in multiple ligament injured knee surgery. In Fanelli, GC, editor. The multiple ligament injured knee: a practical guide to management. 2nd edn. New York: Springer; 2013. (Reprinted with permission).

9 Arthroscopic Transtibial Tunnel Posterior Cruciate Ligament Reconstruction

Gregory C. Fanelli

Introduction

Posterior cruciate ligament (PCL) injuries, in practice, rarely occur as an isolated knee ligament injury. The PCL injuries are most often combined with at least one other knee ligament injury [1, 2]. The reasons for PCL reconstruction surgical failure most commonly are failure to address associated ligament instabilities, failure to address lower extremity malalignment, and incorrect tunnel placement [3]. Identifying the multiple planes of instability in these complex knee ligament injuries is essential for successful treatment of the PCL-injured knee. The PCL disruption will lead to increased posterior laxity at 90° of knee flexion. Recognition and correction of the medial- and/or lateral-side instability is the key to successful posterior and anterior cruciate ligament (ACL) surgery.

There are three different types of instability patterns that have been observed in medial- and lateral-side knee injuries [4–6]. These are, type A (axial rotation instability only), type B (axial rotation instability combined with varus and/or valgus laxity with a firm endpoint), and type C (axial rotation instability combined with varus and/or valgus laxity with little or no endpoint). The axial rotation instability (type A) medial or lateral side is most frequently overlooked. It is also critical to understand that combined medial- and lateral-side instability of different types occur with bicruciate and unicruciate multiple ligament knee injuries. Examples include PCL, ACL, lateral-side type C, and medial-side type A; or PCL, medial-side type B, and lateral-side type A instability patterns.

A combination of careful clinical examination, radiographs, and magnetic resonance tomography (MRI) studies aids in determining the correct diagnosis of multiple ligament knee injuries. Knee examination under anesthesia combined with fluoroscopy, stress radiography, and diagnostic arthroscopy also contributes to accurately diagnosing the multiple planes of instability [7, 8]. Once again, recognition and correction of the medial- and lateral-side instability is the key to successful PCL and ACL surgery. The purpose of this chapter is to describe the arthroscopic transtibial tunnel PCL reconstruction surgical technique.

Operating Room Considerations

PCL-based reconstruction procedures are routinely performed in an outpatient setting unless specific circumstances indicate the necessity of an inpatient environment [9, 10]. The same experienced surgical teams are assembled for these complex surgical procedures. Experienced and familiar teams provide for a smoother operation, shorter surgical times, enhanced patient care, and a greater probability of success in these difficult surgical procedures. Preoperative and postoperative prophylactic antibiotics are routinely used in these complex and time-consuming surgical procedures to decrease the probability of infection.

Graft Selection

My preferred graft for the PCL reconstruction is the Achilles tendon allograft for single-bundle PCL reconstructions, and Achilles tendon (anterolateral bundle) and tibialis anterior (posteromedial bundle) allografts for double-bundle PCL reconstructions. The allograft tissue used is from the same tissue bank with the same methods of tissue procurement and preservation that provides a consistent graft of high quality. It is very important for the surgeon to "know the tissue bank" and to obtain high-quality allograft tissue that will maximize the probability of surgical success.

G. C. Fanelli (✉)
303 Kaseville Road, Danville, PA 17821, USA
e-mail: gregorycfanelli@gmail.com

G. C. Fanelli (ed.), *Posterior Cruciate Ligament Injuries*,
DOI 10.1007/978-3-319-12072-0_9, © Springer International Publishing Switzerland 2015

PCL Reconstruction Surgical Technique

The principles of PCL reconstruction are to identify and treat all pathology, accurately place tunnels to produce anatomic graft insertion sites, utilize strong graft material, mechanical graft tensioning, secure graft fixation, and a deliberate post-operative rehabilitation program [7, 9–15].

The patient is placed on the operating room table in the supine position, and after satisfactory induction of anesthesia, the operative and nonoperative lower extremities are carefully examined [9, 10]. A tourniquet is applied to the upper thigh of the operative extremity but is not routinely inflated, and that extremity is prepped and draped in a sterile fashion. The well leg is supported by the fully extended operating room table, which also supports the surgical leg during medial- and lateral-side surgery. A lateral post is used to control the surgical extremity. An arthroscopic leg holder is not used (Fig. 9.1). Preoperative and postoperative antibiotics are given, and antibiotics are routinely used to help prevent infection in these time-consuming, difficult, and complex cases. Allograft tissue is prepared prior to bringing the patient into the operating room to minimize general anesthesia time for the patient. Autograft tissue is harvested prior to beginning the arthroscopic portion of the procedure. The Biomet Sports Medicine PCL/ACL System (Biomet Sports Medicine, Warsaw, Indiana) are the surgical instruments used for this surgical procedure. Intraoperative radiography and C-arm image intensifier are not routinely used for this surgical procedure.

The arthroscopic instruments are inserted with the inflow through the superolateral patellar portal. Instrumentation and visualization are positioned through inferomedial and inferolateral patellar portals, and can be interchanged as necessary. Additional portals are established as necessary. Exploration of the joint consists of evaluation of the patellofemoral joint, the medial and lateral compartments, medial and lateral menisci, and the intercondylar notch. The residual stumps of the PCLs are debrided; however, the posterior (and ACL when applicable) anatomic insertion sites are preserved to serve as tunnel reference points. The notchplasty for the ACL portion of the procedure in combined PCL–ACL reconstruction cases is performed at this time.

An extracapsular extra-articular posteromedial safety incision is made by creating an incision approximately 1.5–2-cm long starting at the posteromedial border of the tibia approximately 1 in. below the level of the joint line and extending distally (Fig. 9.2). Dissection is carried down to the crural fascia, which is incised longitudinally. An interval is developed between the medial head of the gastrocnemius muscle and the nerves and vessels posterior to the surgeon's finger, and the capsule of the knee joint anterior to the surgeon's finger (Fig. 9.3). The posteromedial safety incision enables the surgeon to protect the neurovascular structures,

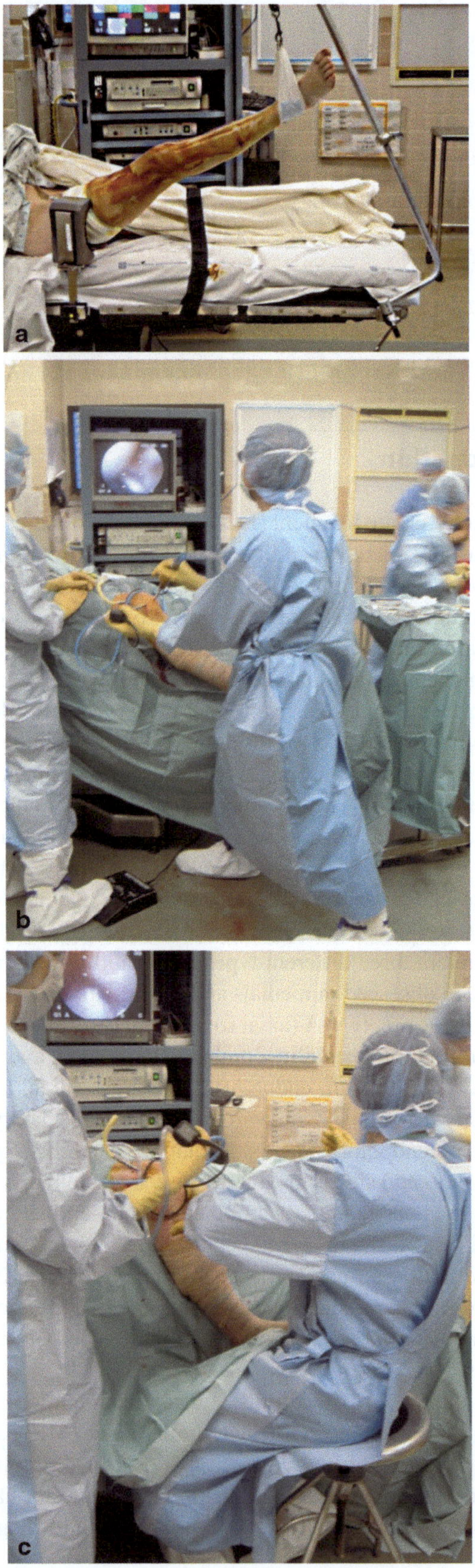

Fig. 9.1 Patient positioning. **a** The patient is positioned on the fully extended operating room table with a lateral post used for control of the surgical extremity. **b** The surgeon stands during the basic arthroscopic

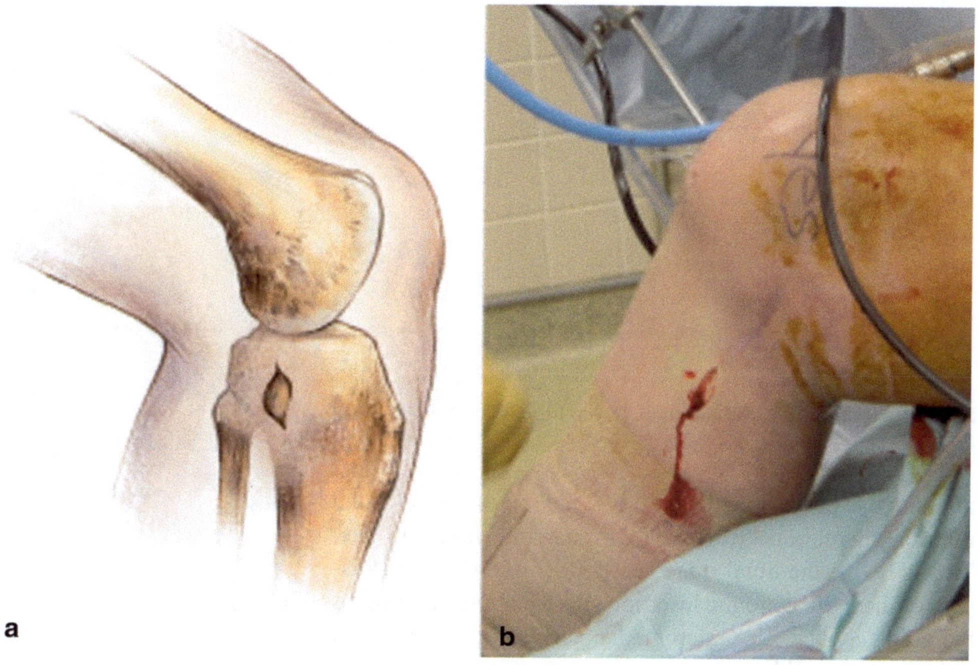

Fig. 9.2 **a** Posteromedial extra-articular extracapsular safety incision. (From Fanelli 2012 [10]). **b** Intraoperative photograph of the posteromedial safety incision. (From Fanelli 2013 [9]. Reprinted with permission)

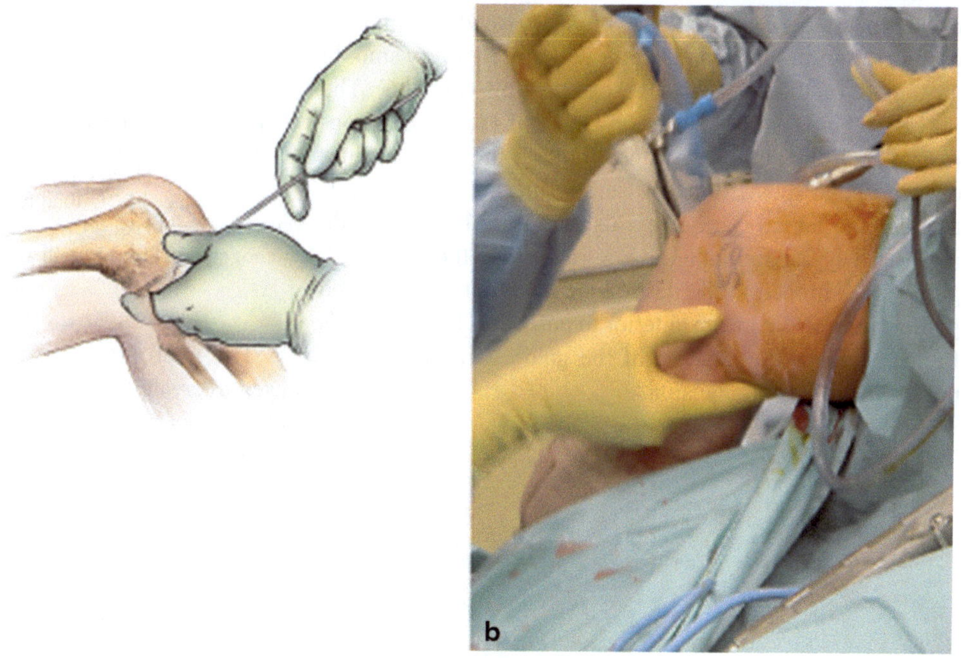

Fig. 9.3 **a** The surgeon is able to palpate the posterior aspect of the tibia through the extracapsular extra-articular posteromedial safety incision. This enables the surgeon to accurately position guide wires, create the tibial tunnel, and protect the neurovascular structures. (From Fanelli 2012 [10]). **b** Intraoperative photograph of posterior instrumentation with the surgeon's finger in the posteromedial safety incision. (From Fanelli 2013 [9]. Reprinted with permission)

confirm the accuracy of the PCL tibial tunnel, and to facilitate the flow of the surgical procedure. The neurovascular structures of the popliteal fossa are in close proximity to the posterior capsule of the knee joint, and are at risk during the transtibial PCL reconstruction. The posteromedial safety incision is very important for the protection of these structures.

portion of the procedure. **c** The surgeon is seated during the PCL, ACL, and lateral-side reconstruction. *PCL* posterior cruciate ligament, *ACL* anterior cruciate ligament. (From Fanelli 2013 [9]. Reprinted with permission)

The curved over-the-top PCL instruments (Biomet Sports Medicine, Warsaw, Indiana) are used to sequentially lyse adhesions in the posterior aspect of the knee and elevate the capsule from the posterior tibial ridge. This will allow accurate placement of the PCL/ACL drill guide and correct placement of the tibial tunnel (Fig. 9.4).

The arm of the PCL/ACL guide (Biomet Sports Medicine, Warsaw, Indiana) is inserted through the inferior me-

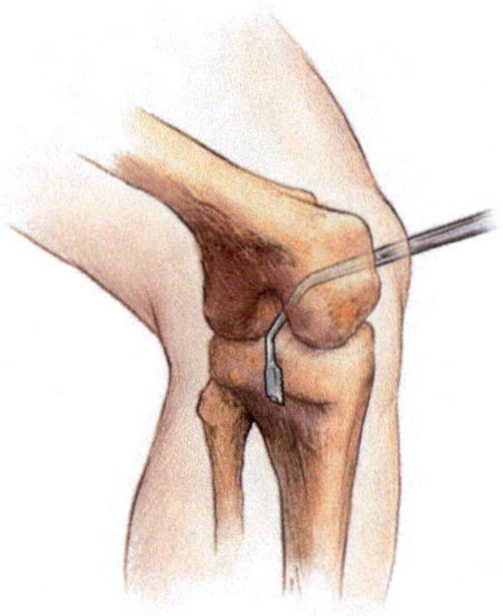

Fig. 9.4 Posterior capsular elevation. (From Fanelli 2012 [10])

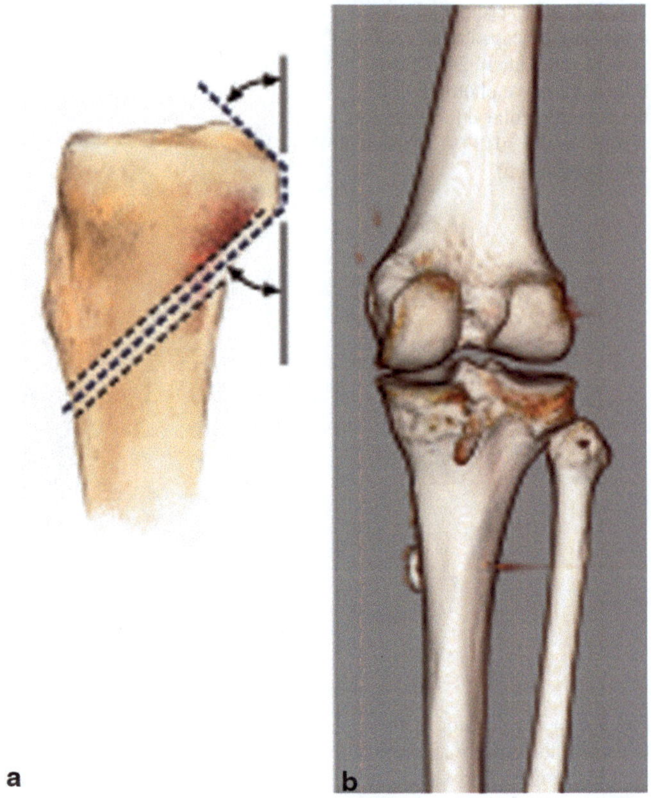

Fig. 9.6 **a** Drawing demonstrating the desired turning angles the PCL graft will make after the creation of the tibial tunnel. (From Fanelli 2012 [10]). **b** Three-dimensional CT scan demonstrating the position of a well placed PCL tibial tunnel. Note the *smooth turning angles* the PCL graft will take. *PCL* posterior cruciate ligament, *CT* computerized tomography. (From Fanelli 2013 [9]. Reprinted with permission)

dial patellar portal. The tip of the guide is positioned at the inferior lateral aspect of the PCL anatomic insertion site. This is below the tibial ridge posterior and in the lateral aspect of the PCL anatomic insertion site. The bullet portion of the guide contacts the anteromedial surface of the proximal tibia at a point midway between the posteromedial border of the tibia and the tibial crest anterior at or just below the level of the tibial tubercle (Fig. 9.5). This will provide an angle of graft orientation such that the graft will turn two very smooth 45° angles on the posterior aspect of the tibia (Fig. 9.6). The tip of the guide, in the posterior aspect of the tibia, is confirmed with the surgeon's finger through the extracapsular extra-articular posteromedial safety incision. Intraoperative AP and lateral X-ray may also be used; however, I do not routinely use intraoperative X-ray. When the PCL/ACL guide is positioned in the desired area, a blunt spade-tipped guide wire is drilled from anterior to posterior. The surgeon's finger confirms the position of the guide wire through the posteromedial safety incision.

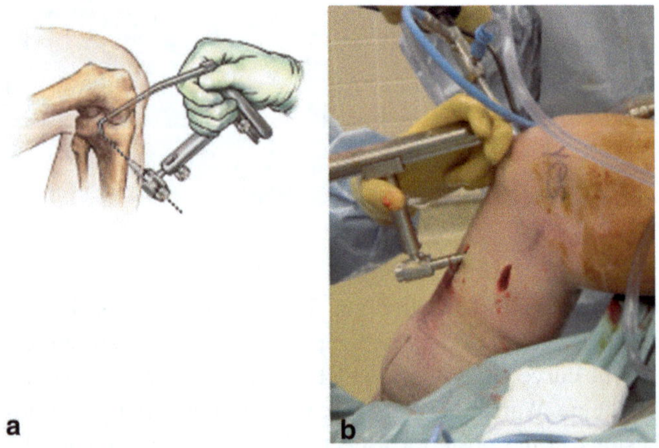

Fig. 9.5 **a** PCL–ACL drill guide positioned to place guide wire in preparation for creation of the transtibial PCL tibial tunnel. (From Fanelli 2012 [10]). **b** Intraoperative photograph of the drill guide positioned to create the PCL tibial tunnel. *PCL* posterior cruciate ligament, *ACL* anterior cruciate ligament. (From Fanelli 2013 [9]. Reprinted with permission)

The appropriately sized standard cannulated reamer is used to create the tibial tunnel. The surgeon's finger through the extracapsular extra-articular posteromedial incision is monitoring the position of the guide wire. When the drill is engaged in bone, the guide wire is reversed, blunt end pointing posterior, for additional patient safety. The drill is advanced until it comes to the posterior cortex of the tibia. The chuck is disengaged from the drill, and completion of the tibial tunnel is performed by hand (Fig. 9.7).

The PCL single- or double-bundle femoral tunnels are made from inside out using the double-bundle aimers or an endoscopic reamer can be used as an aiming device (Biomet Sports Medicine, Warsaw, Indiana). The appropriately sized double-bundle aimer or endoscopic reamer is inserted through a low anterolateral patellar arthroscopic portal to create the PCL anterolateral bundle femoral tunnel with the surgical knee in 90–110° of knee flexion. The double-bundle aimer or endoscopic reamer is positioned directly on the footprint of the femoral anterolateral bundle PCL insertion site (Fig. 9.8). The appropriately sized guide wire is drilled through the aimer or endoscopic reamer, through the bone, and out a small skin incision. Care is taken to prevent any

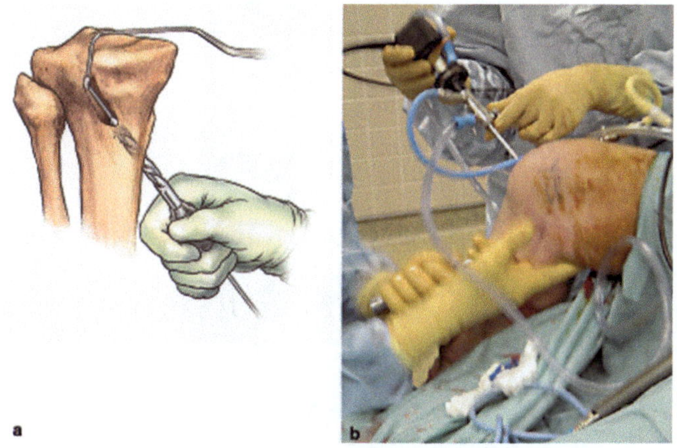

Fig. 9.7 **a** Final PCL tibial tunnel reaming by hand for an additional margin of safety. (From Fanelli 2012 [10]). **b** Intraoperative photograph of hand finishing of the PCL tibial tunnel. *PCL* posterior cruciate ligament. (From Fanelli 2013 [9]. Reprinted with permission)

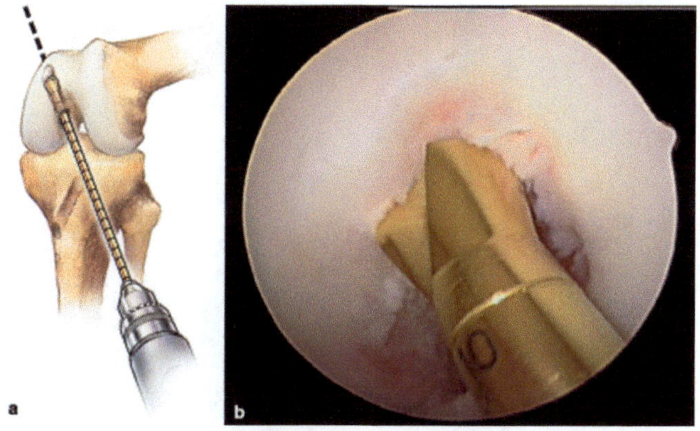

Fig. 9.9 **a** Endoscopic acorn reamer is used to create the PCL anterolateral bundle femoral tunnel through the low anterolateral patellar portal. (From Fanelli 2012 [10]). **b** Intraoperative view of an endoscopic acorn reamer is positioned to create the PCL anterolateral bundle femoral tunnel. *PCL* posterior cruciate ligament. (From Fanelli 2013 [9]. Reprinted with permission)

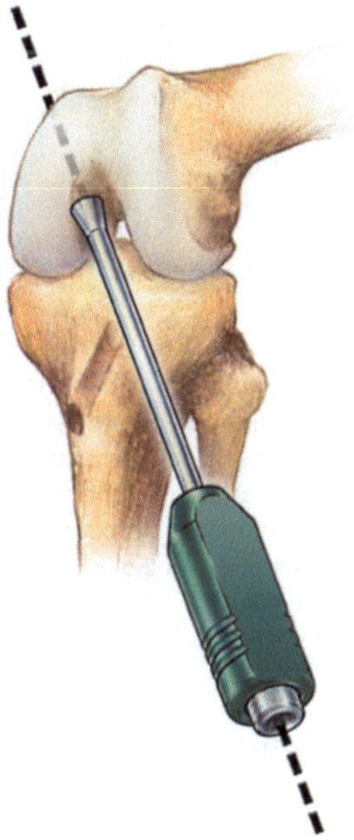

Fig. 9.8 Double-bundle aimer positioned to drill a guide wire for creation of the PCL anterolateral bundle tunnel. *PCL* posterior cruciate ligament. (From Fanelli 2012 [10])

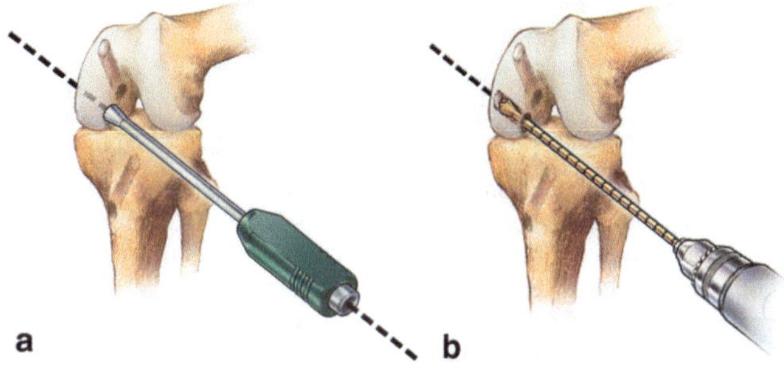

Fig. 9.10 **a** Double-bundle aimer positioned to drill a guide wire for creation of the PCL posteromedial bundle femoral tunnel through the low anterolateral patellar portal. (From Fanelli 2013 [9]. Reprinted with permission). **b** Endoscopic acorn reamer is used to create the PCL posteromedial bundle femoral tunnel. A 5-mm bone bridge is maintained between tunnels. *PCL* posterior cruciate ligament. (From Fanelli 2012 [10])

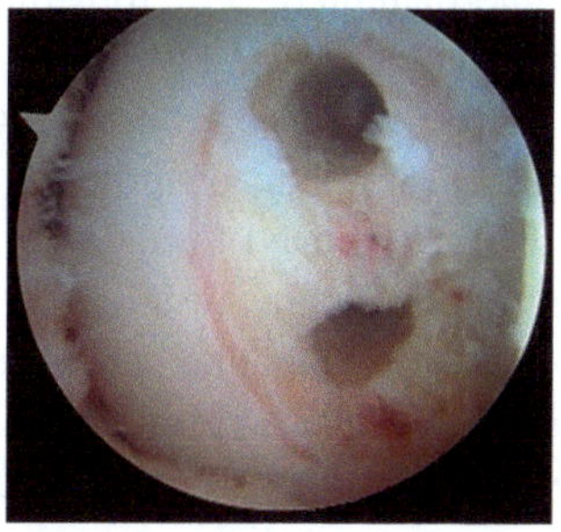

Fig. 9.11 Completed PCL anterolateral and posteromedial bundle tunnels fill the anatomic footprint of the PCL. A 5-mm bone bridge is maintained between the tunnels. *PCL* posterior cruciate ligament. (From Fanelli 2013 [9]. Reprinted with permission)

compromise of the articular surface. The double-bundle aimer is removed, and the endoscopic reamer is used to drill the anterolateral PCL femoral tunnel from inside to outside (Fig. 9.9). When the surgeon chooses to perform a double-bundle double-femoral tunnel PCL reconstruction, the same process is repeated for the posteromedial bundle of the PCL (Fig. 9.10). Care must be taken to ensure that there will be an adequate bone bridge (approximately 5 mm) between the two femoral tunnels prior to drilling. This is accomplished using the calibrated probe, and direct arthroscopic visualization of the PCL femoral anatomic insertion sites (Fig. 9.11).

My preferred surgical technique of PCL femoral tunnel creation from inside to outside is for two reasons. There is a greater distance and margin of safety between the PCL

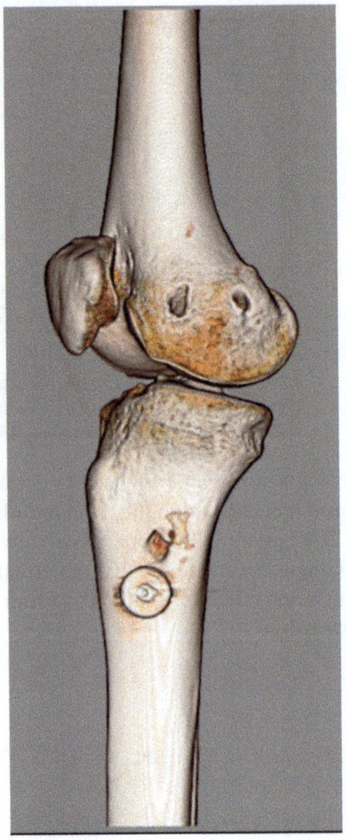

Fig. 9.12 Three-dimensional CT scan showing properly positioned PCL femoral tunnel exit points after inside-to-outside PCL femoral tunnel creation. Note the distance between the femoral tunnel exit points and the distal medial femoral condyle articular surface. *CT* computerized tomography, *PCL* posterior cruciate ligament. (From Fanelli 2013 [9]. Reprinted with permission)

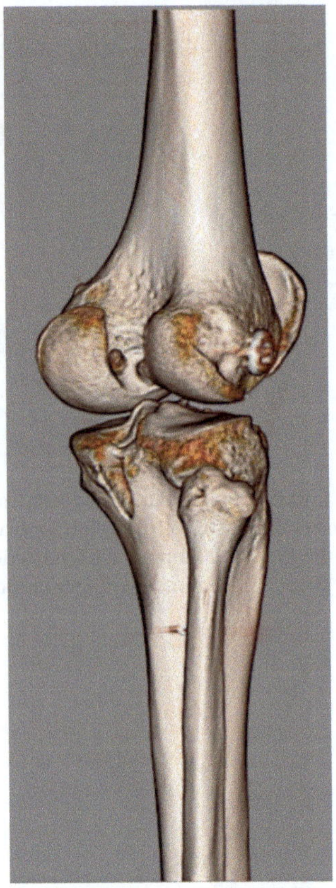

Fig. 9.13 Three-dimensional CT scan showing properly positioned intra-articular PCL femoral tunnel position after inside-to-outside PCL femoral tunnel creation. A more accurate placement of the PCL femoral tunnels is possible because I can place the double-bundle aimer or endoscopic reamer on the anatomic footprint of the anterolateral or posteromedial PCL insertion site under direct visualization. *CT* computerized tomography, *PCL* posterior cruciate ligament. (From Fanelli 2013 [9]. Reprinted with permission)

femoral tunnels and the medial femoral condyle articular surface using the inside-to-outside method (Fig. 9.12). Additionally, a more accurate placement of the PCL femoral tunnels is possible, in my opinion, because I can place the double-bundle aimer or endoscopic reamer on the anatomic footprint of the anterolateral or posteromedial PCL insertion site under direct visualization (Fig. 9.13).

A Magellan suture retriever (Biomet Sports Medicine, Warsaw, Indiana) is introduced through the tibial tunnel into the joint, and retrieved through the femoral tunnel (Fig. 9.14). The traction sutures of the graft material are attached to the loop of the Magellan suture retriever, and the graft is pulled into position. The graft material is secured on the femoral side using a bioabsorbable interference screw for primary aperture opening fixation, and a polyethylene ligament fixation button for backup fixation.

The cyclic dynamic method of graft tensioning using the Biomet graft-tensioning boot is used to tension the PCL and ACL grafts [11]. This tensioning method is discussed in Chap. 21 of this book. Tension is placed on the PCL graft distally using the Biomet graft-tensioning boot (Biomet Sports Medicine, Warsaw, Indiana) (Fig. 9.15). Tension is gradually applied with the knee in 0° of flexion (full extension) reducing the tibia on the femur. This restores the anatomic tibial step off. The knee is cycled through a full range of motion multiple times to allow pretensioning and settling of the graft. The process is repeated until there is no further change in the torque setting on the graft tensioner. The knee is placed in 70–90° of flexion and fixation is achieved on the tibial side of the PCL graft with a bioabsorbable interference screw and backup fixation with a bicortical screw and spiked ligament washer or polyethylene ligament fixation button (Fig. 9.16).

Additional Technical Ideas

The posteromedial safety incision protects the neurovascular structures, confirms the accuracy of the PCL tibial tunnel placement, and enhances the flow of the surgical procedure. We have found it very important to use primary and backup fixation. During cruciate ligament reconstruction, primary aperture fixation is achieved with bioabsorbable interference

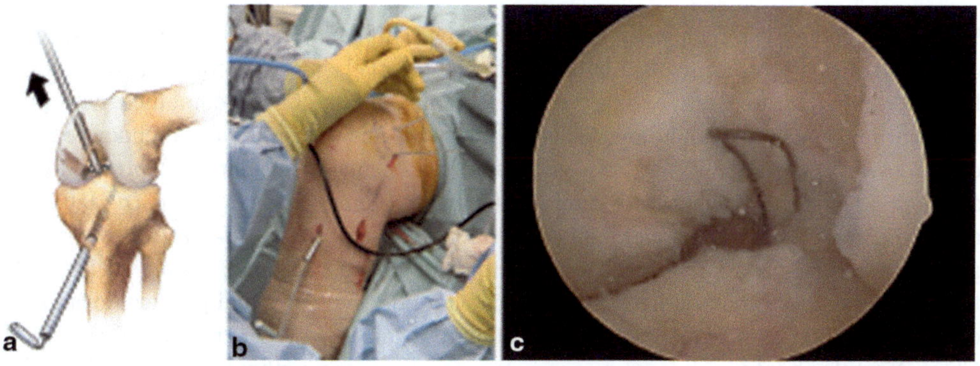

Fig. 9.14 **a** Magellan suture passing device. (From Fanelli 2012 [10]). **b** and **c** Intraoperative external and arthroscopic views demonstrating the positioning of the Magellan suture- and graft-passing device. (From Fanelli 2013 [9]. Reprinted with permission)

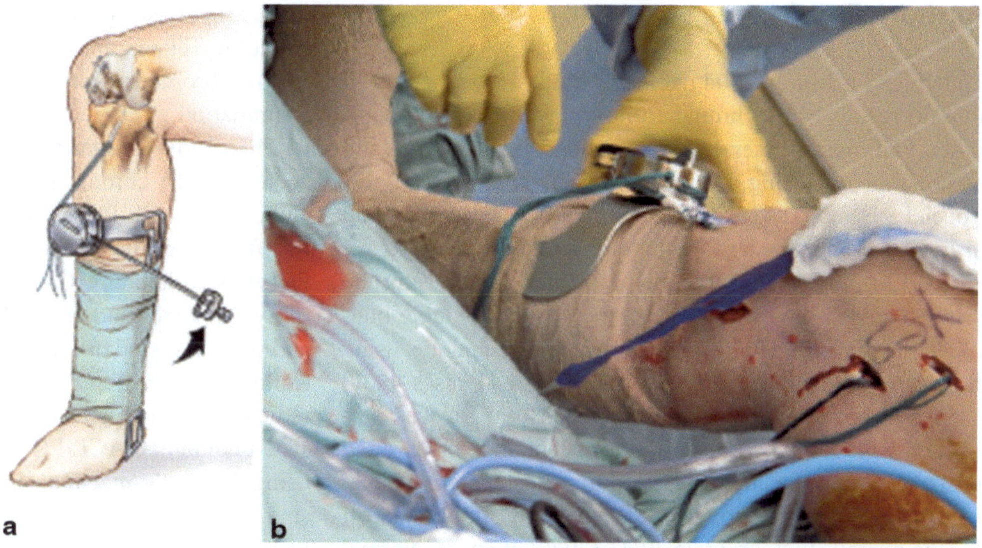

Fig. 9.15 **a** Knee ligament graft-tensioning boot is used to tension the PCL graft. This mechanical tensioning device uses a ratcheted torque wrench device to assist the surgeon during graft tensioning. (From Fanelli 2012 [10]). **b** Intraoperative photograph of Biomet tensioning boot applied to the tibia to tension the PCL reconstruction graft. *PCL* posterior cruciate ligament. (From Fanelli 2013 [9]. Reprinted with permission)

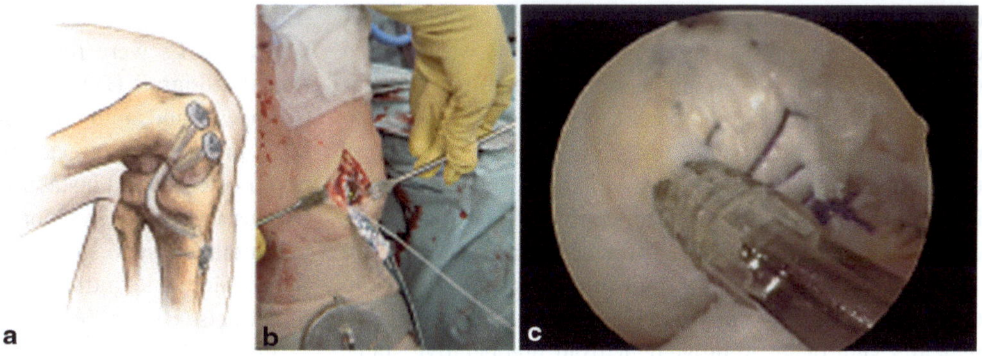

Fig. 9.16 **a** PCL final graft fixation using primary and backup fixation. (From Fanelli 2012 [10]). **b** PCL final tibial fixation. **c** Interference fit fixation of PCL graft in femoral tunnel. *PCL* posterior cruciate ligament. (From Fanelli 2013 [9]. Reprinted with permission)

screws, and backup fixation is performed with a screw and spiked ligament washer and ligament fixation buttons. Secure fixation is critical to the success of this surgical procedure. Mechanical tensioning of the PCL at 0° of knee flexion (full extension) and restoration of the normal anatomic tibial step-off at 70–90° of flexion and fixation of the PCL graft at 70–90° of knee flexion has provided the most reproducible method of establishing the neutral point of the tibia–femoral relationship in our experience. Full range of motion is confirmed on the operating table to assure the knee is not "captured" by the reconstruction.

Postoperative Rehabilitation

The knee is maintained in full extension for 3–5 weeks non-weight bearing. Progressive range of motion occurs during postoperative week 3–5 through 10. Progressive weight bearing occurs at the beginning of postoperative weeks 3 through 5. Progressive closed kinetic chain strength training, proprioceptive training, and continued motion exercises are initiated very slowly beginning at postoperative week 12. The long-leg range-of-motion brace is discontinued after the 10th week. Return to sports and heavy labor occurs after the

9–12th postoperative month when sufficient strength, range of motion, and proprioceptive skills have returned [16–19]. It is very important to carefully observe these complex knee ligament injury patients, and get a feel for the "personality of the knee." The surgeon may need to make adjustments and individualize the postoperative rehabilitation program as necessary. Careful and gentle range of motion under general anesthesia is a very useful tool in the treatment of these complex cases and is utilized as necessary. Our postoperative rehabilitation program is discussed in more detail in Chap. 25 of this book.

Author's Results

Fanelli and Edson in 2004 published the 2–10-year (24–120 month) results of 41 chronic arthroscopically assisted combined PCL/posterolateral reconstructions evaluated pre and postoperatively using Lysholm, Tegner, and Hospital for Special Surgery (HSS) knee ligament rating scales, KT-1000 arthrometer testing, stress radiography, and physical examination [20]. PCL reconstructions were performed using the arthroscopically assisted single-femoral tunnel–single-bundle transtibial tunnel PCL reconstruction technique using fresh-frozen Achilles tendon allografts in all 41 cases. In all 41 cases, posterolateral instability reconstruction was performed with combined biceps femoris tendon tenodesis and posterolateral capsular shift procedures. Postoperative physical exam revealed normal posterior drawer/tibial step-off for the overall study group in 29/41 (70 %) of knees. Normal posterior drawer and tibial step-offs were achieved in 91.7 % of the knees tensioned with the Biomet Sports Medicine mechanical graft tensioner. Posterolateral stability was restored to normal in 11/41 (27 %) of knees, and tighter than the normal knee in 29/41 (71 %) of knees evaluated with the external rotation thigh–foot angle test. Thirty-degree varus stress testing was normal in 40/41 (97 %) of knees, and grade 1 laxity in 1/41 (3 %) of knees. Postoperative KT-1000 arthrometer testing mean side-to-side difference measurements were 1.80 mm (PCL screen), 2.11 mm (corrected posterior), and 0.63-mm (corrected anterior) measurements. This is a statistically significant improvement from preoperative status for the PCL screen and the corrected posterior measurements ($p=0.001$). The postoperative stress radiographic mean side-to-side difference measurement measured at 90° of knee flexion, and 32 lb. of posterior-directed force applied to the proximal tibia using the Telos device was 2.26 mm. This is a statistically significant improvement from preoperative measurements ($p=0.001$). Postoperative Lysholm, Tegner, and HSS knee ligament rating scale mean values were 91.7, 4.92, and 88.7, respectively, demonstrating a statistically significant improvement from preoperative status ($p=0.001$). The authors concluded that chronic combined PCL/posterolateral instabilities can be successfully treated with arthroscopic PCL reconstruction using fresh-frozen Achilles tendon allograft combined with posterolateral corner reconstruction using biceps tendon tenodesis combined with posterolateral capsular shift procedure. Statistically significant improvement is noted ($p=0.001$) from the preoperative condition at 2–10-year follow-up using objective parameters of knee ligament rating scales, arthrometer testing, stress radiography, and physical examination.

Our results of multiple-ligament-injured knee treatment without mechanical graft tensioning are outlined below [21]. This study presented the 2–10-year (24–120 month) results of 35 arthroscopically assisted combined ACL/PCL reconstructions evaluated pre and postoperatively using Lysholm, Tegner, and HSS knee ligament rating scales, KT-1000 arthrometer testing, stress radiography, and physical examination.

This study population included 26 males, 9 females, 19 acute, and 16 chronic knee injuries. Ligament injuries included 19 ACL/PCL/posterolateral instabilities, 9 ACL/PCL/medial collateral ligament (MCL) instabilities, 6 ACL/PCL/posterolateral/MCL instabilities, and 1 ACL/PCL instability. All knees had grade III preoperative ACL/PCL laxity, and were assessed pre- and postoperatively with arthrometer testing, three different knee ligament rating scales, stress radiography, and physical examination. Arthroscopically assisted combined ACL/PCL reconstructions were performed using the single-incision endoscopic ACL technique, and the single-femoral tunnel–single-bundle transtibial tunnel PCL technique. PCLs were reconstructed with allograft Achilles tendon (26 knees), autograft bone patellar tendon bone (BTB; 7 knees), and autograft semitendinosus/gracilis (2 knees). ACLs were reconstructed with autograft BTB (16 knees), allograft BTB (12 knees), Achilles tendon allograft (6 knees), and autograft semitendinosus/gracilis (1 knee). MCL injuries were treated with bracing or open reconstruction. Posterolateral instability was treated with biceps femoris tendon transfer, with or without primary repair, and posterolateral capsular shift procedures as indicated. No Biomet Sports Medicine graft-tensioning boot was used in this series of patients (Biomet Sports Medicine, Warsaw, Indiana).

Postoperative physical examination results revealed normal posterior drawer/tibial step-off in 16/35 (46 %) of knees and Normal Lackman and pivot shift tests in 33/35 (94 %) of knees. Posterolateral stability was restored to normal in 6/25 (24 %) of knees, and tighter than the normal knee in 19/25 (76 %) of knees evaluated with the external rotation thigh–foot angle test. Thirty-degree varus stress testing was normal in 22/25 (88 %) of knees, and grade 1 laxity in 3/25 (12 %) of knees. Thirty-degree valgus stress testing was normal in 7/7 (100 %) of surgically treated MCL tears, and normal in 7/8 (87.5 %) of brace-treated knees. Postoperative KT-1000 arthrometer testing mean side-to-side difference measurements were 2.7 mm (PCL screen), 2.6 mm (corrected posterior), and 1.0 mm (corrected anterior) measurements, a statistically significant improvement from preoperative status ($p=0.001$). Postoperative stress radiographic side-to-side difference measurements measured at 90° of knee flexion, and 32 pounds of posteriorly directed proximal force were 0–3 mm in 11/21 (52.3 %), 4–5 mm in 5/21 (23.8 %), and 6–10 mm in 4/21 (19 %) of knees. Postoperative Lysholm, Tegner, and HSS knee ligament rating scale mean values were 91.2, 5.3, and 86.8 respectively, demonstrating a statistically significant improvement from preoperative status ($p=0.001$). No Biomet graft-tensioning boot was used in this series of patients.

The conclusions drawn from the study were that combined ACL/PCL instabilities could be successfully treated with arthroscopic reconstruction and the appropriate collateral ligament surgery. Statistically significant improvement was noted from the preoperative condition at 2–10-year follow-up using objective parameters of knee ligament rating scales, arthrometer testing, stress radiography, and physical examination.

Our results of multiple-ligament-injured knee treatment using mechanical graft tensioning are outlined below [22]. These data present the 2-year follow-up of 15 arthroscopically assisted ACL–PCL reconstructions using the Biomet graft-tensioning boot (Biomet Sports Medicine, Warsaw, Indiana). This study group consists of 11 chronic and 4 acute injuries. These injury patterns included six ACL/PCL/PLC injuries, four ACL/PCL/MCL injuries, and five ACL/PCL/PLC/MCL injuries. The Biomet graft-tensioning boot was used during the procedures as in the surgical technique described above. All knees had grade III preoperative ACL/PCL laxity, and were assessed pre and postoperatively using Lysholm, Tegner, and HSS knee ligament rating scales, KT-1000 arthrometer testing, stress radiography, and physical examination.

Arthroscopically assisted combined ACL/PCL reconstructions were performed using the single-incision endoscopic ACL technique, and the single-femoral tunnel–single-bundle transtibial tunnel PCL technique. PCLs were reconstructed with allograft Achilles tendon in all 15 knees. ACLs were reconstructed with Achilles tendon allograft in all 15 knees. MCL injuries were treated surgically using primary repair, posteromedial capsular shift, and allograft augmentation as indicated. Posterolateral instability was treated with allograft semitendinosus free graft, with or without primary repair, and posterolateral capsular shift procedures as indicated. The Biomet graft-tensioning boot was used in this series of patients.

Post-reconstruction physical examination results revealed normal posterior drawer/tibial step-off in 13/15 (86.6 %) of knees, Normal Lackman test in 13/15 (86.6 %) knees, and normal pivot shift tests in 14/15 (93.3 %) knees. Posterolateral stability was restored to normal in all knees with posterolateral instability when evaluated with the external rotation thigh–foot angle test (nine knees equal to the normal knee and two knees tighter than the normal knee). Thirty-degree varus stress testing was restored to normal in all 11 knees with posterolateral lateral instability. Thirty- and zero-degree valgus stress testing was restored to normal in all nine knees with medial-side laxity. Postoperative KT-1000 arthrometer testing mean side-to-side difference measurements were 1.6 mm (range 3–7 mm) for the PCL screen, 1.6 mm (range 4.5–9 mm) for the corrected posterior, and 0.5 mm (range 2.5–6 mm) for the corrected anterior measurements, a significant improvement from preoperative status. Postoperative stress radiographic side-to-side difference measurements measured at 90° of knee flexion, and 32 pounds of posteriorly directed proximal force using the Telos stress radiography device were 0–3 mm in 10/15 knees (66.7 %), 0–4 mm in 14/15 (93.3 %), 4 mm in 4/15 knees (26.7 %), and 7 mm in 1/15 knees (6.67 %). Postoperative Lysholm, Tegner, and HSS knee ligament rating scale mean values were 86.7 (range 69–95), 4.5 (range 2–7), and 85.3 (range 65–93) respectively, demonstrating a significant improvement from preoperative status. The study group demonstrates the efficacy and success of using a mechanical graft-tensioning device in PCL and ACL reconstruction procedures.

Our comparison of single- and double-bundle PCL reconstruction in the PCL-based multiple-ligament-injured knee using allograft tissue revealed the following [23]. Ninety consecutive arthroscopic transtibial PCL reconstructions were performed by a single surgeon (GCF). Forty-five single- and double-bundle reconstructions were performed using fresh-frozen Achilles tendon allograft for the anterolateral bundle and tibialis anterior allograft for the posteromedial bundle. Postoperative comparative results were assessed using Telos stress radiography, KT 1000, Lysholm, Tegner, and HSS knee ligament rating scales. Postoperative period ranged from 15 to 72 months.

Three groups of data were analyzed: Single- and double-bundle all; single-bundle PCL collateral and PCL double-bundle collateral; and single-bundle PCL–ACL collateral and double-bundle PCL–ACL collateral.

Mean postoperative side-to-side difference values for Telos, KT PCL screen, KT corrected posterior, and KT corrected anterior measurements for the overall single-bundle group in millimeters were 2.56, 1.91, 2.11, and 0.23, respectively. Mean postoperative side-to-side difference values for Telos, KT PCL screen, KT corrected posterior, and KT corrected anterior measurements for the overall double-bundle group in millimeters were 2.36, 2.46, 2.94, and 0.15, respectively. Mean postoperative values for Tegner, Lysholm, and HSS knee ligament rating scales for the single-bundle group were 5.0, 90.3, and 86.2, respectively. Mean postoperative values for Tegner, Lysholm, and HSS knee ligament rating scales for the double-bundle group were 4.6, 87.6, and 83.3, respectively.

Mean postoperative side-to-side difference values for Telos, KT PCL screen, KT corrected posterior, and KT corrected anterior measurements for the PCL-collateral single-bundle group in millimeters were 2.59, 1.63, 2.03, and 0.25, respectively. Mean postoperative side-to-side difference values for Telos, KT PCL screen, KT corrected posterior, and KT corrected anterior measurements for the PCL-collateral double-bundle group in millimeters were 1.85, 2.03, 2.83, and −0.17, respectively. Mean postoperative values for Tegner, Lysholm, and HSS knee ligament rating scales for the single-bundle PCL-collateral group were 5.4, 90.9, and 87.7, respectively. Mean postoperative values for Tegner, Lysholm, and HSS knee ligament rating scales for the double-bundle PCL-collateral group were 4.9, 89.0, and 86.5, respectively.

Mean postoperative side-to-side difference values for Telos, KT PCL screen, KT corrected posterior, and KT corrected anterior measurements for the PCL–ACL-collateral single-bundle group in millimeters were 2.53, 2.19, 2.19, and 0.22, respectively. Mean postoperative side-to-side difference values for Telos, KT PCL screen, KT corrected posterior, and KT corrected anterior measurements for the PCL–ACL-collateral double-bundle group in millimeters were 3.16, 2.86, 3.09, and 0.41, respectively. Mean postoperative values for Tegner, Lysholm, and HSS knee ligament rating scales for the PCL–ACL-collateral single-bundle group were 4.7, 89.6, and 84.6, respectively. Mean postoperative values for Tegner, Lysholm, and HSS knee ligament rating scales for the PCL–ACL-collateral double-bundle group were 4.3, 86.0, and 79.4, respectively. There was no statistically significant difference between the single- and double-bundle PCL reconstruction in any of the groups compared ($p > 0.05$).

Return to pre-injury level of activity was evaluated between the single- and double-bundle PCL reconstruction groups. The bicruciate single-bundle reconstruction group return to pre-injury level of activity was 73.3 %, and the bicruciate double-bundle reconstruction group return to pre-injury level of activity was 84.0 %. There was no statistically significant difference ($p = 0.572$) between the single- and double-bundle group in the PCL-based multiple-ligament-injured knee. Both single- and double-bundle arthroscopic transtibial tunnel PCL reconstructions provide excellent results in these complex multiple-ligament-injured knee instability patterns. Our results did not indicate that one PCL reconstruction surgical procedure was clearly superior to the other.

Our 2–18-year postsurgical results in combined PCL, ACL, and medial- and lateral-side knee injuries (global laxity) revealed the following information [24]. Forty combined PCL–ACL–lateral–medial-side (global laxity reconstructions were performed by a single surgeon (GCF). Twenty-eight of 40 were available for 2–18-year follow-up (70 % follow-up rate). The patients were evaluated postoperatively with three different knee ligament rating scales for physical examination and functional capacity (HSS, Lysholm, Tegner). Static stability was assessed postoperatively comparing the normal to the injured knee using the KT-1000 knee ligament arthrometer (PCL screen, corrected posterior, corrected anterior, and 30° posterior-to-anterior translation), and stress radiography at 90° of flexion to assess PCL static stability using the Telos device. All measurements are reported as a side-to-side difference in millimeters comparing the normal to the injured knee. Range of motion, varus and valgus stability, and axial rotation stability of the tibia relative to the femur using the dial test are reported comparing the injured to the normal knee. Incidence of degenerative joint disease and return to pre-injury level of function is also reported.

Knee ligament rating scale mean scores were: HSS 79.3/100 (range 56–95), Lysholm 83.8/100 (range 58–100), and Tegner 4/10 (range 2–9). KT-1000 mean side-to-side difference measurements in millimeters were: PCL screen at 90° of knee flexion 2.02 mm (range 0–7 mm), corrected posterior at 70° of knee flexion 2.48 mm (range 0–9 mm), corrected anterior at 70° of knee flexion 0.28 mm (range 3–7 mm), and the 30° of knee flexion posterior-to-anterior translation 1.0 mm (range 6–6 mm). Telos stress radiography at 90° of knee flexion with a posterior displacement force applied to the area of the tibial tubercle mean side-to-side difference measurements in millimeters were 2.35 mm (range 2–8 mm).

Range of motion side-to-side difference mean flexion loss comparing the normal to the injured knee was 14.0° (range 0–38°). There were no flexion contractures. Varus and valgus stability was evaluated on physical examination at hyperextension, 0°, and 30° of knee flexion comparing the injured to the normal knee. Symmetrical varus stability was achieved in 93.3 % of knees, and symmetrical valgus stability was achieved in 92.6 % of knees. The dial test performed at 30° of knee flexion to evaluate axial rotation posterolateral stability comparing the injured to the normal knee was symmetrical in 85.2 %, tighter than the normal knee (less external rotation) in 11.1 %, and more lax (greater external rotation) in 3.7 % of knees. Thus, posterolateral axial rotation instability was corrected or overcorrected in 96.3 % of knees.

Radiographic post-traumatic degenerative joint disease occurred in 29.6 % of injured knees. No degenerative joint disease was found in 70.4 % of the injured knees. Postoperatively, patients were able to return to their pre-injury level of activity in 59.3 % of cases and returned to decreased level of postoperative activity in 40.7 % of cases.

Summary

The goals leading to successful PCL reconstruction surgery include identification and treatment of associated pathology such as posterolateral instability, posteromedial instability, and lower extremity malalignment. The use of strong graft material, properly placed tunnels to as closely as possible, approximate the posterior cruciate ligament insertion sites, and minimization of graft bending also enhance the probability of PCL reconstruction success. In addition, mechanical graft tensioning, primary and backup PCL graft fixation, and the appropriate postoperative rehabilitation program are also necessary ingredients for PCL reconstruction success. Both single- and double-bundle PCL reconstruction surgical techniques are successful when evaluated with stress radiography, KT-1000 arthrometer measurements, and knee ligament rating scales. Indications for double-bundle PCL reconstruction as of this writing include severe hyperextension of the knee and revision PCL reconstruction. Our 2–18-year postsurgical results in combined PCL, ACL, and medial- and lateral-side knee injuries (global laxity) revealed very successful PCL reconstruction using the arthroscopic transtibial tunnel surgical technique.

References

1. Fanelli GC. PCL injuries in trauma patients. Arthroscopy. 1993;9:291–4.
2. Fanelli GC, Edson CJ. PCL injuries in trauma patients, part II. Arthroscopy. 1995;11:526–9.
3. Noyes FR, Barber-Westin SD. Posterior cruciate ligament revision reconstruction, part 1. Causes of surgical failure in 52 consecutive operations. Am J Sports Med. 2005;33(5):646–54.
4. Fanelli GC, Feldmann DD. Management of combined anterior cruciate ligament/posterior cruciate ligament/posterolateral complex injuries of the knee. Oper Tech Sports Med. 1999;7(3):143–9.
5. Fanelli GC, Harris JD. Surgical treatment of acute medial collateral ligament and posteromedial corner injuries of the knee. Sports Med Arthrosc Rev. 2006;14(2):78–83.
6. Fanelli GC, Harris JD. Late MCL (medial collateral ligament) reconstruction. Tech Knee Surg. 2007;6(2):99–105.
7. Fanelli GC, Giannotti BF, Edson CJ. The posterior cruciate ligament: arthroscopic evaluation and treatment. Current concepts review. Arthroscopy. 1994;10(6):673–88.
8. LaPrade RF. Arthroscopic evaluation of the lateral compartment of knees with grade 3 posterolateral knee complex injuries. Am J Sports Med. 1997;25(5):596–602.
9. Fanelli GC. Surgical treatment of combined PCL ACL medial and lateral side injuries (global laxity): acute and chronic. In: Fanelli GC, editor. The multiple ligament injured knee. A practical guide to management. 2nd ed. New York: Springer; 2013. pp. 281–301.
10. Fanelli GC. Rationale and surgical technique for PCL and multiple knee ligament reconstruction. 3rd ed. Warsaw: Biomet Sports Medicine; 2012.
11. Fanelli GC. Mechanical graft tensioning in multiple ligament knee surgery. In: Fanelli GC, editor. The multiple ligament injured knee. A practical guide to management. 2nd ed. New York: Springer; 2013. pp. 323–30.
12. Fanelli GC, Boyd J. How I manage PCL injuries. Oper Tech Sports Med. 2009;17(3):175–93.
13. Fanelli GC, Beck JD, Edson CJ. Double bundle posterior cruciate ligament reconstruction. Surgical technique and results. Sports Med Arthrosc Rev. 2010;18(4):242–8.
14. Fanelli GC, Beck JD, Edson CJ. Arthroscopic trans tibial double bundle PCL reconstruction. J Knee Surg. 2010;23(2):89–94.
15. Fanelli GC, Edson CJ, Reinheimer KN, Garofalo R. Posterior cruciate ligament and posterolateral corner reconstruction. Sports Med Arthrosc Rev. 2007;15(4):168–75.
16. Fanelli GC. Posterior cruciate ligament rehabilitation: how slow should we go? Arthroscopy. 2008;24(2):234–5.
17. Edson CJ, Fanelli GC, Beck JD. Rehabilitation after multiple ligament reconstruction of the knee. Sports Med Arthrosc Rev. 2011;19(2):162–6.
18. Edson CJ, Fanelli GC, Beck JD. Postoperative rehabilitation of the posterior cruciate ligament. Sports Med Arthrosc Rev. 2010;18(4):275–9.
19. Edson CJ, Fanelli GC. Postoperative rehabilitation of the multiple ligament injured knee. In: Fanelli GC, editor. The multiple ligament injured knee. A practical guide to management. 2nd ed. New York: Springer; 2013. pp. 437–42.
20. Fanelli GC, Edson CJ. Combined posterior cruciate ligament-posterolateral reconstruction with Achilles tendon allograft and biceps femoris tendon tenodesis: 2–10 year follow-up. Arthroscopy. 2004;20(4):339–45.
21. Fanelli GC, Edson CJ. Arthroscopically assisted combined ACL/PCL reconstruction. 2–10 year follow-up. Arthroscopy. 2002;18(7):703–14.
22. Fanelli GC, Edson CJ, Orcutt DR, Harris JD, Zijerdi D. Treatment of combined ACL PCL medial lateral side injuries of the knee. J Knee Surg. 2005;28(3):240–8.
23. Fanelli GC, Beck JD, Edson CJ. Single compared to double bundle PCL reconstruction using allograft tissue. J Knee Surg. 2012;25(1):59–64.
24. Fanelli GC, Edson CJ. Surgical treatment of combined PCL, ACL, medial, and lateral side injuries (global laxity): surgical technique and 2 to 18 year results. J Knee Surg. 2012;25(4):307–16.

Further Reading

25. Fanelli GC, editor. The multiple ligament injured knee. A practical guide to management. 2nd ed. New York: Springer; 2013.

Open Tibial Inlay Graft for Posterior Cruciate Ligament Reconstruction

10

S. Mark Heard and Meagan Heard

Development of the Open Tibial Inlay Technique

Due to the poor overall results from early posterior cruciate ligament (PCL) reconstruction techniques, conservative treatment was the standard of care for many years [1]. However, research shows that an untreated PCL-deficient knee leads to significant disability and reduced knee function when compared to an untreated anterior cruciate ligament (ACL)-deficient knee [2]. Clancy facilitated a change in the standard treatment after he published his case series of 23 patients introducing the transtibial tunnel patellar tendon graft PCL reconstruction [3]. The positive results reported by Clancy in both acute and chronic PCL-deficient knees inspired surgeons to pursue this surgical approach. Despite this surgical advance, the transtibial PCL reconstruction still demonstrated a high failure rate [3]. In 1992, Dr. Marc Friedman discussed PCL graft weakening in an instructional course lecture and indicated that it was caused by wear on the graft as it exits the tibial tunnel and passes around the posterior tibia. He coined the phrase, "the killer turn" for this concern [4]. Publications regarding the killer turn with the transtibial tunnel technique have since become more prevalent in the literature [4–10]. In addition, biomechanical studies of PCL reconstructions also suggest this higher rate of graft failure to be due to wearing of the graft at the posterior tibial plateau tunnel exit [7–9].

There is no definitive description of the rationale for the open tibial inlay technique; however, Dr. Jack Hughston published a history of PCL surgery, which speaks to how reconstruction techniques have evolved [1]. For example, it may have developed secondary to positive results with early open reduction and internal fixation of avulsion fractures of the PCL insertion on the tibia. Trickey and Torsisu separately published positive outcomes of open reduction and internal fixation of PCL avulsion fractures on the posterior tibia [11, 12]. The surgical approach and internal fixation used in this technique closely mimic the open tibial inlay technique. Alternately, the open tibial inlay technique may have evolved as a means of addressing late failures, or it may have developed as a solution in the operating room when wrestling a graft around the sharp corner of the tibial plateau.

Jakob and Ruegsegger, followed by Berg were the first surgeons to describe the open tibial inlay technique [4, 10]. These authors described the technique as well as the clinical results they obtained from their initial patients in detail [4, 10]. Bergfeld and Parker from the Cleveland Clinic then published their results on cadaveric open tibial inlay reconstructions and related biomechanical studies [13]. These studies compared the open tibial inlay and transtibial tunnel techniques, demonstrating minimal graft wear and thinning in the open tibial inlay specimens. Drawing on the success of these cadaveric studies, Bergfeld and Parker began performing this procedure in patients [13]. These surgeons are often given credit for popularizing this technique in North America. Around the same time, orthopedic surgeons Benedetto, Jakon, Thomann, and Gaechter started utilizing this procedure in Europe [13].

The open tibial inlay approach has been adopted by surgeons because it addresses the killer turn and initial graft fixation, therefore, managing the two biggest concerns of the tibial tunnel portion of the transtibial technique [4–6,14]. As with all surgical techniques, the open tibial inlay procedure will continue to evolve as surgical instruments, surgical techniques, and intraoperative technologies develop. Researchers have recently published the surgical approach and results of all-arthroscopic tibial inlay techniques [15–18]. The all-arthroscopic tibial inlay techniques address some of the concerns of the open tibial inlay technique by eliminating the

S. M. Heard (✉)
Sport Medicine Orthopaedic Surgery, Banff Sport Medicine,
Suite 207-303 Lynx Street, 1300, Banff, Alberta T1L 1B3, Canada
e-mail: mheard@telusplanet.net

M. Heard
Banff Sport Medicine, Suite 207-303 Lynx Street, 1300, T1L 1B3
Banff, Alberta, Canada
e-mail: heard.meagan@gmail.com

G. C. Fanelli (ed.), *Posterior Cruciate Ligament Injuries*,
DOI 10.1007/978-3-319-12072-0_10, © Springer International Publishing Switzerland 2015

large incision and patient position changes, and reducing the duration of the surgery [15–18]. However, these techniques are very technically demanding and have slightly, though not statistically, weaker initial fixation than the open tibial inlay technique [18]. More analysis will determine whether this technique will produce superior outcomes and gain widespread popularity.

Biomechanical Studies

Biomechanically, the most important aspect of the PCL reconstruction is not how the graft behaves during the surgery at time zero, but rather how the graft behaves during normal use or cyclic loading. It is important to note that there is minimal literature assessing the biomechanics of PCL reconstruction using the open tibial inlay technique. Time-zero cadaveric studies demonstrate no biomechanical advantage to the open tibial inlay technique. However, cyclic loading biomechanical studies suggest that there is some advantage to the open tibial inlay surgical technique [8–10].

Oakes et al. assessed 12 paired male cadaveric knees, with each pair receiving matching patellar tendon allograft reconstructions with an open tibial inlay technique on one side, and a transtibial tunnel technique on the other [7]. The proximal ends of all grafts were pretensioned to restore knee stability at 90° of flexion. No significant differences were seen in the mean graft forces between the two techniques under tibial loads consisting of 100 Newtons (N) of posterior tibial force. However, mean graft forces with both reconstruction techniques were significantly higher than the native PCL with the knee flexed beyond 90°. The authors recommend avoiding flexion of the knee beyond 90° in the early postoperative phase due to the increased forces generated at these angles [7]. Overall, neither of the two surgical techniques demonstrated any statistically significant or clinically relevant advantage with respect to generation of time-zero graft forces.

Similarly, Bergfeld et al. examined six paired cadaveric knees with each pair also receiving matching patellar tendon allograft reconstructions [8]. After cycling each knee 72 times, the transtibial tunnel grafts demonstrated significantly greater laxity than the open tibial inlay grafts. There was evidence of fraying and thinning of the transtibial tunnel grafts at the site of the tunnel exits, as well as mechanical degradation of the graft. The authors concluded that after cycling the knees, the open tibial inlay grafts demonstrated significantly less laxity than the tibial tunnel grafts.

The most enlightening study comparing the transtibial tunnel and open tibial inlay PCL reconstruction techniques was published by Markolf et al. [9]. These authors performed a cadaveric study assessing 62 knees reconstructed with either a transtibial tunnel or open tibial inlay technique, that were subsequently loaded with between 50 and 300 N for 2000 cycles. All of the open tibial inlay grafts survived the testing; however, 10 of 31 transtibial tunnel grafts failed prior to completing 2000 cycles. The surviving transtibial tunnel grafts demonstrated significant thinning with a 40 % loss of cross-sectional area at the tunnel exit, compared to a 12.5 % loss in the open tibial inlay grafts. Both techniques exhibited graft elongation, with the open tibial inlay technique averaging 5.9 mm versus 9.8 mm for the transtibial tunnel technique. On the basis of these studies as well as other biomechanical analyses of PCL reconstruction, there is a definite trend supporting the open tibial inlay technique in terms of graft strength and maintenance of cross-sectional area during cyclic loading [6,7–9,14].

Clinical Studies

Despite cadaveric biomechanical studies favoring the open tibial inlay technique, there is limited high-quality clinical research examining PCL surgical approaches. Studies assessing a large number of open tibial inlay reconstructions, or comparing transtibial tunnel and open tibial inlay PCL reconstructions are lacking. Cooper and Stewart reviewed 41 patients following PCL reconstruction using an open tibial inlay technique, with between 2 and 10 years follow-up [19]. All patients received bone–patellar–bone autograft or allograft, and 85 % of these patients had secondary instabilities that were surgically addressed. All patients demonstrated a preoperative posterior drawer examination of greater than 12 mm posterior translation. About 27 patients had chronic posterior instability and 14 were treated acutely. The postoperative drawer tests were normal in 9 patients, were grade 1+ in 25 patients, and were grade 2+ in 7 patients. Preoperatively, the objective International Knee Documentation Committee (IKDC) scores for all affected knees were "D" or severely abnormal. Postoperatively, 4 affected knees scored "A," 24 scored "B," 11 scored "C," and 2 knees remained at "D." Overall, this study concluded that the open tibial inlay surgical technique was successful for both primary repairs and combined reconstructions.

Two studies comparing PCL reconstructive techniques merit further discussion. Seon and Song studied 43 isolated, chronic PCL tears with a minimum 2-year follow-up [20]. About 21 patients received a transtibial tunnel reconstruction using a quadrupled hamstring autograft, and 22 patients underwent open tibial inlay using a bone–patellar–bone autograft. Postoperatively, both groups demonstrated significant improvement in Lysholm and Tegner scores, but no statistically significant differences were evident between the two groups. Knee laxity was assessed as normal or grade 1 in 19/21 patients in the transtibial tunnel group, and 20/22 in open tibial inlay group. Instrumented posterior laxity testing revealed statistically significant differences in both groups comparing pre- and postoperative measurements but no difference between the groups. Overall, Seon and Song determined that both of these PCL reconstruction techniques produced good clinical results, and are satisfactory PCL reconstruction procedures.

MacGillivray et al. published a retrospective study of 20 patients with a minimum of 2-year follow-up [21]. Thirteen patients underwent a transtibial tunnel reconstruction, while seven patients underwent an open tibial inlay reconstruction, with a mix of graft types in each group. Overall, 90% of the patients were satisfied with their surgical outcome. The postoperative tibial drawer test improved in 5/13 knees in the transtibial tunnel group, and 4/7 knees in the open tibial inlay group, with no statistically significant difference between groups. Postoperatively, corrected KT 1000 measurements were 5.9 mm in the transtibial group, and 5.5 mm in the open tibial inlay group, with no statistically significant difference between groups. Outcome measures, including the Tegner, Lysholm, and the American Academy of Orthopedic Surgery (AAOS) knee scores, all improved compared with preoperative results, but there was no difference between groups. Clinically, neither technique in this study restored anteroposterior stability. The results of these studies must be considered with the knowledge that no concomitant collateral ligament procedures were performed on any patients [20, 21]. Both of these studies serve to highlight the challenges of conducting clinical studies in PCL-deficient patients due to the complex and variable ligament injury patterns that present.

Patient Positioning

It is surgically demanding to access the popliteal fossa and posterior capsule while performing a PCL reconstruction. Therefore, it is not surprising that many combinations of patient positioning are used to complete this task. In his initial publication on the open tibial inlay procedure, Berg described the lateral patient position [1]. However, many surgeons use a supine figure-4, or a prone position for the tibial portion of the procedure, the latter of which requires a position change for the femoral and arthroscopic work. As there is no consensus on the "best" position for this procedure, the three most common patient positions are outlined below.

Lateral Position

The patient is placed in a beanbag or other body positioner, in a lazy lateral position with the surgical leg uppermost, and the pelvis tilted slightly posteriorly (Fig. 10.1a). The hip is externally rotated for the arthroscopy as well as the anterior, medial, and lateral work, and it is internally rotated to access the posterior knee (Fig. 10.1b). This position allows the surgeon to operate with the knee in extension or flexion, which enables selection of the best working angle. The posterior medial or posterior approaches can be performed in this position. The lateral position also allows the surgery to be completed without significant patient-positioning changes. One disadvantage of the lateral position is that access for both the anterior and posterior work is somewhat compromised and awkward.

Supine Figure-4 Position

The patient is positioned in supine, and then rolled 15–20° with a wedge placed under the opposite hip. In order for this position to be used, the patient must have adequate external rotation of the hip; therefore, the figure-4 position is not suitable for a patient with increased femoral anteversion. For all of the anterior and arthroscopic work, the hip is slightly internally rotated and flexed to 90°. The surgical leg may be supported with a lateral post and a foot stop, or it may be flexed over the side of the bed. To access the posterior knee, the knee and hip are externally rotated and flexed to approximately 60°. The foot can then be placed on the opposite thigh, making the "4" position. In addition, tilting the table can aid in the visualization of the posterior knee. Laupattarakasem et al. [22] have also described a novel approach, with the surgeon positioned between the patient's legs to access the posterior knee (Fig. 10.2).

A significant advantage of this position is that it allows the surgeon to complete the entire inlay PCL reconstruction with the patient in the supine position. This supine figure-4 position also allows the surgeon to use either a posteromedial or a posterior approach. However, there are some disadvantages to this patient position. One of the biggest disadvantages is that the degree and angle of knee flexion makes it difficult to obtain adequate lighting of the operative area from the overhead fixtures and therefore the surgical area is often shadowed. Visualization can be aided with the use of a headlamp to correct this concern. Another disadvantage of this position is the increased difficulty of completing an adequate arthrotomy and debridement of the PCL insertion, because the knee is flexed.

Prone Position

Parker and Bergfeld describe their duo-table technique to achieve the prone position for an open tibial inlay technique [13]. The patient starts in the supine position until the femoral tunnels are drilled and any necessary meniscal work is completed [13]. A separate operating room table is used

Fig. 10.1 **a** Lateral position using beanbag body positioner. **b** Lateral position with surgical leg externally rotated for anterior surgical access

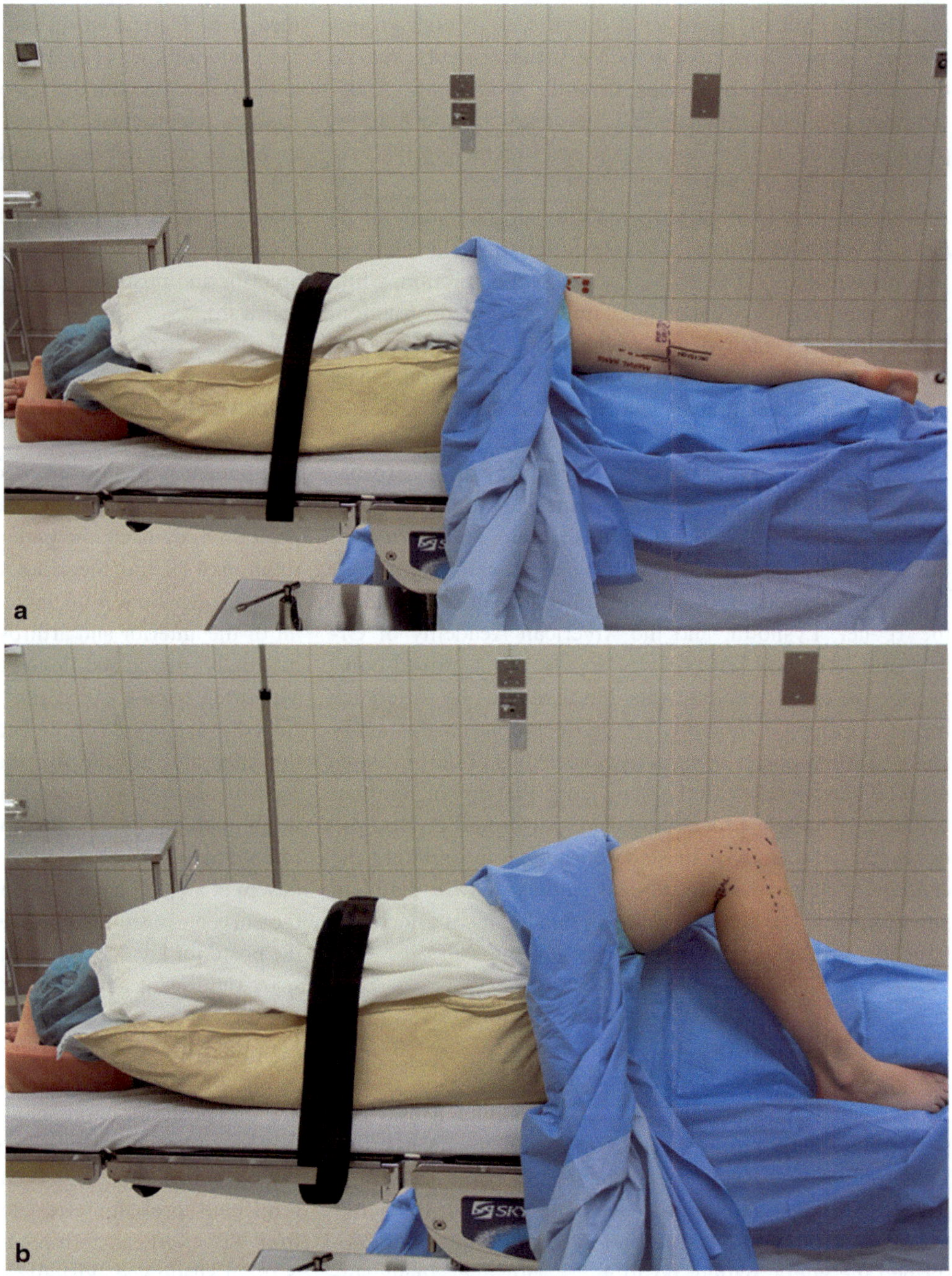

to roll the patient into the prone position and the patient is redraped [13]. The open tibial inlay technique is then completed through a posterior approach. Once the bone block is secured to the tibia, the patient is rolled back into the supine position and redraped [13]. Alternately, after the patient is anesthetized, it is possible to drape, prepare, and perform the posterior work with the patient in the prone position, and while keeping the patient draped and the field sterile, perform a single turn to the supine position for the remainder of the case.

Once the patient is lying face down with his/her arms comfortably out to the side, place a pillow underneath the patient's feet to achieve 20–30° of knee flexion. This slight flexion reduces the tension in both the gastrocnemius and hamstrings muscles, which will facilitate posterior exposure of the knee. Pillows may also be placed under the patient's hips and chest for comfort, and to protect bony prominences. The prone position can be used for either the posterior medial or posterior approaches. The major advantage of the prone position is improved visualization of the posterior knee for the surgical dissection and placement of the tibial inlay graft. The major disadvantage of this position is the time and manpower required to move the patient, along with the risk of contaminating the surgical field during this process.

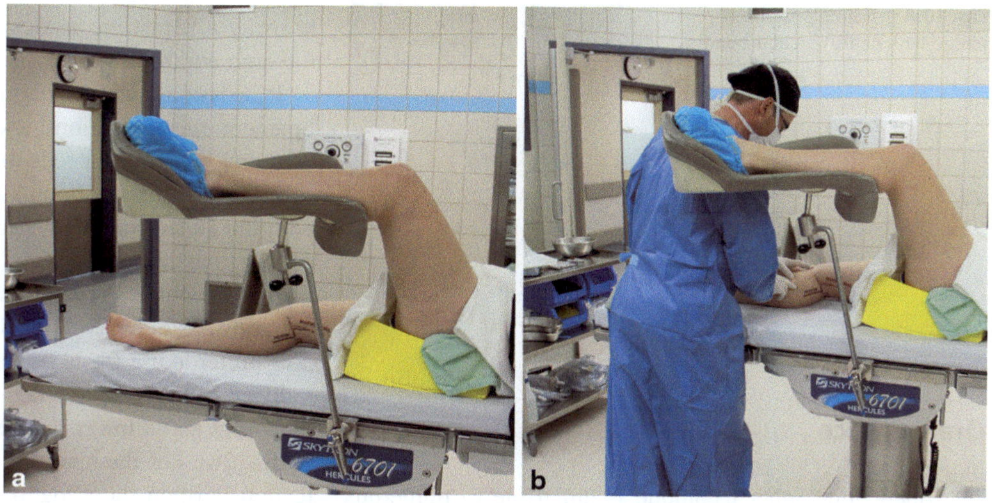

Fig. 10.2 **a** Modified figure-4 position using a surgical foot stirrup. **b** Modified figure-4 position with surgeon placement

Surgical Approaches

Posterior Medial Approach

The posterior medial approach was first described by Berg [4]. This method uses the interval between the distal aspect of the medial hamstrings, and the medial head of gastrocnemius. In the original description, the medial head of the gastrocnemius is detached; however, other surgeons have since described leaving this origin intact and flexing the knee to access the PCL insertion site [4, 8, 23, 24]. The skin incision initiates proximally along the medial border of the semitendinosus, then moves laterally and distally close to the midline at the popliteal skin crease, and ends approximately 10 cm distal to the popliteal skin crease. The proximal interval lies between the medial hamstrings and the neurovascular bundle. More distally, the interval is medial to the medial head of the gastrocnemius, which can be reflected laterally by either detaching the medial head proximally, or flexing the knee to relax the muscle (Fig. 10.3). The popliteus muscle is then reflected laterally and distally, and the medial genicular vessels are exposed and ligated or cauterized. This exposes the PCL footprint and the posterior capsule.

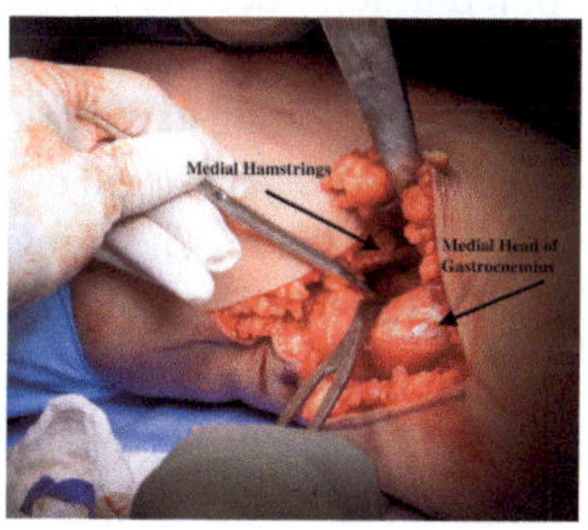

Fig. 10.3 Posterior medial approach

The posterior medial approach can be performed in the lateral, supine figure-4, or prone position. The most positive aspect of this approach is that it provides for protection of the neurovascular bundle with the medial head of gastrocnemius. One of the main challenges for surgeons using this approach is the difficulty in visualizing the posterior capsule and PCL footprint without detaching the medial head of gastrocnemius. This can compromise an adequate arthrotomy, as well as correct positioning of the tibial inlay graft. Additionally, this approach makes it difficult for screw insertion to be perpendicular to the graft bone block, which could potentially compromise the fixation.

Posterior Approach

The posterior approach accesses the posterior capsule and PCL insertion on the tibia directly via the popliteal fossa. Proximally, the interval is located between the medial hamstrings and the neurovascular bundle, and distally between the medial head of gastrocnemius and the neurovascular bundle. This approach is the author's preferred technique and is described in detail later in this chapter.

This approach can be performed with the patient in the lateral, figure-4 or prone position. The advantage of this approach is direct visualization of all the midline posterior structures, specifically the PCL tibial footprint and the posterior capsule (Fig. 10.4). This approach allows for a well-visualized arthrotomy and debridement of remnant PCL fibers. It also enables insertion and solid fixation of a well-docked graft, and facilitates smooth graft passage. The major disadvantages of the posterior approach are the large posterior incision, the amount of dissection, the time-consuming patient position changes, and the proximity to the neurovascular structures.

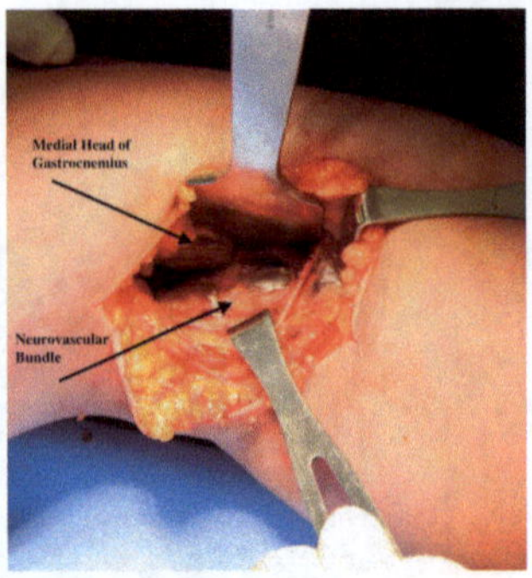

Fig. 10.4 Midline posterior image with neurovascular bundle

Graft Choice

The open tibial inlay technique is amenable to numerous graft options including autografts, allografts, and synthetic grafts. This PCL reconstruction approach was developed during an era when autograft tissue was primarily used for ligament reconstructions [4, 13, 19]. Use of patellar tendon autograft was reported in the early literature [4, 13, 19]. The patellar tendon autograft has many benefits beside the inherent benefit of being autologous. This graft facilitates a bony union at both the tibial and femoral insertions by 4–6 weeks postoperatively, which provides early central stabilization, and may prevent laxity during the more vigorous phases of rehabilitation. The patellar tendon autograft has some disadvantages including the limited amount of soft tissue tendon that can be harvested, (approximately 10–12 mm width and 2–3 mm depth). This amount of tissue is much less than a native PCL. Secondly, the graft length may not allow for the graft to be docked below the crest of the tibial plateau, thus risking proximal migration and/or tilt, if screw fixation loosens during cyclic loading. Lastly, the patellar tendon is not conducive to a double-bundle surgical technique on the femur, limiting this graft type to a single bundle technique.

The quadriceps tendon is another frequently used autograft. It is possible to harvest a large graft, (up to 80 mm length and approximately 6–8 mm depth). Due to the layered structure of this tendon, it can be used in a double-bundle technique on the femoral side. The disadvantages of the quadriceps graft are harvest-site morbidity, including pain, decreased knee function, and reduced quadriceps power [25]. Laupattarakasem et al. described a unique approach using a doubled semitendinosus autograft [22]. The graft is looped over a partially threaded screw, whereby the cortical bone window that was excised for the inlay becomes a washer [22]. The graft is augmented with any remnant posterior PCL fibers and placed under this bony washer [22]. This novel technique is useful for surgeons performing multiligament reconstruction surgery, particularly when allograft tendon is not available, or in a patient with a ruptured patellar tendon. Another advantage of this technique is the biologic bone–tendon–bone healing that it provides. The biggest drawback to using a hamstring autograft is that the size is limited to 6–8 mm width.

PCL reconstructive surgery frequently requires multiple ligament reconstructions and repairs, and therefore more than one graft often needs to be harvested. Considering the substantial degree of trauma that causes PCL injuries, along with the added trauma of harvesting autograft, it is not surprising that allograft tissue has become very popular for these procedures. Preparation and sterilization procedures of allograft tissue have evolved, and the majority of surgeons now prefer to use fresh, frozen, unirradiated allografts. Unirradiated allografts have been reported to produce superior outcomes and a lower failure rate compared with irradiated grafts [26]. For the open tibial inlay technique, the Achilles tendon is often the allograft of choice, but some surgeons use 12–15 mm patellar or quadriceps tendon allografts. The major advantages of allograft tissue are the large graft size as well as reduced harvest site and patient morbidity [27]. In addition, often more than one allograft can be harvested from a single Achilles tendon. The disadvantages of allograft tissue are reduced bone and soft tissue quality, prolonged graft healing, incorporation and remodeling, and the risk of infectious disease transmission [27].

Lastly, there is an option of using synthetic grafts for PCL reconstruction. These are typically completed using a transtibial technique, but some have eyelets that could be secured to the posterior tibia in an inlay fashion. Synthetic grafts may be used to augment native PCL tissue, but are less frequently used in North America than in Europe [28]. These grafts can be useful in the acute multiligament knee injury by enabling the creation of a central joint stabilizer, when other soft tissue damage prohibits multiple ligament repairs.

Author's Preferred Surgical Approach

Surgical Preparation

The patient is anesthetized in the supine position, the surgical leg is shaved, and a tourniquet is applied to the proximal thigh as a safety measure if any vascular injury occurs. The arthroscopic portals, planned incisions, and the knee joint are all injected with 20 cc of 0.25 % Marcaine with 1/400,000 epinephrine to decrease intraoperative bleeding and postoperative pain. Additionally, 2 g of prophylactic, intravenous cefazolin is administered prior to starting the procedure. This surgery can be performed using either a spinal anesthetic or a general anesthetic. The spinal anesthetic offers the advantage of the patient being able to assist with the position changes. If using a general anesthetic, the anesthesiologist should intubate the patient for maximal airway protection.

Before placing the patient into the prone position, the surgeon performs an examination under anesthesia to confirm

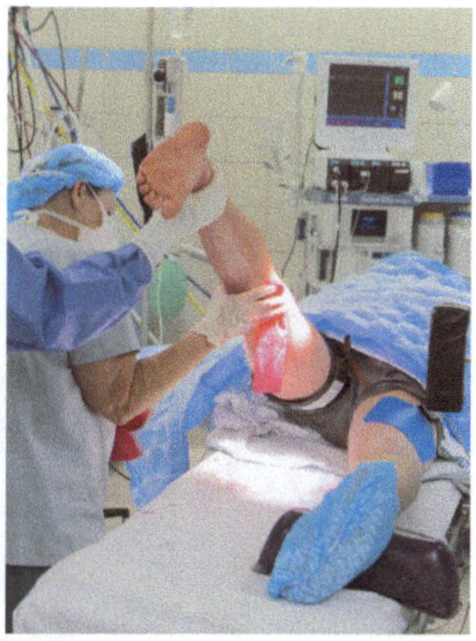

Fig. 10.5 Positioning for preparation of the surgical limb

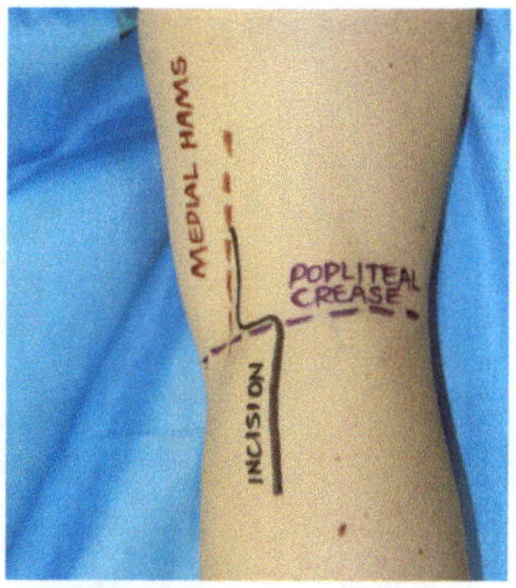

Fig. 10.6 Posterior approach lazy "S" incision

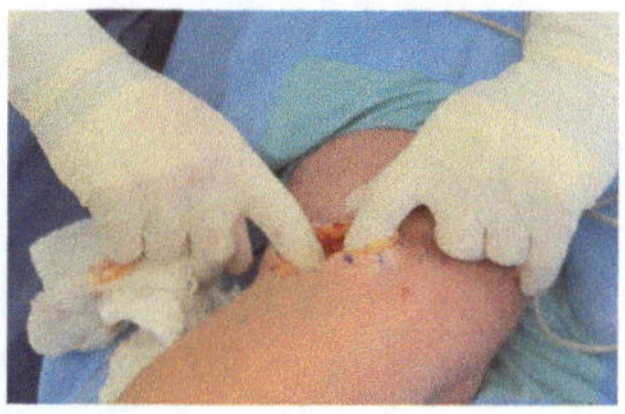

Fig. 10.7 Finger dissection

the diagnosis. The contralateral extremity should also be examined to assess normal knee ligament function. Prior to the skin preparation, the patient is rolled into the prone position. Perform this patient transfer with the surgical leg uppermost, as this transfer will be repeated in the opposite direction later in the procedure. This will ensure that anesthesia lines and monitoring equipment will not become tangled during position changes. Once in the prone position, place a pillow under patient's ankles to achieve 20–30° of knee flexion, which will facilitate relaxation of the hamstrings and gastrocnemius muscles. Pillows may also be placed under the patient's hips and chest for comfort and to protect bony prominences. The patient is prepared for surgery in the prone position. An easy way to assist with the preparation of the entire surgical area is to place one hand under the anterior knee, and to pull the leg up toward the ceiling and away from the body, to ensure the leg stays straight (Fig. 10.5). Once the limb is prepared, drape the patient using a split drape, in addition to a disposable single-hole leg drape, the latter of which will be used during the entire procedure.

Surgical Technique

With the tourniquet deflated and the use of cautery for hemostasis, perform a classic posterior approach to the knee. Make a 10–15-cm lazy "S" shape incision through the popliteal crease, with a slightly longer distal limb (Fig. 10.6). This nonlinear incision prevents a painful scar or flexion contracture. Incise the fascia with a scalpel and extend the fascial incision using scissors. Identify the superficial sural cutaneous nerve and remain medial to this structure. Using blunt finger dissection, dissect through the fat that is lateral to semimembranosus and the medial head of gastrocnemius until the neurovascular bundle is exposed (Fig. 10.7). The popliteal artery can be palpated during this dissection to confirm you are in the correct interval. Frequently, there is a small neurovascular bundle that innervates the medial head of gastrocnemius, which crosses the field obliquely, and can be preserved (Fig. 10.8). Most often, surgeons will be able to complete the procedure proximal to this bundle. However, in some patients, it is necessary to expose distally from this bundle to properly visualize the tibia for placement and fixation of the tibial inlay graft.

A Hohmann, or similarly spiked retractor, can be placed medially to retract the medial head of gastrocnemius along with the medial hamstring tendons. Deep dissection on the tibia begins on the medial side, away from the neurovascular structures. The medial genicular artery is cauterized, after which the popliteus muscle is elevated using a soft tissue elevator and reflected laterally and distally. A second Hohmann is added on the posterior lateral tibial plateau where it is hammered into cancellous bone, 3–4 cm below the joint line. This second retractor serves to protect the neurovascular bundle throughout the remaining dissection. The surgeon

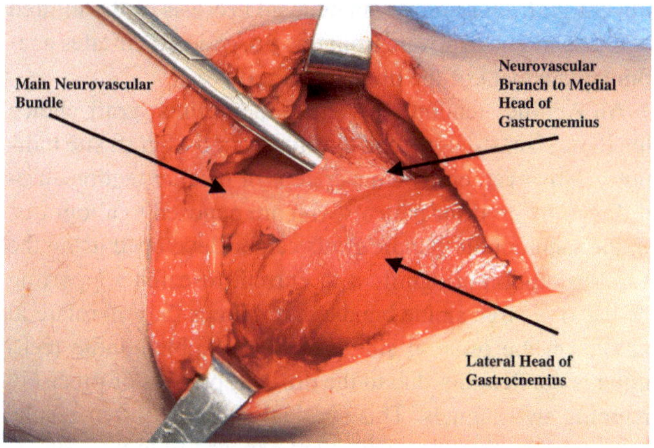

Fig. 10.8 Neurovascular branch to medial head of gastrocnemius

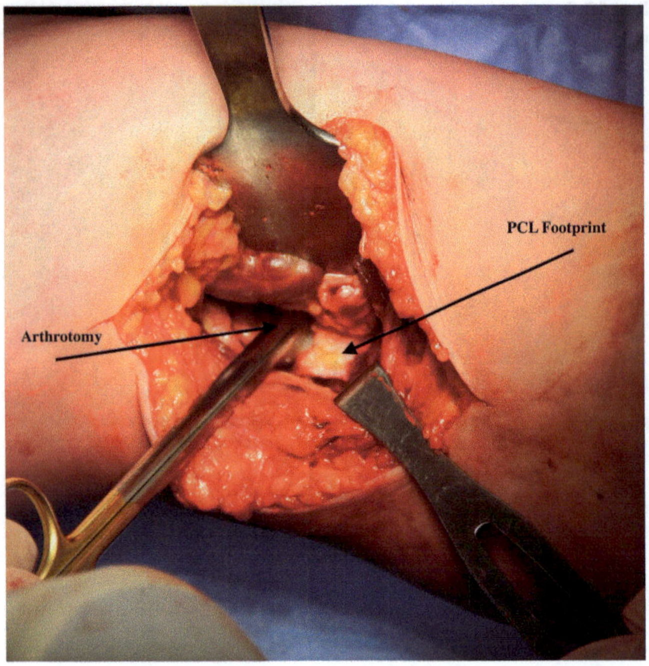

Fig. 10.9 Footprint and insertion point of the native PCL. *PCL* posterior cruciate ligament

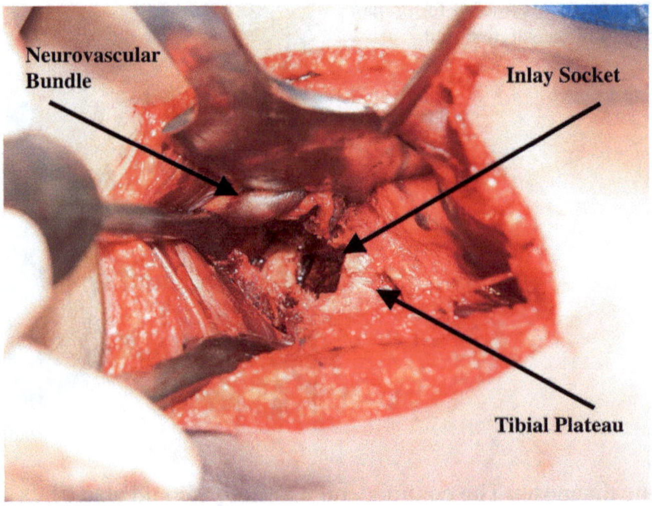

Fig. 10.10 Tibial inlay socket

should now be able to fully visualize the footprint and insertion of the native PCL, along with the posterior capsule (Fig. 10.9).

A formal "L"-shaped arthrotomy is performed on the medial and distal side of the posterior knee joint, away from the neurovascular structures. Often the posterior horn of the medial meniscus can be visualized as a landmark. A medially based arthrotomy also prevents damaging the meniscofemoral ligaments of Wrisberg and Humphrey. The native insertion of the PCL is resected down to its footprint and any remaining bulk of the PCL is excised. If the posteromedial bundle of the PCL is intact, these fibers can be preserved and the tibial inlay graft can be used solely as an anterolateral bundle. These steps allow for easy graft passage, and also prevent graft loosening from delayed necrosis of the injured PCL fibers. The exposure from this dissection facilitates anatomic placement of the tibial inlay graft.

An Achilles tendon allograft is the optimal graft choice due to its size, strength, and the elimination of graft site morbidity. However, either a quadriceps or patellar tendon autograft can be used for patients who are opposed to allografts. Single- and double-bundle grafts can be developed using the Achilles tendon allograft, with current research supporting the use of a large single bundle that mimics the anterolateral bundle on the femoral side [26]. The double-bundle technique is challenging due to the difficult process of precisely mapping two tunnels. This surgical approach often results in two smaller bundles, which are exposed to higher forces, thereby increasing the risk for subsequent graft failure.

An osteotome is used to create an open tibial inlay socket, approximately 1.5 cm in diameter and 3.5 cm in length (Fig. 10.10). Once cancellous bone is exposed, blood will obscure the field, so it is best to start with the technically most difficult distal cut first. Following the distal cut, move laterally next to the neurovascular bundle, finishing with the more straightforward proximal and medial cuts. This sequence minimizes the risk of damaging neurovascular structures after the field becomes bloodied. The placement of the superior aspect of this socket is critical for docking the graft. Ensure that 2–3 mm of solid posterior tibial plateau bone is preserved for this docking process. Proximally, the socket should be 1 cm deep to ensure that the bone block cannot migrate proximally. Distally, it is less important for the socket to be deep, and often the graft is somewhat proud against the tibia. It is important to note that the socket size can vary depending on the size of the patient and the graft being used (Fig. 10.11).

On a sterile preparation table, the Achilles tendon allograft is fashioned into a single bone block for the tibial side, with either a single or double bundle for the femoral side. The bone block is created to preserve the maximum number of fibers from the tendon (Fig. 10.12). This bone block can be wider on the surface and trapezoidal rather than rectangular in shape (Fig. 10.13). It is important to create a perpendicular proximal end of the open tibial inlay bone block so that it docks neatly in the socket and prevents migration until bony union occurs. The cancellous or deep side of the bone block is usually 1.5 cm wide by 3.5 cm long, matching the size of the socket. The final allograft bone block is usually 1.0–1.5 cm deep.

When using an Achilles tendon allograft, if the soft tissue portion is too large for the femoral tunnel, or if additional tissue is required for an ACL or posterolateral corner (PLC) reconstruction, you must carefully identify the superficial

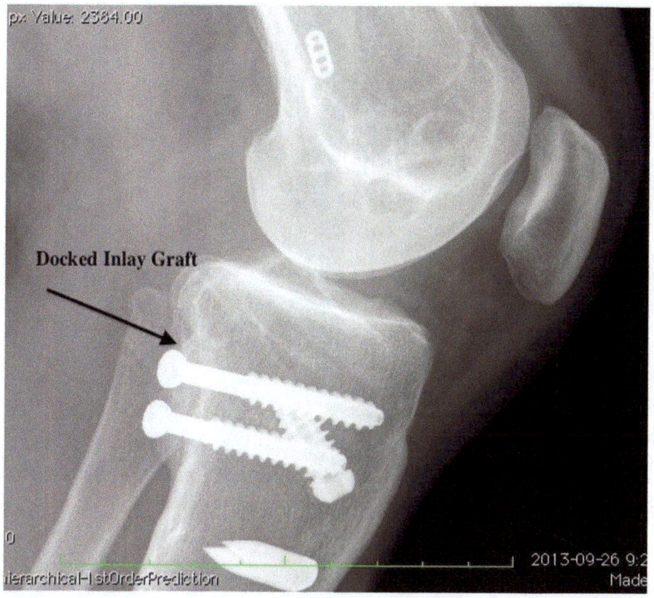

Fig. 10.11 Lateral radiograph showing well-docked, flush bone block proximally and slightly proud on distal margin

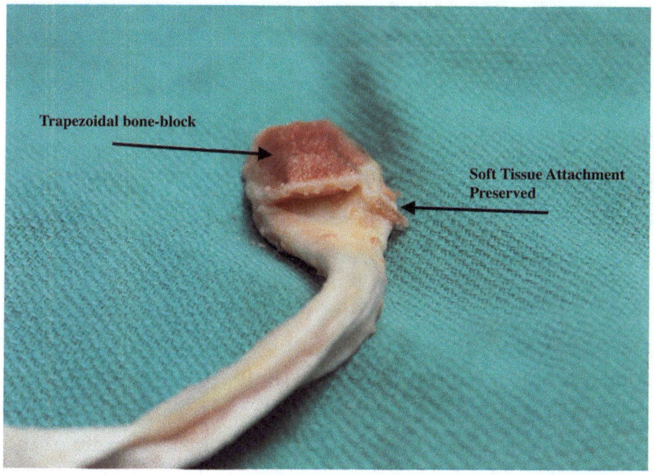

Fig. 10.12 Preservation of soft-tissue/maximal fibers

from the deep fibers (Fig. 10.14a). It is important to preserve the deep fibers inserting on the bone for the PCL allograft as to not dysfunction the soft tissue portion of the graft. In addition, medial and lateral fibers that are wider than the bone block should be retained as wings, which will later scar down to the posterior tibia. Although cutting these fibers away may make the allograft look more streamlined and tidy, this excision could decrease the graft's strength and function (Fig. 10.14b).

Preparing the bone block on the sterile table eliminates the use of power tools in the vicinity of the neurovascular bundle. Two guide wires from a cannulated large fragment screw set are drilled parallel into the bone, 1.5 cm apart (Fig. 10.15). The guide wires are then drilled with a cannulated 4.5 drill

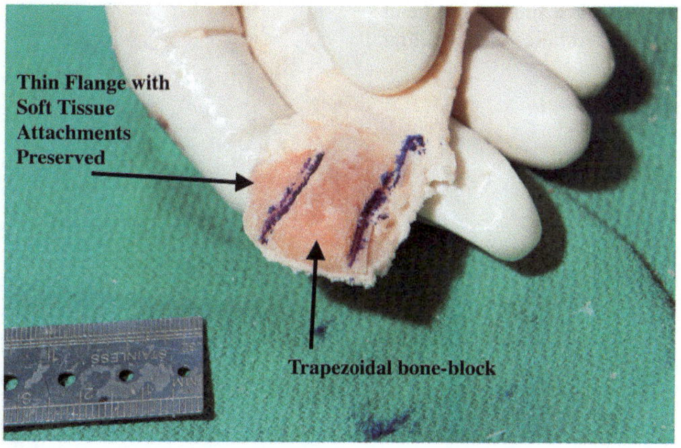

Fig. 10.13 Trapezoidal bone-block and preservation of soft tissue attachments

bit and tapped. The prepared graft is then taken to the knee and docked into the slot. The guide wires can be lightly hammered into the cancellous bone in a slightly distal and lateral direction, and secured with two cannulated 6.5 cancellous screws, the lengths usually being 50 mm for the proximal screw and 45 mm for the distal screw. Aiming slightly lateral and distal is important to avoid interfering with a possible ACL tibial tunnel (Fig. 10.16). There is usually no need to predrill into the cancellous tibial bone, which again enables the surgeon to avoid the use of a power tool in the posterior knee. The soft tissue portion of the graft is then placed in the wound in the posterior aspect of the knee, and a sharp towel clip can be used to hold the skin closed.

Next, while maintaining a draped and sterile surgical field, the patient is moved to the supine position. The surgical knee must move up toward the ceiling, to ensure that the repositioning maneuver is completed correctly and the drapes remain sterile. This repositioning is usually performed with the surgical team controlling the patient's hips and legs, and the circulating team and anesthetist controlling the head, chest, and arms. To allow the circulating team more space during this maneuver, adjust the drape poles down toward the patient's hips. Also, move all of your instruments and cautery to a mayo stand during this procedure. To avoid the drapes becoming tangled, rotate the drape on the thigh once the patient is supine. A second drape can be placed under the limb if a further barrier is desired (Fig. 10.17).

Once the patient is repositioned into the supine position, the femoral footprint of the PCL can be exposed arthroscopically, and the femoral tunnels can be drilled. A single anterolateral tunnel is drilled with a femoral guide using an outside-in technique. The use of an outside-in technique enables the surgeon to consistently and accurately place the tunnel exit at the site of the tubercle on the medial epicondyle, decreasing the angle of the graft at the internal aperture of the femoral tunnel [29]. This method also avoids a tunnel that is too close to the articular cartilage and also ensures the graft

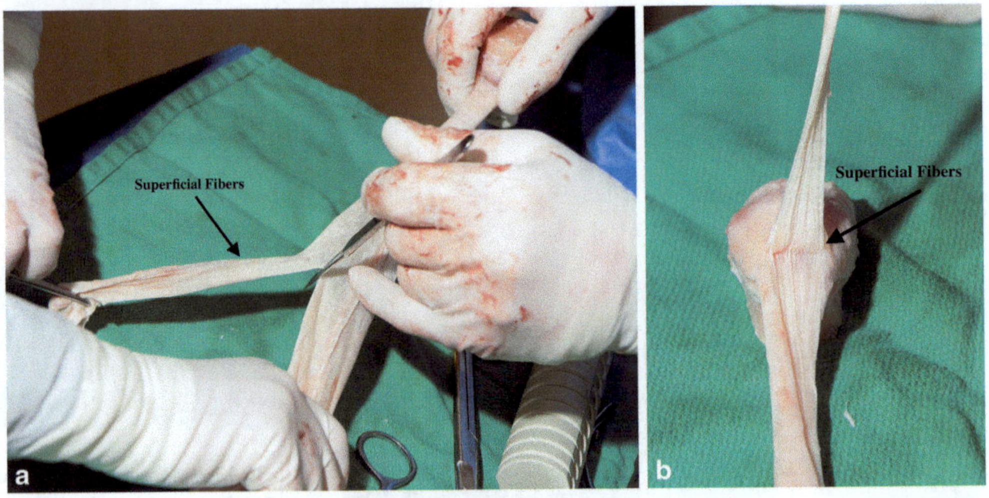

Fig. 10.14 **a** and **b** Superficial fibers of Achilles tendon allograft

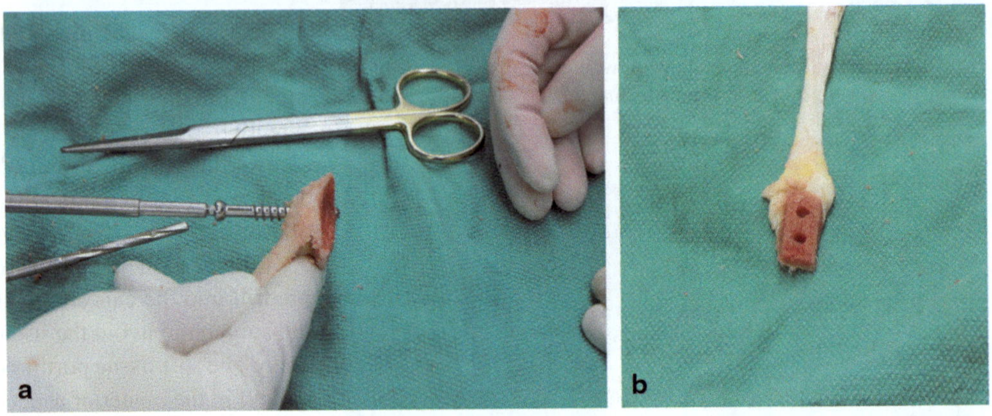

Fig. 10.15 **a** and **b** Drilling of parallel tunnels

exits in an optimal position if the Achilles tendon allograft is extended into a medial collateral ligament (MCL) reconstruction as a single graft (Fig. 10.18).

A looped 18-gauge wire is used to pass the leader sutures of the tendinous portion of the graft from posterior to anterior through the medial portal under arthroscopic guidance (Fig. 10.19). The wire must be visualized as it passes medial to the ACL and then out the arthrotomy in the back of the knee. A finger can be placed into the posterior knee to palpate the wire as it passes through. It is essential to ensure that the wire, as well as the leader sutures of the graft, pass proximal to the oblique neurovascular branch that innervates the medial head of gastrocnemius. To retrieve the graft, a ringed suture grasper is inserted into the femoral tunnel from outside-in, and the leader sutures are brought to the exterior of the knee. The graft is delivered, cycled, tensioned, and the knee restored to the normal anterior step-off in 90° of flexion, and secured with an interference fit screw that can be backed up with a staple if desired.

Consistent with other PCL reconstruction techniques, the open tibial inlay technique is rarely done in isolation. Addressing the secondary instabilities, whether anterior, posterior lateral, and/or posterior medial, are critical to the success of the procedure. It is important to remember that robust tibial fixation is not a substitute for failing to address secondary pathology.

The wound closure of the posterior incision is one of the most awkward steps of this procedure. The leg can be elevated onto a raised mayo stand or an assistant can hold the leg elevated to facilitate wound closure. It is not essential to close the fascia, and interrupted subcutaneous sutures and staples can be used for the skin. For the first 24–48 h, a moist antibiotic-impregnated gauze, along with absorbent gauze, is applied with a tensor bandage. Prior to the patient being discharged from hospital, a sealed sterile dressing that permits showering is applied, and this can remain in place for the first 2–3 weeks.

Postsurgical Care

Postoperatively, 1 g cefazolin is administered every 8 h for three doses, and subcutaneous low molecular weight heparin is prescribed for 21 days. The patient is placed in a

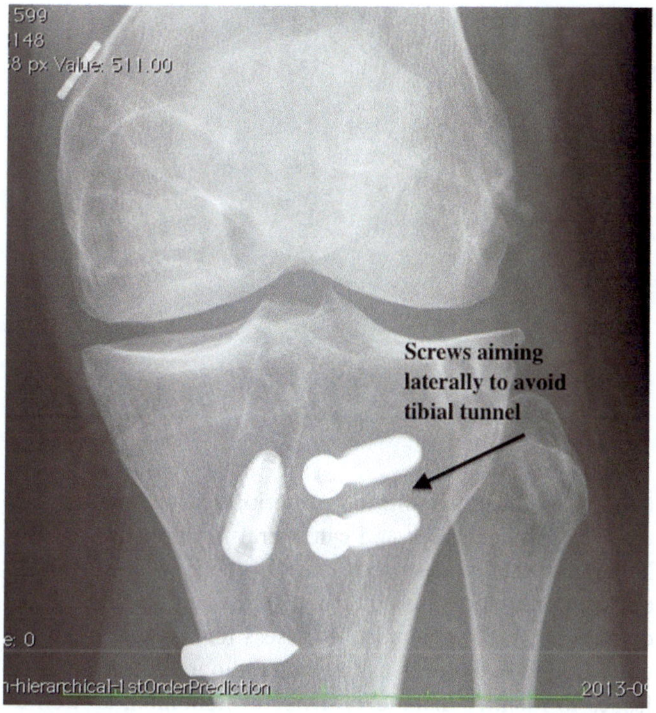

Fig. 10.16 AP radiograph of screw placement and angulation

hinged knee immobilizer locked in extension for 3 weeks, and then gentle closed kinetic motion is permitted. The patient usually requires crutches for protected weight bearing for 6 weeks. Knee flexion beyond 90° is discouraged until 6 weeks postoperative to prevent stress on the graft [7]. In terms of early exercise, quadriceps activation is encouraged, while hamstring activation is discouraged to prevent posterior shearing forces on the graft. Due to the use of allograft tissue and the frequent rate of multiligament reconstruction, progress through rehabilitation is generally slower than with the ACL patient. Plyometrics commence at 6 months and return to regular sporting activities is considered at 1 year.

Procedural Complications

Saltzer et al. reviewed the American Board of Orthopeadic Surgery database, and determined that PCL reconstructive surgery has the highest complication rate at 20.1 % compared to a mean of 4.1 % for all arthroscopic knee procedures [30]. There are a number of complications that the surgeon should review with prospective patients to ensure informed consent; these include: infection, deep vein thrombosis, pulmonary embolism, neurovascular injury, knee stiffness, graft failure, and other medical and anesthetic risks.

Complications and concerns specific to the open tibial inlay graft technique include the incision, hematoma, neurovascular injury, and graft failure. The large posterior incision, which is difficult for patients to see and care for, makes incision breakdown, local infection, and late scar contracture possible complications of this procedure. Also, with deep surgical dissection to access the PCL footprint, a hematoma can develop in the posterior knee and may or may not require surgical drainage. Posterior knee pain and foot dysesthesia are the hallmark signs of this complication, and typically resolve without intervention within a few weeks.

Fig. 10.17 a–c Patient repositioning from prone to supine position

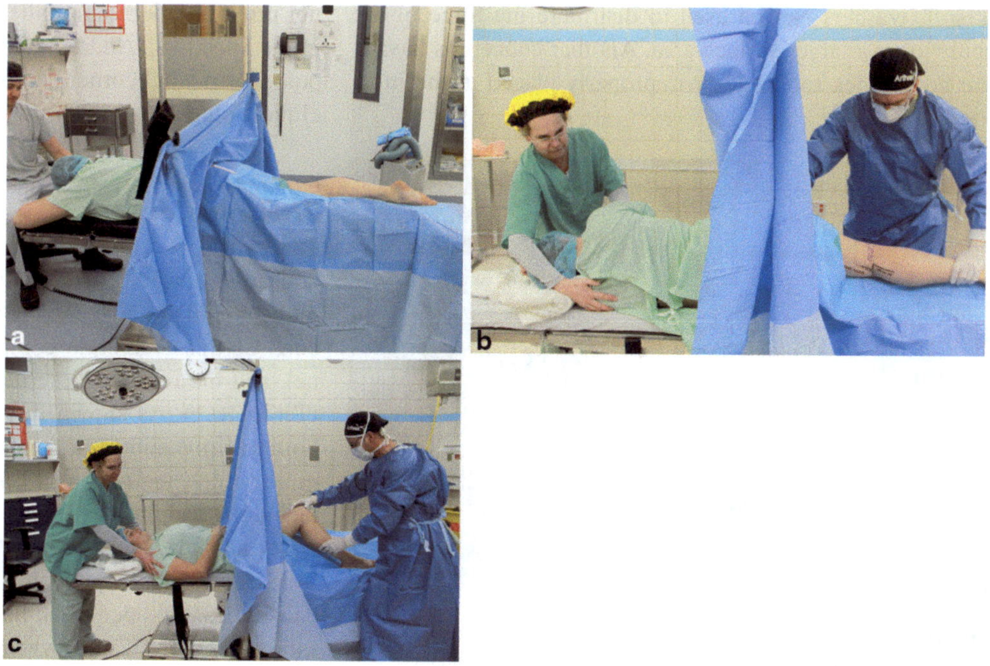

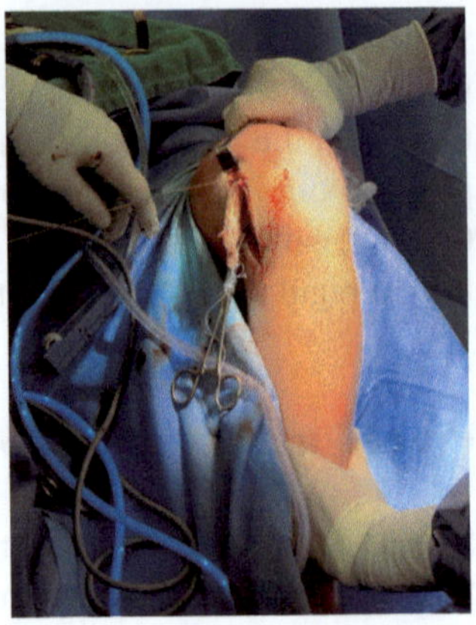

Fig. 10.18 Extension of Achilles tendon allograft for an MCL reconstruction. *MCL* medial collateral ligament

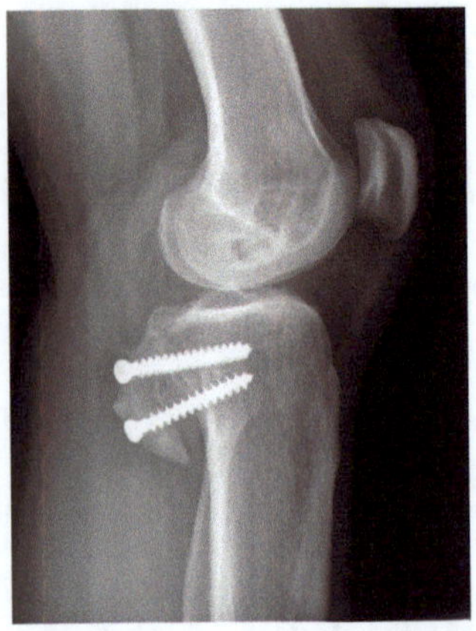

Fig. 10.20 Lateral radiograph showing a bone block that is too large for the inlay tray

Neurovascular injury is always a concern in PCL surgery due to proximity of the tibial nerve, along with the popliteal artery and vein, to the tibial insertion of the PCL [31, 32]. The open tibial inlay technique may actually be safer for the neurovascular bundle than the transtibial tunnel technique because in the latter technique, a guide pin or reamer could slip past protection and cause injury. For the inlay technique, using blunt finger dissection around the neurovascular bundle and avoiding the use of power tools in the posterior aspect of the knee significantly reduces the risk of neurovascular injury. In a patient with an acute traumatic neurovascular injury, an open tibial inlay approach at the time of vascular repair is possibly safer than a delayed arthroscopic approach, and could be considered an indication for this technique.

Graft placement on the tibial footprint and secure fixation are strengths of this technique but can also cause complications. Graft fracture during screw insertion and loss of fixation is the greatest concern. To prevent these issues, two screws are recommended for fixation. If the graft bone block is soft, washers can be used to distribute the force of the screw over a larger surface area. Another concern is having the bone block too large or improperly placed in the inlay trough, and/or extending too posteriorly which can change the PCL biomechanics and cause graft failure (Fig. 10.20). Nonunion, graft reabsorption, and stripping of the soft tissue off the bone block are other potential complications. Postoperatively, the surgeon should assess for bony union of the graft around 4–6 weeks using plain radiographs of the knee. Issues to identify include evidence of nonunion, as well as the graft tilting out distally, which may suggest some loss of distal fixation. Initial conservative postoperative rehabilitation and hinged brace immobilization are regimes that aid in preventing early graft failure prior to bony union [5].

With the tibial inlay technique, an inadequate arthrotomy can cause two problems. With a small arthrotomy, it can be difficult to pass the graft forward to the femoral tunnel. Alternatively, if the arthrotomy is too proximal and does not extend down to the posterior tibia, the graft can be suspended by the capsule and slowly stretch out, resulting in graft laxity. Regardless of technique, the single most important reason for late graft failure following PCL reconstruction is not properly addressing other ligamentous pathology found in the knee [33]. Addressing the posterior lateral corner, the posterior medial corner and/or the ACL is key to improving clinical outcomes in PCL surgery [33, 34].

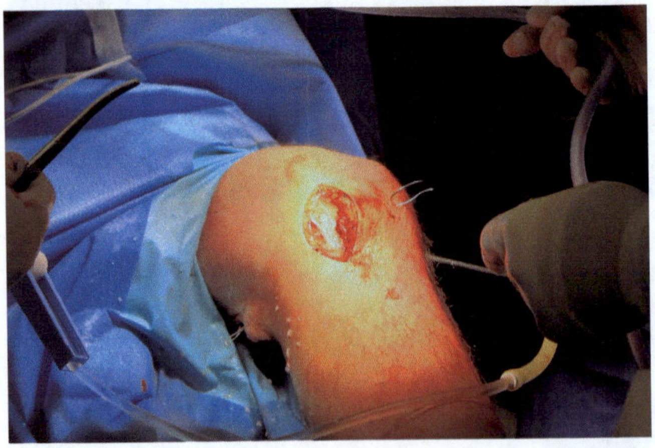

Fig. 10.19 Use of 18-gauge wire to pass leader sutures from posterior to anterior through the medial portal under arthroscopic guidance

Pros and Cons

A chapter on the open tibial inlay PCL reconstruction technique would not be complete without reviewing the pros and cons of this technique compared with the transtibial tunnel, and the recently described arthroscopic inlay approach (Table 10.1). As shown in Table 10.1, each technique has both positive and negative aspects, making it hard to determine which technique is optimal. Therefore, the surgical technique should be selected based on the surgeon's preference and skill level, along with an analysis of technique that is best suited to the patient. Based on cadaveric biomechanical studies, the open tibial inlay technique has demonstrated more favorable results when compared with the transtibial

Table 10.1 Summary comparison of the pros and cons of the open tibial inlay, transtibial tunnel, and arthroscopic inlay techniques

	Open tibial inlay	Transtibial	Arthroscopic tibial inlay
Pros	No tibial tunnels/stress risers	Reduced OR time	No tibial tunnels/stress risers
	PCL footprint visualization	No position change	Reduced OR time
	Potentially reduced neurovascular risk	PCL augmentation/partial PCL tears	No position change
	Biomechanical studies	Cosmetic	Cosmetic
	Revision surgery	Wound care	Wound care
Cons	Prolonged OR time	Tibial tunnels/stress risers	Technically demanding
	Position change	PCL footprint visualization	PCL footprint visualization
	Tibial hardware	Neurovascular risk	Neurovascular risk
	Cosmetics	Biomechanical studies	Graft fixation
	Wound care		
Equal	Clinical results	Clinical results	Clinical results
	Use in multiligament	Use in multiligament	Use in multiligament

PCL posterior cruciate ligament

tunnel technique. However, the limited clinical studies to date have shown no evidence of a difference in outcomes between these two approaches.

The two strongest advantages of the open tibial inlay technique are its secure bone-to-bone fixation on the tibia, and the elimination of the "killer turn" [4–6,14]. This technique is a good choice for revision surgery, especially if the tibial tunnel is in a suboptimal position [23]. The major disadvantages of this technique are the larger surgical dissection, the need for intraoperative repositioning of the patient, and the longer surgical duration [20].

One of the most positive attributes of the transtibial tunnel technique is that it is better suited for multiligament procedures [35]. This technique enables the majority of the surgery to be completed arthroscopically, thereby decreasing soft tissue morbidity; it also allows a shorter surgical duration, and for the surgery to be completed in the supine position [20, 35]. However, cadaveric studies have demonstrated higher rates of graft stretching and weakening using this technique [7–9]. Furthermore, clinical studies, although not statistically significant, have shown a trend toward the open tibial inlay technique demonstrating superior anatomic positioning of grafts in long-term follow-up [7–9, 19–21].

The arthroscopic tibial inlay technique was developed with the goal of bringing the best of the open tibial inlay and transtibial techniques together [15–18]. The greatest positive attributes of this technique are that it addresses the "killer turn," provides bone-to-bone healing of the graft on the tibia, and is completed arthroscopically in the supine position [15–18]. Identified disadvantages include the technical difficulty of this approach, including the more challenging tibial inlay drilling and graft passage as well as the weaker initial fixation of the graft [15–18]. High-quality clinical trials are needed to determine if the arthroscopic inlay technique is as, or more effective than the open tibial inlay and transtibial techniques.

Conclusion

The open tibial inlay technique's attributes of solid, bony tibial fixation, anatomic graft positioning, and elimination of the "killer turn" make it a favorable option for PCL reconstruction. Although all of the PCL reconstruction techniques may be considered technically difficult, when completed successfully, research has shown that good clinical results can be obtained. A challenge for surgeons pursuing high-quality research is the fact that most PCL tears occur concomitantly with other ligamentous and soft-tissue injuries, making technique comparisons difficult. The positive attributes of this surgical approach, along with the strengths of the open tibial inlay technique in revision surgery, ensure this surgical approach is a good addition to a surgeon's toolbox.

Acknowledgments Acknowledging Banff Sport Medicine, Dr. Gregory ML Buchko MD, FRCSC, Dr. Laurie A Hiemstra MD, PhD, FRCSC, and Sarah Kerslake MSc, BPhty.

References

1. Hughston JC. History of posterior cruciate ligament surgery. Oper Tech Sports Med. 1993;1(2):86–8.
2. Aroen A, Sivertsen EA, Owesen C, Engebretsen L, Granan LP. An isolated rupture of the posterior cruciate ligament results in reduced preoperative knee function in comparison with an anterior cruciate ligament injury. Knee Surg Sports Traumatol Arthrosc. 2013;21(5):1017–22.
3. Clancy W. Repair and reconstruction of the posterior cruciate ligament. In: Chapman MW, editor. Operative Orthopaedics. 3. Philadelphia: Lippincott; 1988.
4. Berg EE. Posterior cruciate ligament tibial inlay reconstruction. Arthroscopy. 1995;11(1):69–76.
5. McAllister DR, Hussain SM. Tibial inlay posterior cruciate ligament reconstruction: surgical technique and results. Sports Med Arthrosc Rev. 2010;18(4):249–53.

6. McAllister DR, Markolf KL, Oakes DA, Young CR, McWilliams J. A biomechanical comparison of tibial inlay and tibial tunnel posterior cruciate ligament reconstruction techniques: graft pretension and knee laxity. Am J Sports Med. 2002;30(3):312–7.
7. Oakes DA, Markolf KL, McWilliams J, Young CR, McAllister DR. Biomechanical comparison of tibial inlay and tibial tunnel techniques for reconstruction of the posterior cruciate ligament. Analysis of graft forces. J Bone Joint Surg. 2002;84-A(6):938–44.
8. Bergfeld JA, McAllister DR, Parker RD, Valdevit AD, Kambic HE. A biomechanical comparison of posterior cruciate ligament reconstruction techniques. Am J Sports Med. 2001;29(2):129–36.
9. Markolf KL, Zemanovic JR, McAllister DR. Cyclic loading of posterior cruciate ligament replacements fixed with tibial tunnel and tibial inlay methods. J Bone Joint Surg. 2002;84-A(4):518–24.
10. Jakob RP, Ruegsegger M. Therapy of posterior and posterolateral knee instability. Orthopade. 1993;22(6):405–13.
11. Trickey EL. Rupture of the posterior cruciate ligament of the knee. J Bone Joint Surg Br. 1968;50(2):334–41.
12. Torisu T. Isolated avulsion fracture of the tibial attachment of the posterior cruciate ligament. J Bone Joint Surg. 1977;59(1):68–72.
13. Parker R, Bergfeld J, McAllister D, Calabrese G. Arthroscopically assisted posterior cruciate ligament reconstruction: tibial inlay technique. In: Fanelli GC, editor. Posterior cruciate ligament injuries: a practical guide to management. 1. New York: Springer; 2001. pp. 157–73.
14. Voos JE, Mauro CS, Wente T, Warren RF, Wickiewicz TL. Posterior cruciate ligament: anatomy, biomechanics, and outcomes. Am J Sports Med. 2012;40(1):222–31.
15. Campbell RB, Jordan SS, Sekiya JK. Arthroscopic tibial inlay for posterior cruciate ligament reconstruction. Arthroscopy. 2007;23(12):1356 e1–4.
16. Kim SJ, Kim SH, Kim SG, Kung YP. Comparison of the clinical results of three posterior cruciate ligament reconstruction techniques: surgical technique. J Bone Joint Surg. 2010;92 (Suppl 1 Pt 2):145–57.
17. Mariani PP, Margheritini F. Full arthroscopic inlay reconstruction of posterior cruciate ligament. Knee Surg Sports Traumatol Arthrosc. 2006;14(11):1038–44.
18. Zehms CT, Whiddon DR, Miller MD, Quinby JS, Montgomery SL, Campbell RB, et al. Comparison of a double bundle arthroscopic inlay and open inlay posterior cruciate ligament reconstruction using clinically relevant tools: a cadaveric study. Arthroscopy. 2008;24(4):472–80.
19. Cooper DE, Stewart D. Posterior cruciate ligament reconstruction using single-bundle patella tendon graft with tibial inlay fixation: 2- to 10-year follow-up. Am J Sports Med. 2004;32(2):346–60.
20. Seon JK, Song EK. Reconstruction of isolated posterior cruciate ligament injuries: a clinical comparison of the transtibial and tibial inlay techniques. Arthroscopy. 2006;22(1):27–32.
21. MacGillivray JD, Stein BE, Park M, Allen AA, Wickiewicz TL, Warren RF. Comparison of tibial inlay versus transtibial techniques for isolated posterior cruciate ligament reconstruction: minimum 2-year follow-up. Arthroscopy. 2006;22(3):320–8.
22. Laupattarakasem W, Boonard M, Laupattarakasem P, Kosuwon W. Tibial inlay technique using hamstring graft for posterior cruciate ligament reconstruction and remnant revision. Arthrosc Tech. 2013;2(1):e1–7.
23. Burks RT, Schaffer JJ. A simplified approach to the tibial attachment of the posterior cruciate ligament. Clin Orthop Relat Res. 1990;254:216–9.
24. Lee SH, Jung YB, Lee HJ, Jung HJ, Kim SH. Revision posterior cruciate ligament reconstruction using a modified tibial-inlay double-bundle technique. J Bone Joint Surg. 2012;94(6):516–22.
25. Comley AKJ. Donor site morbidity after quadriceps tendon harvest for rotator cuff repair. The Aust N Z J Surg. 1999;69(11): 808–10.
26. Sun K, Tian S, Zhang J, Xia C, Yu T. Anterior cruciate ligament reconstruction with BPB autograft, irradiated versus non-irradiated allograft: a prospective randomized clinical study. Knee Surg Sports Traumatol Arthrosc. 2009;17:464–74.
27. Montgomery SR, Johnson JS, McAllister DR, Petrigliano FA. Surgical management of PCL injuries: indications, techniques, and outcomes. Curr Rev Musculoskelet Med. 2013;6(2):115–23.
28. Johnson D, Laboureau J. Cruciate Ligament reconstruction with synthetics. In: Fanelli GC, editor. Posterior cruciate ligament injuries : a practical guide to management. 1. New York: Springer; 2001. pp. 189–214.
29. Handy MH, Blessey PB, Kline AJ, Miller MD. The graft/tunnel angles in posterior cruciate ligament reconstruction: a cadaveric comparison of two techniques for femoral tunnel placement. Arthroscopy. 2005;21(6):711–4.
30. Salzler MJ, Lin A, Miller CD, Herold S, Irrgang JJ, Harner CD. Complications after arthroscopic knee surgery. Am J Sports Med. 2014;42(2):292–6.
31. Fanelli GC, Monahan T. Complications in posterior cruciate ligament and posterolateral corner surgery. Oper Tech Sports Med. 2001;9(2):96–9.
32. Zawodny SR, Miller MD. Complications of posterior cruciate ligament surgery. Sports Med Arthrosc Rev. 2010;18(4):269–74.
33. Noyes FR, Barber-Westin SD. Posterior cruciate ligament revision reconstruction, part 1: causes of surgical failure in 52 consecutive operations. Am J Sports Med. 2005;33(5):646–54.
34. Fanelli GC. Posterior cruciate ligament injuries in trauma patients. Arthroscopy. 1993;9(3):291–4.
35. Fanelli GC, Fedmann D. Management of combined anterior cruciate ligament-posterior cruciate ligament-posterolateral complex injuries of the knee. Oper Tech Sports Med. 1999;7(3):143–9.

All-Arthroscopic Tibial Inlay Double-Bundle Posterior Cruciate Ligament Reconstruction

11

Alexander E. Weber and Jon K Sekiya

Introduction

Posterior cruciate ligament (PCL) injuries are relatively rare; however, their treatment remains a challenging problem for the managing orthopedic surgeon. Not all clinical outcomes following PCL rupture are uniformly poor; however, recent studies suggest that the kinematics of the PCL-deficient knee is significantly altered from the intact state [1, 2]. In a similar fashion to the anterior cruciate ligament–deficient knee, PCL deficiency redistributes the forces across the knee joint [1, 2]. The results of which are an increase in pressure in the medial and patellofemoral compartments which may lead to premature and severe arthrosis [2, 3]. Reconstruction of the PCL restores the affected knee to a stability state more similar to the intact knee and it is now accepted that patients with PCL laxity greater than 10 mm compared to the contralateral side have improved outcomes with PCL reconstruction (PCL-R) [4–8].

There are multiple surgical techniques and graft choices for PCL-R with no "gold standard." The purpose of this chapter is to discuss the clinical presentation of PCL injury, the diagnostic approach, and the surgical treatment of PCL rupture. Furthermore, the technical aspect is focused on the double-bundle arthroscopic inlay surgical technique as this is currently the senior author's preferred technique for PCL-R. Pearls and pitfalls of the surgical technique are highlighted during the technical description. Following the technical aspects, a literature review drives a discussion of the advantages of the double-bundle arthroscopic inlay PCL-R and provides evidence as to why this is our advocated and chosen surgical technique for reconstruction of the PCL.

J. K. Sekiya (✉)
Department of Orthopedic Surgery, University of Michigan, Ann Arbor, MI, USA
e-mail: sekiya@med.umich.edu

A. E. Weber
Department of Orthopedic Surgery, University of Michigan Hospital, Ann Arbor, MI, USA

Preoperative Considerations

History

In the case of an acute injury, there is often a history of a direct trauma to the pretibial aspect of the lower extremity or a hyperextension injury to the affected knee. An effusion or swelling is often present with an acute PCL injury; however, the lack thereof does not rule out a PCL injury. A knee dislocation often results in injury to the PCL, which is likely associated with concomitant ligamentous or soft tissue injuries. In the case of severe knee trauma, 95 % of patients with a PCL injury have associated ligamentous injuries. The most common associated injury is disruption of the posterolateral knee structures (approximately 60 %) [9]. High-energy traumas may result in capsular damage and extravasation of the joint effusion, thus the absence of an effusion should not lessen the examiner's suspicion for ligamentous injury. Patients with chronic PCL injuries may complain of pain and instability with activity without additional or associated signs or symptoms.

Physical Examination

It is crucial to fully evaluate and appreciate the extent of the soft tissue and ligamentous injury to the knee. PCL injury may be associated with a knee dislocation that spontaneously reduces prior to presentation. A thorough physical examination of the entire affected lower extremity is appropriate. Remember to assess the presumed intact structures and consistently compare to the contralateral knee.

The first component of the physical examination should be an assessment of the neurovascular status of the affected limb. This is of particular importance if there is suspicion for or history of knee dislocation. Once the neurovascular competence of the injured limb is established, inspection and palpation for a knee effusion is conducted. This is followed by an examination of knee, hip, and ankle range of motion.

G. C. Fanelli (ed.), *Posterior Cruciate Ligament Injuries*,
DOI 10.1007/978-3-319-12072-0_11, © Springer International Publishing Switzerland 2015

With regard to the knee, it should be passively taken through a range of motion and, if the patient is capable, passive range of motion should be compared to active range of motion. With the knee flexed, the relationship of the tibial plateau and femoral condyles as well as the natural tibial step-off can be assessed. In 90° of flexion, the Godfrey test is used to assess for a posterior sag sign (Fig. 11.1). The dynamic posterior drawer test is also performed in 90° of flexion and can evaluate the magnitude of posterior tibial translation. In cases of traumatic PCL injuries, a concomitant posterolateral corner (PLC) injury is present as well. This injury pattern can be assessed with the constellation of a reverse pivot test, a dial test, a posterolateral drawer test, and a varus stress testing at both 30° and 90° of flexion.

Radiography

The initial diagnostic imaging study should be plain radiographs (anteroposterior and lateral) of the knee. These initial radiographs are helpful in that they can rule out a fracture or an unreduced knee in the acute setting. Plain radiographs can be used to assess the medial or patellofemoral compartments for arthrosis in patients who present with a suspected chronic PCL deficiency. Long-leg standing films should be obtained if any fixed or dynamic instability is suspected or if there is evidence of extra-articular deformity. Posterior tibial subluxation may be evaluated on standard lateral radiographs; however, if there is any doubt bilateral stress (weighted) radiographs should be performed (Fig. 11.2).

Other Imaging Modalities

Although not regularly utilized in our current diagnostic algorithm, the extent of degenerative changes in the chronically PCL-deficient knee can be assessed with a bone scan.

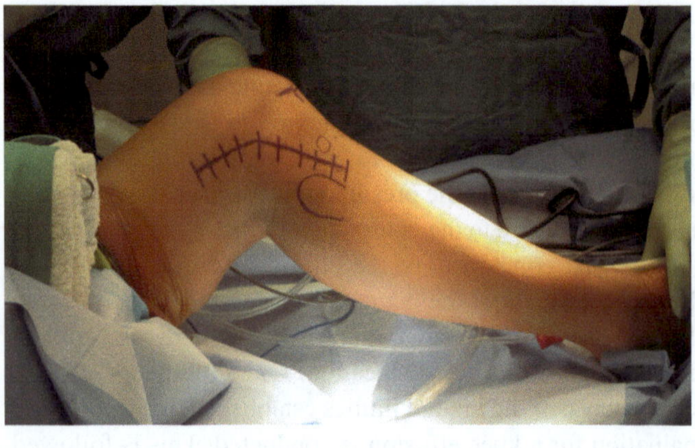

Fig. 11.1 Intraoperative physical exam finding of the PCL-deficient knee; a posterior sag of the right tibia in 90° of flexion

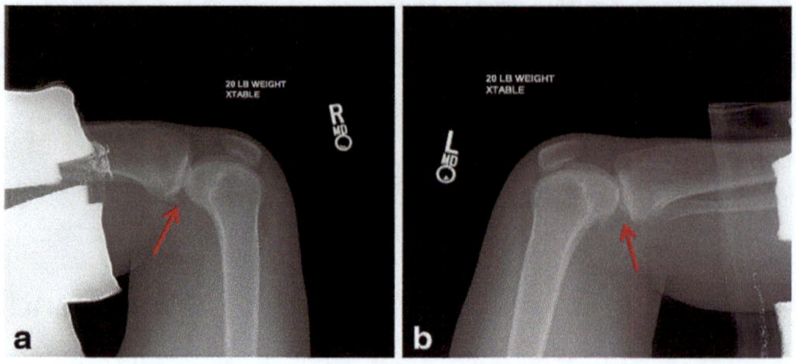

Fig. 11.2 Stress radiographs of the bilateral knees. The normal anatomic position of the tibia in relation to the femur (*arrow*) in a ligamentously intact knee (**a**). Posterior tibial subluxation in relation to the femur (*arrow*) is present in a PCL-deficient knee (**b**)

More commonly, a magnetic resonance imaging (MRI) study is an essential part of the work up of a PCL injury. The MRI serves to confirm the suspected PCL rupture but more importantly provides an assessment of associated ligamentous injuries such as those to the PLC that will affect the preoperative plan, the surgical technique, and ultimately the clinical outcome (Fig. 11.3).

Indications and Contraindications

Patients who sustain acute isolated grade I or II PCL injuries should be treated with nonoperative, protected weight bearing, and progressive rehabilitation. The grade I or II injuries that do not respond well to nonoperative measures and go on to have persistent or recurrent instability may be treated surgically. Grade III isolated PCL tears should be treated with surgical reconstruction, although not all authors agree on the existence of an isolated grade III PCL injury [10–12]. The majority of acute PCL ruptures occur as part of a larger constellation of knee injury, either a multiligamentous knee injury or a knee dislocation. In either case, surgical intervention is advocated for the majority of patients, especially those

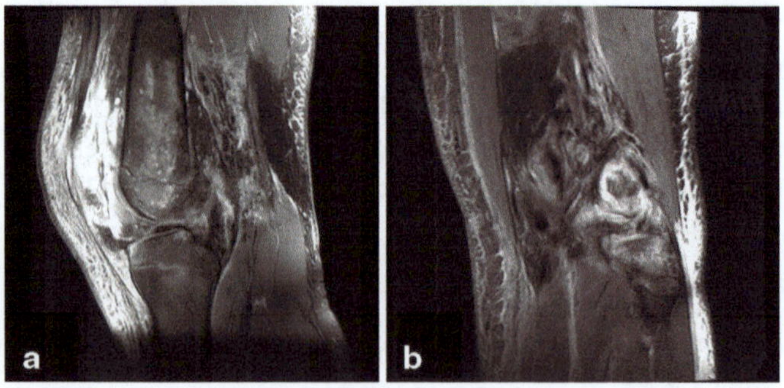

Fig. 11.3 Magnetic resonance imaging of a patient who sustained an acute complete tear of the PCL off the femur (**a**) and a patient with a concomitant PLC injury in the presence of an acute PCL tear (**b**).

patients who are young and active. The timing of intervention remains controversial; however, the literature supports either early or late reconstruction depending on the severity of injury (isolated PCL vs. multiligamentous injury), the surgeon's preference, and the patient's activity level [6, 12–18]. In the presence of an acute bony avulsion, early reconstruction is generally advocated.

There are a number of instances in which an acute PCL-R is contraindicated. In the setting of a traumatic open knee injury or in the presence of a neurovascular injury requiring repair or reconstruction, the PCL-R should be deferred into the late period to allow for resolution of the open injury or nervous insult. Relative contraindications to PCL-R include the presence of a chronic, fixed posteriorly subluxated deformity of the tibia and the PCL-deficient knee in which significant arthrosis is present. In both of the aforementioned scenarios, for the best clinical outcome, the senior author recommends a biplane osteotomy rather than a soft tissue reconstruction.

Surgical Technique

Overview

Once the decision has been made to proceed to the operating room for PCL-R, there are a number of surgical variables to consider, including graft material, number of graft bundles, and surgical technique (transtibial vs. open inlay vs. arthroscopic inlay). First to address the issue of number of graft bundles, recent biomechanical studies and a systematic review of the literature concluded that while there are no clinical studies to suggest an advantage of double-bundle grafts, there are distinct biomechanical advantages to the double-bundle PCL-R [19–21]. Thus, the senior author (JKS) has transitioned to the use of double-bundle grafts in primary PCL-R and when possible in revision PCL-R. The evolution of PCL-R surgical technique has been such that the all-arthroscopic tibial inlay technique has combined the advantages of both the transtibial and open inlay techniques while obviating the disadvantages of each technique [22–24]. For these reasons, the double-bundle arthroscopic inlay technique is our preferred technique for PCL-R and will be presented here.

Anesthesia and Positioning

Preoperative femoral and sciatic nerve catheters may be placed in the preoperative holding area for postoperative pain management. The catheters should not be dosed until a postoperative neurovascular assessment is complete in the recovery room. Following catheter placement, the patient is then transported to the operating room and placed supine on a radiolucent table. The radiolucent table is paramount as fluoroscopic confirmation of tunnel position and orientation will be necessary throughout the case. The patient should undergo general anesthesia and endotracheal intubation, but it is important to communicate with the anesthesia team that no long-acting paralytics should be given to ensure all neurologic stimulation induces a response. Once the patient is anesthetized and intubated, a comprehensive exam under anesthesia is performed to assess the integrity of all ligamentous and soft tissue structures of the knee. The results of the examination under anesthesia often aid in dictating the surgical plan. Once the exam is complete, the patient's nonoperative extremity bony prominences are well padded and a sandbag bump is taped to the bed. The bulk of the surgical work is performed between 45° and 90 ° of flexion and to facilitate these flexion angles, the sandbag is taped to the ipsilateral side of the table roughly at the level of the contralateral heel cord (Fig. 11.4). Additionally, doing the majority of the surgical procedure in flexion is a safety measure as flexion ensures the contents of the popliteal fossa fall away from the posterior tibia to allow for safe arthroscopic dissection of the tibial footprint. Although rarely inflated, a well-padded tourniquet is applied to the ipsilateral proximal thigh. The main advantage to working without the tourniquet is the early detection of a vascular injury if one was to occur. Lastly, when positioning, a flip-down lateral post is placed at the level of the tourniquet and set in a high position to act as a buttress for levering of the leg if a valgus force is necessary for medial compartment work.

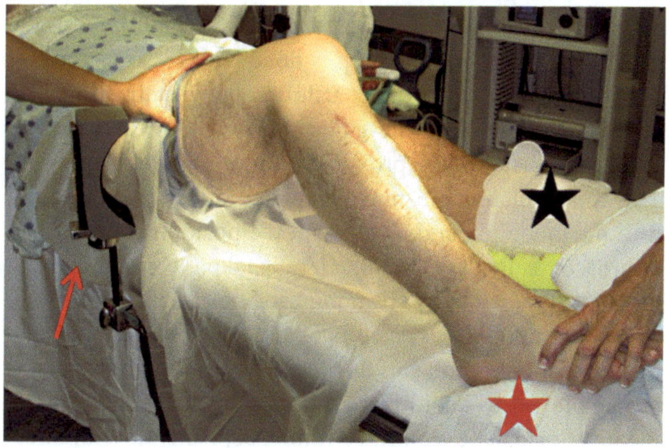

Fig. 11.4 Surgical positioning for the arthroscopic inlay procedure. A sandbag or bump is secured to the radiolucent table to allow the operative knee to be ranged in the flexion arc of 45–90 ° (*red star*). A lateral post is attached to the table at the level of the thigh tourniquet to act as a fulcrum when placing a valgus force on the knee (*red arrow*). The contralateral leg is well padded and a sequential compression device is placed for deep venous thrombus prophylaxis (*black star*)

Portal Placement

Slight adjustments are made to the standard arthroscopic portal locations for the all-arthroscopic tibial inlay double-bundle PCL-R. A standard anterolateral (AL) portal is made, but the anteromedial (AM) portal is altered. The AM portal must be established in closer proximity to the patellar tendon for increased access to the posteromedial joint space. Later in the procedure, at the time of graft passage, the AM portal is extended into a 2-cm parapatellar arthrotomy to facilitate graft passage. The location of the posteromedial working portal is also crucial to prevent surgical struggle and should thus be established under direct visualization. An 18-gauge spinal needle is used to access the posteromedial aspect of the joint on a line between the posteromedial edge of the tibia and the femoral condyle. The posteromedial working portal is first utilized to clear the tibial footprint of the PCL and as such the ideal portal placement is approximately 1 cm cranial to the posteromedial joint line.

Once the three initial portals are created, a thorough diagnostic arthroscopic exam is conducted. The exam should include an evaluation of the integrity of all ligaments, menisci, and chondral surfaces. Injuries to the posteromedial and posterolateral corners are evaluated with increased opening of the medial and lateral compartments respectively under conditions of valgus and varus stress. In either case, a missed corner injury will place undue stress on the PCL-R and lead to increased risk of clinical failure.

Tibial Socket

The tibial socket is created prior to the femoral tunnels. First, a PCL guide pin (Arthrex Inc., Naples, FL, USA) is drilled from the anterior tibial surface into and through the tibial PCL footprint. This step is done with the assistance of fluoroscopy and under direct arthroscopic visualization. The target for insertion of the guide pin is within the footprint and 7 mm distal to the proximal pole of the tibial footprint. The corresponding 3.5-mm cannulated drill is used to over-drill the guide pin and once again the position is confirmed arthroscopically (Fig. 11.5a). Care is taken to avoid altering the tunnel trajectory by changing hand position while drilling and, more importantly, care is taken to avoid plunging into the posterior structures of the knee. Two safety mechanisms are employed to avoid plunging: the first is that the reaming position can be confirmed fluoroscopically or with direct arthroscopic visualization. The second is that the newest iteration of the drill guide has a built-in 13-mm footplate that protects against plunging (Arthrex Inc.). If another drilling system is employed, a straight curette may be placed on top of the guide pin, entering the joint via the AM portal. Once the tunnel is reamed, the tibial socket is ready to be created

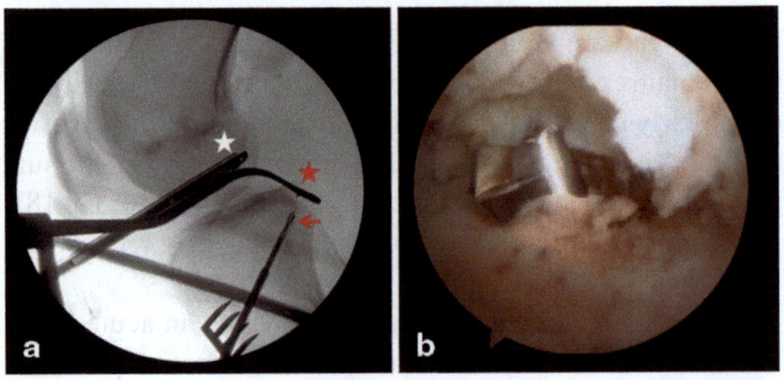

Fig. 11.5 Creation of the tibial socket. Fluoroscopic image demonstrating the PCL guide system (*red star*) and the cannulated drilling of the tibial socket (*red arrow*) (**a**). This step is done under fluoroscopic and direct arthroscopic visualization (*white star*). Arthroscopic view confirming successful insertion and position of the FlipCutter at the tibial footprint of the PCL (**b**)

with the FlipCutter (Arthrex Inc.). The drill and guide pin are removed and replaced by the FlipCutter (Arthrex Inc.), which is advanced through the tibial tunnel until it is visualized intra-articularly with the arthroscope (Fig. 11.5b). Once the working end of the FlipCutter is within the joint, the blade is engaged by "flipping" it into a perpendicular position. The blade is activated and a 13-mm diameter tibial socket to a depth of 10–12 mm is then drilled in a retrograde fashion (Fig. 11.6). The FlipCutter blade is then advanced into the joint and "flipped" back into the upright positioned to enable the device to be withdrawn.

Graft Preparation

In cases of isolated PCL-R autograft, tendon–bone constructs may be considered; however, the majority of operative PCL injuries include additional soft tissue/ligamentous injuries requiring reconstruction, thus allograft is preferred. The current graft of choice is the Achilles tendon allograft with calcaneal bone block. With this technique, there is no clinical outcome study we are aware of to suggest a superiority

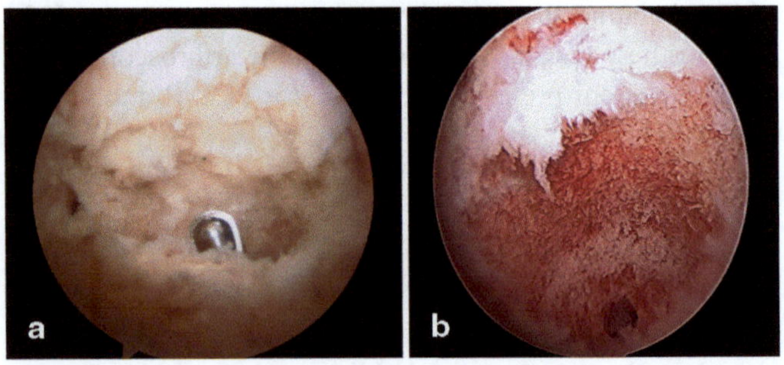

Fig. 11.6 Arthroscopic images of the completed tibial socket reamed by the FlipCutter. Anterior to posterior arthroscopic image with shaver-clearing debride from tibial socket (**a**). Arthroscopic view of the tibial socket; diameter 13 mm, depth 10–12 mm (**b**)

of allograft or autograft; however, the Achilles tendon–bone allograft is a natural graft choice as the anatomic raphe between the superficial and deep fibers facilitates the creation of two bundles (Fig. 11.7a). Sharp dissection is used to develop the interval between deep and superficial Achilles fibers, in line with the longitudinal fibers of the graft to a distance of approximately 1 cm proximal of the calcaneal bone block. The newly created graft bundles are oriented in the anterior-to-posterior orientation with the larger bundle (8–11 mm) for the anterolateral bundle (ALB) and the smaller bundle (6–9 mm) for the posteromedial bundle (PMB). Each bundle of the bifid graft is reinforced with a No. 2 braided, nonabsorbable whipstitch (Fig. 11.7b).

Attention is then turned to trimming and shaping the calcaneal bone plug for a press fit into the tibial socket. The stability of the all-arthroscopic tibial inlay PCL-R technique relies heavily on the press-fit design of the graft [25]. The proper press fit for a 13-mm socket is a cylindrical 12-mm bone plug, which can be either created with the aid of a coring reamer or hand whittled with a rongeur. The coring reamer is the most expedient and accurate method; however, there is a learning curve associated with this technique. Once the outer diameter of the bone plug is established, a central tunnel is created within the bone plug and over-reamed to a diameter of 3.5 mm with a cannulated drill system. The 1 cm of tendon left in continuity is then whipstitched with a No. 2 braided nonabsorbable suture and the free ends of this stitch are passed through the center tunnel of the bone plug from the cortical to cancellous side of the bone plug (Fig. 11.8). The free limbs passing through the bone block aid in guiding the bone plug into position. Once the bone block is seated and the graft is tensioned, the free limbs are tied over a post or button to augment tibial fixation. Recently, we have transitioned to the use of cortical button fixation which we have tested biomechanically in the laboratory and found to be equivalent in strength to post fixation. In addition to equivalent strength and stiffness, the cortical button has ease of use and improved visualization to seat the bone plug fluoroscopically.

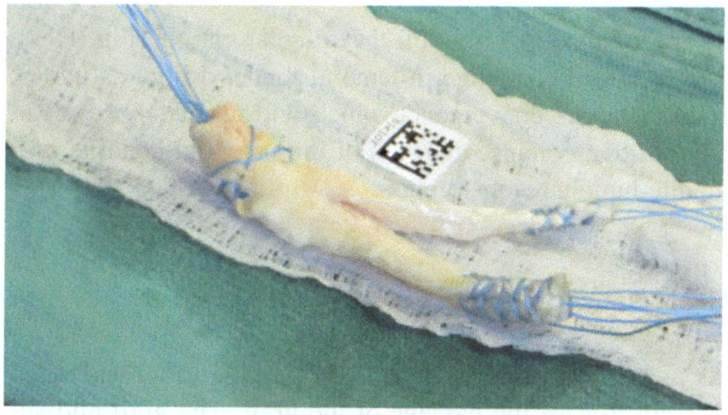

Fig. 11.8 Preparation of the bone segment of the tendon–bone graft. After sculpting the cubed bone block into a cylinder, the central calcaneal aperture is created with the use of a 3.5-mm drill system. The graft is finalized by passing a No. 2 braided, nonabsorbable suture through the remaining 1 cm of intact tendon at the bone plug end of the graft. The free limbs are then shuttled through the bone plug to aid in guiding the bone plug into the tibial socket and ultimately assisting with fixation

Femoral Tunnel

The femoral tunnels may be created inside out or outside in; however, for accuracy of placement we prefer the outside-in technique. A skin incision is made anteromedially overlying the vastus medialis obliquus (VMO) at the level of the medial epicondyle extending in line and anterior to the intermuscular septum. Once the fascia is incised, the VMO is elevated with a Cobb and retracted with a deaver or deaver-like retractor over the anterior femur. The periosteum is then exposed to clearly identify the starting position for the tunnels and ensure accurate tunnel position. The ideal tunnel for the ALB places the anterior edge of the ALB 1–2 mm off the articular margin of the medial femoral condyle at the 11:30 (left) or 12:30 (right) clock position. To create this tunnel, the guide pin is placed approximately 5 mm posterior to the articular margin (Fig. 11.9). For the PMB, the guide pin is placed 7 mm off the articular margin at the 9:00 (left) or 3:00 (right) position. The edge of the drilled tunnel should

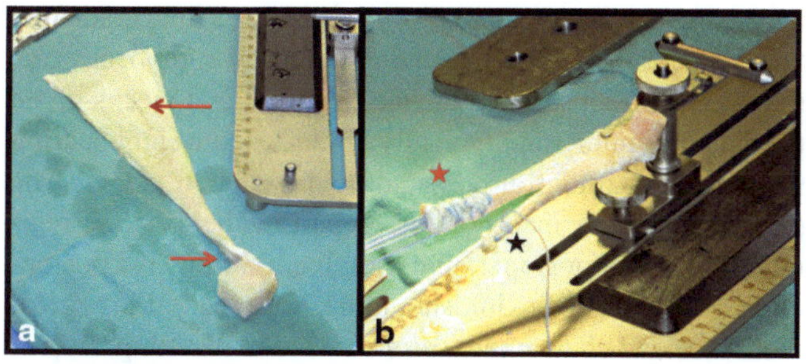

Fig. 11.7 Preparation of the soft tissue segment of the tendon–bone graft. The natural raphe of the Achilles tendon allograft is appreciated (*red arrows*) before sharply dissecting the graft into two limbs (**a**). Each limb is whipstitched and tubularized with a No. 2 braided, nonabsorbable suture; ALB (*red star*) and PMB (*black star*) (**b**)

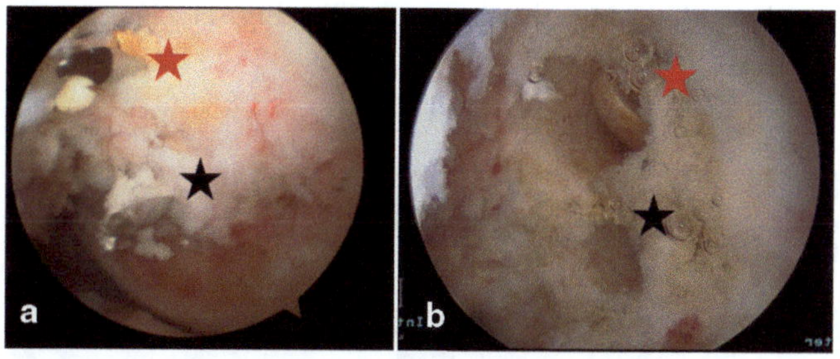

Fig. 11.9 Arthroscopic confirmation of anatomic position of the femoral tunnels. The respective guide pins located in the center of the ALB (*red star*) and PMB footprints (*black star*) (**a**). The guide pins are overdrilled and two tunnels are created with a distinct bone bridge to prevent bone bridge collapse and tunnel convergence (**b**)

lie approximately 3 mm off the articular margin (Fig. 11.9). The technical challenge in femoral tunnel drilling is avoidance of tunnel convergence which will ultimately result in bone bridge collapse and loss of the potential benefits of a double-bundle reconstruction.

Graft Passage/Tibial Fixation

As mentioned previously, the AM portal is often extended 1–2 cm to ease the passage of the graft. The graft and sutures must be cleanly passed through the arthrotomy and fat pad avoiding incarceration of the graft or entanglement of the sutures in the fat pad. The calcaneal bone plug is seated into the tibial socket and the position is confirmed fluoroscopically prior to any fixation (Fig. 11.10). The press-fit security is assessed arthroscopically by probing the interface and once the stability of the construct is deemed adequate, the tibial side of the graft is fixed to the anterior tibial cortex with the cortical button construct. We have recently employed the TightRope as the tibial cortical fixation technique (Arthrex, Inc.).

Femoral Fixation

Once the tibial side of the graft is secure, the femoral-sided suture limbs are retrieved through their respective bone tunnels with a looped 18-gauge wire. Before fixing the AL and PM bundles, the knee and graft are cycled to eliminate laxity in the construct. In a similar fashion to the double-bundle ACL reconstruction, in which the two bundles are preferentially fixed at different flexion angles to recapitulate the native ligament tension in each bundle separately, there is discussion that the two bundles of the PCL-R should also be differentially fixed [26, 27]. However, until these data emerge in the literature, we are currently tensioning both bundles at 90° of flexion [28]. The tensioned bundles are fixed with bioabsorbable interference screws and the fixation is then backed up with postfixation. The graft tension is tested with a probe and visualized arthroscopically (Fig. 11.11).

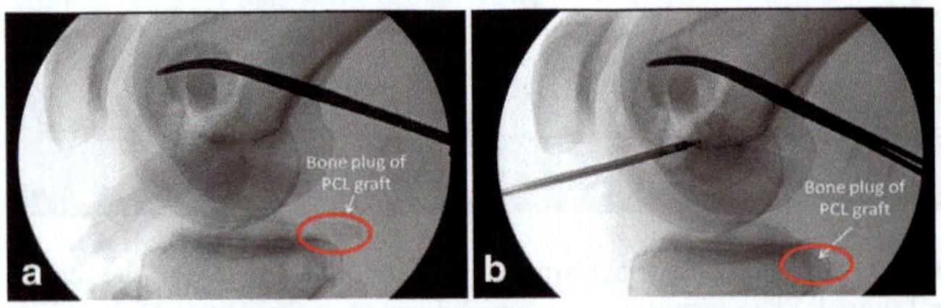

Fig. 11.10 Fluoroscopic confirmation of a well-positioned tibial bone plug (**a**). Once tension is placed on the suture limbs, the seating of the bone plug in the tibial socket is confirmed (**b**) (Adapted from [42])

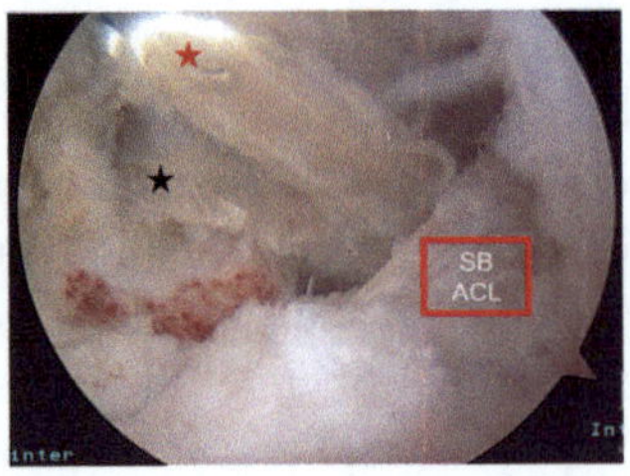

Fig. 11.11 The arthroscopic appearance of a completed double-bundle arthroscopic tibial inlay PCL reconstruction with appropriate graft tension; ALB (*red star*) and PMB (*black star*) are distinct graft bundles. A concomitant single-bundle ACL reconstruction (SB ACL) was also performed in this patient

Postoperative Considerations

Rehabilitation

The overall objective of rehabilitation is to protect the reconstructed knee in the early postoperative period, and then gradually increase gains in motion and strength over time. There are a number of rehabilitation protocols in the literature with demonstrated good to excellent results for both the isolated PCL-R and the multiligament reconstructed knee [6, 29, 30]. A full description of each protocol is outside the scope of this chapter, and will be reviewed later in the text; however, the following is an overview of the preferred rehabilitation protocol.

Cryotherapy and a hinged knee brace locked in full extension are placed on the operative limb at the conclusion of the case. Controlled range of motion exercises and partial weight bearing with the operative extremity locked in extension are permissible in the immediate postoperative period. If chondroplasty, meniscal repair, or fracture fixation is performed at the time of PCL-R, a period of nonweight bearing will occur prior to advancing to partial weight bearing. In the early postoperative period, isometric quadriceps exercises are permitted and electrical muscle stimulation may be used to enhance quadriceps recruitment [31]. Prone passive knee flexion, quadriceps strengthening sets, and patellar mobilization exercises are expected in a progressive and graduated fashion over the 1st postoperative month. Weight bearing as tolerated with an assisted device begins at 2–4 weeks given the extent of injury and typically graduates to weight bearing as tolerated without an assisted device after 6 weeks. The stationary bike is incorporated as part of the exercise regimen in the 2nd postoperative month and in the 3rd postoperative month full flexion should be achieved. Full range of motion closed chain exercises are added in the 4th postoperative month and athletes are returned to straight-line running at 6 months. Between 6 and 9 months, sport-specific activities are initiated in a stepwise fashion. Most athletes return to full sports activities between 9 and 12 months. Currently, there are a number of criteria used to return athletes to full participation, including absence of effusion, satisfactory clinical examination, quadriceps and hamstring strength at or above 90 % of the contralateral leg, one-leg hop and vertical jump at or above 90 % of the contralateral leg, full-speed run, shuttle run, and figure-of-eight running without a limp, and ability to perform squat and rise without difficulty [12, 32].

Complications

Although complications associated with PCL-R are rare events, they do occur, in part, due to the proximity of the ligament to vital neurovascular structures. As with any surgical procedure, complications may be divided into preoperative, intraoperative, and postoperative events. The major preoperative complication encounter is neuropraxia secondary to poor or improper positioning of the contralateral leg or bilateral arms. Intraoperatively, the most pressing concern is damage to the popliteal neurovascular structures. These structures are at greatest risk during tibial-sided drilling. The all-arthroscopic tibial inlay technique innately provides some decreased risk due to the lack of popliteal fossa dissection. In addition, the current instrumentation: a tibial guide with a plunge blocking insert and retrograde socket drilling with the FlipCutter both provide additional safety features. Likewise, the all-arthroscopic inlay technique affords arthroscopic visualization and fluoroscopic confirmation of drill position at all times. Intermittent checks of thigh and calf tone are important to ensure that compartment syndrome does not develop in response to fluid extravasation into the soft tissue. This is especially important when operating in the early postoperative period in a multiligament-injured knee or knee dislocation in which the joint capsule may be damaged. Iatrogenic cartilage damage or subsequent avascular necrosis of the medial femoral condyle can be avoided by placing the starting and exiting points for the femoral tunnels clear of the subchondral bone. Graft-tensioning errors are made intraoperatively but oftentimes not recognized until the postoperative period. Over-constraint of the knee is possible with excessive graft tensioning or poor graft position. Conversely, under tensioning the graft can lead to residual laxity and subsequently the development of early arthrosis. In the postoperative period, overaggressive or overly cautious rehabilitation may lead to graft failure or knee stiffness, respectively.

Discussion

While there are limited clinical data regarding the success of the double-bundle all-arthroscopic tibial inlay PCL-R, this technique is a natural progression in the evolution of the treatment of PCL injury and is grounded in sound biomechanical evidence [11, 22, 24, 33, 34]. The use of a double-bundle graft is supported by a number of in vitro biomechanical studies which have found the double-bundle PCL-R to more closely reproduce normal knee biomechanics and kinematics [20, 21, 33, 35]. A recent systematic review of the literature supported the biomechanical basis for use of the double-bundle graft. In particular, the systematic review found that there may not be a definitive advantage to double-bundle PCL-R in regard to anteroposterior stability; however, there is a distinct advantage of double-bundle PCL-R in regard to rotational stability in the setting of unrecognized or untreated PLC injury [19]. Most recently, in a controlled biomechanical study, Wijdicks et al. [20] rebuffed the equivalence of the single-bundle graft to anteroposterior stability and suggested that the double-bundle graft is superior to resisting posterior translation at all flexion angles greater than 0°. In addition, these authors found comparable results to previous studies in that the double-bundle PCL-R restored rotational stability to a significantly greater degree than did the single-bundle PCL-R [20]. Although the time-zero biomechanical data suggest superiority of a double-bundle graft, there are currently no high-level clinical studies that support the use of double-bundle reconstruction over single-bundle reconstruction or vice versa [19].

While there is no "gold standard" surgical technique for reconstruction of the PCL, the biomechanical advantages of the tibial inlay technique (either open or arthroscopic) have been documented. The inlay technique avoids the "killer turn" and subsequent graft elongation or failure which has been demonstrated in cadaveric studies [36, 37]. The arthroscopic inlay approach is biomechanically comparable to the open inlay approach at time zero and avoids the morbidity associated with a posterior approach to the knee and violation of the posteromedial joint capsule [22, 24, 38]. We are aware of four clinical or functional outcome studies involving the double-bundle all-arthroscopic tibial inlay PCL-R technique, all with promising results [27, 39–41]. In 2005 and 2006, the short-term results of the all-arthroscopic double-bundle tibial inlay PCL-R were documented to be comparable to historical controls [27, 40]. More recently, Kim et al. [39] compared cohorts of isolated PCL injuries undergoing either single-bundle transtibial reconstructions, single-bundle arthroscopic tibial inlay reconstructions, or double-bundle arthroscopic tibial inlay reconstructions. The authors found that the mean Lysholm and range of motion at final follow-up were equivalent between all groups; however, the single-bundle transtibial reconstructions had significant increased laxity as compared to the double-bundle arthroscopic inlay group [39]. The results of the Kim et al. study [39] suggest some functional advantage of the all-arthroscopic tibial inlay double-bundle PCL-R in the isolated PCL-injured knee. Until recently, the clinical and functional results of this technique in the multiligamentous injured knee were largely unknown. Recent work from our institute implementing this surgical technique in a multiligament-injured patient cohort suggests that at greater than 2 years following surgery, this technique is clinically, functionally, and radiographically comparable to the transtibial and open tibial inlay techniques in a similar patient population [41].

Conclusion

Although injury to the PCL is less frequent than ACL injury, incorrect management of PCL ruptures can ultimately lead to a cascade of events similar to that of ACL injury, thus resulting in knee joint arthrosis. Multiple surgical techniques exist for the reconstruction of the PCL, including transtibial drilling, open tibial inlay, and arthroscopic tibial inlay. Arthroscopic tibial inlay circumvents the potential for graft failure associated with the "killer turn" in transtibial PCL-R, and eliminates the potential morbidity accompanying an open surgical approach to the posterior knee associated with open tibial inlay. Furthermore, double-bundle PCL-R more closely recapitulates the normal knee kinematics following PCL injury. Lastly, the emerging clinical results for the all-arthroscopic tibial inlay double-bundle PCL-R are comparable if not superior to the alternative surgical techniques. For all these reasons, we recommend the all-arthroscopic tibial inlay double-bundle PCL-R.

References

1. Logan M, Williams A, Lavelle J, Gedroyc W, Freeman M. The effect of posterior cruciate ligament deficiency on knee kinematics. Am J Sports Med. 2004;32(8):1915–22.
2. Van de Velde SK, Bingham JT, Gill TJ, Li G. Analysis of tibiofemoral cartilage deformation in the posterior cruciate ligament-deficient knee. J Bone Joint Surg Am. 2009;91(1):167–75.
3. Boynton MD, Tietjens BR. Long-term followup of the untreated isolated posterior cruciate ligament-deficient knee. Am J Sports Med. 1996;24(3):306–10.
4. Bianchi M. Acute tears of the posterior cruciate ligament: clinical study and results of operative treatment in 27 cases. Am J Sports Med. 1983;11(5):308–14.
5. Clancy WG, Jr., Pandya RD. Posterior cruciate ligament reconstruction with patellar tendon autograft. Clin Sports Med. 1994;13(3):561–70.
6. Fanelli GC, Edson CJ. Arthroscopically assisted combined anterior and posterior cruciate ligament reconstruction in the multiple ligament injured knee: 2- to 10-year follow-up. Arthroscopy. 2002;18(7):703–14.
7. LaPrade RF. Arthroscopic evaluation of the lateral compartment of knees with grade 3 posterolateral knee complex injuries. Am J Sports Med. 1997;25(5):596–602.
8. Sekiya JK, Whiddon DR, Zehms CT, Miller MD. A clinically relevant assessment of posterior cruciate ligament and posterolateral corner injuries. Evaluation of isolated and combined deficiency. J Bone Joint Surg Am. 2008;90(8):1621–7.
9. Fanelli GC, Edson CJ. Posterior cruciate ligament injuries in trauma patients: Part II. Arthroscopy. 1995;11(5):526–9.
10. Fanelli GC, Giannotti BF, Edson CJ. The posterior cruciate ligament arthroscopic evaluation and treatment. Arthroscopy. 1994;10(6):673–88.
11. Sekiya JK, Haemmerle MJ, Stabile KJ, Vogrin TM, Harner CD. Biomechanical analysis of a combined double-bundle posterior cruciate ligament and posterolateral corner reconstruction. Am J Sports Med. 2005;33(3):360–9.
12. Sekiya JK, West RV, Ong BC, Irrgang JJ, Fu FH, Harner CD. Clinical outcomes after isolated arthroscopic single-bundle posterior cruciate ligament reconstruction. Arthroscopy. 2005;21(9): 1042–50.
13. Cooper DE, Stewart D. Posterior cruciate ligament reconstruction using single-bundle patella tendon graft with tibial inlay fixation: 2- to 10-year follow-up. Am J Sports Med. 2004;32(2):346–60.
14. Fanelli GC, Beck JD, Edson CJ. Single compared to double-bundle PCL reconstruction using allograft tissue. J Knee Surg. 2012;25(1):59–64.
15. Harner CD, Waltrip RL, Bennett CH, Francis KA, Cole B, Irrgang JJ. Surgical management of knee dislocations. J Bone Joint Surg Am. 2004;86-A(2):262–73.
16. Levy BA, Dajani KA, Whelan DB, Stannard JP, Fanelli GC, Stuart MJ et al. Decision making in the multiligament-injured knee: an evidence-based systematic review. Arthroscopy. 2009;25(4):430–8.
17. MacGillivray JD, Stein BE, Park M, Allen AA, Wickiewicz TL, Warren RF. Comparison of tibial inlay versus transtibial techniques for isolated posterior cruciate ligament reconstruction: minimum 2-year follow-up. Arthroscopy. 2006;22(3):320–8.
18. Mook WR, Miller MD, Diduch DR, Hertel J, Boachie-Adjei Y, Hart JM. Multiple-ligament knee injuries: a systematic review of the timing of operative intervention and postoperative rehabilitation. J Bone Joint Surg Am. 2009;91(12):2946–57.
19. Kohen RB, Sekiya JK. Single-bundle versus double-bundle posterior cruciate ligament reconstruction. Arthroscopy. 2009;25(12):1470–7.
20. Wijdicks CA, Kennedy NI, Goldsmith MT, Devitt BM, Michalski MP, Aroen A et al. Kinematic analysis of the posterior cruciate ligament, part 2: a comparison of anatomic single- versus double-bundle reconstruction. Am J Sports Med. 2013;41(12):2839–48.
21. Whiddon DR, Zehms CT, Miller MD, Quinby JS, Montgomery SL, Sekiya JK. Double compared with single-bundle open inlay posterior cruciate ligament reconstruction in a cadaver model. J Bone Joint Surg Am. 2008;90(9):1820–9.
22. Campbell RB, Jordan SS, Sekiya JK. Arthroscopic tibial inlay for posterior cruciate ligament reconstruction. Arthroscopy. 2007;23(12):1356 e1–4.
23. Jordan SS, Campbell RB, Sekiya JK. Posterior cruciate ligament reconstruction using a new arthroscopic tibial inlay double-bundle technique. Sports Med Arthrosc. 2007;15(4):176–83.
24. Zehms CT, Whiddon DR, Miller MD, Quinby JS, Montgomery SL, Campbell RB et al. Comparison of a double bundle arthroscopic inlay and open inlay posterior cruciate ligament reconstruction using clinically relevant tools: a cadaveric study. Arthroscopy. 2008;24(4):472–80.
25. Ruberte Thiele RA, Campbell RB, Amendola A, Sekiya JK. Biomechanical comparison of figure-of-8 versus cylindrical tibial inlay constructs for arthroscopic posterior cruciate ligament reconstruction. Arthroscopy. 2010;26(7):977–83.
26. Anderson CJ, Westerhaus BD, Pietrini SD, Ziegler CG, Wijdicks CA, Johansen S et al. Kinematic impact of anteromedial and posterolateral bundle graft fixation angles on double-bundle anterior cruciate ligament reconstructions. Am J Sports Med. 2010;38(8):1575–83.
27. Kim SJ, Park IS. Arthroscopic reconstruction of the posterior cruciate ligament using tibial-inlay and double-bundle technique. Arthroscopy. 2005;21(10):1271.
28. Harner CD, Janaushek MA, Ma CB, Kanamori A, Vogrin TM, Woo SL. The effect of knee flexion angle and application of an anterior tibial load at the time of graft fixation on the biomechanics of a posterior cruciate ligament-reconstructed knee. Am J Sports Med. 2000;28(4):460–5.

29. Edson CJ, Feldman DD. Rehabilitation of posterior cruciate ligament injuries. In: Fanelli GC, editor. Posterior cruciate ligament injuries: a practical guide to management. New York: Springer; 2001. pp. 267–89.
30. Noyes FR, Barber-Westin SD. Reconstruction of the anterior and posterior cruciate ligaments after knee dislocation. Use of early protected postoperative motion to decrease arthrofibrosis. Am J Sports Med. 1997;25(6):769–78.
31. Kim KM, Croy T, Hertel J, Saliba S. Effects of neuromuscular electrical stimulation after anterior cruciate ligament reconstruction on quadriceps strength, function, and patient-oriented outcomes: a systematic review. J Orthop Sports Phys Ther. 2010;40(7):383–91.
32. Chu BI, Martin RL, Carcia CR, et al. Surgical techniques and postoperative rehabilitation for isolated posterior cruciate ligament injuries. Orthop Phys Ther Pract. 2007;19(4):185–9.
33. Harner CD, Janaushek MA, Kanamori A, Yagi M, Vogrin TM, Woo SL. Biomechanical analysis of a double-bundle posterior cruciate ligament reconstruction. Am J Sports Med. 2000;28(2):144–51.
34. Tsukada H, Ishibashi Y, Tsuda E, Fukuda A, Yamamoto Y, Toh S. Biomechanical evaluation of an anatomic double-bundle posterior cruciate ligament reconstruction. Arthroscopy. 2012;28(2):264–71.
35. Race A, Amis AA. PCL reconstruction. In vitro biomechanical comparison of 'isometric' versus single and double-bundled 'anatomic' grafts. J Bone Joint Surg Br. 1998;80(1):173–9.
36. Bergfeld JA, McAllister DR, Parker RD, Valdevit AD, Kambic HE. A biomechanical comparison of posterior cruciate ligament reconstruction techniques. Am J Sports Med. 2001;29(2):129–36.
37. Markolf KL, Zemanovic JR, McAllister DR. Cyclic loading of posterior cruciate ligament replacements fixed with tibial tunnel and tibial inlay methods. J Bone Joint Surg Am. 2002;84-A(4):518–24.
38. Campbell RB, Torrie A, Hecker A, Sekiya JK. Comparison of tibial graft fixation between simulated arthroscopic and open inlay techniques for posterior cruciate ligament reconstruction. Am J Sports Med. 2007;35(10):1731–8.
39. Kim SJ, Kim TE, Jo SB, Kung YP. Comparison of the clinical results of three posterior cruciate ligament reconstruction techniques. J Bone Joint Surg Am. 2009;91(11):2543–9.
40. Mariani PP, Margheritini F. Full arthroscopic inlay reconstruction of posterior cruciate ligament. Knee Surg Sports Traumatol Arthrosc. 2006;14(11):1038–44.
41. Weber AE, Bissell B, Wojtys EM, Sekiya JK. All-arthroscopic tibial inlay double-bundle PCL-R in multiligamentous knee reconstructions: Early results with 2-year follow-up. Clin Orthops Relat Res. 2014; provisionally accepted.
42. Weber AE, Sekiya JKS. Arthroscopic double-bundle tibial inlay posterior cruciate ligament reconstruction. In: Cole BJ, Sekiya JK, editors. Surgical techniques of the shoulder, elbow, and knee in sports medicine, 2nd Edition. Philadelphia: Elsevier. 2013. pp. 861–870.

All-Inside Posterior Cruciate Ligament Reconstruction

12

William M. Engasser, Paul L. Sousa, Michael J. Stuart and Bruce A. Levy

Introduction

The incidence of posterior cruciate ligament (PCL) injury has been reported with significant variability in the literature. A review by Shelbourne et al. [1] demonstrated a PCL disruption incidence of 1–44 % in acute knee injuries [2–7]. This large variation appears to be dependent on the specific population being studied. For example, Miyasaka [6] reported a 3 % incidence of PCL injury in the general population, and Fanelli [7] reported a 38 % incidence of PCL injury in patients with hemarthrosis of the knee at a regional trauma center. The literature provides clinicians with an estimation of PCL injury risk, but the true incidence remains elusive due to unreported injuries.

The mechanism of PCL injury typically involves a traumatic, posteriorly directed force to the tibia with the knee in a flexed position. This mechanism commonly occurs during a motor vehicle collision or when an athlete falls on their knee with the foot plantarflexed [8,9]. Additional implicated mechanisms include hyperflexion, hyperextension, and extreme rotation [10–12].

Although PCL tears can occur in isolation, they are more commonly seen in the setting of the multiple-ligament-injured knee [11,13–16]. In a recent study by Becker et al. [17], 65 of 82 patients (79 %) presenting with a multiple-ligament knee injury had evidence of PCL injury on MRI. Whether isolated or combined, PCL injuries must be evaluated with an in-depth history, detailed physical examination, and advanced imaging. Treatment options include nonoperative management, repair, or reconstruction. This chapter focuses on the initial management of PCL injuries and evidence to support our preferred all-inside PCL reconstruction technique.

Physical Examination

The physical examination begins with a thorough neurovascular assessment. Many of these injuries occur from high-energy mechanism, and exclusion of a compartment syndrome is important. A full lower-extremity assessment is then performed, including knee range of motion, limb alignment, gait, and ligament stability.

Three physical exam tests determine the integrity of the PCL: posterior drawer, posterior sag, and quadriceps active. The posterior drawer maneuver is the most effective with a sensitivity of 90 % and a specificity of 99 % [18,19]. This maneuver is performed by applying a posterior force to the tibia with the knee flexed at 90°and the hip flexed at 45°. The amount of tibial translation on the femur determines the test grade: grade 1 = less than 5 mm, grade 2 = 5–10 mm, and grade 3 = greater than 10 mm. The anterior margin of the tibial condyles lies approximately 10 mm anterior to the femoral condyles anatomically when the knee is flexed to 90°. A grade 2 posterior sag (grade 2 PCL injury) is diagnosed when the tibial condyles are flush with the femoral condyles, and a grade 3 posterior sag is present if the tibial condyles translate posterior to the femoral condyles. The quadriceps active test is performed with the patient in a supine position with the knee flexed to 90°. The examiner then applies a counter force to the patient's ankle in order to resist knee extension while the patient contracts their quadriceps muscles. Anterior translation of the tibia during this maneuver suggests a PCL injury, since the initial posterior tibial translation is reduced by quadriceps contraction.

PCL disruption frequently occurs in the setting of the multi-ligament-injured knee [11,13–16]. Assessment of the anterior cruciate ligament (ACL) with a PCL injury is challenging. The examiner must pay attention to the position of the tibia relative to the femoral condyles when performing

B. A. Levy (✉) · M. J. Stuart
Orthopedic Surgery, Mayo Clinic, Rochester, MN, USA

W. M. Engasser · P. L. Sousa
Sports Medicine, Orthopedic Surgery, Mayo Clinic, Rochester, MN, USA

G. C. Fanelli (ed.), *Posterior Cruciate Ligament Injuries*,
DOI 10.1007/978-3-319-12072-0_12, © Springer International Publishing Switzerland 2015

the Lachman's test and pivot shift tests. The increased posterior translation of the tibia relative to the femur in a PCL-deficient knee may cause false-positive examination maneuvers. The examiner must focus on the tibial start point and endpoint during both the pivot shift and Lachman tests. Increased anterior tibial translation with a firm endpoint suggests an intact ACL, whereas increased anterior tibial translation with a soft endpoint is consistent with both disruption of the ACL and PCL.

Assessment of posterolateral corner (PLC), integrity involves a variety of examination maneuvers including the dial test at 30° and 90°, external rotation recurvatum test, external rotation drawer test, and reverse pivot shift test. The dial test is performed by examining the lateral movement of the tibial tubercle with an external rotation force at both 30° and 90° of knee flexion. Increased tibial tubercle external rotation of greater than 10° compared to the contralateral side denotes a significant difference. A positive dial test at 90° of knee flexion indicates PCL injury and at 30° of flexion indicates PLC injury. The external rotation recurvatum test is performed with the patient supine and both knees fully extended. With the patient fully relaxed, the examiner lifts the patient's legs off the table by grasping the foot. Relative hyperextension combined with external rotation of the tibia indicates a positive exam. The external rotation drawer test is performed with the patient supine and the injured knee flexed to 90°. The examiner externally rotates the tibia and applies a posterior force similar to a posterior drawer test. Posterior displacement or increased step-off of the tibial plateau indicates a positive exam finding. The reverse pivot shift test is performed with the patient supine. The examiner begins with the knee flexed, applies valgus and external rotational forces, and slowly extends the knee. Reduction of the posteriorly subluxated lateral tibial plateau is considered a positive test.

Imaging

Plain radiographs and magnetic resonance imaging (MRI) are utilized when assessing a PCL-injured knee. Anteroposterior (AP) and supine lateral radiographs of the knee are used to assess for posterior tibiofemoral subluxation, fractures, asymmetry of the joint spaces, and bony avulsion of the tibial insertion of the PCL. A fibular head avulsion fracture with posterior tibiofemoral subluxation on the supine lateral view suggests both PCL and PLCinjuries.

Numerous studies have demonstrated the benefit of stress radiographs in the evaluation of the PCL-injured knee [20–22]. Shulz et al. [21] found that greater than 8 mm of posterior displacement on stress radiograph demonstrates isolated PCL injury, whereas greater than 12 mm of posterior displacement represents combined PCL and PLC injuries. A cadaveric sectioning study by Sekiya et al. [22] correlated stress radiograph displacement and posterior drawer examination findings in isolated PCL-sectioned and combined PCL- and PLC-sectioned knees. The authors found an average of 9.8 mm of posterior tibial displacement on stress radiograph and a grade 2 posterior drawer test when only the PCL was sectioned. This posterior displacement increased to an average of 19.4 mm and a grade 3 posterior drawer test when both the PCL and the PLC structures were sectioned. Thus, it was concluded that greater than 10 mm of posterior displacement on lateral supine stress radiograph and a grade 3 posterior drawer test indicates injury to the PCL and PLC.

MRI is the best imaging modality to assess the PCL in an injured knee. Complete disruption or signal change within the PCL can be seen, but it is critical to correlate the imaging findings with physical examination. 3-Tesla MRI scanners are most useful when evaluating the ligaments and other soft tissue structures, including menisci, chondral surfaces, tendons, muscles, and capsular structures.

Indications for PCL Reconstruction

Management of both isolated and combined PCL injuries is still being debated within the orthopedic literature. Several studies have demonstrated successful clinical and functional outcomes after nonoperative management of isolated PCL injuries [1,11,15,23,24] using bracing and physical therapy. A natural history study on isolated PCL injuries by Parolie et al. [5] revealed that 80 % of patients were satisfied with their knee function and 84 % had returned to their sport prior to injury at a mean follow-up of 6.2 years.

Patel et al. [25] retrospectively reviewed 58 knees with isolated PCL injuries treated without surgery. Within this series, 24 % of patients had grade A (partial tear), 76 % grade B (complete tear), and 0 % grade C (tibia is displaced behind the femur) on posterior drawer testing. The authors found that 90 % of knees had mild or no pain, 93 % did not demonstrate any swelling, and only 8 % of patients reported episodes of giving way. The mean Lysholm score was 85.2 with 92 % of knees reporting as good or excellent. No correlation was found between degree of laxity and final outcome score.

Shelbourne et al. [1,15,24] have since performed a prospective case series looking at both short- and long-term outcomes after acute, isolated PCL injuries treated nonoperatively. In the most recent publication of this series, 68 patients at a mean follow-up of 17.6 years reported an International Knee Documentation Committee (IKDC) [26] score of 73.4. Furthermore, they found no correlation between PCL laxity grades and outcome measures. Of the 68 patients in this cohort, 44 had both subjective and objective measures available. This subset of patients had a mean follow-up of 14.3 years (range, 10–21 years). Mean muscle strength in the injured knee was found to be 97 % compared to the uninvolved leg with all patients demonstrating normal range of motion. The overall grade of radiographs was normal in 59 % of patients, nearly normal in 30 %, abnormal in 9 %, and severely abnormal in 1 % at long-term follow-up. Additionally, 11 % of patients had medial joint space narrowing greater than 2 mm. The grade of radiographically measured osteoarthritis, however, was not significant in any knee compartment based on PCL laxity. A major limitation of this long-term study was that none of the 44 patients had an initial PCL injury greater than grade 2.

The successful results seen from nonoperative treatment in the previously mentioned studies are likely skewed because only grade 1 and 2 isolated PCL injuries were studied. We therefore, only recommend nonoperative management for these lower-grade injuries. In higher-grade PCL tears, we recommend surgical management. Operative indications for the PCL-injured knee include:

- Avulsion fracture of the PCL tibial insertion (open reduction and internal fixation)
- Acute or chronic isolated grade 3 PCL injury (ligament reconstruction)
- PCL insufficiency in the setting of the multiple-ligament-injured knee (ligament reconstruction)

Scientific Rationale

There are a variety of different PCL reconstruction techniques that have been developed including arthroscopic transtibial, open inlay, and arthroscopic inlay. Bone tunnel creations in these techniques have used "inside-out," "outside-in," and "all-inside" techniques. PCL reconstruction graft construct options include anterolateral (AL), single-bundle or AL and posteromedial (PM) bundle, double-bundle reconstructions using either allograft or autograft. The all-inside PCL reconstruction is our preferred technique based on current evidence in the literature.

Transtibial Versus Inlay

The arthroscopic transtibial technique is performed by drilling a tunnel from the anterior portion of the tibia to the footprint of the PCL. As the graft passes through the tibia, it is forced to make the "killer turn" around the posterior tibial margin. In a biomechanical study by Markolf et al. [27], the authors compared the transtibial and tibial inlay PCL reconstruction techniques using a bone–patellar tendon–bone (BTB) allograft. Each graft construct was placed through 2000 cycles of 50–300 N tensile force. Ten of the 31 knees (32 %) in the transtibial technique group failed before completing 2000 cycles and none of the 31 knees (0 %) failed in the inlay technique group. The location of graft failure in all of these cases occurred at the point of the "killer turn" along the posterior aspect of the tibia at the level of the PCL facet. Additionally, when comparing change in graft thickness of the 21 paired grafts that survived, they found that the transtibial group had greater graft attrition than the inlay group. The authors did note, however, that both groups had significant graft damage and increase in graft length after 2000 cycles. The authors concluded that while both techniques demonstrated graft attrition and lengthening, the inlay technique had significantly less graft failure.

In another study by McAllister et al. [28], the authors compared 12 cadaveric knees fixed with either the transtibial or inlay PCL reconstruction techniques. The knees underwent AP tibial loading of 200 N for 50 cycles. Two of the 12 (17 %) grafts fixed by the transtibial technique failed prior to completing 50 cycles, but none of the 12 (0 %) failed in the inlay reconstruction group. The graft failures occurred at the point of the "killer turn." The authors also found that both groups had a significant increase in mean AP laxity at 90°after 50 cycles, but found no difference between the two groups in this regard.

In a more recent cadaveric study comparing these two techniques, Margheritini et al. [20] measured posterior tibial displacement at various knee angles in ten knees. The knees were tested in both the PCL-intact and PCL-deficient states, and were then reconstructed with either the transtibial or inlay techniques. The authors found that both reconstruction techniques reduced the posterior tibial displacement at all knee flexion angles, but found no significant difference between the two reconstruction groups.

While the biomechanical studies demonstrate lower failure rates when using the inlay versus the transtibial technique, the clinical data cloud this debate. We performed a systematic review of the literature [29] and found no important advantage of one technique over the other. Satisfactory subjective and objective outcomes were seen in both types of reconstruction. The mean score for patients reconstructed with the transtibial technique was found to be 77.8 with 77.7 % normal and nearly normal responses in the objective IKDC scoring system. The mean IKDC score for patients reconstructed with the inlay technique was 75.1 with 100 % normal and nearly normal response. Additionally, both techniques had equivalent results on posterior stress radiographic measurements. The transtibial technique demonstrated a mean difference of 3.5 mm and the inlay technique demonstrated a mean difference of 4.3 mm when compared to the contralateral knee. Furthermore, arthrometer measurements showed no significant difference between the two groups.

While a few studies have attempted to directly compare the transtibial and inlay techniques, the results are difficult to interpret because graft selection and number of bundles reconstructed were inconsistent. Regardless, each of these studies demonstrated that both techniques produced similar clinical and functional outcomes.

Campbell et al. [30] published the first arthroscopic inlay technique in 2007 utilizing a BTB allograft and a RetroDrill (Arthrex, Naples, FL, USA) to create the tibial socket. This technique has the benefit of avoiding the "killer turn" while eliminating the morbidity associated with a large posterior incision and capsulotomy. Bovid et al. [31] presented a case report using the arthroscopic inlay technique in a skeletally immature patient. This technique enabled the tibial socket to be created without violating the physis. At 17 months postoperatively, the patient returned to full function, however, no long-term follow-up has been presented to date.

Salata and Sekiya [32] published a further modification of the Campbell and Bovid techniques using a FlipCutter (Arthrex, Naples, FL, USA) in order to create the tibial socket. In their technique, a PCL guide was used to drill a guide wire posteriorly toward the tibial footprint of the PCL. Then, a 3.5-mm cannulated drill is reamed over the guide pin. Next, the FlipCutter was advanced through the created tunnel and was deployed once exiting the cortex. The authors then performed retrograde drilling of the tibial socket using the FlipCutter. The authors argue that the anatomic position of the tibial insertion of the PCL in this technique avoids the killer turn, similar to the Campbell and Bovid techniques. The FlipCutter is more easily positioned, however, and it avoids intra-articular assembly seen with the RetroDrill.

Single Bundle Versus Double Bundle

Both single-bundle and double-bundle PCL reconstructions have demonstrated satisfactory clinical outcomes [33–39]. While authors who support the double-bundle technique argue that it restores native PCL biomechanics and anatomy, clinical studies have thus far shown equivalent results with both reconstruction techniques.

The native PCL complex consists of the AL bundle, PM bundle, and the anterior and posterior meniscofemoral ligaments (AMFL, PMFL). The weaker PM bundle tightens when the knee is flexed to approximately 20–30°. The stronger AL bundle tightens at 80–90°of knee flexion and is the primary constraint to posterior tibial displacement [40]. As such, the AL bundle is reconstructed during single-bundle PCL reconstruction.

Markolf et al. [41] performed a biomechanical study that sought to compare single- and double-bundle PCL reconstruction. In this cadaveric study, the authors measured AP laxity and PCL forces at various angles of knee flexion. The measurements were obtained with the PCL intact, sectioned, reconstructed with a single-bundle technique, and reconstructed with a double-bundle technique. The authors found that the single-bundle technique restored native PCL forces better than the double-bundle technique. The double-bundle reconstruction created higher than normal PM graft forces, which could not be explained. However, the authors did find that the mean AP laxity of the single-bundle reconstructions was 1.1–2.0 mm greater than the double-bundle technique at 0–30°of flexion. They questioned whether this increase in force would eventually cause elongation of the graft and eventually gain more AP tibial laxity.

Whiddon et al. [42] compared single-bundle and double-bundle PCL reconstruction in the presence of a PLC injury using ten cadaveric knees. The authors first examined each knee with an intact PCL using the posterior drawer and dial test exam maneuvers, as well as stress radiographs. The PCL and PLC of each knee were disrupted. This was accomplished by sectioning the PCL and by removing the FCL and popliteus femoral attachments with an osteotome creating a large bone block. The authors then performed single-bundle and double-bundle PCL reconstruction with and without the PLC fixed back to the lateral femur. The authors found that in the setting of a disrupted PLC, the double-bundle PCL reconstruction showed less posterior tibial displacement. However, when the PLC was restored, no difference in posterior tibial displacement was noted between the single- or double-bundle techniques. The authors concluded that because PLC reconstructions tend to stretch out, the double-bundle technique may be superior in the setting of combined PCL and PLC injuries.

Similar to the biomechanical data, clinical studies continue to demonstrate equivalent results when directly comparing single- versus double-bundle PCL reconstruction techniques. Wang et al. [36] performed a prospective study in which they reconstructed 19 patients with single AL bundle reconstructions and compared them to 16 patients with double-bundle reconstructions. Lysholm, Tegner, and IKDC scores were utilized to measure functional outcomes. Radiographic examination and ligamentous laxity were also measured. The authors found no significant difference in all of these parameters measured between the single- and double-bundle PCL reconstruction groups.

Yoon et al. [43] also performed a prospective randomized trial comparing arthroscopic single- versus double-bundle PCL reconstruction. A single surgeon performed 25 single-bundle reconstructions and 28 double-bundle reconstructions in patients with isolated PCL injuries. An Achilles tendon allograft was used in all cases. Both the single- and double-bundle reconstructions were performed using an arthroscopic transtibial technique for the tibial portion and "outside-in" femoral tunnel placement. The authors found that the double-bundle reconstruction had 1.4 mm less posterior tibial displacement and higher IKDC scores than the single-bundle construct. All other measures of evaluation, including range of motion, stress radiographs, and Tegner and Lysholm scores, demonstrated no difference between the two groups.

Fanelli et al. [44] published a series of 90 consecutive patients (45 single- and 45 double-bundle reconstructions) in an effort to compare the two reconstruction techniques. All of the patients in this series had PCL-based multiple-ligament-injured knees. The surgical technique was identical for the single- and double-bundle groups, except the double-bundle group had a second tunnel created on the femur for the PM bundle. All patients had a minimum of 2-year follow-up and evaluation, including stress radiography, KT-1000 arthrotomy, Tegner, Lysholm, and Hospital for Special Surgery outcome scores. The author found no difference between the single- and double-bundle PCL reconstructions.

Our preferred technique is a single AL bundle reconstruction because it reduces surgery time and clinical evidence demonstrates no advantage to performing a double-bundle reconstruction.

Femoral Tunnel: "Outside-In" Versus "Inside-Out"

For the femoral side of the PCL reconstruction, both "outside-in" and "inside-out" techniques have been developed. The "outside-in" technique is performed by creating an incision on the medial side of the knee with dissection through the vastus medialis oblique (VMO) muscle. A tunnel is then drilled from the medial cortex of the femur to the intercondylar notch using an arthroscopically placed PCL femoral footprint guide. The "inside-out" technique is performed by creating an accessory inferolateral portal. Through this portal, with the knee flexed to approximately 100°, a guide pin is inserted into the femoral footprint and then over-reamed through the femoral cortex.

A proposed advantage of the "outside-in" technique is the avoidance of the second so-called killer turn, otherwise called the "critical corner," which is prevalent with the "inside-out" technique. Much like the "killer turn" in the tibial tunnel, many authors believe that too large of an angle can cause graft lengthening and even failure. In their biomechanical study, Handy et al. sought to measure the "critical corner" angle in both "outside-in" and "inside-out" techniques using nine cadaveric knees. The authors found that the "outside-in" group had graft/femoral tunnel angles of 50° with the knee in flexion and −14° in extension. The "inside-out" group had graft/femoral tunnel angles of 87° in flexion and 27° in extension. It was concluded that the "outside-in" technique reduces the angle of the "critical corner."

In another biomechanical study by Schoderbek Jr. et al. [45], the authors sought to compare the "critical corner" of the "outside-in" and "inside-out" techniques with the knee flexed at 90° and 120°. The authors found that the mean graft/femoral tunnel angle was significantly less at both of these flexion points using the "outside-in" method. Therefore, the authors recommend the use of the "outside-in" technique because it creates smaller angles for the PCL graft. Tompkins et al. [46] recently performed a study comparing the ability of the "outside-in" and "inside-out" techniques to place tunnels into the anatomic femoral footprint of the PCL. The authors found that both techniques were equal in the ability to correctly place the femoral tunnel. While the biomechanical studies may show an increased risk of graft failure with the "inside-out" technique due to the increased "critical corner" angulation, clinical studies have shown successful outcomes with both techniques [35–37,39,43,44]. We have performed several revision PCL cases where the previous surgeons used an "outside-in" technique and reamed right through the femoral articular cartilage. Although we have used both techniques in the past, we currently prefer the "inside-out" technique because it allows us to use the reamer as a guide placed directly onto the PCL femoral footprint thereby, decreasing the risk of articular cartilage blowout.

AutograftVersus Allograft

A wide variety of graft types have been used for reconstruction of the PCL. While some authors prefer allograft due to decreased surgery time, less donor-site morbidity, and adequate graft length, others prefer using autograft due to graft availability and decreased risk of disease transmission or rejection. We performed a systematic review comparing the use of [47] allograft and autograft in PCL reconstruction. At minimum 2-year follow-up, both graft constructs produced satisfactory clinical and functional outcomes as measured by Lysholm, IKDC, and Tegner scoring systems. Additionally, we found no statistically significant difference between allograft and autograft with stress radiograph measurements and arthrometer testing.

Because the majority of PCL reconstructions are performed in the setting of multiple-ligament surgery, we currently use allograft tissue for the reasons mentioned above. In order to perform the all-inside technique with current fixation strategies, a minimum 36-cm-long graft is required. It would be extremely difficult to find an autograft option for a graft of this length. Therefore, our preferred graft choice is a tibialis anterior or peroneus longus nonirradiated allograft when performing the all-inside PCL reconstruction technique.

All-Inside PCL Reconstruction Surgical Technique

Patient Positioning

With the patient supine, a bilateral knee examination under anesthesia is performed to assess ligament integrity. The limb is then positioned, prepped, and draped.

Graft Preparation

The graft is prepared using a graft preparation board, which maintains tension on both femoral and tibial TightRopes (Arthrex, Naples, FL, USA). The graft is folded in a quadruple-looped fashion and sewn together with a number #2 FiberWire suture (Fig. 12.1). The graft is then marked with a sterile pen at 25 mm from both the femoral and tibial sides for intraoperative assessment of graft position in the tibial and femoral sockets. The prepared total graft length should be 95–100 mm.

Tibial Preparation

After a standard diagnostic arthroscopy, an accessory PM portal is placed in order to expose the PCL tibial footprint between the mamillary bodies. The PCL guide is inserted through the anteromedial (AM) portal and positioned at the base of the PCL facet (Fig. 12.2). Proper placement of the guide can be confirmed with fluoroscopy as needed (Fig. 12.3). A FlipCutter (Arthrex, Naples, FL, USA) is then drilled from anterior to posterior through the tibia until the drill tip penetrates the posterior cortex (Fig. 12.4). The PCL guide is used to protect the FlipCutter from plunging into the posterior neurovascular structures. The FlipCutter is then deployed and used to create the tibial socket with a depth of at least 35–40 mm (Fig. 12.5). The tibial socket is then

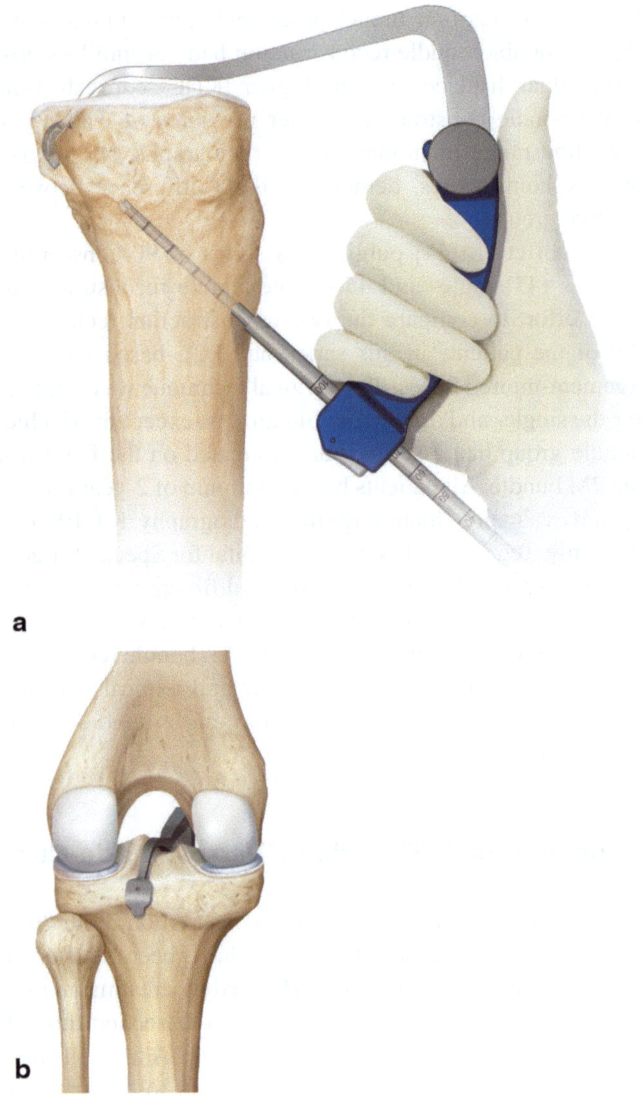
a

b

Fig. 12.2 **a** PCL guide positioned for the creation of the tibial tunnel. **b** Posterior view of PCL guide positioned just proximal to the distal edge of the posterior facet

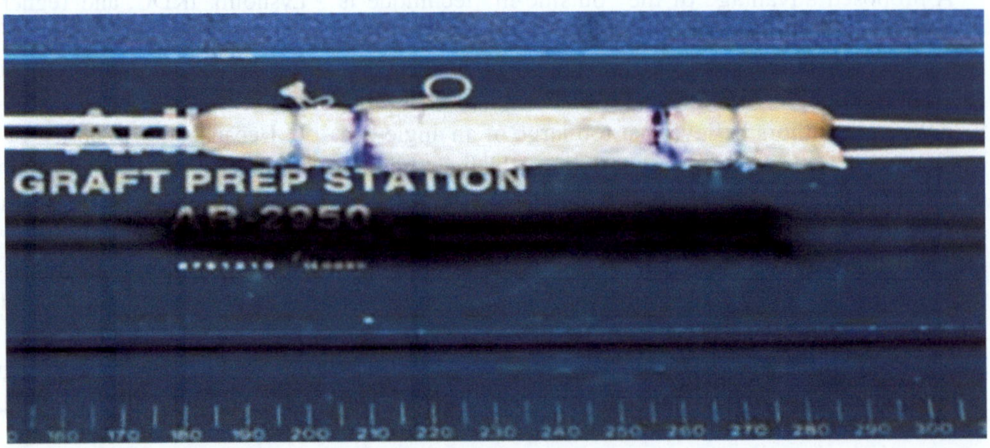

Fig. 12.1 Prepared tibialis anterior allograft under tension on a GraftLink preparation board (Arthrex, Naples, FL, USA) for PCL reconstruction

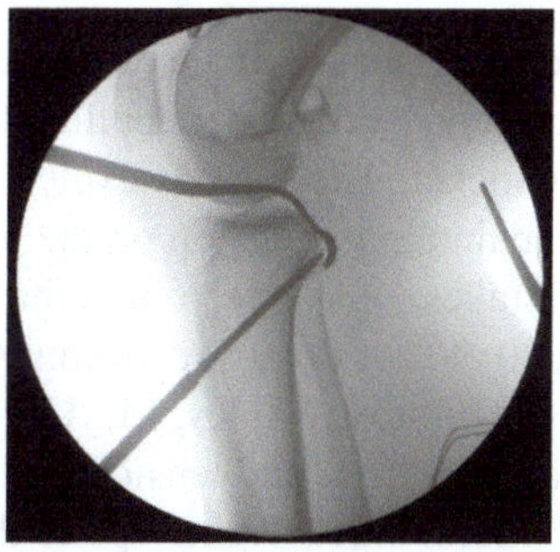

Fig. 12.3 Lateral fluoroscopic image showing proper placement of the PCL guide at the base of the PCL facet

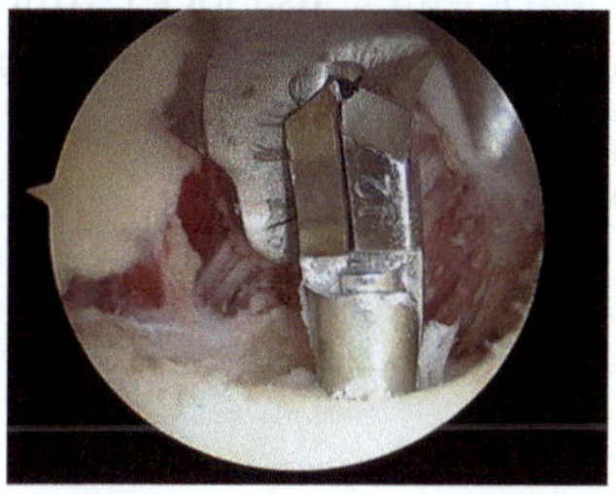

Fig. 12.4 Intraoperative arthroscopic image of the 12-mm FlipCutter (Arthrex, Naples, FL, USA) penetrating the posterior tibial cortex. The PCL guide acts to protect the neurovascular bundle while drilling. View from the AM portal

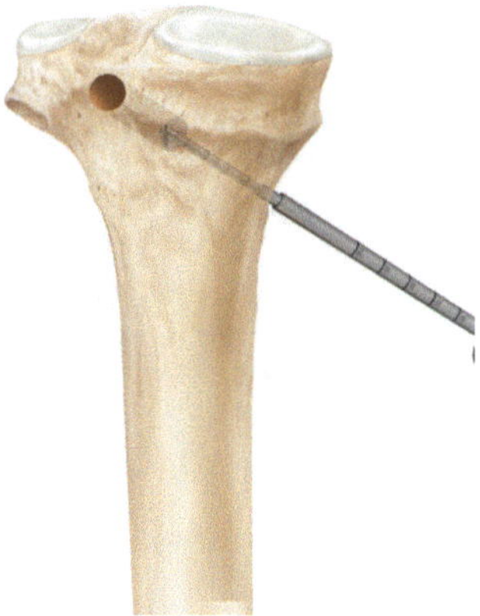

Fig. 12.5 The FlipCutter (Arthrex, Naples, FL, USA) is used to back-ream to a depth of at least 35–40 mm when making the tibial tunnel

cleaned out using a shaver. Passing sutures are then placed into the socket and pulled through the joint out of the AM or AL portals (Figs. 12.6 and 12.7).

Femoral Preparation

The native femoral AL bundle footprint of the PCL is exposed and some of the fibers are preserved to aid placement of the femoral socket. A guide wire is placed through an accessory, distal inferolateral portal and inserted into the center of the anatomic footprint. An 11- or 12-mm reamer is then passed over a guide wire and positioned at the most distal and anterior margins of the footprint. This avoids the risk of cartilage blowout as the reamer basically acts as a guide. The femoral socket is then reamed to a depth of at least 25 mm (Fig. 12.8a). Similar to the tibial side, a passing suture is then placed for eventual graft passage (Fig. 12.8b).

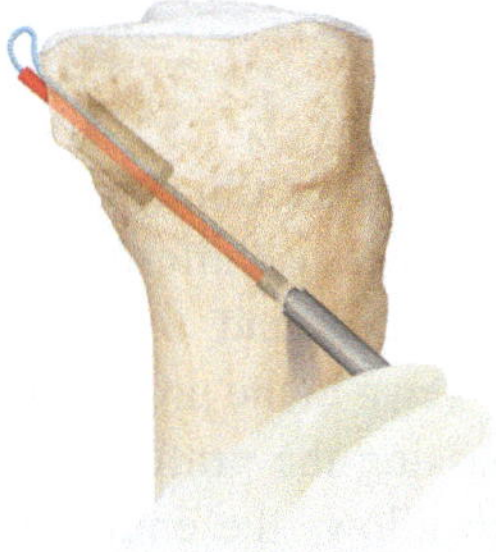

Fig. 12.6 A passing suture is placed through the drill sleeve into the joint for graft passage purposes

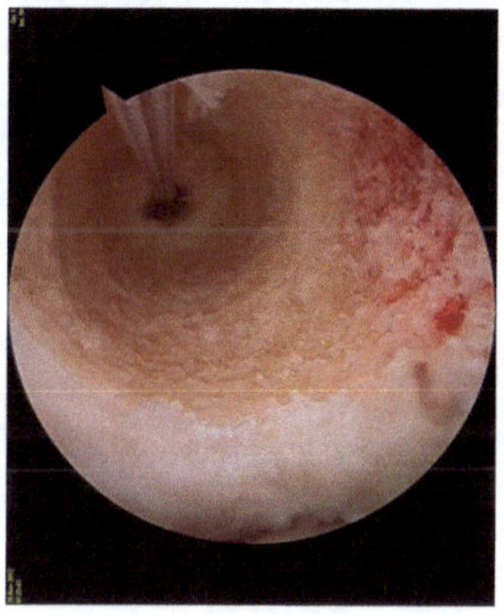

Fig. 12.7 Intraoperative arthroscopic image of passing sutures within the tibial socket. View from the PM portal

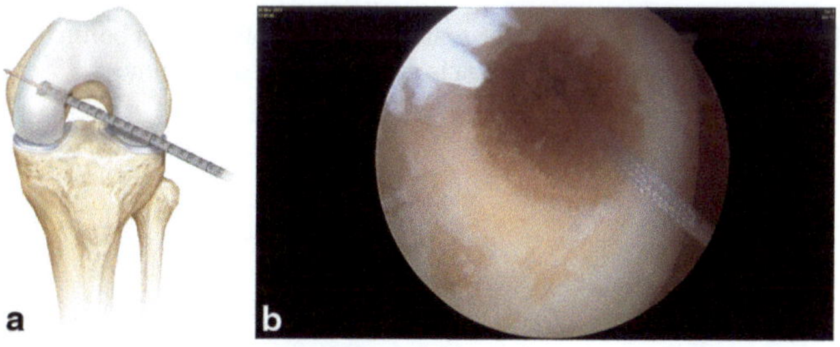

Fig. 12.8 **a** Creation of the femoral socket using an r eventual graft passage. The femoral socket should be drilled to at least 25 mm. **b** Intraoperative arthroscopic image of passing sutures within the femoral socket. View from the AM portal

Securing the Graft

The passing sutures on both the tibial and femoral sides are first pulled through an accessory inferolateral portal. These sutures should be looped around the TightRope sutures, which were previously sewn to the prepared graft. In our experience, we prefer passing the graft into the tibial socket first (Fig. 12.9), which allows the entire graft to be inside the knee joint before completing the reconstruction. We then pull graft into the femoral socket (Fig. 12.10) while maintaining tension on the tibial TightRope sutures. It is important to maintain counter-tension on the femoral side of the graft as the TightRope device is deployed. The TightRope sutures should be tensioned in order to seat the graft to a depth of approximately 20 mm in the femoral socket. The arthroscope is then placed into the PM portal and the tibial portion of the graft is visualized to ensure that at least 20 mm of graft is in the tibial socket. If there is excess length, the femoral TightRope can be tightened, pulling the graft further into the femoral socket. The knee is cycled with 20 cycles of knee flexion, maintaining tension on the tibial TightRope (Fig. 12.11). This takes some creep out of the graft construct. With the knee at 80–90° of flexion, a 16-mm Attachable Button System (ABS; Arthrex, Naples, FL, USA) button is secured to the tibial TightRope and tensioned (Fig. 12.12). Retensioning the femoral-sided TightRope is the final step in securing the PCL graft in both the femoral and tibial sockets (Fig. 12.13). If desired, secondary fixation on the tibial side can be performed. Our preferred technique is to secure the tibial sutures with a 5.5-mm push lock (Arthrex, Naples, FL, USA). Tying the sutures around a post is another viable option. A final AP radiograph of the all-inside PCL GraftLink technique is shown (Fig. 12.14).

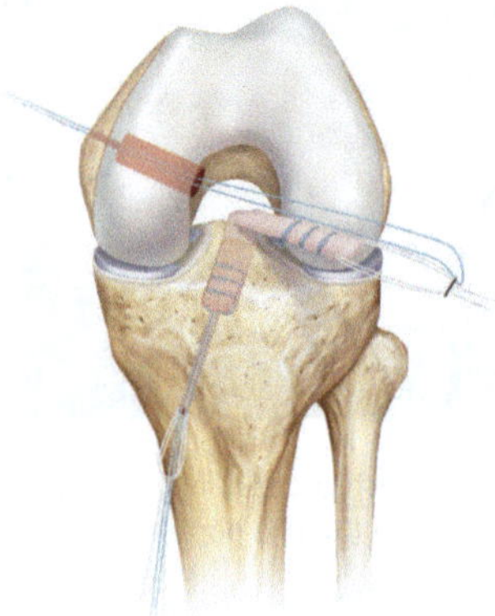

Fig. 12.9 The tibial side of the graft is pulled into the socket before the femoral side. Final tibial fixation is not performed at this time

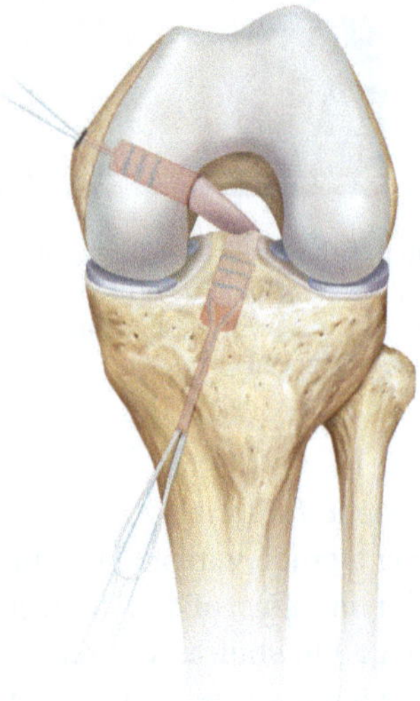

Fig. 12.10 The femoral side of the graft is pulled into the socket and is secured with a TightRope cortical button while maintaining tension on the tibial side of the graft

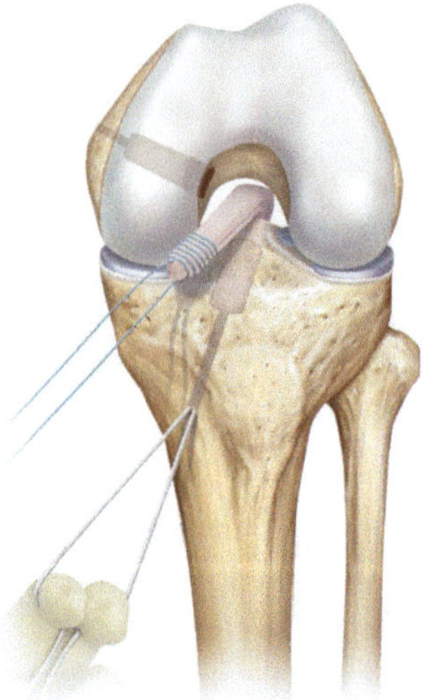

Fig. 12.11 Tensioning of the tibial sutures

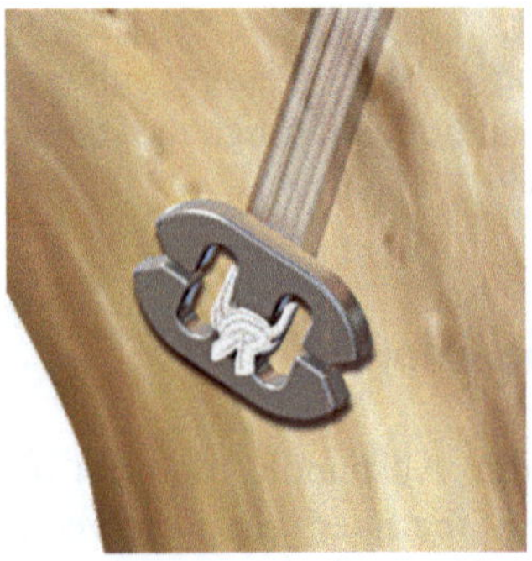

Fig. 12.12 ABS tibial TightRope button (Arthrex, Naples, FL, USA) is secured and sutures are cut

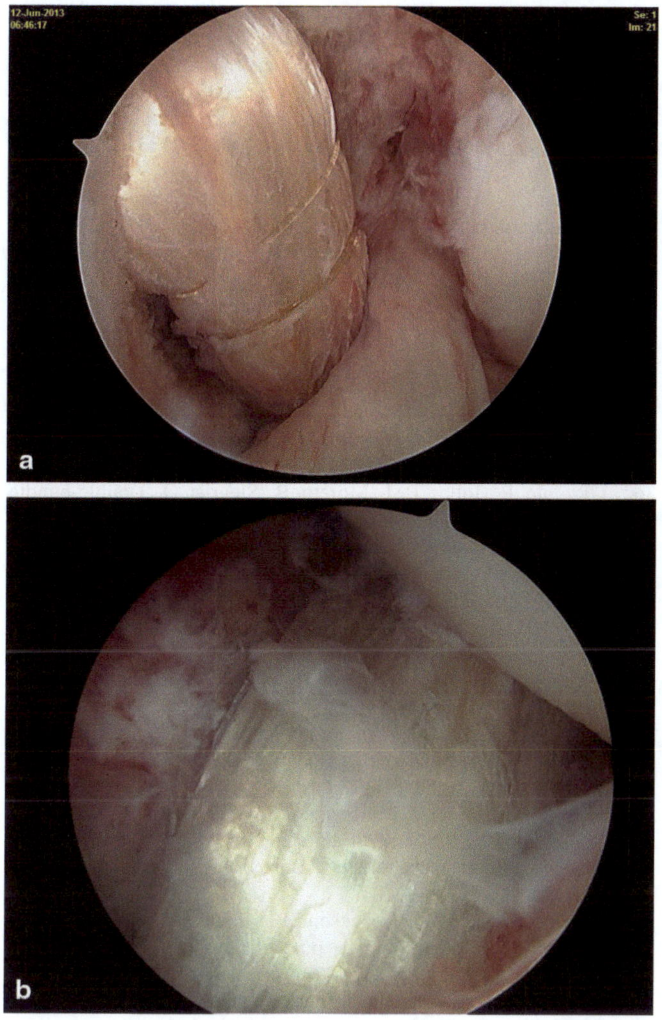

Fig. 12.13 **a** Intraoperative arthroscopic image with the femoral side of the graft in position. View from the AL portal. Note the intact ACL. **b** Intraoperative arthroscopic image with the tibial side of the graft in position. At least 20 mm of graft should be seated within the tibial socket. View from the PM portal

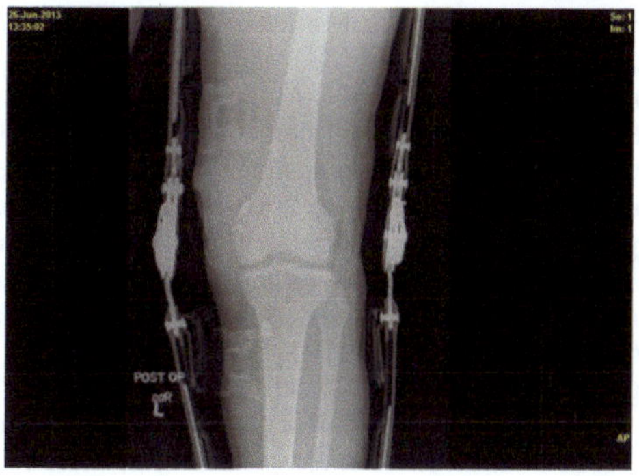

Fig. 12.14 Anteroposterior postoperative radiographs of PCL reconstruction using the all-inside technique. Patient also underwent posterolateral corner reconstruction

Conclusion

Numerous surgical techniques for PCL reconstruction have demonstrated successful clinical and functional outcomes [29–39,43,44]. These techniques include arthroscopic transtibial, open inlay, and arthroscopic inlay. Advances in surgical technique and instrumentation have led to the development of a novel all-inside PCL reconstruction. This technique utilizes suspensory fixation in both tibial and femoral sockets and allows for either allograft or autograft to be used. This reconstruction avoids the "killer turn" seen with the transtibial technique, which may decrease the chance of graft attrition while delivering decreased morbidity and excellent visualization using an all-arthroscopic approach. While early results using this technique are promising, long-term clinical and functional outcome studies are needed to validate this novel PCL reconstruction.

References

1. Shelbourne KD, Davis TJ, Patel DV. The natural history of acute, isolated, nonoperatively treated posterior cruciate ligament injuries. A prospective study. Am J Sports Med. 1999 May–Jun;27(3):276–83.
2. Fanelli GC, Giannotti BF, Edson CJ. The posterior cruciate ligament arthroscopic evaluation and treatment. Arthroscopy. 1994 Dec;10(6):673–88.
3. Hughston JC, Degenhardt TC. Reconstruction of the posterior cruciate ligament. Clin Orthop Relat Res. 1982 Apr; (164):59–77.
4. O'Donoghue DH. Surgical treatment of injuries to ligaments of the knee. JAMA. 1959 Mar 28;169(13):1423–31.
5. Parolie JM, Bergfeld JA. Long-term results of nonoperative treatment of isolated posterior cruciate ligament injuries in the athlete. Am J Sports Med. 1986 Jan–Feb;14(1):35–8.
6. Miyasaka KC, Daniel DM, Stone ML, Hirshman P. The incidence of knee ligament injuries in the general population. Am J Knee Surg. 1991;4:6.
7. Fanelli GC, Edson CJ. Posterior cruciate ligament injuries in trauma patients: Part II. Arthroscopy. 1995 Oct;11(5):526–9.
8. Clancy WG Jr, Shelbourne KD, Zoellner GB, Keene JS, Reider B, Rosenberg TD. Treatment of knee joint instability secondary to rupture of the posterior cruciate ligament. Report of a new procedure. J Bone Joint Surg Am. 1983 Mar;65(3):310–22.
9. Cooper DE, Warren RF, Warner JP. The posterior cruciate ligament and posterolateral structures of the knee: anatomy, function and patterns of injury. Am Acad Orthop Surg. 1991;40:1.
10. Fowler PJ, Messieh SS. Isolated posterior cruciate ligament injuries in athletes. Am J Sports Med. 1987 Nov–Dec;15(6):553–7.
11. Rubinstein RA Jr, Donald Shelbourne K. Diagnosis of posterior cruciate ligament injuries and indications for nonoperative and operative treatment. Oper Tech Sports Med. 1993;1(2):99–103.
12. Kim SJ, Kim TW, Kim SG, Kim HP, Chun YM. Clinical comparisons of the anatomical reconstruction and modified biceps rerouting technique for chronic posterolateral instability combined with posterior cruciate ligament reconstruction. J Bone Joint Surg Am. 2011 May 4;93(9):809–18.
13. Matava MJ, Ellis E, Gruber B. Surgical treatment of posterior cruciate ligament tears: an evolving technique. J Am Acad Orthop Surg. 2009 Jul;17(7):435–46.

14. Shelbourne KD, Muthukaruppan Y. Subjective results of nonoperatively treated, acute, isolated posterior cruciate ligament injuries. Arthroscopy. 2005 Apr;21(4):457–61.
15. Veltri DM, Warren RF. Isolated and combined posterior cruciate ligament injuries. J Am Acad Orthop Surg. 1993 Nov;1(2):67–75.
16. Becker EH, Watson JD, Dreese JC. Investigation of multiligamentous knee injury patterns with associated injuries presenting at a level I trauma center. J Orthop Trauma. 2013 Apr;27(4):226–31.
17. Esmaili Jah AA, Keyhani S, Zarei R, Moghaddam AK. Accuracy of MRI in comparison with clinical and arthroscopic findings in ligamentous and meniscal injuries of the knee. Acta Orthop Belg. 2005 Apr;71(2):189–96.
18. Rubinstein RA Jr, Shelbourne KD, McCarroll JR, VanMeter CD, Rettig AC. The accuracy of the clinical examination in the setting of posterior cruciate ligament injuries. Am J Sports Med. 1994 Jul–Aug;22(4):550–7.
19. Margheritini F, Mancini L, Mauro CS, Mariani PP. Stress radiography for quantifying posterior cruciate ligament deficiency. Arthroscopy. 2003 Sep;19(7):706–11.
20. Schulz MS, Steenlage ES, Russe K, Strobel MJ. Distribution of posterior tibial displacement in knees with posterior cruciate ligament tears. J Bone Joint Surg Am. 2007 Feb;89(2):332–8.
21. Sekiya JK, Whiddon DR, Zehms CT, Miller MD. A clinically relevant assessment of posterior cruciate ligament and posterolateral corner injuries. Evaluation of isolated and combined deficiency. J Bone Joint Surg Am. 2008 Aug;90(8):1621–7.
22. Dandy DJ, Pusey RJ. The long-term results of unrepaired tears of the posterior cruciate ligament. J Bone Joint Surg Br. 1982;64(1):92–4.
23. Shelbourne KD, Clark M, Gray T. Minimum 10-year follow-up of patients after an acute, isolated posterior cruciate ligament injury treated nonoperatively. Am J Sports Med. 2013 Jul;41(7):1526–33.
24. Patel DV, Allen AA, Warren RF, Wickiewicz TL, Simonian PT. The nonoperative treatment of acute, isolated (partial or complete) posterior cruciate ligament-deficient knees: an intermediate-term follow-up study. HSS J. 2007 Sep;3(2):137–46.
25. Hefti F, Muller W, Jakob RP, Staubli HU. Evaluation of knee ligament injuries with the IKDC form. Knee Surg Sports Traumatol Arthrosc. 1993;1(3–4):226–34.
26. Markolf KL, Zemanovic JR, McAllister DR. Cyclic loading of posterior cruciate ligament replacements fixed with tibial tunnel and tibial inlay methods. J Bone Joint Surg Am. 2002 Apr;84-A(4):518–24.
27. McAllister DR, Markolf KL, Oakes DA, Young CR, McWilliams J. A biomechanical comparison of tibial inlay and tibial tunnel posterior cruciate ligament reconstruction techniques: graft pretension and knee laxity. Am J Sports Med. 2002 May–Jun;30(3):312–7.
28. May JH, Gillette BP, Morgan JA, Krych AJ, Stuart MJ, Levy BA. Transtibial versus inlay posterior cruciate ligament reconstruction: an evidence-based systematic review. J Knee Surg. 2010 Jun;23(2):73–9.
29. Campbell RB, Jordan SS, Sekiya JK. Arthroscopic tibial inlay for posterior cruciate ligament reconstruction. Arthroscopy. 2007 Dec;23(12):1356. e1–4.
30. Bovid KM, Salata MJ. Vander Have KL, Sekiya JK. Arthroscopic posterior cruciate ligament reconstruction in a skeletally immature patient: a new technique with case report. Arthroscopy. 2010 Apr;26(4):563–70.
31. Salata MJ, Sekiya JK. Arthroscopic posterior cruciate ligament tibial inlay reconstruction: a surgical technique that may influence rehabilitation. Sports Health. 2011 Jan;3(1):52–8.
32. Cooper DE, Stewart D. Posterior cruciate ligament reconstruction using single-bundle patella tendon graft with tibial inlay fixation: 2- to 10-year follow-up. Am J Sports Med. 2004 Mar;32(2):346–60.
33. Hermans S, Corten K, Bellemans J. Long-term results of isolated anterolateral bundle reconstructions of the posterior cruciate ligament: a 6- to 12-year follow-up study. Am J Sports Med. 2009 Aug;37(8):1499–507.
34. Sekiya JK, West RV, Ong BC, Irrgang JJ, Fu FH, Harner CD. Clinical outcomes after isolated arthroscopic single-bundle posterior cruciate ligament reconstruction. Arthroscopy. 2005 Sep;21(9):1042–50.
35. Wang CJ, Chen HS, Huang TW. Outcome of arthroscopic single bundle reconstruction for complete posterior cruciate ligament tear. Injury. 2003 Oct;34(10):747–51.
36. Garofalo R, Jolles BM, Moretti B, Siegrist O. Double-bundle transtibial posterior cruciate ligament reconstruction with a tendon-patellar bone-semitendinosus tendon autograft: clinical results with a minimum of 2 years' follow-up. Arthroscopy. 2006 Dec;22(12):1331–8. e1.
37. Yoon KH, Bae DK, Song SJ, Lim CT. Arthroscopic double-bundle augmentation of posterior cruciate ligament using split Achilles allograft. Arthroscopy. 2005 Dec;21(12):1436–42.
38. McGuire DA, Hendricks SD. Comparison of anatomic versus nonanatomic placement of femoral tunnels in Achilles double-bundle posterior cruciate ligament reconstruction. Arthroscopy. 2010 May;26(5):658–66.
39. Forsythe B, Harner C, Martins CA, Shen W, Lopes OV Jr, Fu FH. Topography of the femoral attachment of the posterior cruciate ligament. Surgical technique. J Bone Joint Surg Am. 2009 Mar 1;91(Suppl 2 Pt 1):89–100.
40. Markolf KL, Feeley BT, Jackson SR, McAllister DR. Biomechanical studies of double-bundle posterior cruciate ligament reconstructions. J Bone Joint Surg Am. 2006 Aug;88(8):1788–94.
41. Whiddon DR, Zehms CT, Miller MD, Quinby JS, Montgomery SL, Sekiya JK. Double compared with single-bundle open inlay posterior cruciate ligament reconstruction in a cadaver model. J Bone Joint Surg Am. 2008 Sep;90(9):1820–9.
42. Yoon KH, Bae DK, Song SJ, Cho HJ, Lee JH. A prospective randomized study comparing arthroscopic single-bundle and double-bundle posterior cruciate ligament reconstructions preserving remnant fibers. Am J Sports Med. 2011 Mar;39(3):474–80.
43. Fanelli GC, Beck JD, Edson CJ. Single compared to double-bundle PCL reconstruction using allograft tissue. J Knee Surg. 2012 Mar;25(1):59–64.
44. Schoderbek RJ Jr, Golish SR, Rubino LJ, Oliviero JA, HartJM, MillerMD. The graft/femoral tunnel angles in posterior cruciate ligament reconstruction: a comparison of 3 techniques for femoral tunnel placement. J Knee Surg. 2009 Apr;22(2):106–10.
45. Tompkins M, Keller TC, Milewski MD, Gaskin CM, Brockmeier SF, Hart JM, et al. Anatomic femoral tunnels in posterior cruciate ligament reconstruction: inside-out versus outside-in drilling. Am J Sports Med. 2013 Jan;41(1):43–50.
46. Hudgens JL, Gillette BP, Krych AJ, Stuart MJ, May JH, Levy BA. Allograft versus autograft in posterior cruciate ligament reconstruction: an evidence-based systematic review. J Knee Surg. 2013 Apr;26(2):109–15.

The All-Inside Technique: Surgical Technique and Outcomes

13

Ranjodh Dhami, Robby S. Sikka, Ryan P. Dunlay and Joel L. Boyd

Introduction

In recent years, two distinct segments of the posterior cruciate ligament (PCL) have been described: the anterolateral and the posteromedial (PM) bundle. These bundles are based on variations in the tension of the fibers at different degrees of flexion, with the anterolateral bundle having more tension under flexion than extension, and with the converse being true for the PM bundle [1]. The relative positions of these bundles with respect to the tibia and femur are pivotal for any surgical technique.Edwards et al. [2] eloquently described the anatomy of these bundles using 39 articulated cadaveric knees. They found that the center of the anterolateral bundle measured a distance from the medial tibial edge which was, on average, 48 ± 4 % of the total maximum width of the tibial plateau. Similarly, the PM bundle was found to have a value of 48 ± 5 %. In contrast, the femoral PCL attachment showed greater variability. Takahashi et al. corroborated these findings and found similar averages for the tibial attachments of the anterolateral and PM bundles at 51 and 50 %, respectively.Additionally, the femoral attachments again showed much greater variation [3] (Tables 13.1 and 13.2). Additionally, in a normal range of motion, Papannagari et al. [4] used a dual-orthogonal fluoroscopic system to demonstrate a synergistic function of the two bundles, as both experienced an increase in length with degrees of flexion ranging from 0°to 120 °.

The importance of graft location and placement on the restoration of function has been a matter of ongoing research (Figs. 13.1 and 13.2). Gill et al. demonstrated that restoration of rotational properties depends heavily on the tibial placement of the PCL graft [5]. Mannor et al. demonstrated that varying the position of the femoral tunnel alters the tension of the graft and subsequently the biomechanical properties of the knee [6]. Markolf et al. also investigated the effect of tunnel placement on knee biomechanics [7]. In a study of ten cadaveric knees, they tested graft positions which were medially and laterally displaced from the tibial footprint by 5 mm. There was no significant change in knee laxities or rotational forces when compared to an anatomically placed tunnel, though the medially displaced graft exhibited greater forces under flexion angles greater than 65°. These studies underline the importance of establishing the femoral and tibial tunnels in an anatomic position and form the basis for future investigation into the clinical impact of PCL graft positioning.

With the aim of determining reference points for reconstruction, subsequent studies have investigated possible bony landmarks for the PCL femoral insertion.In a study of 20 cadavers, Lopes et al. located an osseous prominence proximal to the femoral footprint of the PCL in 18/20 (90 %) and coined the term "medial intercondylar ridge."Additionally, in 8/20 of the specimen, an osseous bridge and obvious change in slope between the AL and PM bundle footprints was noted [8]. Clinically, these anatomical landmarks may be of great utility in finding the anatomically correct placement of the PCL footprint on the femur during reconstruction.

Controversy remains in regard to the degree to which function can be restored through various surgical techniques. Gill et al. showed that under normal physiologic loads, single-bundle reconstruction restores the anteroposterior laxity of the PCL at flexion angles up to 90° [5]. Additionally, Gill et al. showed a nonstatistically significant reduction of external rotation in single-bundle repaired knees [5]. However, the success of single-bundle reconstructions in restoring the rotational component of PCL function is still a matter of contention. In studies by Race et al. [9], Harner et al.

J. L. Boyd (✉)
Orthopaedic Surgery, University of Minnesota, Bloomington, MN, USA
e-mail: joel.boyd@tria.com

R. Dhami
Penn State Hershey Medical Center, Hershey, PA, USA

R. S. Sikka
TRIA Orthopaedic Center, Minneapolis, MN, USA

R. P. Dunlay
Orthopaedic Surgery, ORA Orthopedics, Bettendorf, IA, USA

G. C. Fanelli (ed.), *Posterior Cruciate Ligament Injuries*,
DOI 10.1007/978-3-319-12072-0_13, © Springer International Publishing Switzerland 2015

Table 13.1 Tibial attachment data summary

	Mean measurement ± SD (mm) AL	PM
Anteroposterior length	8±2	6±1
Width	9±2	10±2
Center from posterior tibial axis (posteroanterior)	7±2	3±1
Center from medial tibial edge	37±4	38±5

SD standard deviation, *PM* posteromedial, *AL* anterolateral

Table13.2 Femoral attachment data summary

	AL	PM
Parallel to femoral longaxis		
Clock position	9–12 (center: 10:20±30)	7:30–10:30 (center: 8:30±30)
Distance from cartilage edge (mm) ± SD	7±2	10±3
Parallel to Blumensaat's Line		
Clock position	9–12:30 (center:11:20±20)	7:30–12:00 (center: 9:45±30)
Distance from cartilage edge (mm) ± SD	6±1	12±3

PM posteromedial, *AL* anterolateral, *SD* standard deviation

[10], and Whiddon et al. [11], in vitro double-bundle PCL reconstruction more closely restored the function of the native PCL. Wijdicks et al. were also able to demonstrate significantly less internal rotation with double-bundle repair at angles of 90 ° or greater [12]. Bergfeld et al., however, found no definitive advantage of double-bundle repair [13].

Indications for Surgery

Though studies have shown mixed results, the general consensus has been that isolated PCL tears can be managed well conservatively.Shelbourne et al. prospectively examined a group of patients with isolated PCL injuries who were treated nonoperatively [14]. With a minimum follow-up of 10 years, radiographically patients were normal or near normal in 89 % of cases. Additionally, the mean International Knee Documentation Committee (IKDC) grade was 73.4.Parolie and Bergfeld examined 25 patients with isolated PCL tears treated nonoperatively and 68 % returned to at least the same level of sport with 80% reporting satisfactory results [15]. In contrast, Boynton and Titjens et al. showed that in their population of 50 patients with isolated PCL tears treated nonoperatively, 20 % had disabling instability or meniscus pathology [16]. Keller et al. similarly reported poor results in 40 patients with isolated PCL tears. They noted that 90 % had knee pain, 65 % had limited activity secondary to the PCL-deficient knee, and 43 % reported difficulty walking [17]. The mixed results demonstrated by these studies for PCL injuries treated nonoperatively continue to confound recommendations for treatment.

Currently, there is consensus that PCL-deficient knees exhibit a higher incidence of arthrosis and meniscus tears. In a long-term follow-up study, Dejour et al. reported that 89 % of PCL-deficient knees had persistent pain and 50 % had recurrent effusions at 15 years after initial injury [18]. At 25 years, the vast majority of these knees showed degenerative changes, especially in the medial and patellofemoral compartments. With these results, the question persists as to which subtype of PCL tears are best treated with reconstruction and which are those that can be safely treated nonoperatively with minimal risk for negative long-term sequela.

Most PCL tears occur in the context of multi-ligamentous injury. Sekiya et al. demonstrated in a cadaveric study that a grade 3 posterior drawer on physical examination correlated with the presence of a posterolateral corner injury in addition to a complete disruption of the PCL [19]. With isolated transection of the PCL, posterior translation of the tibia relative to the femur was only grade 2, measuring <10 mm of displacement. This evidence demonstrates that in patients presenting with clinically unstable knees in the face of a grade III injury, other concomitant ligamentous injuries deserve consideration. This underscores the necessity to consider other ligamentous pathology prior to embarking on PCL reconstruction and considering specific surgical techniques.

More agreed-upon indications for surgical reconstruction of PCL injuries include avulsion fractures, a decrease in tibial step-off of 8 mm or greater, and PCL tears with concomitant ligamentous or structural injury [20]. Additionally, for chronic PCL tears, surgery is indicated when the injury becomes symptomatic, or the patient has failed nonoperative treatment with functional instability. In the multi-trauma patient, the vascular status of the injury, the skin condition, the nature of concomitant injuries, as well as the stability of the reduction and the patient all may play a role in operative, nonoperative, and delayed operative intervention.

The All-Inside Technique

The core goals of PCL reconstruction remain the same: to accurately reconstruct the PCL within the footprint, recreate the normal anatomy, restore ligament stability, and restore knee range of motion and function. In respect to these factors, the all-inside PCL reconstruction technique holds multiple distinct advantages over its historic open tibial inlay counterpart. By use of smaller incisions, the all-inside technique can be much less invasive and can avoid additional operative time through use of arthroscopic assisted placement of the tibial tunnel [21]. Furthermore, the all-inside technique is particularly useful in multi-ligamentous reconstruction [21]. The all-inside technique allows the surgeon to drill away from neurovascular structures by use of a reverse-drill technique which leads to less bone removal through potential creation of a socket as opposed to the traditional tunnel. This allows for greater retention of normal host bone and also yields a smaller potential for graft migration.Research has also shown that retrograde socket drilling is more accurate than antegrade drilling. In a study of cadaveric knees, Lubowitz et al. demonstrated that 3.5-mm tibial retrograde socket drilling was significantly more accurate than 2.4-mm antegrade pin placement in approximating the anterior cruciate ligament (ACL) footprint [22].

The strength of the all-inside techniques compared to the open inlay technique is one area of concern. However, with ongoing advancements in arthroscopic technique as well as improved instrumentation, this concern has diminished. Zehms et al. demonstrated in a cadaveric model that a novel arthroscopic double-bundle PCL inlay reconstruction using all-inside techniques provides comparable stability to its open counterpart [23]. Additionally, Kim et al. have demonstrated positive results in employing the all-inside inlay technique [24]. In their study of evaluating all-inside double-bundle reconstruction, they showed less than 3 mm of side-to-side difference in posterior translation.

With the open tibial inlay technique, there is evidence that the posterior capsulotomy may increase the clinical laxity. This is thought to be secondary to violation of the posterior capsular restraint.In a study of 14 cadaveric knees, Ritchie et al. demonstrated an average increase of 0.59 mm in posterior translation after PM capsular sectioning [25]. Park et al. similarly found that the violation of the posterior capsule necessary to perform the open tibial inlay technique increased posterior translation by 0.97 mm at 0° of flexion and 0.94 mm at 120° of knee flexion [26]. Though these increases in tibial translation are relatively small, they deserve attention for the possibility of introducing laxity when a posterior approach is considered.

While there is not sufficient evidence to indicate better PCL stability or improved clinical outcomes with the all-inside techniques, there are many tangible benefits for the surgeon. For instance, by making use of a PM portal, the all-inside techniques allow the ability to fully visualize the distal extent of the PCL tibial insertion. Additionally, as is the case with the open technique, patient positioning and the necessity to retract muscle and the neurovascular structures are eliminated, yielding a more confident and clear visualization of the footprint.

Author's Preferred Technique

A soft tissue graft is prepared by folding the TightRope® Attachable Button System (ABS) implant and stitching the tails together with #2 FiberLoop® after quadrupling the graft (GraftLink technique video—link http://www.arthrex.com/resources/video/y_WtppuzPE64CAFGbc-3LA/all-inside-pcl-reconstruction-using-the-pcl-graftlink).The graft is prepared to the appropriate length and the ends can be tapered with a stitch to ease graft passage.

An accessory PM portal may first be localized with a spinal needle. Once established, a 2 cm incision is made and screw-in cannula placed under direct visualization in an "outside-in" fashion. An alternative approach would be to make use of the knee obturator for posterior portals device and create the PM portal in an "inside-out" fashion.

The soft tissue still remaining on the PCL footprint is gently debrided with a shaver and/or radiofrequency ablator device placed through the PM portal to expose the full extent of the PCL footprint on the tibia. Care should be taken to protect the neurovascular structures that lie just posterior to the capsule.

The mamillary bodies at the posterior aspect of the tibia can be palpated through the PM portal to confirm anatomic placement. The PCL should be positioned directly between these two bodies and distal on the tibia. The side-specific Anatomic Contour PCL Guide is placed over the back of the tibia through the anteromedial portal and positioned between the mamillary bodies. The arthroscope can be placed in the PM portal to best visualize the footprint. (Fig. 13.1). Fluoroscopic guidance may be used to confirm correct positioning of the posterior guide in the "over-the-top" position and assist with drill trajectory. When in position, the marking hook will guide the FlipCutter® to the ideal location and angle for transtibial PCLR.A small 2–3 cm incision is made in this location and the guide is gently tapped to confirm that it is in cortical bone. Before drilling the FlipCutter®, make note of the osseous length as read by the drill sleeve markings as it enters the guide handle (Fig. 13.2).

Place the FlipCutter® into the drill sleeve and move the rubber grommet back to a distance equal to the interosseous length. This will give an indication of drill depth. With the arthroscope in the PM portal, drill the FlipCutter® until it is visualized just in the joint. Remove the guide and confirm

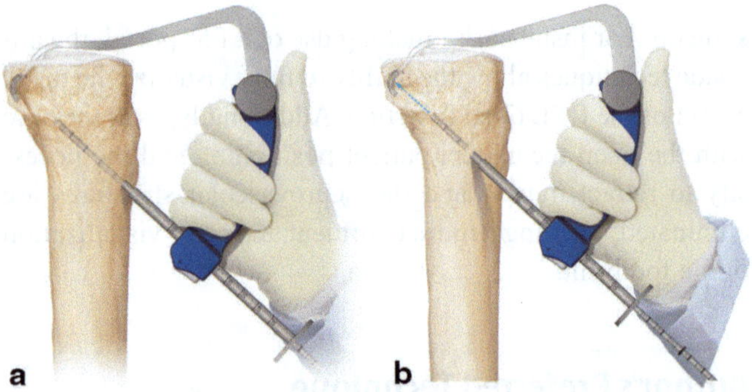

Fig. 13.1 **a** and **b** Place the tibial PCL reconstruction guide through the AM portal and over the PCL footprint. The 11 mm marking hook may be used to visually reproduce the footprint, or the 12 and 13 mm *laser line* markings may be referenced off the anterior edge of the footprint. Choose a FlipCutter II equal to the size according to the measured diameter of your prepared GraftLink soft tissue graft. Insert the FlipCutter until the tip contacts the anterior cortex. Slowly drill the FlipCutter and visualize arthroscopically for posterior cortex penetration (Images provided courtesy of Arthrex, Inc.)

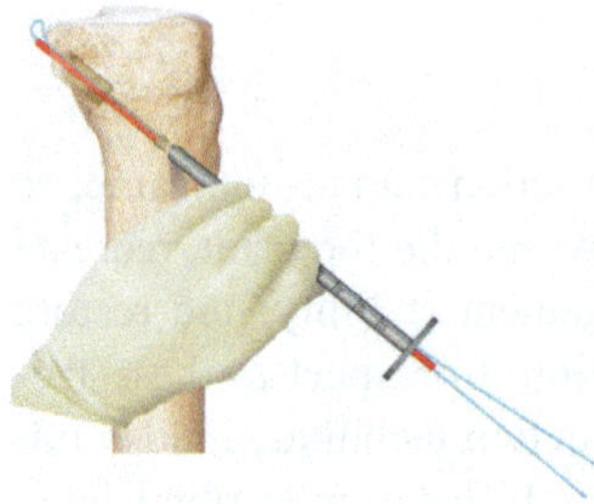

Fig. 13.3 Pass a #2 FiberStick™ through the drill sleeve and into the joint for retrieval. Temporarily secure the tibial passing suture until femoral socket preparation has been completed. (Image provided courtesy of Arthrex, Inc.)

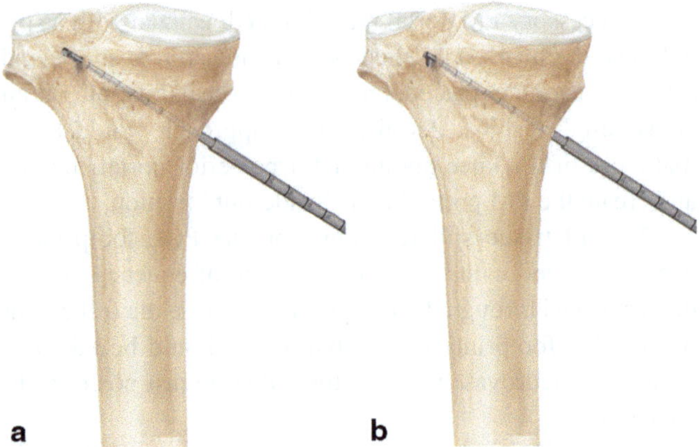

Fig. 13.2 **a** and **b** Once the FlipCutter has been confirmed to exit the posterior cortex either arthroscopically or with a combination of arthroscopy and fluoroscopy, push the button on the blue hub, and slide forward to flip the cutting tip into retrograde reaming position. Use a mallet to tap the 7 mm tip of the stepped drill sleeve into bone to facilitate passing suture after the tibial socket has been created. Once the drill sleeve is secure and the appropriate tibial footprint position has been confirmed, reverse-ream a socket of the appropriate depth (depending on graft length) (Images provided courtesy of Arthrex, Inc.)

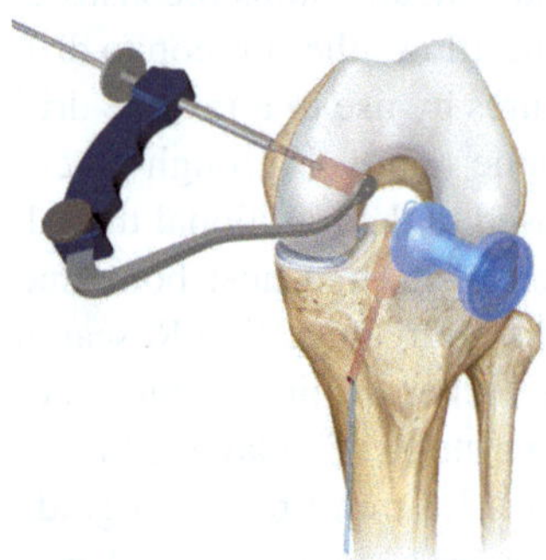

Fig. 13.4 Femoral socket preparation. Depending on preference, an inside-out technique or outside-in technique may be utilized for femoral socket creation. If an inside-out technique is chosen, then a low anterolateral portal is necessary to facilitate correct trajectory for the PCL footprint on the femur. Conversely, a FlipCutter can be used in an outside-in fashion. A standard or PCL-specific femoral guide may be used and placed in the anatomic center of the PCL footprint on the femur. Once confirmed, a small stab incision is made inferior to the vastus medialis, and the guide for the flip cutter is secured flush with the medial femoral condyle. The FlipCutter is subsequently drilled into position and confirmed arthroscopically. Similar to the tibia, the FlipCutter is transitioned to the reverse-ream position and a mallet is used to secure the stepped drill sleeve. The femoral socket is reverse-reamed to the appropriate depth. The FlipCutter is transitioned to its standard forward position and removed. A FiberStick loaded with a #2 FiberWire suture is passed into the joint from outside in through the stepped drill sleeve

that the FlipCutter® is in the center of the PCL footprint. Tap in the stepped drill sleeveand slide down the rubber grommet until it is flush with the drill guide. "Flipcut" the socket to a depth of at least 20 mm as indicated by the distance on the drill sleeve. After completing the socket, "unflip" the FlipCutter® and remove it from the drill sleeve.Place a #2 FiberStick™ up the sleeve and into the joint for future graft passage (Fig. 13.3).

Place the arthroscope back into the anteromedial portal and visualize the femoral footprint of the PCL.Place the All-Inside PCL Femoral Guide in the center of the anterolateral bundle.Drill the FlipCutter® from outside-in, and "FlipCut" the socket to a depth of at least 20 mm as indicated by the distance on the drill sleeve (Fig. 13.4). Place a #2 FiberStick™ down the sleeve and into the joint for future graft passage.Alternatively, the femoral socket can be drilled with a standard reamer from inside-out and a Beath pin used to pass suture retrograde for future graft passage.

The #2 FiberStick™ sutures are retrieved through the anterior portal.The graft is introduced through the portal and the TightRope® ABS is passed into the tibia using the passing suture (Fig. 13.5). The graft is advanced all the way to the bottom of the tibial socket by pulling on the inner loop of the implant, without shortening the loop.The #2 FiberStick™ from the femoral socket is next retrieved and the graft is pulled into the femoral socket.The femoral end of the graft can be tensioned with the knee at 20–90° of knee flexion (Fig. 13.6).Once both the femoral and tibial sides are secured and tensioned, a knot may be tied over the button

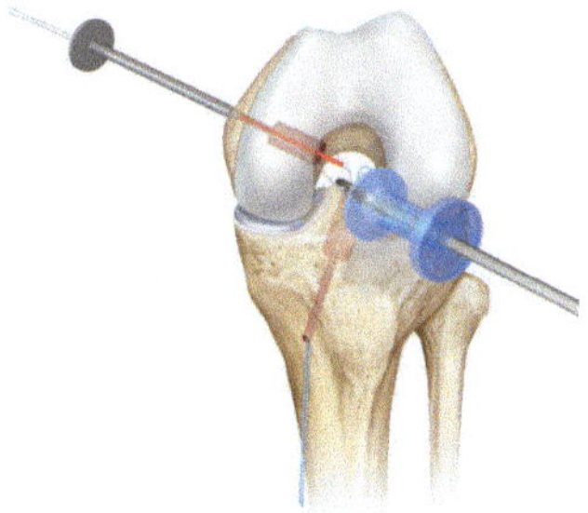

Fig. 13.5 The looped end of the femoral passage suture and the looped end of the tibial passage suture are simultaneously retrieved out the anteromedial portal so as avoid a suture bridge. (Images provided courtesy of Arthrex, Inc.)

to act as another form of fixation.Alternatively, the excess suture can be used for further backup fixation or the excess cut for removal (Fig. 13.7).

A cold compressive dressing is placed atop the wound and the patient is placed in a knee immobilizer until quad function adequately returns. The patient is typically made weight bearing as tolerated with range of motion as tolerated.

Outcomes

The degree to which all-inside single-bundle reconstruction can restore proper function of the knee is unclear. Results from all-inside single-bundle PCL reconstruction outcome studies within the past 10 years are summarized in Table 13.3 [27–35]. In general, satisfactory postoperative restoration of function is achieved, as indicated by the Lysholm and IKDC scores. Of particular note, in a long-term study with a minimum follow-up of 60 months, Wu et al. showed a good or excellent Lysholm knee score in 86% of patients [32]. In another long-term study, with mean follow-up of 4.1 years, Boutefnouchet et al. similarly showed good or excellent Lysholm knee scores in 93% of patients with single-

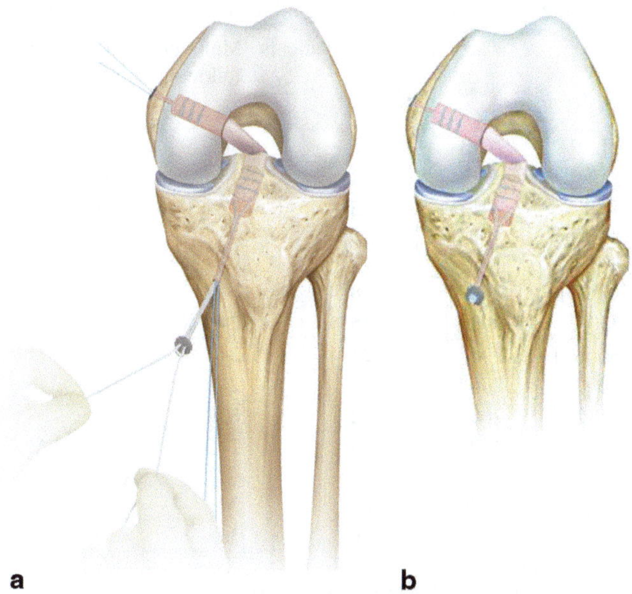

a b

Fig. 13.7 **a**, **b** Once the graft is at the appropriate depth in the femoral socket, secure the ABS button to the tibial sutures and tension the tibial side of the graft with the knee in 90° of flexion. Make sure to tension the strands symmetrically and remove any slack buildup created by one strand, while pulling on the other (avoid spreading sutures during tensioning). Once the button is seated, pull on the graft to confirm complete fixation. Once the graft is seated, the tensioning strands may be cut.Note: A knot may be tied before cutting the sutures to protect the implant during cutting and to act as backup fixation. (Images provided courtesy of Arthrex, Inc.)

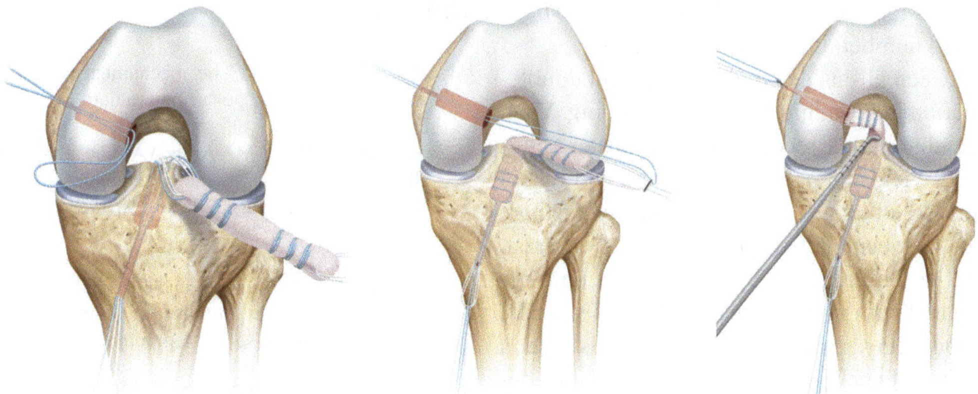

a b c

Fig. 13.6 Graft Passage. **a**, **b**, **c** Push the graft posteriorly until it reaches the tibial socket. To assist passage, place a blunt trocar through the lateral portal as a pulley while visualizing through the anteromedial portal, inferior to the graft. Hold light tension on the implant (not the tensioning strands) to guide the graft into position. A trocar may be placed in the posteromedial portal and use as a pulley to direct the graft into the socket. Once the graft has reached the socket, fully seat the graft in the socket without finally securing the graft on the anterior cortex with the ABS button. This will facilitate passage of the graft into the femoral socket. Pass the TightRope into the femoral socket.Begin to tight then femoral TightRope to bring the graft into the socket, making sure that adequate graft remains in the tibial socket

Table 13.3 Studies of all-inside single-bundle PCL reconstruction within the past 10 years

Author	Year	# of Patients	Minimum follow-up	Graft tendon	IKDC grade (%)				Lysholm
					A	B	C	D	
Lin [27]	2013	25	36	Q	16	68	16	0	92
Lin [27]	2013	34	36	H	35	59	6	0	94
Boutefnouchet [28]	2013	15	12	H	67	27	6	0	91
Kim [29]	2009	8	24	A	–	–	–	–	87
Li [30]	2009	15	24	H	53	20	20	7	85
Zhao [31]	2007	21	24	H	52	24	19	5	83
Zhao [31]	2007	22	24	H[a]	64	27	9	0	92
Wu [32]	2007	22	60	Q	23	64	13	0	89
MacGillivray [33]	2006	13	24	Q and A	–	–	–	–	81
Seon [34]	2006	21	24	H	–	–	–	–	91
Chan [35]	2006	20	36	H	25	60	10	5	93

[a] 7-strand graft
Q = Quadriceps; H = Hamstring; A = Achilles
IKDC International Knee Documentation Committee

bundle repair [28]. In a systematic review of arthroscopic single-bundle transtibial PCL reconstruction, YM Kim et al. concluded that this technique can improve posterior knee laxity by one grade, with 75 % of patients reaching normal or near-normal outcomes [36].

Common complications may include knee pain and instability. Li et al. encountered one patient with anterior knee pain, and two with paraesthesias which resolved in 6 months [30]. One patient required arthroscopic lysis and manipulation of the knee for treatment of arthrofibrosis [30]. This was also seen in one patient by Wu et al. [32]. Zhao et al. had five total patients with medial knee discomfort with flexion [31]. This was corrected at 1-year postoperation by removing the tape knots and mini-plate of the femoral fixation. Hardware removal and complex regional pain syndrome have also been described in a small number of patients [28, 32, 35].

The debate between all-inside single-bundle and double-bundle reconstruction in the clinical setting is ongoing. Yoon et al. found that double-bundle reconstruction using an Achilles tendon allograft yielded a better IKDC score and objective stability than single-bundle. However, subjectively, there was no difference between the two groups [37]. In contrast, Wang et al. found no difference in the clinical outcome between patients treated with single-bundle and double-bundle PCL reconstruction with semitendinosis and gracilis tendon grafts [38]. Similarly, Fanelli et al. found no difference between single-bundle and double-bundle reconstruction with regard to Lysholm, Tegner, or Hospital for Special Surgery ratings [39]. In a study comparing PCL reconstruction via arthroscopic tibial inlay single-bundle, arthroscopic tibial inlay double-bundle, and conventional transtibial single-bundle technique, SJ Kim et al. demonstrated that between the tibial inlay groups, the double-bundle group had a statistically significant difference in mean side-to-side difference [29]. However, this statistically significant difference did not apply to the transtibial single-bundle group. In another study of patients requiring concurrent reconstruction of the lateral collateral ligament and popliteus tendon, SJ Kim et al. found no significant difference between single-bundle and double-bundle PCL reconstruction in regard to posterior translation, posterolateral rotary instability, and IKDC and Lysholm knee scores [40]. Ultimately, the all-inside single-bundle reconstruction technique exhibits satisfactory outcomes in comparison to the double-bundle reconstruction technique for both isolated and multi-ligamentous PCL injury.

References

1. Race A, Amis AA. The mechanical properties of the two bundles of the human posterior cruciate ligament. J Biomech. 1994 Jan;27(1):13–24.
2. Edwards A, Bull AMJ, Amis AA. The attachments of the fiber bundles of the posterior cruciate ligament: an anatomic study. Arthrosc J Arthrosc Relat Surg Off Publ Arthrosc Assoc N Am Int Arthrosc Assoc. 2007 Mar;23(3):284–90.
3. Takahashi M, Matsubara T, Doi M, Suzuki D, Nagano A. Anatomical study of the femoral and tibial insertions of the anterolateral and posteromedial bundles of human posterior cruciate ligament. Knee Surg Sports Traumatol Arthrosc Off J ESSKA. 2006 Nov;14(11):1055–9.
4. Papannagari R, DeFrate LE, Nha KW, Moses JM, Moussa M, Gill TJ, et al. Function of Posterior Cruciate Ligament Bundles During In Vivo Knee Flexion. Am J Sports Med. 2007 Sep 1;35(9):1507–12.
5. Gill TJ, DeFrate LE, Wang C, Carey CT, Zayontz S, Zarins B, et al. The biomechanical effect of posterior cruciate ligament reconstruction on knee joint function. Kinematic response to simulated muscle loads. Am J Sports Med. 2003 Aug;31(4):530–6.

6. Mannor DA, Shearn JT, Grood ES, Noyes FR, Levy MS. Two-bundle posterior cruciate ligament reconstruction. An in vitro analysis of graft placement and tension. Am J Sports Med. 2000 Dec;28(6):833–45.
7. Markolf KL, McAllister DR, Young CR, McWilliams J, Oakes DA. Biomechanical effects of medial-lateral tibial tunnel placement in posterior cruciate ligament reconstruction. J Orthop Res Off Publ Orthop Res Soc. 2003 Jan;21(1):177–82.
8. Lopes OV Jr, Ferretti M, Shen W, Ekdahl M, Smolinski P, Fu FH. Topography of the femoral attachment of the posterior cruciate ligament. J Bone Joint Surg Am. 2008 Feb;90(2):249–55.
9. Race A, Amis AA. PCL reconstruction. In vitro biomechanical comparison of "isometric" versus single and double-bundled "anatomic" grafts. J Bone Joint Surg Br. 1998 Jan;80(1):173–9.
10. Harner CD, Janaushek MA, Kanamori A, Yagi M, Vogrin TM, Woo SL. Biomechanical analysis of a double-bundle posterior cruciate ligament reconstruction. Am J Sports Med. 2000 Apr;28(2): 144–51.
11. Whiddon DR, Zehms CT, Miller MD, Quinby JS, Montgomery SL, Sekiya JK. Double Compared with Single-Bundle Open Inlay Posterior Cruciate Ligament Reconstruction in a Cadaver Model. J Bone Jt Surg. 2008 Sep 1;90(9):1820–9.
12. Wijdicks CA, Kennedy NI, Goldsmith MT, Devitt BM, Michalski MP, Årøen A, et al. Kinematic analysis of the posterior cruciate ligament, part 2: a comparison of anatomic single- versus double-bundle reconstruction. Am J Sports Med. 2013 Dec;41(12):2839–48.
13. Bergfeld JA, Graham SM, Parker RD, Valdevit ADC, Kambic HE. A biomechanical comparison of posterior cruciate ligament reconstructions using single- and double-bundle tibial inlay techniques. Am J Sports Med. 2005 Jul;33(7):976–81.
14. Shelbourne KD, Clark M, Gray T. Minimum 10-year follow-up of patients after an acute, isolated posterior cruciate ligament injury treated nonoperatively. Am J Sports Med. 2013 Jul;41(7):1526–33.
15. Parolie JM, Bergfeld JA. Long-term results of nonoperative treatment of isolated posterior cruciate ligament injuries in the athlete. Am J Sports Med. 1986 Feb;14(1):35–8.
16. Boynton MD, Tietjens BR. Long-term followup of the untreated isolated posterior cruciate ligament-deficient knee. Am J Sports Med. 1996 Jun;24(3):306–10.
17. Keller PM, Shelbourne KD, McCarroll JR, Rettig AC. Nonoperatively treated isolated posterior cruciate ligament injuries. Am J Sports Med. 1993 Feb;21(1):132–6.
18. Dejour H, Walch G, Peyrot J, Eberhard P. The natural history of rupture of the posterior cruciate ligament. Rev Chir Orthopédique Réparatrice Appar Mot. 1988;74(1):35–43.
19. Sekiya JK, Whiddon DR, Zehms CT, Miller MD. A clinically relevant assessment of posterior cruciate ligament and posterolateral corner injuries. Evaluation of isolated and combined deficiency. J Bone Joint Surg Am. 2008 Aug;90(8):1621–7.
20. Fanelli GC, Beck JD, Edson CJ. Current concepts review: the posterior cruciate ligament. J Knee Surg. 2010 Jun;23(2):61–72.
21. Noyes FR. Noyes' Knee Disorders: Surgery, Rehabilitation, Clinical Outcomes. Elsevier Health Sciences; 2009:4415.
22. Lubowitz JH, Konicek J. A 3.5-mm-diameter anterior cruciate ligament tibial retrograde socket drilling pin is more accurate than a 2.4-mm-diameter pin. Arthrosc J Arthrosc Relat Surg. 2011 May;27(5):666–71.
23. Zehms CT, Whiddon DR, Miller MD, Quinby JS, Montgomery SL, Campbell RB, et al. Comparison of a double bundle arthroscopic inlay and open inlay posterior cruciate ligament reconstruction using clinically relevant tools: a cadaveric study. Arthrosc J Arthrosc Relat Surg Off Publ Arthrosc Assoc N Am Int Arthrosc Assoc. 2008 Apr;24(4):472–80.
24. Kim S-J, Park I-S. Arthroscopic reconstruction of the posterior cruciate ligament using tibial-inlay and double-bundle technique. Arthrosc J Arthrosc Relat Surg Off Publ Arthrosc Assoc N Am Int Arthrosc Assoc. 2005 Oct;21(10):1271.
25. Ritchie JR, Bergfeld JA, Kambic H, Manning T. Isolated sectioning of the medial and posteromedial capsular ligaments in the posterior cruciate ligament-deficient knee. Influence on posterior tibial translation. Am J Sports Med. 1998 Jun;26(3):389–94.
26. Park SE, Stamos BD, DeFrate LE, Gill TJ, Li G. The effect of posterior knee capsulotomy on posterior tibial translation during posterior cruciate ligament tibial inlay reconstruction. Am J Sports Med. 2004 Sep;32(6):1514–9.
27. Lin Y-C, Chen S-K, Liu T-H, Cheng Y-M, Chou PP-H. Arthroscopic transtibial single-bundle posterior cruciate ligament reconstruction using patellar tendon graft compared with hamstring tendon graft. Arch Orthop Trauma Surg. 2013 Apr;133(4):523–30.
28. Boutefnouchet T, Bentayeb M, Qadri Q, Ali S. Long-term outcomes following single-bundle transtibial arthroscopic posterior cruciate ligament reconstruction. Int Orthop. 2013 Feb;37(2):337–43.
29. Kim S-J, Kim T-E, Jo S-B, Kung Y-P. Comparison of the clinical results of three posterior cruciate ligament reconstruction techniques. J Bone Joint Surg Am. 2009 Nov;91(11):2543–9.
30. Li B, Wen Y, Wu H, Qian Q, Wu Y, Lin X. Arthroscopic single-bundle posterior cruciate ligament reconstruction: retrospective review of hamstring tendon graft versus LARS artificial ligament. Int Orthop. 2009 Aug;33(4):991–6.
31. Zhao J, Huangfu X. Arthroscopic single-bundle posterior cruciate ligament reconstruction: Retrospective review of 4- versus 7-strand hamstring tendon graft. The Knee. 2007 Aug;14(4):301–5.
32. Wu C-H, Chen AC-Y, Yuan L-J, Chang C-H, Chan Y-S, Hsu K-Y, et al. Arthroscopic Reconstruction of the posterior cruciate ligament by using a quadriceps tendon autograft: A minimum 5-year follow-up. Arthrosc J Arthrosc Relat Surg. 2007 Apr;23(4):420–427.e2.
33. MacGillivray JD, Stein BES, Park M, Allen AA, Wickiewicz TL, Warren RF. Comparison of tibial inlay versus transtibial techniques for isolated posterior cruciate ligament reconstruction: minimum 2-year follow-up. Arthrosc J Arthrosc Relat Surg Off Publ Arthrosc Assoc N Am Int Arthrosc Assoc. 2006 Mar;22(3):320–8.
34. Seon J-K, Song E-K. Reconstruction of isolated posterior cruciate ligament injuries: a clinical comparison of the transtibial and tibial inlay techniques. Arthrosc J Arthrosc Relat Surg Off Publ Arthrosc Assoc N Am Int Arthrosc Assoc. 2006 Jan;22(1):27–32.
35. Chan Y-S, Yang S-C, Chang C-H, Chen AC-Y, Yuan L-J, Hsu K-Y, et al. Arthroscopic reconstruction of the posterior cruciate ligament with use of a quadruple hamstring tendon graft with 3- to 5-year follow-up. Arthrosc J Arthrosc Relat Surg. 2006 Jul;22(7):762–70.
36. Kim Y-M, Lee CA, Matava MJ. Clinical results of arthroscopic single-bundle transtibial posterior cruciate ligament reconstruction: a systematic review. Am J Sports Med. 2011 Feb;39(2):425–34.
37. Yoon KH, Bae DK, Song SJ, Cho HJ, Lee JH. A prospective randomized study comparing arthroscopic single-bundle and double-bundle posterior cruciate ligament reconstructions preserving remnant fibers. Am J Sports Med. 2011 Mar;39(3):474–80.
38. Wang C-J, Weng L-H, Hsu C-C, Chan Y-S. Arthroscopic single- versus double-bundle posterior cruciate ligament reconstructions using hamstring autograft. Injury. 2004 Dec;35(12):1293–9.
39. Fanelli GC, Beck JD, Edson CJ. Single compared to double-bundle PCL reconstruction using allograft tissue. J Knee Surg. 2012 Mar;25(1):59–64.
40. Kim S-J, Jung M, Moon H-K, Kim S-G, Chun Y-M. Anterolateral transtibial posterior cruciate ligament reconstruction combined with anatomical reconstruction of posterolateral corner insufficiency: Comparison of single-bundle versus double-bundle posterior cruciate ligament reconstruction over a 2- to 6-year follow-up. Am J Sports Med. 2011 Mar;39(3):481–9.

Arthroscopic Primary Repair of Posterior Cruciate Ligament Injuries

14

Dominique D. Nieves, Micah J. Lissy and Gregory S. DiFelice

Introduction

Posterior cruciate ligament (PCL) injuries can either be isolated or associated with a multiple-ligament-injured knee (MLIK). They can be midsubstance tears, soft tissue avulsion "peel off" type tears, or associated with avulsion fractures (typically off the tibia) [1–4]. Most PCL injuries are managed conservatively with bracing and rehabilitation. As discussed in other chapters, surgical intervention regarding PCL injuries is largely focused on the treatment of isolated PCL injuries with symptomatic 3+ posterior laxity, or high-grade PCL injuries in the setting of the MLIK [5–8]. Historically, there was a large amount of interest in open primary repair of the anterior cruciate ligament (ACL) that spilled over to the PCL [9–13]. In comparison to the ACL, however, symptomatic PCL injuries requiring surgical intervention are dramatically less frequent; thus, there is a limited amount of clinical outcomes research on open primary PCL repair [7, 14–16]. It is well known that the disappointing mid- and long-term ACL primary repair results in the 1980s resulted in a collective change of focus towards reconstruction [17–20]. In parallel to this, as the surgical focus on arthroscopic ACL reconstruction became the gold standard, interest in and focus on arthroscopic PCL reconstruction followed.

This book is testament to the wide variety of opinion regarding the optimal surgical treatment for PCL injuries. It is clear from a review of the larger body of current clinical evidence regarding PCL reconstruction that there is little consensus regarding the optimal surgical technique and graft choice [21]. In addition, systematic reviews of PCL reconstruction studies have shown that while patients are subjectively and functionally satisfied, there is usually some residual posterior laxity in comparison to the opposite knee. Bowman et al. note "Clinical results after PCL reconstruction have not been as predictable as other reconstructions in the knee in eliminating the abnormal laxity" [22].

Although the historic course of events described above changed the collective surgical mindset regarding the optimal treatment for surgical PCL injuries, there are many theoretical benefits of repair over reconstruction. Repair minimizes morbidity about an already traumatized knee [23]. In the MLIK, it maintains bone "real estate" for reconstruction of other ligaments injured [24]. It also preserves anatomy by maintaining the exact footprint of one end of the ligament. Repair also maximizes native blood supply and has the possibility of preserving proprioception in the knee [25, 26]. Lastly, it does not burn any bridges in case revision is necessary.

These are the theoretic benefits of repair in general, however, if combined with the benefits of arthroscopic minimally invasive techniques, then the advantages may be even more dramatic. It is intriguing to note that despite a near-universal acceptance of reconstruction as the gold standard of treatment, a recent meta-analysis looking at outcomes of primary repair versus reconstruction of cruciate ligaments in open treatment of the MLIK noted, "No significant difference in clinical outcomes" [27].

Despite the theoretical benefits of repair, and the tremendous technical advances in our arthroscopic abilities that the past several decades have witnessed, there is a paucity of research discussing arthroscopic primary PCL repair in the literature. Much of the discussion in the PCL literature regarding arthroscopic repair of the ligament has mainly been focused on the treatment of avulsion fractures, and could more accurately be described as fracture fixation. These avulsion fractures more commonly occur at the tibial PCL insertion than at the femoral origin, and techniques for arthroscopic reduction and fixation using screws, staples, wires, and sutures are described. Although technically analogous to primary repair, this type of procedure is not discussed in this chapter.

G. S. DiFelice (✉) · D. D. Nieves
Orthopaedics, Hospital for Special Surgery, 535 E. 70th St., New York, NY 10021, USA
e-mail: difeliceg@hss.edu

M. J. Lissy
Sports Medicine, UHS, Binghamton, NY, USA

G. C. Fanelli (ed.), *Posterior Cruciate Ligament Injuries*,
DOI 10.1007/978-3-319-12072-0_14, © Springer International Publishing Switzerland 2015

This chapter focuses on arthroscopic primary PCL repair of soft tissue avulsions at the origin or insertion of the ligament. It is generally accepted that attempts at primary repair of midsubstance PCL ruptures would be of little clinical benefit, and should currently be considered irreparable. Recently, both our diagnostic capabilities regarding advances in magnetic resonance imaging (MRI) technology, and our technical capabilities regarding advances in arthroscopic instrumentation, have allowed increasing clinical discussion of arthroscopic PCL primary soft tissue repairs in carefully selected clinical situations [28–30]. It should be noted that the relative rarity of surgical PCL injuries, taken in combination with the fact that avulsion type tears with the potential to be repaired are only a small subset of this population, limits the ability to accumulate a large clinical experience in any one center. Most, if not all, of the literature in this regard is limited to small retrospective cohorts detailing promising clinical outcomes at short- to mid-term follow-up [31–33]. Common to all of the described techniques is the passage of locking stitches into the ligament remnant using a variety of suture-passing devices, with subsequent fixation back to the bony attachment either through drill holes or with suture anchors.

There are significant limitations to the applicability of this technique. First and foremost, the technique is only applicable to proximal and distal soft tissue type avulsions (avulsion fractures are excluded here as mentioned above). The likelihood of having successful surgical outcomes utilizing arthroscopic PCL repair will be intuitively maximized with acute surgical intervention (<3 weeks), although for numerous reasons this is not always possible. Finally, the quality of soft tissue of the ligament remnant ultimately dictates whether primary repair is possible or if more involved reconstructive techniques will be necessary.

Indications

The technique of arthroscopic primary PCL repair may be considered when:

1. Avulsion or "peel off" tears are noted on MRI in isolated injuries or in the MLIK setting.
2. The injury is roughly within the acute (<3 weeks) injury setting.
3. Adequate tissue quality and length are present on initial evaluation during diagnostic arthroscopy.
4. The patient would maximally benefit from the minimally invasive nature of the technique.

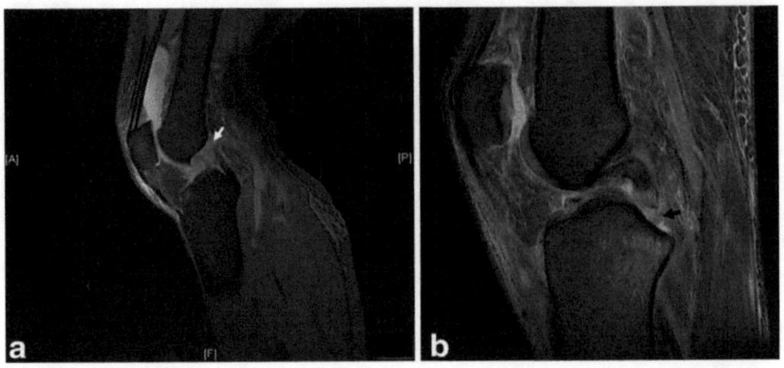

Fig. 14.1 Sagittal view of the preoperative PCL. **a** Top MRI reveals the proximal avulsion, the ligament is still intact at the tibia but avulsed from the femur (*white arrow*). **b** Bottom MRI shows distal avulsion, the ligament is still intact at the femur but avulsed from the tibia (*black arrow*). *PCL* posterior cruciate ligament, *MRI* magnetic resonance imaging. (From Lissy et al. 2012 [33, p. 195]. Reprinted with permission)

Indications and Imaging

MRI is the gold standard for imaging and can reliably detect proximal and distal avulsion or "peel off" type tears (Fig. 14.1). The tear type should be visualized in multiple planes (sagittal, axial, and coronal) to determine the exact nature of the tear. Proximal, or femoral, avulsions are significantly more common than distal, or tibial, avulsions. In fact, in the senior author's 15 years of clinical experience, tibial avulsions are rather rare in comparison.

When reading the MRI, in general, one end of the ligament will appear rather normal at its insertion to bone, and have a large percentage of the ligament that has a relatively "normal" homogeneous signal appearance. It is not uncommon for there to be significant heterogeneity of signal with proximity to the zone of injury at the avulsed end. Unfortunately, no standard has been established as to exactly what appearance is predictive of possible repair. An MRI evaluation will simply give the surgeon an idea that primary repair may be possible at surgery. Ultimately, tissue length and quality at surgery will determine if this procedure has a chance of success. Anecdotally, the MRI is only moderately predictive of which tears will eventually be reparable.

Senior Author's Preferred Surgical Technique

It should be noted that the description of this technique will discuss the repair of a femoral soft tissue avulsion. This is the more common and technically easier repair to perform.

Prior to entering the operating room (OR), the surgeon must assure that the proper equipment is available. Standard knee arthroscopy equipment complimented by some select equipment from the shoulder arthroscopy sets will be required. In particular, large bore, malleable cannulas

(PassPort-Arthrex, Naples, FL, USA), a reloadable suture-passing device (Scorpion FastPass-Arthrex, Naples, FL, USA) and/or other suture-passing devices, and a high-grade polyester suture (#2 Fiberwire-Arthrex, Naples, FL, USA). Depending on the choice of fixation, the surgeon would also need knotless suture anchors (4.75 BioComposite Swivelock-Arthrex, Naples, FL, USA) with their associated punches and taps, or a cannulated drill (RetroDrill-Arthrex, Naples, FL, USA) and a standard ligament button.

The setup does not necessitate a deviation from the surgeon's preferred arthroscopy setup as long as access to the knee is not limited. A leg holder for the opposite leg, however, does help in allowing access to accessory posterior portals that are necessary if addressing tibial-sided avulsions. Standard arthroscopic portals are created and a diagnostic tour of the knee is initiated. The PCL stump must be identified and mobilized by gently freeing it from any scar tissue (Fig. 14.2) that typically will form to the ACL or its remnant depending on the injury pattern. Once mobilized, the surgeon must ensure that there is adequate length for repair and that the ligament tissue is of sufficient quality to hold the stitches. It is important to utilize a broad grasper (Cuff Grasper, Arthrex, Naples, FL, USA) when assessing the ligament so as to avoid further damage to the ligament remnant (Fig. 14.3). When assessing length, it is critical to remember to reduce the knee so that the anterior tibia is 1 cm anterior to the femoral condyles when the knee is flexed at 90°. If the tibia is sagging posteriorly as is common, and the tibia is not reduced, then the PCL will give the appearance that it does not have the appropriate length to reach the wall for primary repair. With a tibial reduction maneuver, a more accurate assessment of length can be made. Once a decision has been made to attempt a primary repair, and prior to passing sutures through the ligament, it is advisable to dilate the medial portal and insert the malleable cannula. It should also be noted that if addressing a tibial avulsion, posteromedial and/or posterolateral accessory portals will be necessary.

The next, and generally the most technically demanding aspect of the procedure, is suture passage through the remnant. Using a reloadable suture-passing device, as would be utilized for a rotator cuff repair, high-tensile suture is passed through the ligament stump and autoretrieved via the trapdoor mechanism on the opposite jaw (Fig. 14.4). It is important to start the first pass as close as possible to intact insertion of the ligament stump so as to maximize the number of locking throws that can be placed into the ligament. Once the first pass is made, the suture is retrieved and the suture limbs are equalized. Each limb of the suture is then passed back through the ligament; alternating suture limbs and the direction of the suture pass gradually progressing along the length of the stump towards the avulsion. This creates an interlocking suture pattern akin to the Bunnell stitch. It is imperative that the previously passed suture is not cut during subsequent passes. This is avoided by monitoring tissue resistance. If resistance is encountered on an attempted pass, the pass should be aborted. The suture passer can then be repositioned and another attempt can be made. There should be little resistance during passage through the tissue.

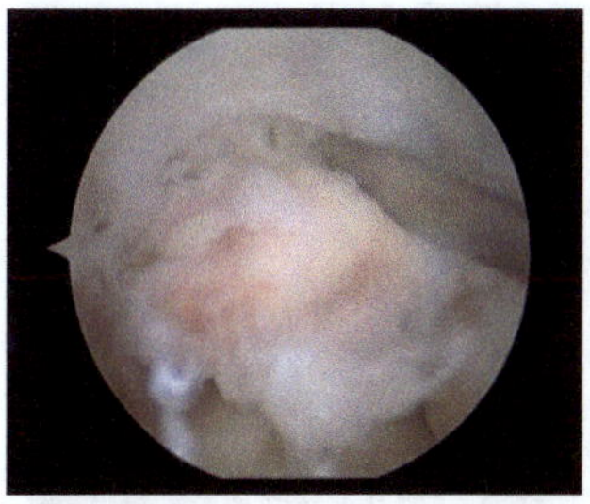

Fig. 14.2 Initial arthroscopic view of the PCL stump prior to debridement. *PCL* posterior cruciate ligament

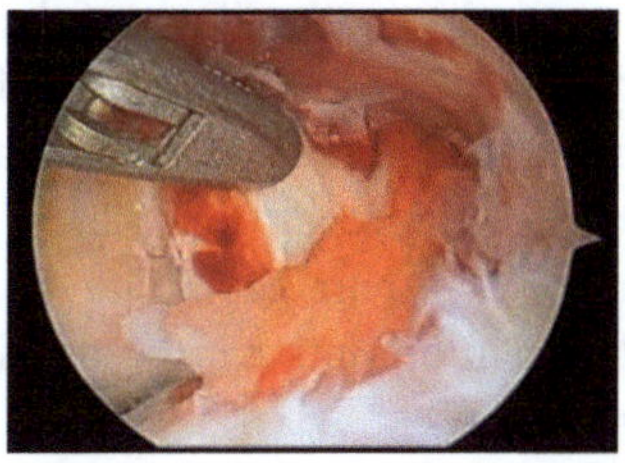

Fig. 14.3 Assessment of the ligament length

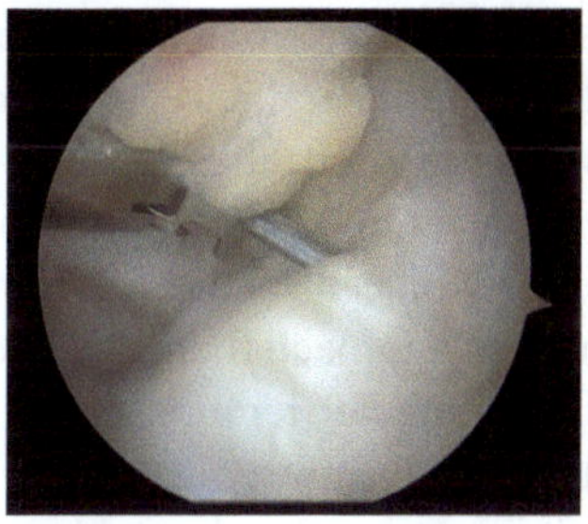

Fig. 14.4 The Scorpion® (Arthrex, Naples, FL, USA) suture passer is used to pass the #2 Fiberwire (Arthrex, Naples, FL, USA) into the PCL. *PCL* posterior cruciate ligament

If individual bundles are identified and isolated, they may be addressed separately; otherwise, the sutures are passed without regard to bundles. Effort should be expended on having the final suture passes exit the torn end of the tendon towards the wall. Typically, two high-tensile sutures are passed per repair resulting in four free limbs of suture exiting the avulsed end of the tendon. Occasionally, with larger patients, it is possible to get two sutures into each bundle, resulting in eight free limbs for repair (Fig. 14.5). Meticulous suture management, utilizing accessory portals, and the malleable cannula are necessary to avoid tangles and soft tissue bridges.

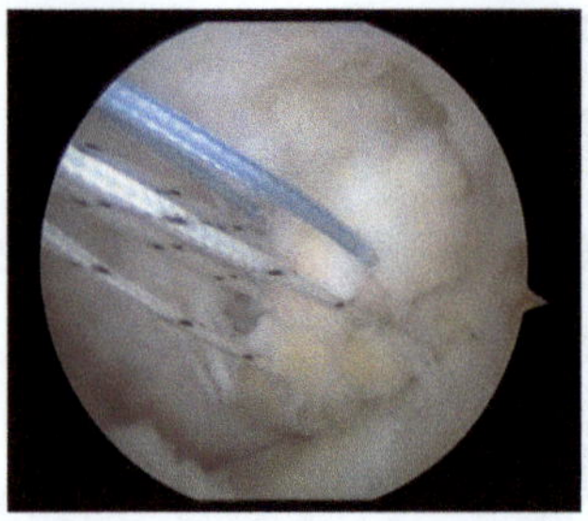

Fig. 14.5 An arthroscopic view of a double-bundle repair of the PCL with sutures passed, prior to fixation. *PCL* posterior cruciate ligament

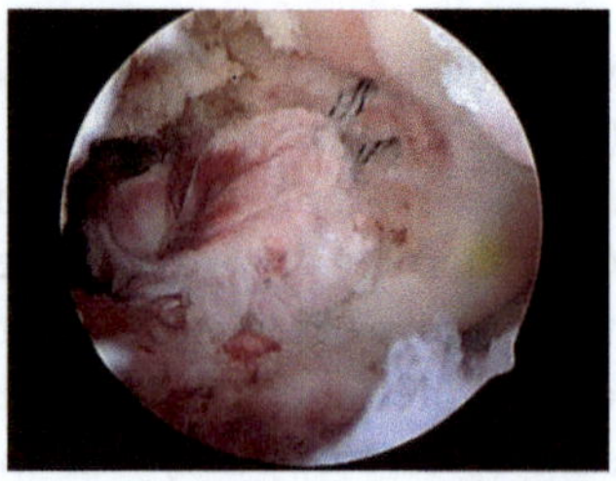

Fig. 14.6 PCL repair through drill holes prior to tensioning. *PCL* posterior cruciate ligament. (From Lissy et al. 2012 [33, p. 205]. Reprinted with permission)

With the suture limbs "parked" out of the way, either out an accessory portal or outside the cannula, they can be gently tensioned to retract the ligament remnant and protect it during preparation of the repair bed. Then, using either an arthroscopic shaver or a burr according to surgeon preference, the insertional footprints can be debrided to create a bed of bleeding bone.

At this point, the technique deviates depending on the choice for fixation. However, regardless of the technique, a precise understanding of the insertional footprint is critical. The goal is to attempt to recreate the anatomic attachments of both the anterolateral and posteromedial bundles. If knotless anchors are used, the steps are slightly different than if the repair is to be tied over a button. First, the arthroscope must be placed in the anteromedial portal to facilitate the angle of approach that is necessary for placing the anchors into the medial femoral condyle from lateral. Next, coming through the anterolateral portal the first anchor hole is made into the anterolateral bundle origin using a drill, awl, and/or tap according to bone quality and surgeon preference. The appropriate sutures are then inserted into the knotless anchor and the anchor is deployed into the medial femoral condyle in standard fashion reapposing the anterolateral bundle to the bone. The knee is held at 90° with an anterior drawer force on the tibia during fixation. This process is then repeated to place the anchor reattaching the posteromedial bundle origin.

If fixation is to be performed by tying over a bone bridge, then the procedure is slightly different. A PCL femoral guide is placed through the medial portal and used to guide the cannulated drill into the origin of the anterolateral bundle. A small incision is made medially over the femoral condyle to advance the guide down to bone. Once the drill is passed, a nitinol-passing wire is shuttled through the cannulation of the drill, retrieved out of the cannula, and used to shuttle the appropriate repair stitches through the femoral condyle (Fig. 14.6). This procedure is then repeated for the posteromedial bundle. After shuttling all of the suture limbs out their respective bone tunnels, they are passed through the ligament button and tied with an anterior drawer force being applied to the tibia. Alternatively, a 2.4-mm drill bit and spinal needles can be used to pass the nitinol wire, or the suture limbs can be tied to a post depending on surgeon preference. Reduction of the ligament to its insertion during fixation with the knee in 90° of flexion should be visualized with the arthroscope. Once fixation is completed, the ligament should be gently probed to confirm integrity of the repair, and a gentle posterior drawer can be performed to evaluate the improvement in posterior laxity afforded by the repair.

Postoperative Management

Postoperative management will be variable and depend on whether this was an isolated repair or in conjunction with a multiligament reconstruction. Confidence in the PCL repair will determine the duration of immobilization prior to beginning range of motion (ROM) exercises. Typically, a hinged knee brace locked in extension is placed in the operating room. Protected weight bearing is recommended with crutches and close attention is paid to edema control and cold therapy. Immediate quadriceps isometrics in extension are encouraged to restore control of the limb. Gentle progressive ROM exercises can be initiated between 2 and 4 weeks postoperatively, again depending on surgeon preference and confidence in the repair. Progression will be dictated by the clinical situation. Active hamstrings should be avoided for 4–6 months.

Case Examples

Case #1: Repair of a PCL Femoral Avulsion in a 67-Year-Old Female with a Knee Dislocation-3 Lateral MLIK

A 67-year-old female suffered an isolated, low-energy, KD-3 lateral knee dislocation after a trip and fall. She was manually reduced in the emergency room (ER), and throughout her post-injury course she had normal neurovascular exams. She was splinted and admitted for neurovascular checks. An MRI revealed that her injury pattern included what appeared to be complete proximal avulsions of both cruciates, and an

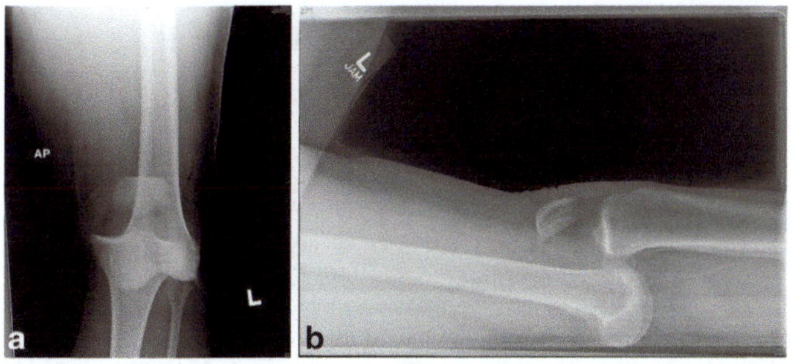

Fig. 14.7 **a** and **b** AP and lateral injury radiographs showing anterior knee dislocation. *AP* anteroposterior

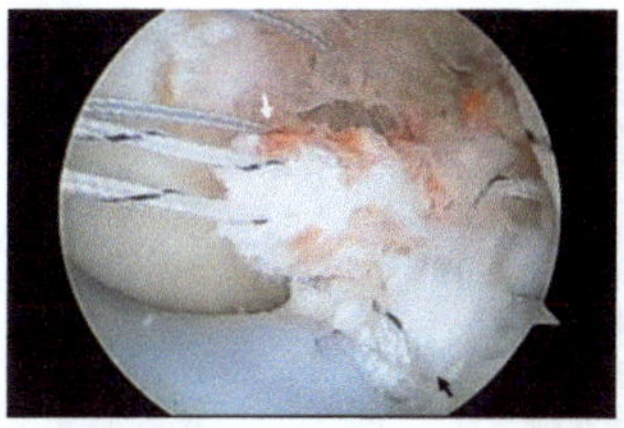

Fig. 14.8 Sutures pull the PCL (*white arrow*) beside the primarily repaired ACL (*black arrow*). Reduction of the knee reveals there is sufficient length of intact PCL to allow primary repair. *PCL* posterior cruciate ligament, *ACL* anterior cruciate ligament

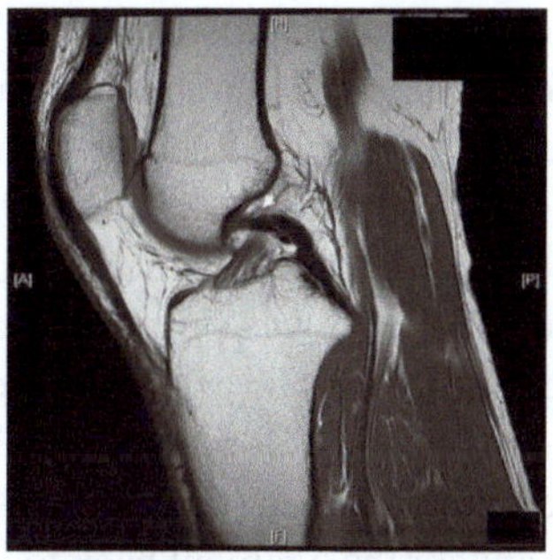

Fig. 14.9 Sagittal plane MRI shows area of abnormal stretch of the PCL highly suspicious for anterolateral bundle PCL avulsion off the femur (*arrow*). Suspicion was raised by isolated 3 uspicion was raised by isolated 3 (f the femur (PCL highly sus*PCL* posterior cruciate ligament, *MRI* magnetic resonance imaging

arcuate fracture resulting in gross laxity in multiple planes on clinical exam (Fig. 14.7).

After several days of observation, the patient was discharged in a locked hinged knee brace. She was allowed protected weight bearing and instructed in edema control. Close follow-up confirmed maintenance of neurovascular stability and gross instability of the knee to anterior and posterior drawer and to varus in extension. Surgical intervention was recommended with a plan for attempted arthroscopic open repair versus allograft reconstruction of the cruciates, and open repair versus allograft augmentation/reconstruction for the lateral side. Given the injury patterns, and her age, the hope was to minimize the surgical insult by primarily repairing the injured structures wherever possible (Fig. 14.8). Surgery was performed at 2.5 weeks post injury.

At surgery, it was felt that the tissue quality and length of both cruciates made it feasible to attempt arthroscopic primary bicruciate repair. The procedure described for the PCL was also successfully performed on the ACL. Suture anchors were used as described for both repairs with excellent restoration of anterior–posterior laxity on exam. In addition, an open lateral-sided primary repair to suture anchors in the fibular head was performed restoring stability to varus loading.

The surgical intervention yielded excellent subjective and objective outcomes. At 1-year follow-up, the patient is thoroughly pleased with her results and her self-reported outcome scores confirm this. Her Lysholm score was 99, her modified Cincinnati score was 97, her Knee injury and Osteoarthritis Outcome Score (KOOS) was 92.9, and her Single Assessment Numeric Evaluation (SANE) score was 98 %. The ROM was symmetric to the opposite side. A physical exam revealed trace to 1+ posterior drawer test with negative anterior drawer and negative Lachman; 1+ opening to varus at full extension and 30° that is symmetric to her opposite knee, and valgus stability.

Case #2: Repair of an Isolated Anterolateral Bundle Avulsion with Grade III Posterior Laxity on Exam

A 34-year-old male sustained a grade III avulsion of the anterolateral bundle of his PCL when he was thrown from his racing bike in a motor vehicle crash. The official radiologic interpretation was read as normal regarding the PCL. However, the results of the patient's physical exam (isolated 3+ posterior drawer), combined with the sagittal MRI of the PCL (Fig. 14.9), raised a high level of suspicion for anterolateral bundle PCL avulsion off the femur. The MRI also revealed an osteochondral defect involving the medial aspect of the medial femoral condyle and thus gave us incentive to evaluate the patient arthroscopically.

The preoperative plan was for a left knee diagnostic arthroscopy and possible attempted PCL repair of one or both bundles depending on what we found at surgery. Evaluation of his laxity pattern, along with the acute nature of the injury, and its particular qualities on MRI, suggested that repair could be successful and improve the resting point positioning of his tibia and long-term function of his knee. A thorough discussion of the uniqueness of this situation was frankly discussed with the patient and he wished to proceed according to this plan. Surgery was performed 1 month after

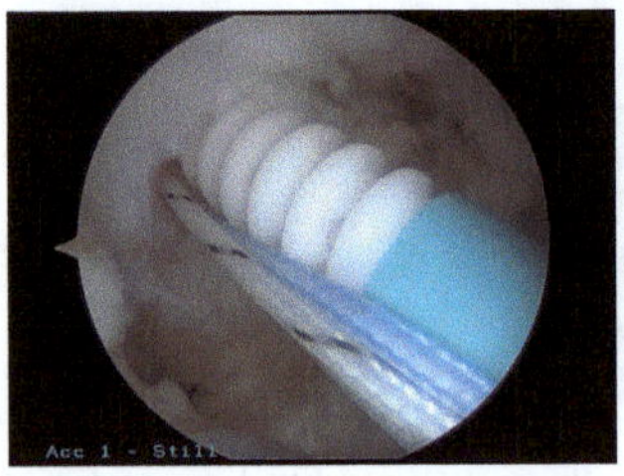

Fig. 14.10 Anterolateral bundle repair stitches being tensioned and fixed using a 4.75 BioComposite SwiveLock

the accident because the patient also suffered from and was initially treated for a high-grade concussion that delayed his presentation for evaluation of his knee.

At surgery, it appeared that the anterolateral bundle was avulsed in isolation. On initial evaluation, it appeared intact, but once the synovial sheath was probed it was clear that it was avulsed. After exposing and isolating the anterolateral bundle avulsion, two locking Bunnell stitches of #2 FiberWire were placed in the ligament as described above. These were then used to anchor the ligament back to its origin using a 4.75 BioComposite SwiveLock (Fig. 14.10). The chondral defect was mechanically debrided. At 8 months follow-up, the patient was noted to have full ROM, a grade 1 posterior drawer, and otherwise negative exam. By using an arthroscopic PCL repair approach, we successfully converted the patient's knee from grade III to grade I laxity.

Case #3: Repair of a PCL Femoral Avulsion in a 17-Year-Old Male with a KD-2 MLIK

A 17-year-old male sustained a closed anterior KD without neurovascular injury after landing awkwardly while jumping on a trampoline. The patient's knee was reduced at another institution and he was transferred for definitive management. An MRI revealed a soft tissue avulsion of the PCL from the femur and a midsubstance ACL rupture. The initial treatment plan was for ACL and PCL reconstruction at 2 weeks after injury, but this plan was altered based on his preoperative examination under anesthesia that revealed less than 90° of flexion was possible despite considerable force being applied. Furthermore, the diagnostic arthroscopy revealed substantial hemorrhagic synovitis (Fig. 14.11). Thus, due to a heightened concern for postoperative arthrofibrosis, the surgical plan was changed to a minimalist approach and a decision was made to only attempt an arthroscopic primary repair of the PCL (Fig. 14.12). It was felt that a delayed ACL reconstruction could be performed if symptomatic anterior laxity was present after recuperation from the initial surgery.

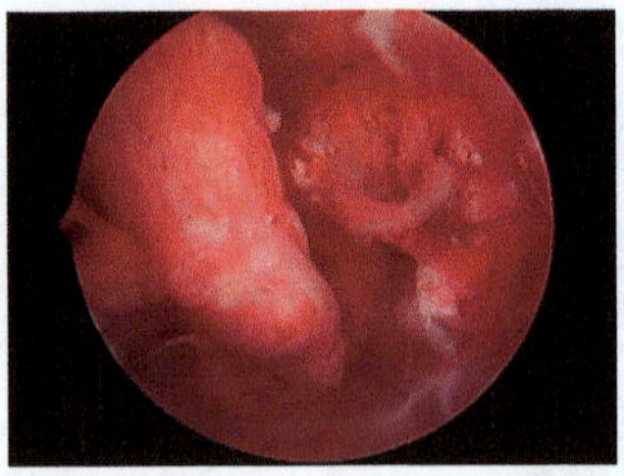

Fig. 14.11 Initial arthroscopic view of the notch in case #3. Significant hemorrhagic synovitis is noted. (From Lissy et al. 2012 [33, p. 203]. Reprinted with permission)

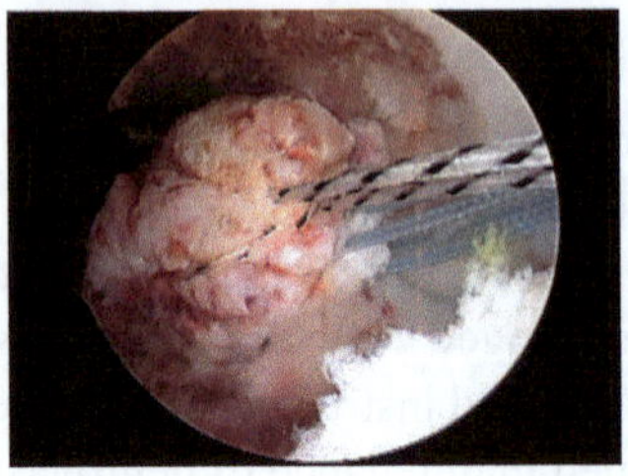

Fig. 14.12 Arthroscopic view of the PCL showing repair stitches passed but prior to fixation. *PCL* posterior cruciate ligament. (From Lissy et al. 2012 [33, p. 204]. Reprinted with permission)

Given the large body habitus and good tissue quality, we were able to place two stitches into each bundle and this afforded us a double-bundle repair. Two drill holes were made into each bundle footprint using a 2.4-mm drill bit, and then spinal needles were used to pass nitinol retrieval wires. These were then used to sequentially draw the repair stitches up into their respective tunnels. The tibial was held reduced with the knee at as close to 90° as we could achieve and then each pair of bundle stitches was tied over its respective bone bridge using alternating half-hitches. This restored his posterior laxity to normal. As a side note, the ACL remnant was resected to avoid any scar tissue formation to the PCL that might encourage arthrofibrosis.

After surgery, the patient was placed in a hinged knee brace locked in extension. This was unlocked for ROM 0–90° at 2 weeks. Isometric quadriceps exercises in extension were started immediately postoperatively. The patient progressed rapidly with physical therapy, and ultimately achieved full ROM. The initial plan for delayed ACL reconstruction was ultimately deferred because the patient achieved excellent stability due to capsular scarring and an excellent functional recovery. Follow-up after 5 years showed symmetric full-knee ROM, a negative posterior drawer examination, and a grade 1A Lachman examination. The Lysholm knee score was 95, and modified Cincinnati knee score was 96. The patient resumed competition in recreational sport without limitation.

Conclusions

There is a wide variety of opinion regarding the indications for surgical management of PCL injuries, whether in isolation or in association with a MLIK. Systematic reviews of the literature have confirmed that although patients seem to do well clinically with surgical reconstruction, there tends to be residual posterior laxity in the knee with modern-day reconstructive techniques. In light of the advances in MRI and our technical abilities in surgery, it may be possible to preoperatively identify a subset of patients that have soft tissue avulsions of the PCL from either the femur or tibia that may be amenable to arthroscopic primary repair of the ligament. This procedure significantly limits the morbidity to the patient in comparison to reconstruction. In addition, it preserves the native tissues including blood supply and potentially proprioception. Although experience with this technique has been limited due to the low incidence of PCL ruptures in general, and such reparable tears specifically, outcomes have been uniformly good. Further research to investigate such a procedure that can possibly minimize morbidity to the patient while improving outcomes is certainly warranted.

References

1. Chen C, Chen W, Shih C. Fixation of small tibial avulsion fracture of the posterior cruciate ligament using the double bundles pull-through suture method. J Trauma. 1999;46(6):1036–8.
2. Inoue M, Yasuda K, Kondo E, Saito K, Ishibe M. Primary repair of posterior cruciate ligament avulsion fracture: the effect of occult injury in the midsubstance on postoperative instability. Am J Sports Med. 2004;32:1230–7.
3. Kim Y, Lee C, Matava M. Clinical results of arthroscopic single-bundle transtibial posterior cruciate ligament reconstruction: a systematic review. Am J Sports Med. 2011;39(2):425–34. (Epub 2010/08/13).
4. Zhao J, He Y, Wang J. Arthroscopic treatment of acute tibial avulsion fracture of the posterior cruciate ligament with suture fixation technique through Y-shaped bone tunnels. Arthroscopy. 2006;22(2):172–81. (Epub 2006/02/07).
5. King J, Cerynik D, Blair J, Harding S, Tom J. Surgical outcomes after traumatic open knee dislocation. Knee Surg Sports Traumatol Arthrosc. 2009;17:1027–32.
6. Levy B, Dajani K, Whelan D, Stannard J, Fanelli G, Stuart M, et al. Decision making in the multiligament-injured knee: an evidence-based systematic review. Arthroscopy. 2009;25:430–8.
7. Levy B, Fanelli G, Whelan D, Stannard J, MacDonald P, Boyd J, et al. Controversies in the treatment of knee dislocations and multiligament reconstruction. J Am Acad Orthop Surg. 2009;17:197–206.
8. Mariani P, Margheritini F, Christel P, Bellelli A. Evaluation of posterior cruciate ligament healing: a study using magnetic resonance imaging and stress radiography. Arthroscopy. 2005;21(11):1354–61. (Epub 2005/12/06).
9. Meyers M, Moore T, HarveyJr J. Traumatic dislocation of the knee joint. J Bone Joint Surg Am. 1975;57(3):430–3.
10. Hughston J, Bowden J, Andrews J, Norwood L. Acute tears of the posterior cruciate ligament. Results of operative treatment. J Bone Joint Surg. 1980;62:438–50.
11. Moore H, Larson R. Posterior cruciate ligament injuries: results of early surgical repair. Am J Sports Med. 1980;8(2):68–78.
12. Pournaras J, Symeonides P. The results of surgical repair of acute tears of the posterior cruciate ligament. Clin Orthop Relat Res. 1991;267:103–7.
13. Strand T, Molster A, Engesaeter L, Raugstad T, Alho A. Primary repair in posterior cruciate ligament injuries. Acta Orthop Scand. 1984;55(5):545–7.
14. Engebretsen L, Risberg M, Robertson B, Ludvigsen T, Johansen S. Outcome after knee dislocations: a 2–9 years follow-up of 85 consecutive patients. Knee Surg Sports Traumatol Arthrosc. 2009;17(9):1013–26.
15. Howells NR1, Brunton LR, Robinson J, Porteus AJ, Eldridge JD, Murray JR. Acute knee dislocation: an evidence based approach to the management of the multiligament injured knee. Injury. 2011;42(11):1198–204. doi: 10.1016/j.injury.2010.11.018. Epub 2010 Dec 14.
16. Rihn J, Groff Y, Harner C, Cha P. The acutely dislocated knee: evaluation andmanagement. J Am Acad Orthop Surg. 2004;12(5):334–6.
17. FeaginJR J, Curl W. Isolated tear of the anterior cruciate ligament: 5 year follow-up stdy. Am J Sport Med. 1976;4(3):95–100.
18. Feagin J, Abbot H, Rokous J. The isolated tear of the anterior cruciate ligament. J Bone Joint Surg. 1972;54A:1340–1.
19. Warren R. Primary repair of the anterior cruciate ligament. Clin Orthop Relat Res. 1983;172:65–70.
20. Sherman M, Lieber L, Bonamo J, Podesta L, Reiter I. The long-term follow up primary anterior cruciate ligament repair—Defining rationale for augmentation. Am J Sport Med. 1991;19(3):243–55.
21. Hammoud S, Reinhardt K, Marx R. Outcomes of posterior cruciate ligament treatment: a review of the evidence. Sports Med Arthrosc Rev. 2010;18(4):280–91.
22. Bowman K, Sekiya J. Anatomy and biomechanics of the posterior cruciate ligament and other ligaments of the knee. Oper Techn Sport Med. 2009;17(3):126–34.
23. Richmond J. Complications associated with treatment of multiligament-injured/dislocated knee. Sports Med Arthrosc Rev. 2001;9:255–60.
24. Levy B, Stuart M. Management of the posterior cruciate ligament-based multiligament-injured knee. Oper Techn Sport Med. 2009;17(3):141–7.
25. Mariani P, Santoriello P, Iannone S, Condello V, Adriani E. Comparison of surgical treatments for knee dislocation. Am J Knee Surg. 1999;12(4):200–14.
26. Owens B, Neault M, Benson E, Busconi B. Primary repair of knee dislocations: results in 25 patients (28 knees) at a mean follow-up of four years. J Orthop Trauma. 2007;21:92–6.
27. Frosch KH, Preiss A, Heider S, Stengel D, Wohlmuth P, Hoffmann MF, et al. Primary ligament sutures as a treatment option of knee dislocations: a meta-analysis. Knee Surg Sports Traumatol Arthrosc. 2013;21(7):1502–9. (Epub 2012/08/08).
28. Bellelli A, Mancini P, Polito M, David V, Mariani P. Magnetic resonance imaging of posterior cruciate ligament injuries: a new classification of traumatic tears. Radiol Med. 2006;111(6):828–35. (Epub 2006/08/10).
29. Gross M, Grover J, Bassett L, Seeger L, Finerman G. Magnetic resonance imaging of the posterior cruciate ligament: clinical use to improve diagnostic accuracy. Am J Sports Med. 1992;20(6):732–7.
30. Sonin A, Fitzgerald S, Hoff F, Friedman H, Bresler M. MR imaging of the posterior cruciate ligament: normal, abnormal, and associated injury patterns. Radiographics. 1995;15(3):551–61.

31. DiFelice G, Lissy M. When to arthroscopically repair the torn posterior cruciate ligament. Clin Orthop Relat Res. 2011;470:861–8.
32. Wheatley W, Martinez A, Sacks T, Schurhoff M, Uribe J, Hechtman K, et al. Arthroscopic posterior cruciate ligament repair. Arthroscopy. 2002;18(7):695–702.
33. Lissy M, Dy C, Ranawat A, DiFelice G. Arthroscopic primary cruciate repair in the multiligament injured knee. In: Fanelli G, editor. The multiple ligament injured knee: a practical guide to management. New York: Springer; 2012.

15 Combined PCL, ACL, Posteromedial, and Posterolateral Reconstruction

Gregory C. Fanelli

Introduction

The multiple-ligament-injured knee is a severe injury that may also involve neurovascular injuries and fractures [1]. Surgical treatment offers good functional results documented in the literature by physical examination, arthrometer testing, stress radiography, and knee ligament rating scales. Mechanical tensioning devices are helpful with cruciate ligament tensioning. Some low-grade medial collateral ligament (MCL) complex injuries may be amenable to brace treatment, while high-grade medial-side injuries require repair–reconstruction. Lateral posterolateral injuries are most successfully treated with surgical repair–reconstruction. Surgical timing in acute multiple-ligament-injured knee cases depends upon the ligaments injured, injured extremity vascular status, skin condition of the extremity, degree of instability, and the patients' overall health. Allograft tissue is preferred for these complex surgical procedures. Delayed reconstruction of 2–3 weeks may decrease the incidence of arthrofibrosis, and it is important to address all components of the instability. Currently, there is no conclusive evidence that double-bundle posterior cruciate ligament (PCL) reconstruction provides superior results to single-bundle PCL reconstruction in the multiple-ligament-injured knee.

The purpose of this chapter is to discuss my surgical technique for combined PCL and anterior cruciate ligament (ACL), medial- and lateral-side reconstructions in acute and chronic multiple-ligament-injured knees with global laxity [1–6]. This chapter focuses on recognizing and defining the instability pattern, the use of external fixation, surgical timing, graft selection and preparation, the author's preferred surgical technique, mechanical graft tensioning, perioperative antibiotics, specialized operating teams, postoperative rehabilitation, and our results of treatment in these complex surgical cases.

G. C. Fanelli (✉)
303 Kaseville Road, 17821 Danville, PA, USA

G. C. Fanelli (ed.), *Posterior Cruciate Ligament Injuries*,
DOI 10.1007/978-3-319-12072-0_15,

Surgical Timing

Surgical timing in the acute bicruciate multiple-ligament-injured knee is dependent upon the vascular status of the involved extremity, the collateral ligament injury severity, the degree of instability, and the postreduction stability. Delayed or staged reconstruction of 2–3 weeks post injury has demonstrated a lower incidence of arthrofibrosis in our experience [7, 8].

Surgical timing in acute ACL–PCL-lateral-side injuries is dependent upon the lateral-side classification [9]. Arthroscopic combined ACL–PCL reconstruction with lateral-side repair and reconstruction with allograft tissue is performed within 2–3 weeks post injury in knees with types A and B lateral posterolateral instability. Type C lateral posterolateral instability combined with ACL–PCL tears is often treated with staged reconstruction. The lateral posterolateral repair and reconstruction with allograft tissue is performed within the 1st week after injury, followed by arthroscopic combined ACL–PCL reconstruction 3–6 weeks later.

Surgical timing in acute ACL–PCL-medial-side injuries is also dependent on the medial-side classification. Some medial-side injuries will heal with 4–6 weeks of brace treatment, provided that the tibiofemoral joint is reduced in all planes. Other medial-side injuries require surgical intervention. Types A and B medial-side injuries are repaired–reconstructed as a single-stage procedure with combined arthroscopic ACL–PCL reconstruction. Type C medial-side injuries combined with ACL–PCL tears are often treated with staged reconstruction. The medial posteromedial repair–reconstruction augmented with allograft tissue is performed within the first 2 weeks after injury, followed by arthroscopic combined ACL–PCL reconstruction 3–6 weeks later [7, 8, 10–13].

Surgical timing may be affected by modifiers beyond the surgeon's control, and may cause the surgical treatment to be performed either earlier or later than desired. The surgical timing modifiers include the injured

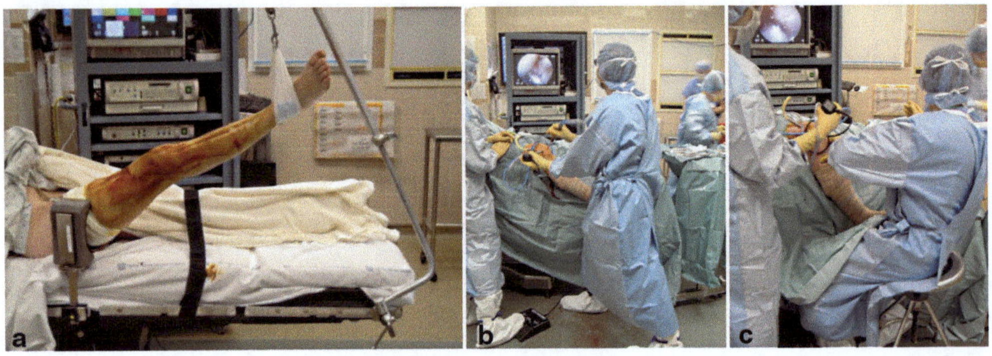

Fig. 15.1 Patient positioning. **a** The patient is positioned on the fully extended operating room table with a lateral post used for control of the surgical extremity. The surgeon stands during the basic arthroscopic portion of the procedure (**b**), and the surgeon is seated during the PCL, ACL, and lateral-side reconstruction (**c**). (From Fanelli 2013 [1]). *PCL* posterior cruciate ligament, *ACL* anterior cruciate ligament.

extremity vascular status, open wounds, reduction stability, skin conditions, multiple system injuries, other orthopedic injuries, and meniscus and articular surface injuries [10, 11]. When delayed or staged reconstruction techniques are used, it is very important to document maintained reduction of the tibiofemoral and patellofemoral articulations with radiographs.

Chronic bicruciate multiple ligament knee injuries often present to the orthopedic surgeon with functional instability, and possibly, some degree of post-traumatic arthrosis. Considerations for treatment require the determination of all structural injuries. These structural injuries may include various ligament injuries, meniscus injuries, bony malalignment, articular surface injuries, and gait abnormalities. Surgical procedures under consideration may include proximal tibial or distal femoral osteotomy, ligament reconstruction, meniscus transplant, and osteochondral grafting.

Graft Selection

My preferred graft for the PCL reconstruction is the Achilles tendon allograft for single-bundle PCL reconstructions, and Achilles tendon and tibialis anterior allografts for double-bundle PCL reconstructions. We prefer Achilles tendon allograft or other allograft for the ACL reconstruction. The preferred graft material for the lateral posterolateral reconstruction is allograft tissue combined with a primary repair, and posterolateral capsular shift procedure. My preferred method for medial-side injuries is a primary repair of all injured structures combined with posteromedial capsular shift and allograft tissue supplementation–augmentation as needed.

Combined PCL–ACL Reconstruction Surgical Technique

The principles of reconstruction in the multiple-ligament-injured knee are to identify and treat all pathology, accurate tunnel placement, anatomic graft insertion sites, utilize strong graft material, mechanical graft tensioning, secure graft fixation, and a deliberate postoperative rehabilitation program [1, 2, 6, 14–20].

The patient is placed on the operating room table in the supine position, and after satisfactory induction of anesthesia, the operative and nonoperative lower extremities are carefully examined [6]. A tourniquet is applied to the upper thigh of the operative extremity, and that extremity is prepped and draped in a sterile fashion. The well leg is supported by the fully extended operating room table, which also supports the surgical leg during medial- and lateral-side surgery. A lateral post is used to control the surgical extremity. An arthroscopic leg holder is not used (Fig. 15.1). Preoperative and postoperative antibiotics are given, and antibiotics are routinely used to help prevent infection in these time-consuming, difficult, and complex cases. Allograft tissue is prepared prior to bringing the patient into the operating room. Autograft tissue is harvested prior to beginning the arthroscopic portion of the procedure.

The arthroscopic instruments are inserted with the inflow through the superolateral patellar portal. Instrumentation and visualization are positioned through inferomedial and inferolateral patellar portals, and can be interchanged as necessary. Additional portals are established as necessary. Exploration of the joint consists of evaluation of the patellofemoral joint, the medial and lateral compartments, medial and lateral menisci, and the intercondylar notch. The residual stumps of both the anterior and PCL are debrided; however, the posterior and ACL anatomic insertion sites are preserved to serve

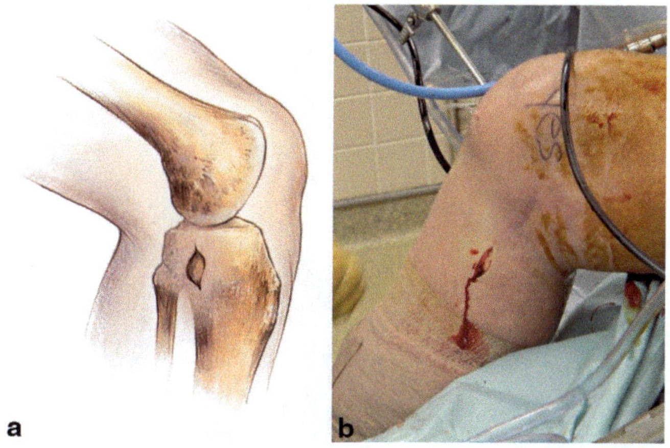

Fig. 15.2 **a** Posteromedial extra-articular extracapsular safety incision. (From Fanelli 2012 [6]). **b** Intraoperative photograph of the posteromedial safety incision. (From Fanelli 2013 [1])

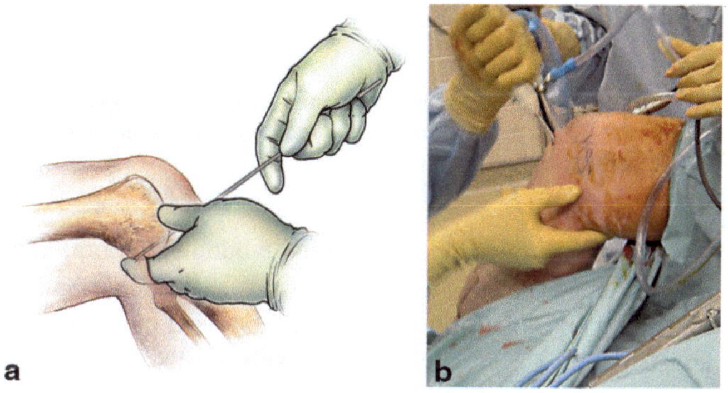

Fig. 15.3 **a** The surgeon is able to palpate the posterior aspect of the tibia through the extracapsular extra-articular posteromedial safety incision. This enables the surgeon to accurately position guide wires, create the tibial tunnel, and to protect the neurovascular structures. (From Fanelli 2012 [6]). **b** Intraoperative photograph of posterior instrumentation with the surgeon's finger in the posteromedial safety incision. (From Fanelli 2013 [1])

as tunnel reference points. The notchplasty for the ACL portion of the procedure is performed at this time.

An extracapsular extra-articular posteromedial safety incision is made by creating an incision approximately 1.5–2 cm long starting at the posteromedial border of the tibia approximately 1 in. below the level of the joint line and extending distally (Fig. 15.2). Dissection is carried down to the crural fascia, which is incised longitudinally. An interval is developed between the medial head of the gastrocnemius muscle and the nerves and vessels posterior to the surgeon's finger, and the capsule of the knee joint anterior to the surgeon's finger (Fig. 15.3). The posteromedial safety incision enables the surgeon to protect the neurovascular structures, confirm the accuracy of the PCL tibial tunnel, and to facilitate the flow of the surgical procedure.

The curved over-the-top PCL instruments (Biomet Sports Medicine, Warsaw, IN, USA) are used to sequentially lyse adhesions in the posterior aspect of the knee, and elevate the capsule from the posterior tibial ridge. This will allow accurate placement of the PCL/ACL drill guide and correct placement of the tibial tunnel (Fig. 15.4).

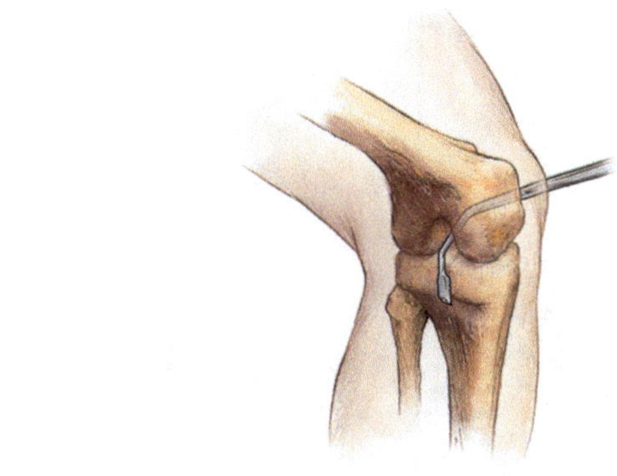

Fig. 15.4 Posterior capsular elevation. (From Fanelli 2012 [6])

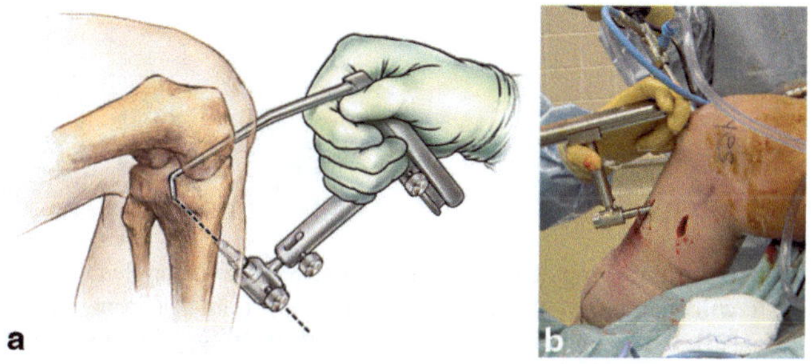

Fig. 15.5 **a** PCL–ACL drill guide positioned to place guide wire in preparation for creation of the transtibial PCL tibial tunnel. (From Fanelli 2012 [6]). **b** Intraoperative photograph of the drill guide positioned to create the PCL tibial tunnel. (From Fanelli 2013 [1]). *PCL* posterior cruciate ligament, *ACL* anterior cruciate ligament

The arm of the PCL/ACL guide (Biomet Sports Medicine, Warsaw, IN, USA) is inserted through the inferior medial patellar portal. The tip of the guide is positioned at the inferior lateral aspect of the PCL anatomic insertion site. This is below the tibial ridge posterior and in the lateral aspect of the PCL anatomic insertion site. The bullet portion of the guide contacts the anteromedial surface of the proximal tibia at a point midway between the posteromedial border of the tibia, and the tibial crest anterior at or just below the level of the tibial tubercle (Fig. 15.5). This will provide an angle of graft orientation such that the graft will turn two very smooth 45° angles on the posterior aspect of the tibia (Fig. 15.6). The tip of the guide in the posterior aspect of the tibia is confirmed with the surgeon's finger through the extracapsular extra-articular posteromedial safety incision. Intraoperative AP and lateral X-ray may also be used; however, I do not routinely use intraoperative X-ray. When the PCL/ACL guide is positioned in the desired area, a blunt spade-tipped guide wire is drilled from anterior to posterior. The surgeon's finger confirms the position of the guide wire through the posterior medial safety incision.

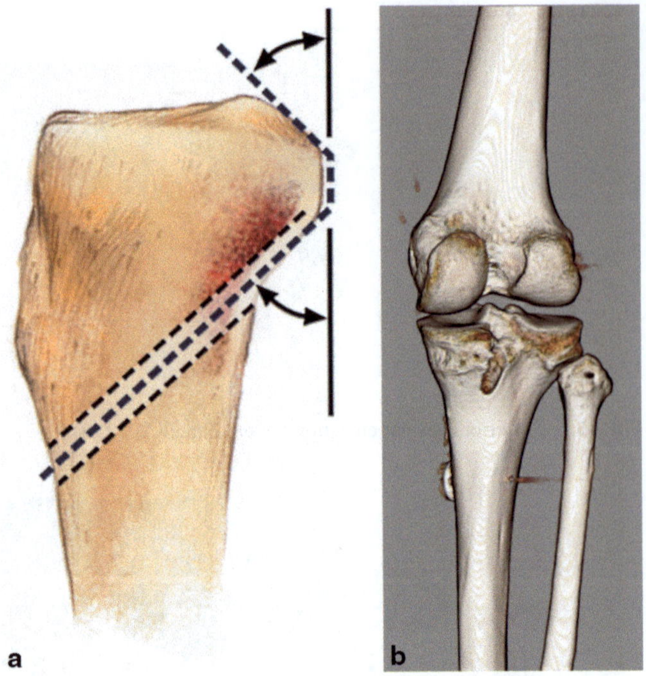

Fig. 15.6 **a** Drawing demonstrating the desired turning angles the PCL graft will make after the creation of the tibial tunnel. (From Fanelli 2012 [6]). **b** Three-dimensional CT scan demonstrating the position of a well-placed PCL tibial tunnel. Note the smooth turning angles the PCL graft will take. (From Fanelli 2013 [1]). *PCL* posterior cruciate ligament, *CT* computed tomography

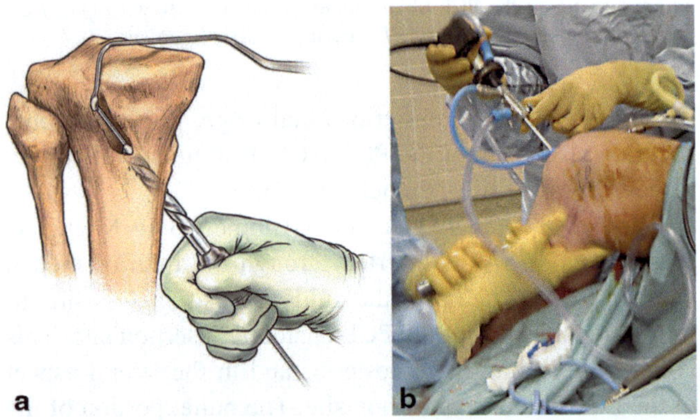

Fig. 15.7 **a** Final PCL tibial tunnel reaming by hand for an additional margin of safety. (From Fanelli 2012 [6]). **b** Intraoperative photograph of hand finishing of the PCL tibial tunnel. (From Fanelli 2013 [1]). *PCL* posterior cruciate ligament

The appropriately sized standard cannulated reamer is used to create the tibial tunnel. The surgeon's finger through the extracapsular extra-articular posteromedial incision monitors the position of the guide wire. When the drill is engaged in bone, the guide wire is reversed, blunt end pointing posterior, for additional patient safety. The drill is advanced until it comes to the posterior cortex of the tibia. The chuck is disengaged from the drill, and completion of the tibial tunnel is performed by hand (Fig. 15.7).

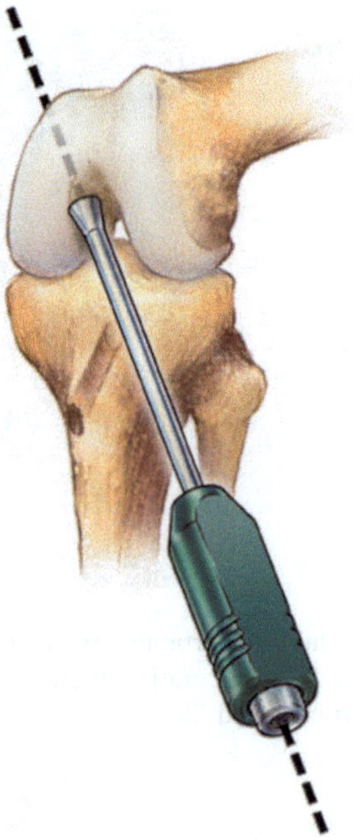

Fig. 15.8 Double-bundle aimer positioned to drill a guide wire for creation of the PCL anterolateral bundle tunnel. (From Fanelli 2012 [6]). *PCL* posterior cruciate ligament

The PCL single-bundle or double-bundle femoral tunnels are made from inside out using the double-bundle aimers, or an endoscopic reamer can be used as an aiming device (Biomet Sports Medicine, Warsaw, IN, USA). The appropriately sized double-bundle aimer or endoscopic reamer is inserted through a low anterior lateral patellar arthroscopic portal to create the PCL anterior lateral bundle femoral tunnel. The double-bundle aimer or endoscopic reamer is positioned directly on the footprint of the femoral anterior lateral bundle PCL insertion site (Fig. 15.8). The appropriately sized guide wire is drilled through the aimer or endoscopic reamer, through the bone, and out a small skin incision. Care is taken to prevent any compromise of the articular surface. The double-bundle aimer is removed and the endoscopic reamer is used to drill the anterior lateral PCL femoral tunnel from inside to outside (Fig. 15.9). When the surgeon chooses to perform a double-bundle double-femoral tunnel PCL reconstruction, the same process is repeated for the posterior medial bundle of the PCL (Fig. 15.10). Care must be taken to ensure that there will be an adequate bone bridge (approximately 5 mm) between the two femoral tunnels prior to drilling. This is accomplished using the calibrated probe, and direct arthroscopic visualization of the PCL femoral anatomic insertion sites (Fig. 15.11).

My preferred surgical technique of PCL femoral tunnel creation from inside to outside is for two reasons. There is a greater distance and margin of safety between the PCL femoral tunnels and the medial femoral condyle articular surface using the inside-to-outside method (Fig. 15.12). In addition, a more accurate placement of the PCL femoral tunnels

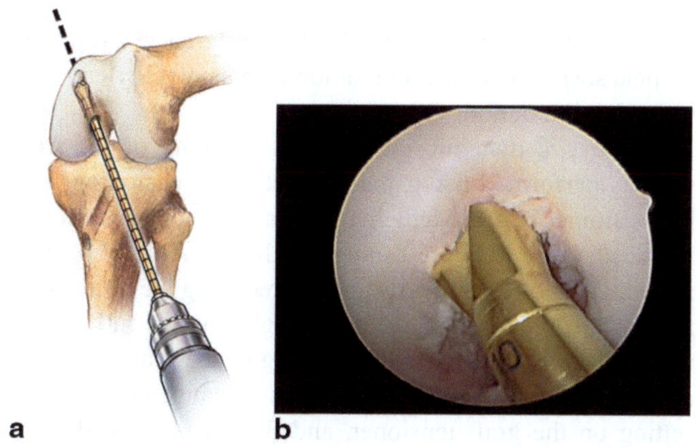

Fig. 15.9 **a** Endoscopic acorn reamer is used to create the PCL anterolateral bundle femoral tunnel through the low anterolateral patellar portal. (From Fanelli 2012 [6]). **b** Intraoperative view of an endoscopic acorn reamer is positioned to create the PCL anterolateral bundle femoral tunnel. (From Fanelli 2013 [1]). *PCL* posterior cruciate ligament

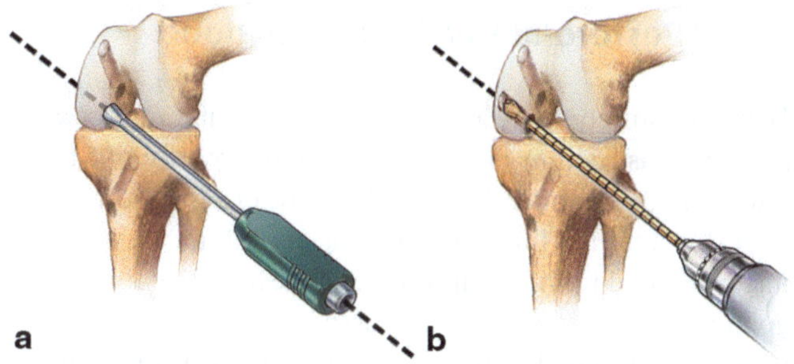

Fig. 15.10 **a** Double-bundle aimer positioned to drill a guide wire for creation of the PCL posteromedial bundle femoral tunnel through the low anterolateral patellar portal. (From Fanelli 2013 [1]). **b** Endoscopic acorn reamer is used to create the PCL posteromedial bundle femoral tunnel. A 5-mm bone bridge is maintained between tunnels. (From Fanelli 2012 [6]). *PCL* posterior cruciate ligament

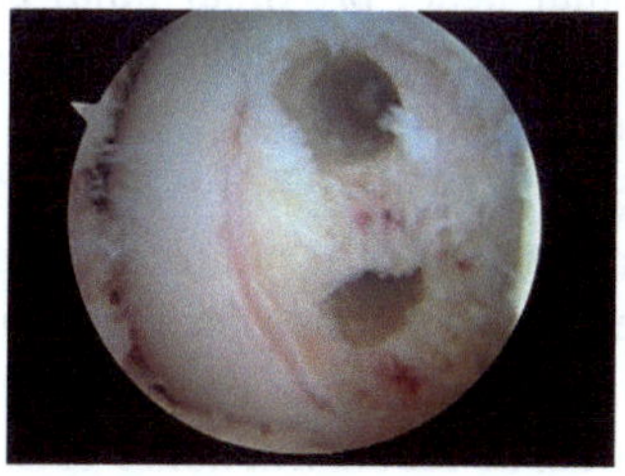

Fig. 15.11 Completed PCL anterolateral and posteromedial bundle tunnels fill the anatomic footprint of the posterior cruciate ligament. A 5-mm bone bridge is maintained between the tunnels. (From Fanelli 2013 [1]). *PCL* posterior cruciate ligament

is possible, in my opinion, because I can place the double-bundle aimer or endoscopic reamer on the anatomic footprint of the anterior lateral or posterior medial PCL insertion site under direct visualization (Fig. 15.13).

A Magellan suture retriever (Biomet Sports Medicine, Warsaw, IN, USA) is introduced through the tibial tunnel into the joint, and retrieved through the femoral tunnel

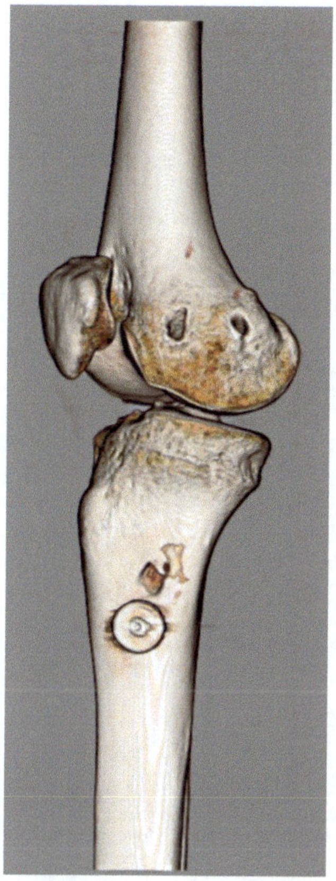

Fig. 15.12 Three-dimensional CT scan showing properly positioned PCL femoral tunnel exit points after inside-to-outside PCL femoral tunnel creation. Note the distance between the femoral tunnel exit points and the distal medial femoral condyle articular surface. (From Fanelli 2013 [1]). *PCL* posterior cruciate ligament, *CT* computed tomography

(Fig. 15.14). The traction sutures of the graft material are attached to the loop of the Magellan suture retriever and the graft is pulled into position. The graft material is secured on the femoral side using a bioabsorbable interference screw for primary aperture opening fixation, and a polyethylene ligament fixation button for backup fixation.

The cyclic dynamic method of graft tensioning using the Biomet graft-tensioning boot is used to tension the posterior and ACL grafts [21]. This tensioning method is discussed in Chap. 21. Tension is placed on the PCL graft distally using the Biomet graft-tensioning boot (Biomet Sports Medicine, Warsaw, IN, USA; Fig. 15.15). Tension is gradually applied with the knee in 0° of flexion (full extension) reducing the tibia on the femur. This restores the anatomic tibial step-off. The knee is cycled through a full range of motion multiple times to allow pretensioning and settling of the graft. The process is repeated until there is no further change in the torque setting on the graft tensioner. The knee is placed in 70–90° of flexion, and fixation is achieved on the tibial side of the PCL graft with a bioabsorbable interference screw, and backup fixation with a bicortical screw and spiked ligament washer or polyethylene ligament fixation button (Fig. 15.16).

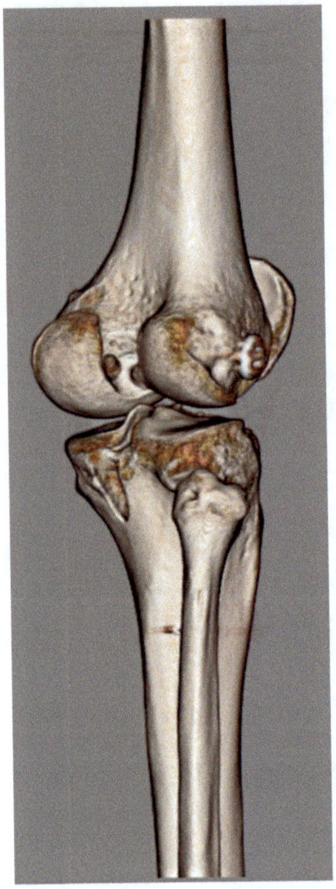

Fig. 15.13 Three-dimensional CT scan showing properly positioned intra-articular PCL femoral tunnel position after inside-to-outside PCL femoral tunnel creation. A more accurate placement of the posterior cruciate ligament femoral tunnels is possible because I can place the double-bundle aimer or endoscopic reamer on the anatomic footprint of the anterior lateral or posterior medial posterior cruciate ligament insertion site under direct visualization. (From Fanelli 2013 [1]). *PCL* posterior cruciate ligament, *CT* computed tomography

With the knee in approximately 90° of flexion, the ACL tibial tunnel is created using a drill guide. My preferred method of ACL reconstruction is the transtibial femoral tunnel endoscopic surgical technique. The arm of the drill guide enters the knee joint through the inferior medial patellar portal (Fig. 15.17). The bullet of the drill guide contacts the anterior medial proximal tibia externally at a point midway between the posterior medial border of the tibia, and the anterior tibial crest just above the level of the tibial tubercle. A 1-cm bone bridge or greater exists between the PCL and ACL tibial tunnels. The guide wire is drilled through the guide and positioned so that after creating the ACL tibial tunnel, the graft will approximate the tibial anatomic insertion site of the ACL. A standard cannulated reamer is used to create the tibial tunnel.

With the knee in approximately 90–100° of flexion, an over-the-top femoral aimer is introduced through the tibial tunnel, and used to position a guide wire on the medial wall of the lateral femoral condyle to create a femoral tunnel approximating the anatomic insertion site of the ACL (Fig. 15.18). The ACL graft is positioned, and fixation achieved on the femoral side using a bioabsorbable interference screw, and cortical suspensory backup fixation with a polyethylene ligament fixation button.

The cyclic dynamic method of tensioning of the ACL graft is performed using the Biomet graft-tensioning boot [21] (Biomet Sports Medicine, Warsaw, IN, USA). Traction is placed on the ACL graft sutures with the knee in 0° of flexion, and tension is gradually applied reducing the tibia on the femur. The knee is then cycled through multiple full flexion and extension cycles to allow settling of the graft. The process is repeated until there is no further change in the torque setting on the graft tensioner, and the Lachman and pivot shift tests are negative. The knee is placed in approximately 30° of flexion, and fixation is achieved on the tibial side of the ACL graft with a bioabsorbable interference screw, and backup fixation with a polyethylene ligament fixation button (Fig. 15.19).

Lateral Posterolateral Reconstruction

My most commonly utilized surgical technique for posterolateral reconstruction is the free graft figure-of-eight technique utilizing semitendinosus allograft, or other soft tissue allograft material (Fig. 15.20). This procedure requires an intact proximal tibiofibular joint, and the absence of a severe hyperextension external rotation recurvatum deformity. This technique combined with capsular repair and posterolateral capsular shift procedures mimics the function of the popliteofibular ligament and lateral collateral ligament, tightens the posterolateral capsule, and provides a post of strong allograft tissue to reinforce the posterolateral corner (PLC). When there is a disrupted proximal tibiofibular joint, or severe hyperextension external rotation recurvatum deformity, a two-tailed (fibular head, proximal tibia) posterior lateral reconstruction is performed in addition to the posterolateral capsular shift procedure (Fig. 15.21).

In acute cases, primary repair of all lateral-side injured structures is performed with suture anchors, screws and washers, and permanent sutures through drill holes as indicated (Fig. 15.22). The primary repair is then augmented with an allograft tissue reconstruction. Posterolateral reconstruction with the free graft figure-of-eight technique utilizes semitendinosus or other soft tissue allograft. A curvilinear incision is made in the lateral aspect of the knee extending from the interval between Gerdy's tubercle and the fibular head to the lateral epicondyle and then proximal following the course of the iliotibial band. A peroneal nerve neurolysis is performed and the peroneal nerve is protected throughout the procedure. The fibular head is identified and a tunnel is created in an anterior-to-posterior direction at the area of maximal fibular head diameter. The tunnel is created by passing a guide pin followed by a standard cannulated drill 7 mm in diameter. The peroneal nerve is protected during

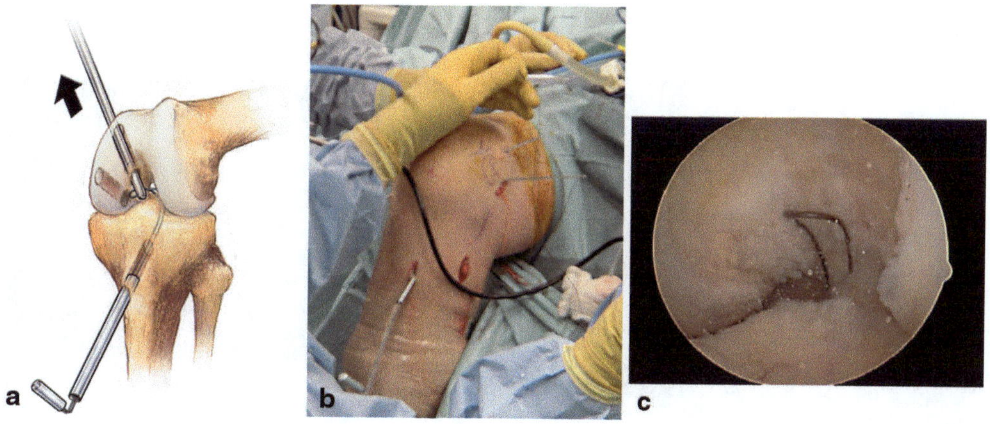

Fig. 15.14 **a** Magellan suture-passing device. (From Fanelli 2012 [6]). **b** and **c** Intraoperative external and arthroscopic views demonstrating the positioning of the Magellan suture and graft-passing device. (From Fanelli 2013 [1])

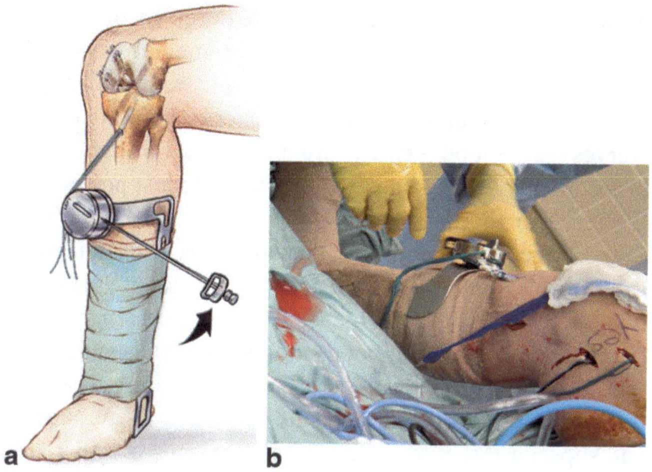

Fig. 15.15 **a** Knee ligament graft-tensioning boot is used to tension the PCL graft. This mechanical tensioning device uses a ratcheted torque wrench device to assist the surgeon during graft tensioning. (From Fanelli 2012 [6]). **b** Intraoperative photograph of Biomet tensioning boot applied to the tibia to tension the PCL reconstruction graft. (From Fanelli 2013 [1]). *PCL* posterior cruciate ligament

tunnel creation, and throughout the procedure. The free tendon graft is passed through the fibular head drill hole. An incision is made in the iliotibial band in line with the fibers exposing the lateral femoral epicondyle area of the distal femur. The graft material is passed medial to the iliotibial band for the fibular collateral ligament limb, and medial to the common biceps tendon and iliotibial band for the popliteus tendon popliteofibular ligament limb. The limbs of the graft are crossed to form a figure of eight with the fibular collateral ligament component being lateral to the popliteus tendon component. A 3.2-mm drill hole is made to accommodate a 6.5-mm diameter fully threaded cancellous screw that is approximately 30–35 mm in length. The drill hole is positioned in the lateral epicondylar region of the distal lateral femur so that after seating a 17–20-mm washer with the abovementioned screw, the washer will precisely secure the two limbs of the allograft tissue at the respective anatomic insertion sites of the fibular collateral ligament and popliteus tendon on the distal lateral femoral condyle. This drill hole is approximately 1 cm anterior to the fibular collateral ligament femoral insertion. A longitudinal incision is made in the lateral capsule just posterior to the fibular collateral ligament. The graft material is tensioned at approximately 30–40° of knee flexion, secured to the lateral femoral epicondylar region with a screw and spiked ligament washer at the aforementioned point. The posterolateral capsule that had been previously incised is then shifted and sewn into the strut of the figure-of-eight graft tissue material to eliminate posterolateral capsular redundancy (Fig. 15.23). The anterior and posterior limbs of the figure-of-eight graft material are sewn to each other to reinforce and tighten the construct. The final graft-tensioning position is approximately 30–40° of knee flexion with a slight valgus force applied and slight internal tibial rotation. The iliotibial band incision is closed. The procedures described are designed to eliminate posterolateral axial rotation and varus rotational instability. Number two ethibond suture is used to sew the tails of the graft together proximal to the washer to prevent slipping, and also to sew the allograft to the deep capsular layers for additional reinforcement.

When there is a disrupted proximal tibiofibular joint, or hyperextension external rotation recurvatum deformity, a two-tailed (fibular head, proximal tibia) posterior lateral reconstruction is utilized combined with a posterolateral capsular shift. A 7- or 8-mm drill hole is made over a guide wire approximately 2 cm below the lateral tibial plateau. A tibialis anterior or other soft tissue allograft is passed through this tibial drill hole and follows the course of the popliteus tendon to its anatomic insertion site on the lateral femoral epicondylar region. Nerves and blood vessels must be protected. The tibialis anterior or other soft tissue allograft is secured with a suture anchor, and multiple number two braided nonabsorbable sutures at the popliteus tendon anatomic femoral insertion site. The knee is cycled through multiple sets

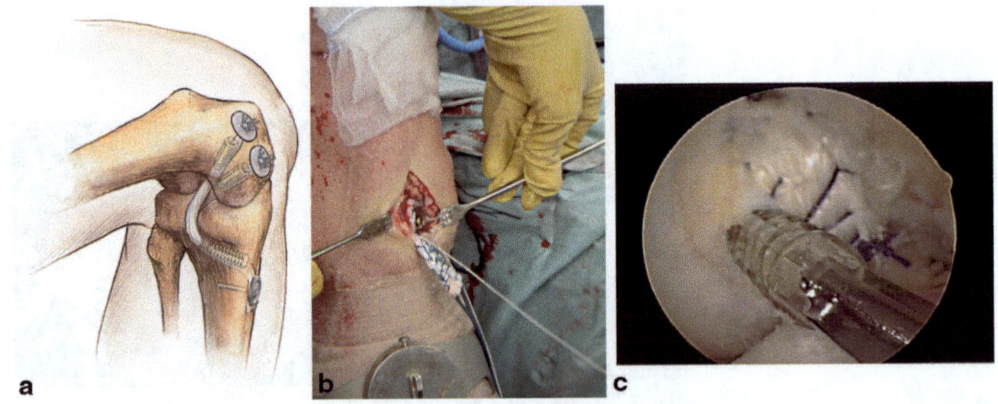

Fig. 15.16 **a** PCL final graft fixation using primary and backup fixation. (From Fanelli 2012 [6]). **b** PCL final tibial fixation. **c** Interference fit fixation of PCL graft in femoral tunnel. (From Fanelli 2013 [1]). *PCL* posterior cruciate ligament

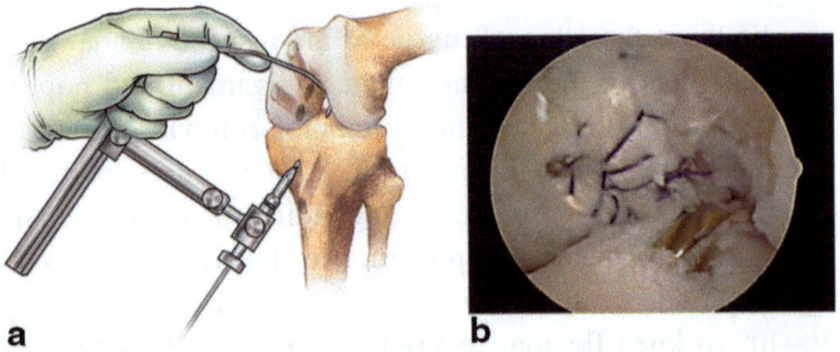

Fig. 15.17 **a** The PCL–ACL drill guide is positioned to create ACL tibial tunnel. (From Fanelli 2012 [6]). **b** ACL tibial tunnel orientation and position to approximate the tibial and femoral anatomic insertion sites of the anterior cruciate ligament. (From Fanelli 2013 [1]). *PCL* posterior cruciate ligament, *ACL* anterior cruciate ligament

of full flexion and extension cycles, placed in 90° of flexion, the tibia slightly internally rotated, slight valgus force applied to the knee, and the graft tensioned, and secured in the tibial tunnel with a bioabsorbable interference screw, and polyethylene ligament fixation button. The fibular-head-based reconstruction and posterolateral capsular shift procedures are then carried out as described above. Number two ethibond suture is used to sew the tails of the graft together proximal to the washer to prevent slipping, and also to sew the allograft to the deep capsular layers for additional reinforcement.

Medial Posteromedial Reconstruction

The surgical leg positioned on the extended operating room table in a supported flexed knee position, posteromedial and medial reconstructions are performed through a medial curved incision taking care to maintain adequate skin bridges between incisions. In acute cases, primary repair of all medial-side injured structures is performed with suture anchors, screws and washers, and permanent sutures through drill holes as indicated. The primary repair is then augmented with an allograft tissue reconstruction (Fig. 15.24). In chronic cases of posteromedial reconstruction, the sartorius fascia is incised and retracted exposing the superficial MCL and the posterior medial capsule. Nerves and blood vessels are protected throughout the procedure. A longitudinal incision is made just posterior to the posterior border of the superficial MCL (Fig. 15.25). Care is taken not to damage the medial meniscus during the capsular incision. Avulsed capsular structures are primarily repaired using bioabsorbable suture anchors and permanent braided number two ethibond sutures. The interval between the posteromedial capsule and medial meniscus is developed. The posteromedial capsule is shifted in an anterior and superior direction. The medial meniscus is repaired to the new capsular position, and the shifted capsule is sewn into the MCL using three number two permanent braided ethibond sutures in a horizontal mattress fashion, and that suture line is reinforced using a running number two ethibond suture.

When superficial MCL reconstruction is indicated, this is performed using allograft tissue after completion of the primary capsular repair, and posteromedial capsular shift procedures are performed as outlined above (Fig. 15.26). This graft material is attached at the anatomic insertion sites of the superficial MCL on the femur and tibia using a screw and spiked ligament washer, or suture anchors. The final graft-tensioning position is approximately 30–40° of knee flexion. It is my preference to secure the tibial insertion site first, and to perform the final tensioning and fixation of the allograft tissue on the femoral side. Number two ethibond suture is used to sew the tails of the graft together proximal to the washer to prevent slipping, and also to sew the allograft to the deep capsular layers for additional reinforcement.

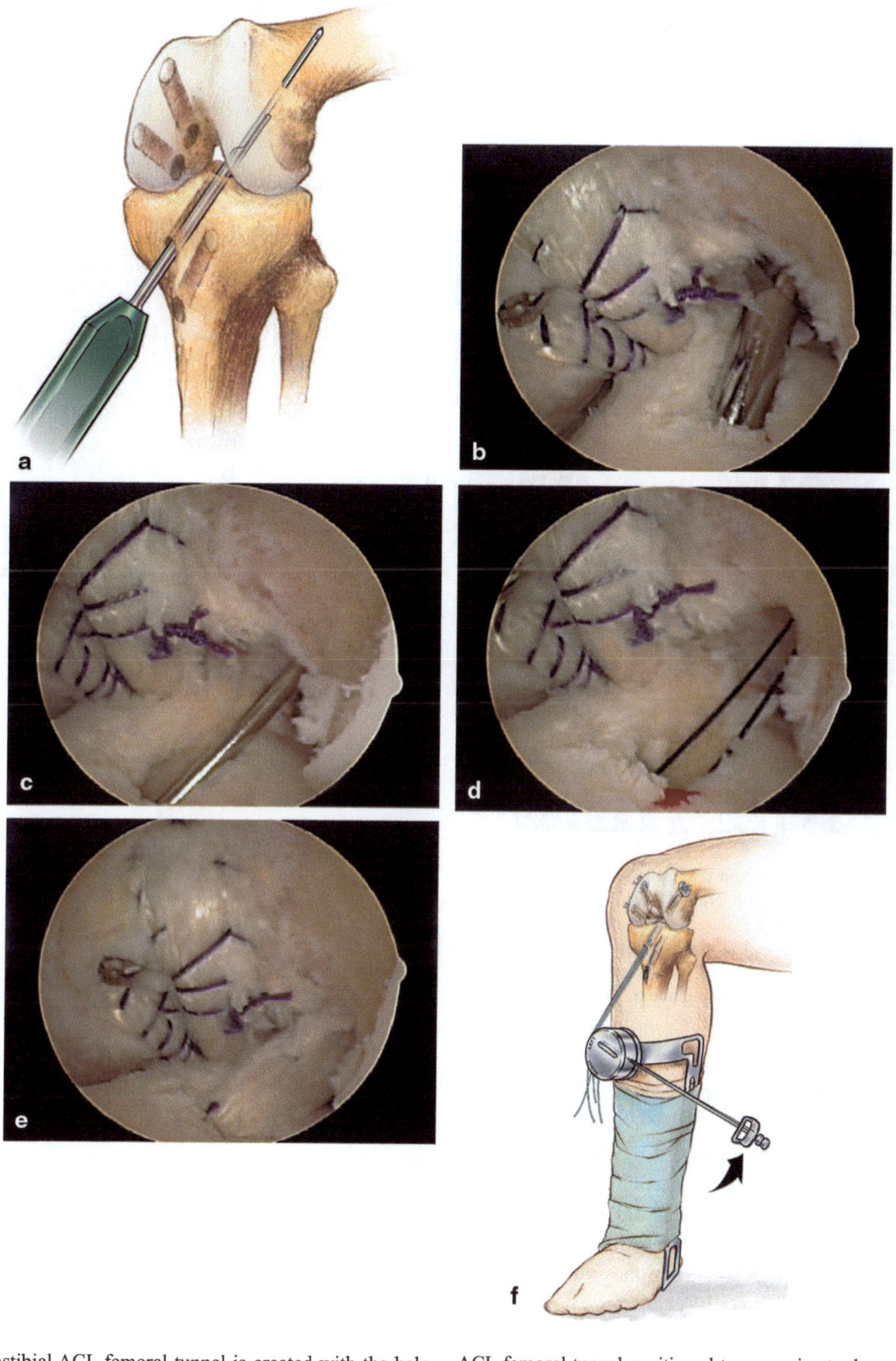

Fig. 15.18 **a** Transtibial ACL femoral tunnel is created with the help of an over-the-top femoral aimer to approximate the ACL femoral insertion site. (From Fanelli 2012 [6]). **b** Arthroscopic view of an over-the-top femoral aimer positioning a guide wire for ACL femoral tunnel creation. **c** Guide wire positioned for ACL femoral tunnel creation. **d** ACL femoral tunnel positioned to approximate the anatomic insertion of the anterior cruciate ligament. **e** Anterior cruciate ligament graft in final position. (From Fanelli 2013 [1]). **f** Final tensioning of the ACL graft using the Biomet graft-tensioning boot. (From Fanelli 2008 [27]). *ACL* anterior cruciate ligament

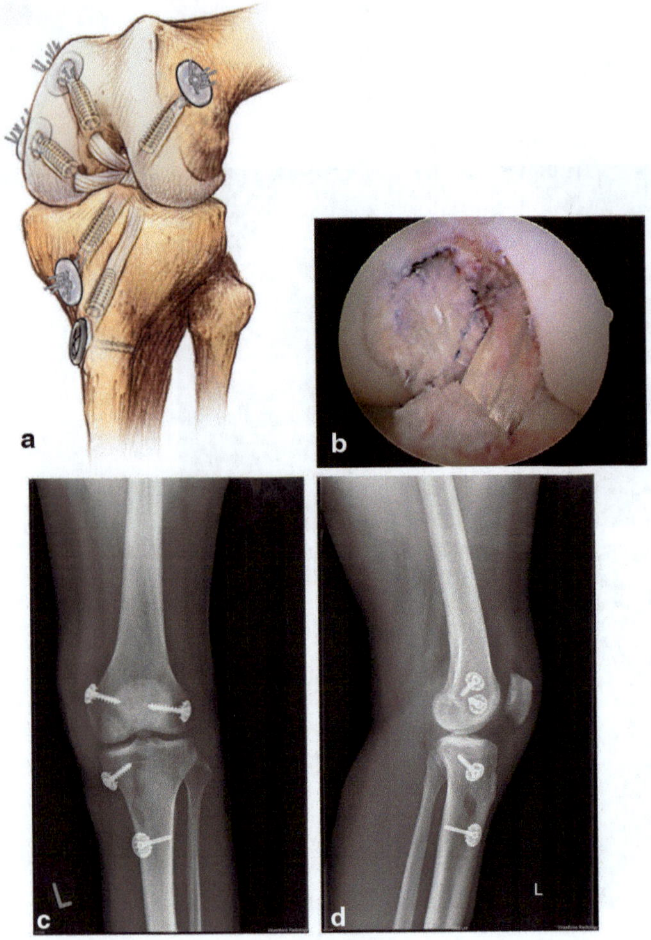

Fig. 15.19 **a** Drawing of final fixation of PCL and ACL grafts. Note primary and backup fixation of each graft. (From Fanelli 2012 [6]). **b** Arthroscopic view of completed PCL–ACL reconstruction. **c** and **d** Postoperative anterior posterior and lateral radiographs of completed combined PCL, ACL, lateral, and medial-side reconstructions. (From Fanelli 2013 [1]). *PCL* posterior cruciate ligament, *ACL* anterior cruciate ligament

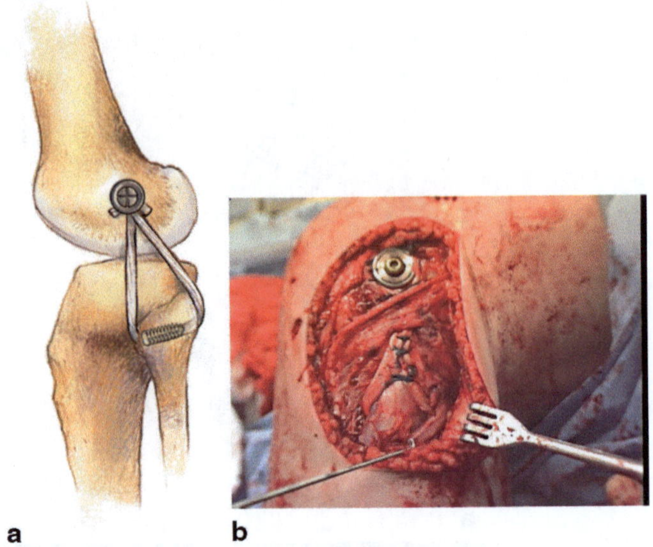

Fig. 15.20 **a** Posterolateral reconstruction using fibular-head-based figure-of-eight allograft tissue. (From Fanelli 2012 [6]). **b** Intraoperative photograph of fibular-head-based posterolateral reconstruction using semitendinosus allograft. Probe is pointing to peroneal nerve neurolysis, a very important part of the procedure. (From Fanelli 2013 [1])

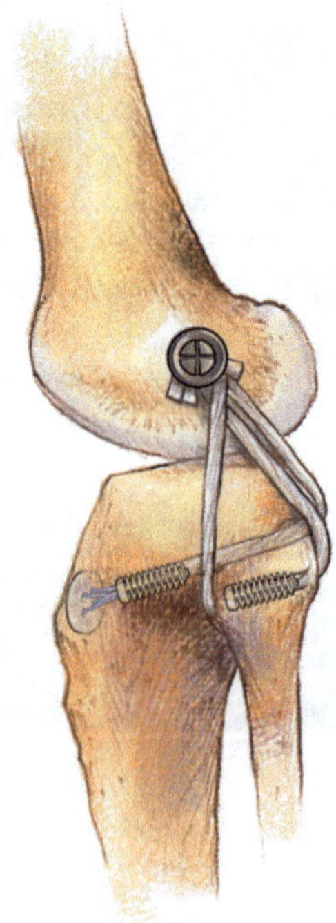

Fig. 15.21 Posterolateral reconstruction using fibular-head-based figure-of-eight allograft tissue combined with tibial-based popliteus tendon allograft reconstruction. (From Fanelli 2012 [6])

Graft Tensioning and Fixation

The PCL is reconstructed first followed by the ACL reconstruction followed by the lateral posterolateral reconstruction, and finally the medial posteromedial reconstruction. Final fixation has been performed on the femoral side of the posterior and ACL reconstruction grafts. Tension is placed on the PCL graft distally using the Biomet knee ligament-tensioning device (Biomet Sports Medicine, Warsaw, IN, USA). This reduces the tibia on the femur in full extension, and restores the anatomic tibial step-off. The knee is cycled through a full range of motion multiple times to allow pretensioning and settling of the graft. The knee is placed in 70–90° of flexion, and fixation is achieved on the tibial side of the PCL graft with a bioabsorbable interference screw, and screw and spiked ligament washer or polyethylene ligament fixation button. The Biomet knee ligament-tensioning device (Biomet Sports Medicine, Warsaw, IN, USA) is next applied to the ACL graft, and tension is gradually applied at full extension reducing the tibia on the femur. The knee is cycled through a full range of motion multiple times to allow pretensioning and settling of the graft. The knee is

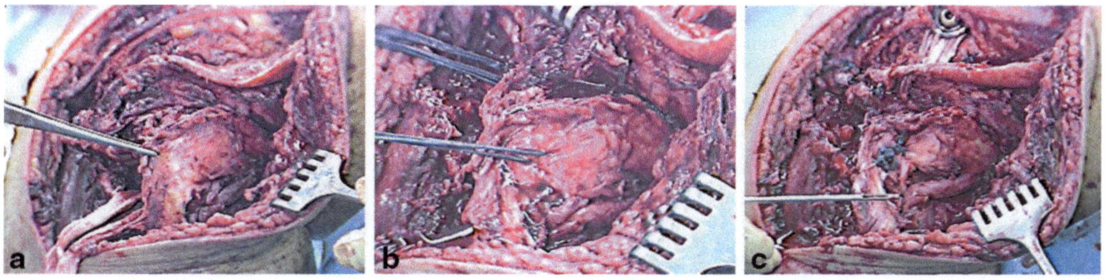

Fig. 15.22 **a** Acute severe lateral-side injury. **b** Lateral posterolateral primary repair with a combination of suture anchors and transosseous sutures. **c** Augmentation of acute lateral posterolateral primary repair with fibular-head-based figure-of-eight allograft semitendinosus lateral posterolateral reconstruction. Probe is pointing to peroneal nerve neurolysis, a very important part of the procedure. (From Fanelli 2013 [1])

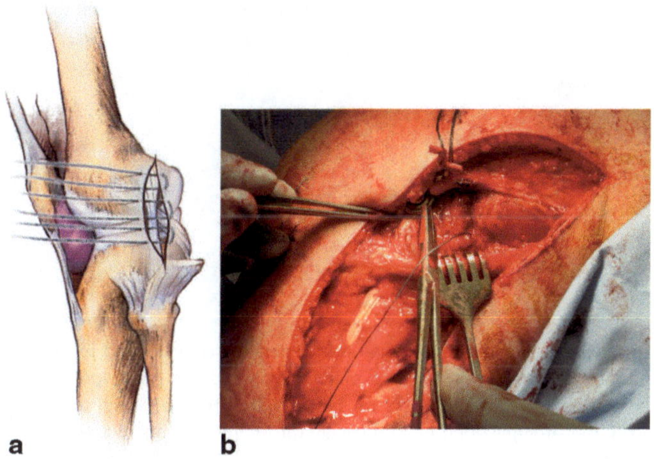

a b

Fig. 15.23 **a** Posterolateral capsular shift is used to decrease redundant posterolateral capsular volume in combination with posterolateral allograft reconstruction. (From Fanelli 2012 [6]). **b** Intraoperative photograph of posterolateral shift using number two ethibond suture material. (From Fanelli 2013 [1])

placed in 30° of flexion, and final fixation is achieved of the ACL graft with a bioabsorbable interference screw, and polyethylene ligament fixation button. The posterior and ACL incisions are thoroughly irrigated and closed in layers. Attention is now turned to the lateral side of the knee where lateral posterolateral reconstruction, tensioning, and fixation are performed as outlined above. The lateral-side incision is thoroughly irrigated and closed in layers. Finally, the medial posteromedial reconstruction, tensioning, and fixation are performed as outlined above. Full range of motion is confirmed on the operating table to assure the knee is not "captured" by the reconstructions.

Additional Technical Ideas

The posteromedial safety incision protects the neurovascular structures, confirms the accuracy of the PCL tibial tunnel placement, and enhances the flow of the surgical procedure. It is important to be aware of femoral and tibial tunnel directions, and to have adequate bone bridges between tunnels. This will reduce the possibility of tibial fracture. We have found it very important to use primary and backup fixation. During cruciate ligament reconstruction, primary aperture fixation is achieved with bioabsorbable interference screws, and backup fixation is performed with a screw and spiked ligament washer, and ligament fixation buttons. Secure fixation is critical to the success of this surgical procedure. The medial- and lateral-side reconstruction primary fixation is achieved with screws and spiked ligament washers, and backup fixation is achieved with multiple number two ethibond reinforcing sutures. Mechanical tensioning of the cruciates at 0° of knee flexion (full extension), and restoration of the normal anatomic tibial step-off at 70–90° of flexion has provided the most reproducible method of establishing the neutral point of the tibial–femoral relationship in our experience. Full range of motion is confirmed on the operating table to assure the knee is not "captured" by the reconstruction.

Postoperative Rehabilitation

The knee is maintained in full extension for 5 weeks non-weight bearing. Progressive range of motion occurs during postoperative weeks 6 through 10. Progressive weight bearing occurs at the beginning of postoperative week 6 progressing at a rate of 20 % body weight per week during postoperative weeks 6 through 10. Progressive closed kinetic chain strength training, proprioceptive training, and continued motion exercises are initiated very slowly beginning at postoperative week 11. The long leg range of motion brace is discontinued after the 10th week and the patient wears a global laxity functional brace for all activities for additional protection. Return to sports and heavy labor occurs after the 9th postoperative month when sufficient strength, range of motion, and proprioceptive skills have returned [4, 5, 22–24]. It is very important to carefully observe these complex knee ligament injury patients, and get a feel for the "personality of the knee." The surgeon may need to make adjustments and individualize the postoperative rehabilitation program as necessary. Careful and gentle range of motion under

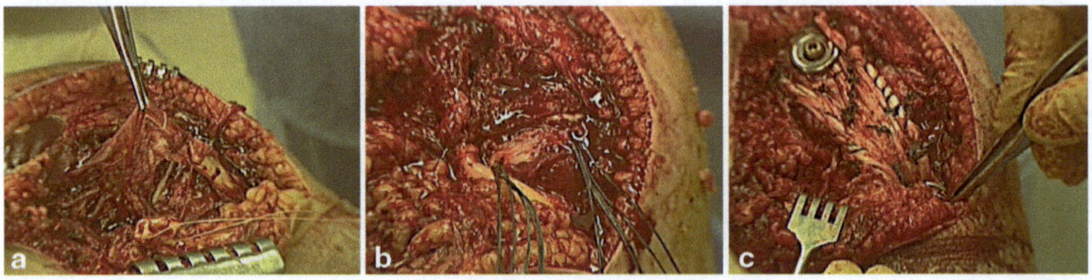

Fig. 15.24 **a** Acute severe medial-side injury. **b** Medial posteromedial primary repair with a combination of suture anchors and transosseous sutures. **c** Augmentation of acute medial posteromedial primary repair with allograft medial posteromedial reconstruction. (From Fanelli 2013 [1])

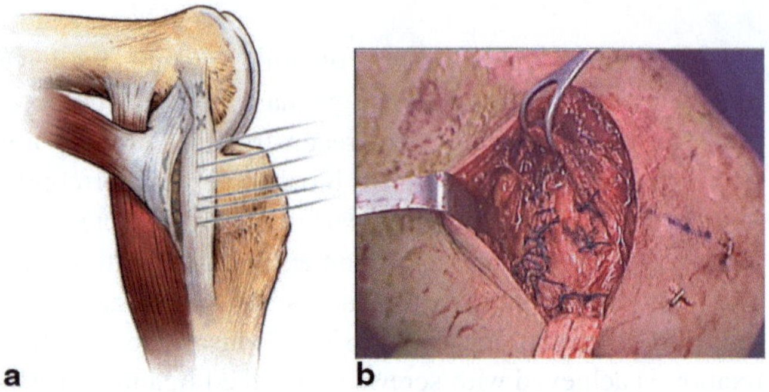

Fig. 15.25 **a** Posteromedial capsular shift utilized in medial posteromedial reconstruction. (From Fanelli 2012 [6]). **b** Intraoperative photograph of posteromedial capsular shift procedure using number two ethibond. (From Fanelli 2013 [1])

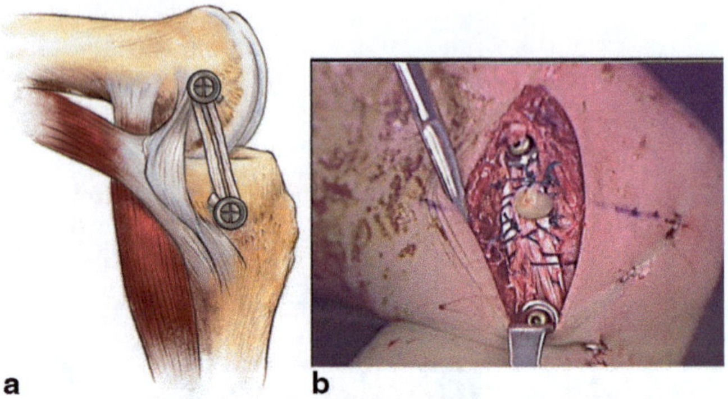

Fig. 15.26 **a** Allograft medial-side reconstruction is used in combination with posteromedial capsular shift procedures for severe medial posteromedial instability. (From Fanelli 2012 [6]). **b** Allograft reconstruction of superficial medial collateral ligament. This reconstruction combined with the posteromedial capsular shift procedure controls valgus and axial rotation instability. (From Fanelli 2013 [1])

general anesthesia is a very useful tool in the treatment of these complex cases, and is utilized as necessary. Our postoperative rehabilitation program is discussed in more detail in Chap. 25.

Author's Results

Our results of multiple-ligament-injured knee treatment without mechanical graft tensioning are outlined below [8]. This study presented the 2–10-year (24–120-month) results of 35 arthroscopically assisted combined ACL/PCL reconstructions evaluated pre- and postoperatively using Lysholm, Tegner, and Hospital for Special Surgery (HSS) knee ligament rating scales, knee laxity testing device KT 1000 knee ligament arthrometer testing, stress radiography, and physical examination.

This study population included 26 males, 9 females, 19 acute, and 16 chronic knee injuries. Ligament injuries included 19 ACL/PCL/posterolateral instabilities, 9 ACL/PCL/MCL instabilities, 6 ACL/PCL/posterolateral/MCL instabilities, and 1 ACL/PCL instability. All knees had grade III preoperative ACL/PCL laxity and were assessed pre- and postoperatively with arthrometer testing, three different knee ligament rating scales, stress radiography, and physical examination. Arthroscopically assisted combined ACL/PCL reconstructions were performed using the single-incision endoscopic ACL technique, and the single-femoral tunnel single-bundle transtibial tunnel PCL technique. PCLs were reconstructed with allograft Achilles tendon (26 knees), autograft bone–patellar tendon–bone (BTB; 7 knees), and autograft semitendinosus/gracilis (2 knees). ACLs were reconstructed with autograft BTB (16 knees), allograft BTB (12 knees), Achilles tendon allograft (6 knees), and autograft semitendinosus/gracilis (1 knee). MCL injuries were treated with bracing or open reconstruction. Posterolateral instability was treated with biceps femoris tendon transfer, with or without primary repair, and posterolateral capsular shift procedures as indicated. No Biomet Sports Medicine graft-tensioning boot was used in this series of patients (Biomet Sports Medicine, Warsaw, IN, USA).

Postoperative physical examination results revealed normal posterior drawer/tibial step-off in 16/35 (46 %) of knees. Normal Lachman and pivot shift tests were conducted in 33/35 (94 %) of knees. Posterolateral stability was restored to normal in 6/25 (24 %) of knees, and tighter than the normal knee in 19/25 (76 %) of knees evaluated with the external rotation thigh–foot angle test. Thirty-degree varus stress testing was normal in 22/25 (88 %) of knees and grade 1 laxity in 3/25 (12 %) of knees. Thirty-degree valgus stress testing was normal in 7/7 (100 %) of surgically treated MCL tears, and normal in 7/8 (87.5 %) of brace-treated knees. Postoperative KT 1000 arthrometer testing mean side-to-side difference measurements were 2.7 mm (PCL screen), 2.6 mm (corrected posterior), and 1.0 mm (corrected anterior) measurements, a statistically significant improvement from preoperative status ($p=0.001$). Postoperative stress radiographic side-to-side difference measurements measured at 90° of knee flexion, and 32 pounds of posteriorly directed proximal force were 0–3 mm in 11/21 (52.3 %), 4–5 mm in 5/21 (23.8 %), and 6–10 mm in 4/21 (19 %) of knees. Postoperative Lysholm, Tegner, and HSS knee ligament rating scale mean values were 91.2, 5.3, and 86.8, respectively, demonstrating a statistically significant improvement from preoperative status ($p=0.001$). No Biomet graft-tensioning boot was used in this series of patients.

The conclusions drawn from the study were that combined ACL/PCL instabilities could be successfully treated with arthroscopic reconstruction and the appropriate collateral ligament surgery. Statistically significant improvement was noted from the preoperative condition at 2–10-year follow-up using objective parameters of knee ligament rating scales, arthrometer testing, stress radiography, and physical examination.

Our results of multiple-ligament-injured knee treatment using mechanical graft tensioning are outlined below [11]. These data present the 2-year follow-up of 15 arthroscopic-assisted ACL–PCL reconstructions using the Biomet graft-tensioning boot (Biomet Sports Medicine, Warsaw, IN, USA). This study group consisted of 11 chronic and 4 acute injuries. These injury patterns included six ACL–PCL–PLC injuries, four ACL–PCL–MCL injuries, and five ACL–PCL–PLC–MCL injuries. The Biomet graft-tensioning boot was used during the procedures as in the surgical technique described above. All knees had grade III preoperative ACL/PCL laxity and were assessed pre- and postoperatively using Lysholm, Tegner, and HSS knee ligament rating scales, KT 1000 arthrometer testing, stress radiography, and physical examination.

Arthroscopically assisted combined ACL/PCL reconstructions were performed using the single-incision endoscopic ACL technique, and the single-femoral tunnel- single-bundle transtibial tunnel PCL technique. PCLs were reconstructed with allograft Achilles tendon in all 15 knees. ACLs were reconstructed with Achilles tendon allograft in all 15 knees. MCL injuries were treated surgically using primary repair, posteromedial capsular shift, and allograft augmentation as indicated. Posterolateral instability was treated with allograft semitendinosus free graft, with or without primary repair, and posterolateral capsular shift procedures as indicated. The Biomet graft-tensioning boot was used in this series of patients.

Post-reconstruction physical examination results revealed normal posterior drawer/tibial step-off in 13/15 (86.6 %) of knees. Normal Lachman test were conducted in 13/15 (86.6 %) knees, and normal pivot shift tests in 14/15 (93.3 %) knees. Posterolateral stability was restored to normal in all knees with posterolateral instability when evaluated with the external rotation thigh–foot angle test (nine knees equal to the normal knee, and two knees tighter than the normal knee). Thirty-degree varus stress testing was restored to normal in all 11 knees with posterolateral lateral instability. Thirty- and zero-degree valgus stress testing was restored to normal in all nine knees with medial-side laxity. Postoperative KT-1000 arthrometer testing mean side-to-side difference measurements were 1.6 mm (range 3–7 mm) for the PCL screen, 1.6 mm (range 4.5–9 mm) for the corrected posterior, and 0.5 mm (range 2.5 to 6 mm) for the corrected anterior measurements; a significant improvement from preoperative status. Postoperative stress radiographic side-to-side difference measurements measured at 90° of knee flexion and 32 pounds of posteriorly directed proximal force using the Telos stress radiography device were 0–3 mm in 10/15 knees (66.7 %), 0–4 mm in 14/15 (93.3 %), 4 mm in 4/15 knees (26.7 %), and 7 mm in 1/15 knees (6.67 %). Postoperative Lysholm, Tegner, and HSS knee ligament rating scale mean values were 86.7 (range 69–95), 4.5 (range 2–7), and 85.3 (range 65–93), respectively, demonstrating a significant improvement from preoperative status. The study group demonstrates the efficacy and success of using a mechanical graft-tensioning device in posterior and ACL reconstruction procedures.

Our comparison of single-bundle and double-bundle PCL reconstruction in the PCL-based multiple-ligament-injured knee revealed the following [2, 3, 5, 25]. Ninety consecutive arthroscopic transtibial PCL reconstructions were performed by a single surgeon (GCF). Forty-five single-bundle and 45 double-bundle reconstructions were performed using fresh-frozen Achilles tendon allograft for the anterolateral bundle, and tibialis anterior allograft for the posteromedial bundle. Postoperative comparative results were assessed using Telos stress radiography, KT 1000, Lysholm, Tegner, and HSS knee ligament rating scales. Postoperative period ranged from 15 to 72 months.

Three groups of data were analyzed: single and double bundle all; single-bundle PCL-collateral and PCL double-bundle-collateral; and single-bundle PCL–ACL-collateral and double-bundle PCL–ACL-collateral.

Mean postoperative side-to-side difference values for Telos, KT PCL screen, KT-corrected posterior, and KT-corrected anterior measurements for the overall single-bundle group in millimeters were 2.56, 1.91, 2.11, and 0.23, respectively. Mean postoperative side-to-side difference values for Telos, KT PCL screen, KT-corrected posterior, and KT-corrected anterior measurements for the overall double-bundle group in millimeters were 2.36, 2.46, 2.94, and 0.15, respectively. Mean postoperative values for Tegner, Lysholm, and

HSS knee ligament rating scales for the single-bundle group were 5.0, 90.3, and 86.2, respectively. Mean postoperative values for Tegner, Lysholm, and HSS knee ligament rating scales for the double-bundle group were 4.6, 87.6, and 83.3, respectively.

Mean postoperative side-to-side difference values for Telos, KT PCL screen, KT-corrected posterior, and KT-corrected anterior measurements for the PCL-collateral single-bundle group in millimeters were 2.59, 1.63, 2.03, and 0.25, respectively. Mean postoperative side-to-side difference values for Telos, KT PCL screen, KT-corrected posterior, and KT-corrected anterior measurements for the PCL-collateral double-bundle group in millimeters were 1.85, 2.03, 2.83, and −0.17, respectively. Mean postoperative values for Tegner, Lysholm, and HSS knee ligament rating scales for the single-bundle PCL-collateral group were 5.4, 90.9, and 87.7, respectively. Mean postoperative values for Tegner, Lysholm, and HSS knee ligament rating scales for the double-bundle PCL-collateral group were 4.9, 89.0, and 86.5, respectively.

Mean postoperative side-to-side difference values for Telos, KT PCL screen, KT-corrected posterior, and KT-corrected anterior measurements for the PCL–ACL-collateral single-bundle group in millimeters were 2.53, 2.19, 2.19, and 0.22, respectively. Mean postoperative side-to-side difference values for Telos, KT PCL screen, KT-corrected posterior, and KT-corrected anterior measurements for the PCL–ACL-collateral double-bundle group in millimeters were 3.16, 2.86, 3.09, and 0.41, respectively. Mean postoperative values for Tegner, Lysholm, and HSS knee ligament rating scales for the PCL–ACL-collateral single-bundle group were 4.7, 89.6, and 84.6, respectively. Mean postoperative values for Tegner, Lysholm, and HSS knee ligament rating scales for the PCL–ACL-collateral double-bundle group were 4.3, 86.0, and 79.4, respectively. There was no statistically significant difference between the single-bundle and the double-bundle PCL reconstruction in any of the groups compared ($p > 0.05$).

Return to the pre-injury level of activity was evaluated between the single- and double-bundle PCL reconstruction groups. The bicruciate single-bundle reconstruction group return to the pre-injury level of activity was 73.3 % and the bicruciate double-bundle reconstruction group return to the pre-injury level of activity was 84.0 %. There was no statistically significant difference ($p = 0.572$) between the single-bundle and double-bundle group in the PCL-based multiple-ligament-injured knee. Both single-bundle and double-bundle arthroscopic transtibial tunnel PCL reconstructions provide excellent results in these complex multiple-ligament-injured knee instability patterns. Our results did not indicate that one PCL reconstruction surgical procedure was clearly superior to the other.

Our 2–18-year postsurgical results in combined PCL, ACL, medial- and lateral-side knee injuries (global laxity) revealed the following information [26]. Forty combined PCL–ACL-lateral–medial side (global laxity) reconstructions were performed by a single surgeon (GCF). Twenty-eight of 40 were available for 2–18-year follow-up (70 % follow-up rate). The patients were evaluated postoperatively with three different knee ligament rating scales for physical examination and functional capacity (HSS, Lysholm, and Tegner). Static stability was assessed postoperatively comparing the normal to the injured knee using the KT 1000 knee ligament arthrometer (PCL screen, corrected posterior, corrected anterior, and 30° posterior-to-anterior translation), and stress radiography at 90° of flexion to assess PCL static stability using the Telos device. All measurements are reported as a side-to-side difference in millimeters comparing the normal to the injured knee. Range of motion, varus and valgus stability, and axial rotation stability of the tibia relative to the femur using the dial test are reported comparing the injured to the normal knee. Incidence of degenerative joint disease and return to pre-injury level of function is also reported.

Knee ligament rating scale mean scores were: HSS 79.3/100 (range 56–95), Lysholm 83.8/100 (range 58–100), and Tegner 4/10 (range 2–9). KT 1000 mean side-to-side difference measurements in millimeters were: PCL screen at 90° of knee flexion 2.02 mm (range 0–7 mm), corrected posterior at 70° of knee flexion 2.48 mm (range 0–9 mm), corrected anterior at 70° of knee flexion 0.28 mm (range −3 to 7 mm), and the 30° of knee flexion posterior-to-anterior translation 1.0 mm (range −6 to 6 mm). Telos stress radiography at 90° of knee flexion with a posterior displacement force applied to the area of the tibial tubercle mean side-to-side difference measurements in millimeters were 2.35 mm (range −2 to 8 mm).

Range of motion side-to-side difference mean flexion loss comparing the normal to the injured knee was 14.0° (range 0–38°). There were no flexion contractures. Varus and valgus stability was evaluated on physical examination at hyperextension, 0°, and 30° of knee flexion comparing the injured to the normal knee. Symmetrical varus stability was achieved in 93.3 % of knees and symmetrical valgus stability was achieved in 92.6 % of knees. The dial test performed at 30° of knee flexion to evaluate axial rotation posterolateral stability comparing the injured to the normal knee was symmetrical in 85.2 %, tighter than the normal knee (less external rotation) in 11.1 %, and more lax (greater external rotation) in 3.7 % of knees. Thus, posterior lateral axial rotation instability was corrected or overcorrected in 96.3 % of knees.

Radiographic post-traumatic degenerative joint disease occurred in 29.6 % of injured knees. No degenerative joint disease was found in 70.4 % of the injured knees. Postoperatively, patients were able to return to their pre-injury level of activity in 59.3 % of cases and returned to a decreased level of postoperative activity in 40.7 % of cases.

Summary

The multiple-ligament-injured knee is a severe injury that may also involve neurovascular injuries and fractures. Surgical treatment offers good functional results documented in the literature by physical examination, arthrometer testing, stress radiography, and knee ligament rating scales. Mechanical tensioning devices are helpful with cruciate ligament tensioning. Some low-grade MCL complex injuries may be amenable to brace treatment while high-grade medial-side injuries require repair and reconstruction. Lateral posterolateral injuries are most successfully treated with surgical repair and reconstruction. Surgical timing in acute multiple-ligament-injured knee cases depends upon the ligaments injured, the injured extremity vascular status, skin condition of the extremity, degree of instability, and the patient's overall health. Allograft tissue is preferred for these complex surgical procedures. Delayed reconstruction of 2–3 weeks may decrease the incidence of arthrofibrosis, and it is important to address all components of the instability. Currently, there is no conclusive evidence that double-bundle PCL reconstruction provides superior results to single-bundle PCL reconstruction in the multiple-ligament-injured knee.

References

1. Fanelli GC. Surgical treatment of combined PCL ACL medial and lateral side injuries (global laxity): acute and chronic. In: Fanelli GC, editor. The multiple ligament injured knee. A practical guide to management. 2nd ed. New York: Springer-Verlag; 2013. pp. 281–301.
2. Fanelli GC, Beck JD, Edson CJ. Double bundle posterior cruciate ligament reconstruction. Surgical technique and results. Sports Med Arthrosc. 2010;18(4):242–8.
3. Fanelli GC, Beck JD, Edson CJ. Combined PCL ACL lateral and medial side injuries: treatment and results. Sports Med Arthrosc. 2011;19(2):120–30.
4. Fanelli GC, Boyd J. How I manage PCL injuries. Oper Tech Sport Med. 2009;17(3):175–93.
5. Fanelli GC, Beck JD, Edson CJ. How I manage the multiple ligament injured (dislocated) knee. Oper Tech Sport Med. 2010;18(4):198–210.
6. Fanelli GC. Rationale and surgical technique for PCL and multiple knee ligament reconstruction. 3rd ed. Biomet Sports Medicine, Warsaw: Indiana; 2012.
7. Fanelli GC, Gianotti BF, Edson CJ. Arthroscopically assisted combined anterior and posterior cruciate ligament reconstruction. Arthroscopy. 1996;12(1):5–14.
8. Fanelli GC, Edson CJ. Arthroscopically assisted combined ACL/PCL reconstruction. 2–10 year follow-up. Arthroscopy. 2002;18(7):703–14.
9. Fanelli GC, Feldmann DD. Management of combined anterior cruciate ligament/posterior cruciate ligament/posterolateral complex injuries of the knee. Oper Tech Sport Med. 1999;7(3):143–9.
10. Fanelli GC, Orcutt DR, Edson CJ. The multiple-ligament injured knee: evaluation, treatment, and results. Arthroscopy. 2005;21(4):471–86.
11. Fanelli GC, et al. Treatment of combined anterior cruciate-posterior cruciate ligament-medial-lateral side knee injuries. J Knee Surg. 2005;18(3):240–8.
12. Fanelli GC, Harris JD. Surgical treatment of acute medial collateral ligament and posteromedial corner injuries of the knee. Sports Med Arthrosc. 2006;14(2):78–83.
13. Fanelli GC, Harris JD. Late MCL (medial collateral ligament) reconstruction. Tech knee surg. 2007;6(2):99–105.
14. Fanelli GC, Edson CJ, Reinheimer KN, Garofalo R. Posterior cruciate ligament and posterolateral corner reconstruction. Sports Med Arthrosc. 2007;15(4):168–75.
15. Fanelli GC, Feldmann DD. Arthroscopically assisted combined anterior cruciate ligament/posterior cruciate ligament reconstruction. In: Fanelli GC, editor. Posterior cruciate ligament injuries: a practical guide to management. New York: Springer-Verlag; 2001. pp. 215–36.
16. Fanelli GC. Combined ACL PCL medial lateral side injuries of the knee. In: Fanelli GC, editor. The multiple ligament injured knee. A practical guide to management. New York: Springer-Verlag; 2004. pp. 111–31.
17. Fanelli GC, Edson CJ, Reinheimer KN. Evaluation and treatment of the multiple ligament injured knee. Instr Course Lect. 2009;58:389–95.
18. Levy B, Dajani KA, Whalen DB, Stannard JP, Fanelli GC, Stuart MJ, Boyd JL, MacDonald PA, Marx RG. Decision making in the multiple ligament injured knee: an evidence based systematic review. Arthroscopy. 2009;25(4):430–8.
19. Fanelli GC, Stannard JP, Stuart MJ, MacDonald PB, Marx RG, Whelan DB, Boyd JL, Levy BA. Management of complex knee ligament injuries. J Bone Joint Surg. 2010;92-A(12):2235–46.
20. Levy B, Fanelli GC, Whalen D, Stannard J, MacDonald P, Boyd J, Marx R, Stuart M. Modern perspectives for the treatment of knee dislocations and multiligament reconstruction. J Am Acad Orthop Surg. 2009;17(4):197–206.
21. Fanelli GC. Mechanical graft tensioning in multiple ligament knee surgery. In: Fanelli GC, editor. The multiple ligament injured knee: a practical guide to management. 2nd ed. Chapter 22 (currently in production).
22. Fanelli GC. Posterior cruciate ligament rehabilitation: how slow should we go? Arthroscopy. 2008;24(2):234–5.
23. Edson CJ, Fanelli GC, Beck JD. Rehabilitation after multiple ligament reconstruction of the knee. Sports Med Arthrosc. 2011;19(2):162–6.
24. Edson CJ, Fanelli GC, Beck JD. Postoperative rehabilitation of the posterior cruciate ligament. Sports Med Arthrosc. 2010;18(4):275–9.
25. Fanelli GC, Beck JD, Edson CJ. Single compared to double bundle PCL reconstruction using allograft tissue. J Knee Surg. 2012;25(1):59–64.
26. Fanelli GC, Edson CJ. Surgical treatment of combined PCL, ACL, medial, and lateral side injuries (global laxity): surgical technique and 2 to 18 year results. J Knee Surg. 2012;25(4):307–16.
27. Fanelli GC. Rationale and surgical technique for PCL and multiple knee ligament reconstruction. 2nd ed. Biomet Sports Medicine, Warsaw, Indiana, 2008.

Further Reading

28. Fanelli GC. The multiple ligament injured knee. A practical guide to management. 2nd ed. New York: Springer-Verlag; 2013.

Surgical Treatment of Combined PCL/Lateral-Sided Injuries

16

Christopher J. Wahl and Paul C. Chin

Introduction

In the first edition of this book, Roger Larson and Michael Metcalf discussed surgical treatment of posterolateral instability of the knee. In the ensuing 13 years, there have been multiple advances in our appreciation of the knee with combined posterior cruciate ligament (PCL) and lateral-sided injuries, and we now have enhanced awareness of their interdependence [1, 2]. Injuries to the PCL and lateral side of the knee can be devastating injuries that can often miss detection during the acute setting. In one study, trauma patients with hemarthroses and PCL tears were more likely to have associated posterolateral corner (PLC) injuries than medial-sided injuries or isolated PCL tears by factors of four and ten, respectively [3, 4]. The natural history of chronic PCL injuries demonstrates a high percentage of medial-sided chondral injuries, medial meniscus tears, and eventual degenerative radiographic change [5, 6]. Moreover, combined PCL- and PLC-deficient knees demonstrate a significantly increased rate of medial femoral condyle degenerative changes [7]. It is generally accepted that injuries to the PCL and PLC complex should be treated concomitantly; however, there is disagreement regarding multiple factors associated with repair of these structures. Ultimately, the surgeon must weigh dogmatism versus pragmatism with respect to the principles surrounding the treatment of PCL/lateral-sided injuries. There is still much controversy with respect to the optimal timing of surgery, staged versus single-stage treatment, repair versus augmented repair versus delayed reconstruction, graft choice, postoperative rehabilitation, and, of course, the ideal surgical technique. Each injury has a unique "personality," and the nature of the injury must be factored into the age, activity, and expectations of the individual patient to assure an optimal outcome.

Anatomy and Biomechanics

Posterior Cruciate Ligament

The PCL anatomy has been extensively investigated. The lateral aspect of the medial femoral condyle serves as the broad origin of the PCL, and the central posterior tibia, distal to the medial and lateral plateau articular surfaces, serves as the insertion of PCL. The length of the PCL is roughly 32–38 mm while the cross-sectional area is 11 mm [8]. The PCL has broad origin and insertion that are three times wider than its midsubstance. Because the synovium from the posterior capsule lines its surfaces, the PCL is considered to be extrasynovial. Although the PCL is typically described as having anterolateral and posteromedial bundles [9], in reality the anatomy of the PCL is complex with fibers forming a continuous confluence with different lengths and attachments that control the microkinematics of the knee.

Biomechanically, the PCL is the primary restraint to posterior translation while serving as a secondary restraint to external tibial rotation [10]. While investigations sought to define definitive roles for the anterolateral and posteromedial bundles, recent studies have supported a codominant rather than reciprocal relationship throughout knee range of motion (ROM) [8, 11–13].

Lateral Structures

Some authors have described the lateral ligamentous complex as the "dark side of the knee" because of its inconsistent nomenclature throughout the literature, anatomic variation, and frequent finding that elegant pictorial descriptions seldom

C. J. Wahl (✉)
Orthopaedic Physician Associates 3216 Northeast 45th Place #304
Seattle, Washington USA 98105
e-mail: wahlmd@gmail.com

P. C. Chin
San Diego Arthroscopy and Sports Medicine Fellowship, San Diego, CA, USA

G. C. Fanelli (ed.), *Posterior Cruciate Ligament Injuries*,
DOI 10.1007/978-3-319-12072-0_16, © Springer International Publishing Switzerland 2015

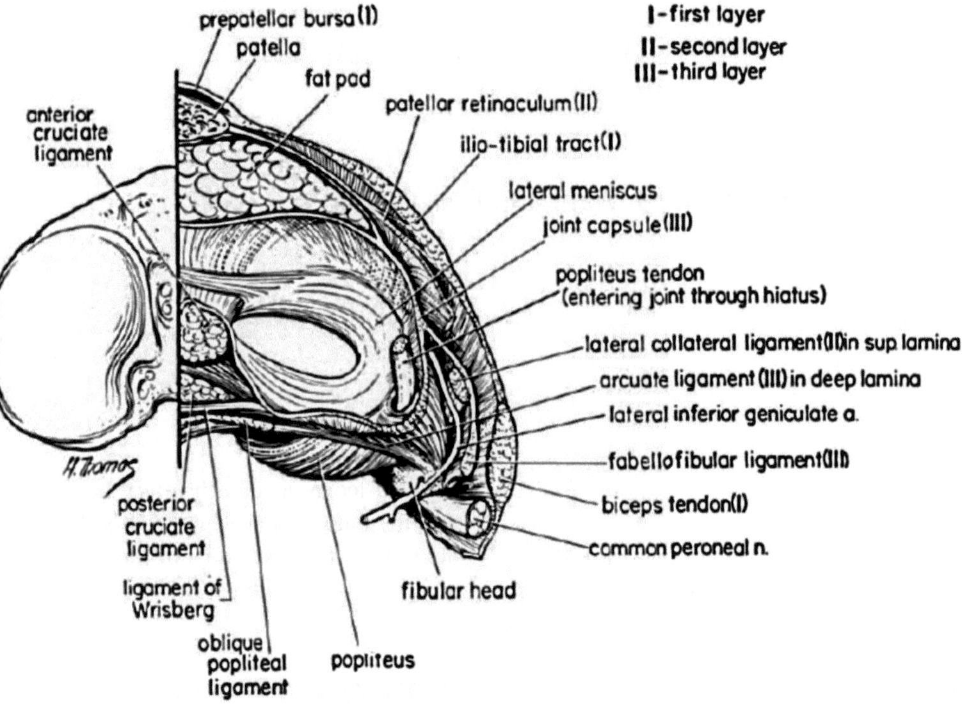

Fig. 16.1 A view of the right knee joint from above after removal of the right femur. Note the three layers of the lateral side and the division of the posterior part of the capsule (*layer III*) into deep and superficial laminae which are separated by the lateral inferior genicular vessels. (From [16]. Reprinted with permission from JBJS/Rockwater Inc.)

resemble actual surgical dissection [14, 15]. Contributing to these enigmatic structures is the fact that a key contributor to lateral-sided stability, the popliteofibular ligament (PFL), was mistakenly omitted from anatomic and orthopedic descriptions for nearly half a century. For descriptive purposes, the lateral side of the knee can be envisioned in three layers, according to Seebacher [16] (Fig. 16.1). The superficial layer is composed of the iliotibial band inserting on Gerdy's tubercle and the biceps femoris inserting on the fibular head. In the middle layer, the quadriceps retinaculum is anterior and the patellofemoral ligaments are posterior. The deep layer consists of the lateral joint capsule and coronary ligaments, the popliteus (and PFL), the lateral collateral ligament (LCL), and the fabellofibular (when present) and arcuate ligaments. The LCL originates slightly posterior and proximal to the lateral epicondyle of the femur and inserts on the lateral aspect of the fibular head [17]. The popliteus musculotendinous complex originates on the proximal posterior tibia, courses superolaterally, and enters the joint as it courses through the popliteus hiatus of the lateral meniscus. The location is consistently distal and anterior to the LCL origin (by 18.5 mm) [17]. The PFL was rediscovered in the orthopedic literature by Staubli and Birrer in 1990 [18]. The PFL courses from the musculotendinous junction of the popliteus with anterior and posterior divisions to a prominence on the posterosuperior fibular head.

Biomechanically, the LCL is the primary static stabilizer to varus opening from 0° to 30° of knee flexion [19]. The perplexing history of the PFL and contributions to posterolateral stability were detailed by Maynard in 1996 revealing it as a static stabilizer of the posterolateral aspect of the knee that resists varus, external tibial rotation, and posterior translation [20]. Finally, the popliteus tendon is assumed to be a dynamic stabilizer of posterolateral knee with variable muscle activation characteristics [21].

Combined injuries to the PCL and PLC lead to altered stability of the knee in posterior translation and rotation. Cadaver investigations that sequentially sectioned components of the PCL and PLC have demonstrated that the PCL is the principal restraint to posterior translation, but restricts, in combination with the PLC, varus rotation and external tibial rotation [10, 22]. These experiments led the way for biomechanical studies that questioned the influence of PLC deficiency on a PCL graft. LaPrade et al. demonstrated that significant force increases occurred in a PCL graft after sectioning of posterolateral structures and recommended concurrent reconstruction to decrease risk of graft failure [23]. Furthermore, Sekiya et al. demonstrated that combined reconstruction of a double-bundle PCL and PLC can restore knee kinematics to a state near intact ligaments [24]. Subsequent experiments by Apsingi et al. demonstrated that a double-bundle PCL graft along with a PLC reconstruction was unnecessary to restore posterior drawer, external rotation, and varus laxity to normal [25]. Unfortunately, agreement is lacking on graft type or technique with either PCL or PLC to recommend one reconstruction over another.

Initial Evaluation and Management

Although knee dislocations are uncommon injuries with a reported incidence of 0.2–2% of all orthopedic injuries, the severity of injury presents multiple challenges to treatment [26]. A systematic approach to management of knee dislocations and their sequelae may avoid missed injuries and devastating complications [27]. The initial encounter with a patient with a PCL and lateral-sided injury may occur after a high-impact injury such as motor-vehicle collision, motorcycle collision, motor–pedestrian collision, fall from height or sporting injury, but it may also occur after a low-impact ground level fall, especially in obese patients. By definition, multiligament knee injuries are high-energy injuries, but may occur via high, low, or ultralow velocity mechanisms. If the encounter occurs in the trauma bay or on the playing field, Advanced Trauma Life Support (ATLS) protocol should be followed. As with any initial patient encounter, a thorough history of the accident will yield information as to the mechanism of injury and the velocity of the injury. A large majority of multiple ligament knee injuries stem from knee dislocations that often spontaneously reduce. Because concomitant and potentially devastating neurovascular injuries are common, a high suspicion for a multiple ligament knee injury must always be maintained. It will be important to obtain information from emergency responders, family, and perhaps on-field physicians who may have witnessed the injury and an observation that "the leg was bent the wrong way" [27]. Obvious physical findings of combined sagittal and coronal plane instabilities are diagnostic of polyligamentous injuries.

If a knee dislocation presents unreduced, the first step should be prompt assessment of neurovascular status and immediate reduction, repeat assessment of neurovascular status, and splinting. The common peroneal nerve may be injured in up to 40% of all knee dislocations; therefore, the neurologic status is a key step in evaluation [28]. Furthermore, the association of arterial injury after knee dislocation with peroneal neuropraxia or permanent peroneal injury can be as high as 62% [27]. Thus, any nerve palsy warrants a high index of suspicion for vascular injury.

A thorough assessment of vascular status is a vital step in the evaluation of a known knee dislocation or multiple-ligament-injured knee as up to 64% of patients may have a vascular injury involving either the artery, vein, or both [26]. Although published reports note that serial physical exams (over a 24-h period) and selective arteriography are a safe practice after knee dislocations [29], most authors recommend assessment of ankle–brachial index (ABI) as a diagnostic predictor of vascular injury after knee dislocation [30–32]. Published reports note 95–100% sensitivity and 97–100% specificity of ABI in detecting arterial damage in the absence of hard signs (active hemorrhage, expanding hematoma, absent pulse, distal ischemia, or bruit) [30–32]. The senior author (C.J.W.) has previously published an algorithm for diagnosis of vascular injuries in knee dislocations or multiple-ligament-injured knees (Fig. 16.2) [33]. Even after normal ABIs, suspected knee dislocations should be admitted for serial ABIs (every 4–6 h) for 24 h to detect the formation of thrombus resulting from intimal injury or pseudoaneurysm. If the ABI is <0.9, then either the "gold standard" arteriogram or a computed tomography (CT) angiogram should be obtained to discover the location and extent of vascular injury. Recent evidence demonstrates that CT angiogram may replace arteriogram as the "gold standard" due to availability and lower cost profile [34].

A detailed physical exam will reveal additional objective characteristics of the knee injury. This begins with inspection for effusions, abrasions, ecchymosis, skin dimples, or lacerations. Multiple studies have documented that an acute traumatic knee hemarthrosis often indicates severe structural damage [3, 4, 35–37]. Fanelli found at arthroscopy that PCL injuries occurred in 38–44% of knees with traumatic hemarthrosis, and of those injuries more than 90% occurred in the presence of other knee ligament injuries [3, 4]. Following inspection, ROM and ligament stability testing will reveal any limitation to normal motion and uncover suspicions of ligament injury. Ligament stability tests include posterior sag sign, Lachman's test, posterior drawer test, pivot shift test, reverse pivot shift test, varus recurvatum test, and the dial test [38]. Combined injuries to the PCL and PLC are suggested by a grade III posterior drawer test, increased rotational laxity of the dial test at both 30° and 90° of flexion, positive varus recurvatum test, and a large reverse pivot shift test [8, 38–40].

Radiographs can be very important in the documentation of knee injuries when abnormalities are present, but normal radiographs do not preclude the presence of a severe injury. Findings of capsular avulsions, marginal tibial plateau fractures, large Segond fractures, or proximal fibula fractures may be harbingers of ligamentous injuries [27]. These findings are distinct from typical tibial plateau fractures (which are less commonly associated with neurovascular injuries). Stress radiographs can be useful to further characterize injuries to the PCL and PLC [40–42]. For chronic injuries, full-length films may uncover limb alignment abnormalities that when corrected may improve sagittal stability [43, 44]. Multiple authors have highlighted the importance of assessing the posterior tibial slope in treating chronic PCL and PLC injuries. Finally, MRI of the injured extremity will confirm suspected ligament damage and provide information regarding additional intraarticular pathology. In addition, MRI can help to indicate the "personality" and energy of the injury,

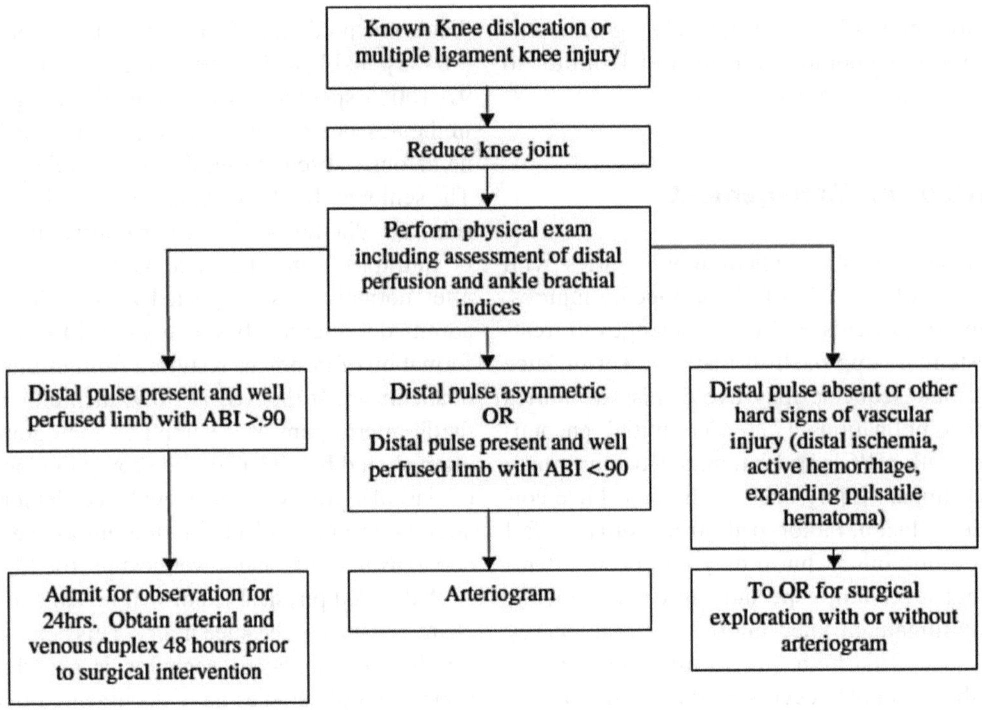

Fig. 16.2 Algorithm for diagnosis of vascular injuries after multiple-liga-ment-injured knees. (From [68]. Reprinted with permission from Springer)

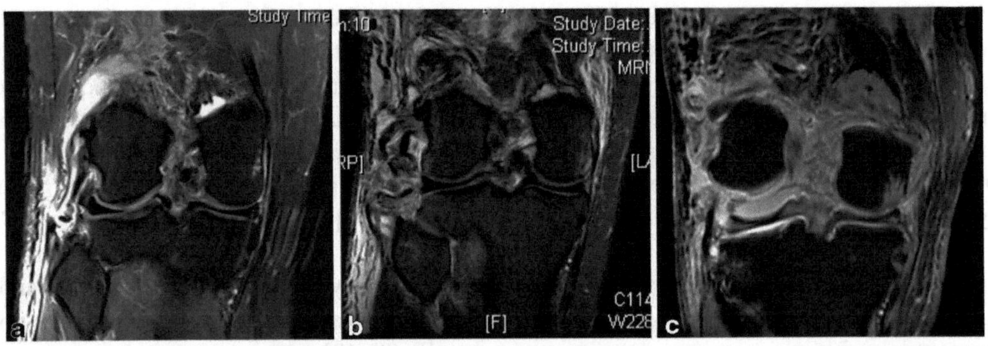

Fig. 16.3 Magnetic resonance images of three injuries that would be classified as KD-3L by the Schenk and Wascher classification system (ACL, PCL, and PLC disruption). **a** A low-velocity injury. Note the small bony avulsion of the distal fibular collateral ligament from the fibula. There is relatively little surrounding soft tissue edema. **b** An intermediate-velocity/high-energy injury. There has been significant disruption with bony avulsions of the lateral capsule and fibular collateral ligament, and avulsion of the popliteus tendon. Substantial surrounding soft tissue injury is present. **c** A high-velocity, extreme-energy injury. Note that lateral anatomic structures are nearly unidentifiable, severe soft tissue edema is present, and gross instability is exemplified by persistent deformity

give the surgeon an indication of the location and extent of injured structures (Fig. 16.3).

Postreduction radiographs should demonstrate a concentric reduction. Hinged knee braces locked in extension stabilize the knee with padding placed in the brace to assist with reduction as necessary. After approximately 1 week of immobilization to permit tissues to stabilize, patients begin gentle ROM. Unstable fractures or vascular injuries may warrant external fixation, but otherwise reestablishing ROM of the injured knee should be the goal. In the senior author's experience, multiligament knee injuries that have undergone extensive immobilization or external fixation not infrequently develop what we term the "FLASCID" knee syndrome (flexion loss with axial, sagittal, and coronal instability after dislocation). This syndrome is characterized by a woody, stiff knee with highly abnormal translation/rotation kinematics at the tibiofemoral articulation. The FLASCID knee is extremely difficult to treat.

There is much debate regarding management of multiple-ligament-injured knees. The Knee Dislocation Study Group reported on many controversies, including nonoperative versus operative treatment, repair versus reconstruction, open versus arthroscopic, early versus late repair, autograft versus allograft, external fixation versus hinged knee bracing, graft fixation, and rehabilitation [45]. Unfortunately, most treatment decisions are based on lower-quality evidence because published high-quality evidence (levels 1 and 2 randomized controlled trials) is scarce. In general, operative treatment is preferred over nonoperative treatment because of improvements in postoperative outcome scores, and reconstruction is preferred over repair [45–48]. Recently, Stannard et al. published a level I randomized controlled trial comparing postoperative treatment of multiple-ligament-injured knees with hinged external fixator versus hinged knee brace [49]. This report noted that reconstructions that were supplemented with a hinged external fixator had fewer ligament reconstruction failures than those supplemented with a hinged knee brace. However, hinged external fixators can be technically demanding to apply and maintain in the hands of surgeons who are unfamiliar with the device. Furthermore, there are often confounding management issues, including medical condition, obesity, concomitant fractures, extensor mechanism disruption, alignment, and social factors that further complicate treatment decisions [50]. Another factor to consider for PCL injuries is its notable healing capacity. In one study, the authors found that more than one third of MRI grade III PCL injuries (complete discontinuity) are clinically stable at the time of repair, and thus the clinical exam of the PCL at the time of surgery should dictate treatment [51].

In general, we advocate an "all-or-none" approach to surgical management of PCL and lateral-sided structures. This recommendation is based on evidence that the PCL and PLC are codominant in controlling posterior translation, external rotation, and varus, so it is ideal to perform concomitant repairs/augmentations/reconstructions so that all repairs are healing in a kinematic environment that is as close to normal as possible. After an acute presentation, the goal is to address injuries in a window from 14 to 21 days after injury. The scheduled delay provides time for an injured capsule to heal, allows the patient to regain knee ROM, and allows for the repair of torn structures before extensive scarring, shortening, and distortion of normal anatomy has taken place. If surgery is not possible within 3 weeks after injury or the patient presents after 3 weeks, it is typical to delay surgery until at least 6 weeks after injury, when the acute inflammatory response has settled, the knee has quieted, and improved ROM has been restored. Prior to delayed reconstruction, a supervised protocol of motion, ice, and compression will help decrease inflammation and "woodiness" of the injured limb. Attempted reconstruction in the maximally inflamed 3–6-week interval after a high-energy injury is often hampered by difficult anatomic dissection secondary to dense fibrotic tissue, protracted ROM recovery, and arthrofibrosis.

Chronic presentation of PCL and PLC injuries can be mired by loss of ROM as a result of extended periods of immobilization. It is crucial to eliminate a bucket-handle meniscus tear, incarcerated cruciate stump, or unreduced tibial eminence fracture as a cause of loss of ROM before instituting a physical therapy program. If a formal course of therapy fails to improve ROM, arthroscopic lysis of adhesions in the suprapatellar pouch, gutters, and the anterior and posterior compartments of the knee as well as manipulation may be required. Delayed reconstructions can be performed to address residual instabilities once the patient has reestablished a more normal knee ROM.

Instruments and Implants

The following instruments/implants can be helpful and should be available:

- 5-lb bean bag or knee flexion/extension limb positioner (preferred)
- Vessel loops (to identify/protect the peroneal nerve)
- Retractors (Weitlaner, Gelpi, Army–Navy, Richardson)
- Hewson suture retriever or arthroscopic suture manipulator
- Long slotted Beath reamer guide pins
- Straight cannulated reamers (6–9 mm)
- ENDOBUTTON™ (Smith & Nephew, Andover, MA) or similar depth gauge
- Flexible guide pin and reamer system: flexible slotted guide pins, curved guide, flexible reamers (for modified LaPrade). (e.g., CLANCY™, Smith & Nephew, Andover, MA)
- Braided nonabsorable, high-tensile strength suture material (suture passage and graft end preparation)
- Small fragment fracture reduction instruments and implants (for fibular fractures or significant
- Double-loaded, self-tapping metal rotator cuff suture anchors (repair of FCL or popliteus avulsions)
- Smith & Nephew ENDOBUTTON CL™ Suspensory fixation soft tissue device in various loop sizes (usually 25–30 mm for modified LaPrade) (e.g., ENDOBUTTON CL™, Smith & Nephew, Andover, MA)
- Cannulated interference screws (various diameter and length)

Surgical Technique

Of primary importance to the success of any operation is a knowledgeable operating room team that has experience with the planned procedures. The surgeon, of course, should be prepared for the intended surgery but also unexpected complications that may occur. Patients are positioned supine with the popliteal fossa at the flexion break. The bed should be equipped with a lateral leg post and variable-flexion positioner to support the leg at various flexion angles. Fluoroscopy should be positioned on the opposite side of the bed to confirm radiographic landmarks during reconstruction.

Generally, the sterile C-arm is placed in a "rainbow" configuration, so it can be slid into or out of the operative field for fluoroscopic viewing during PCL elevation and PCL/PLC tunnel drilling. The proximal thigh should have a tourniquet for safety but should only be inflated in the absence of arterial injury, and then, only for short periods as necessary. The contralateral limb is often prepped to allow comparative exam as well as a source of potential autografts.

The following steps are generally adhered to for PCL and lateral-sided injuries:

1. Bilateral knee exam under anesthesia (EUA)
2. Dissection of the lateral side and identification of posterolateral structures to be repaired and augmented
3. Diagnostic arthroscopy
4. Address meniscal and cartilage pathology
5. PCL/central pivot reconstruction—restores the central pivot of sagittal and coronal stability
6. Primary repair of injured posterolateral structures
7. Graft augmentation of LCL and PLC structures

Exam Under Anesthesia

The EUA is an integral part in creation of the surgical planning. As discussed above, the PCL has a remarkable healing capacity, thus a PCL and PLC reconstruction should only be undertaken with clear examination evidence of incompetence. PCL and PLC injury is apparent with a positive varus recurvatum test, unstable posterolateral drawer test, positive dial test, and reverse pivot test. The intraoperative exam can assist the surgeon in selecting the most appropriate reconstruction option (Fig. 16.4). In the absence of recurvatum or excessive external rotatory deformity, it is possible to obtain successful results using a modification of Larson's technique as described by Arciero [52]. However, when gross disruption of the posterolateral capsule and supporting ligamentous structures is present (evidenced by a positive recurvatum-varus test), it is the author's preference to utilize a modification of the reconstruction technique originally described by LaPrade [53].

Even in the absence of gross sagittal plane instability, it is the author's preference to reconstruct/augment the PCL if clinical grade II (B) or worse instability is present (when the tibial plateau lies flush with the femoral condyles on draw testing). In cases where varus/valgus instability is appreciated, a careful comparison to the other extremity is useful. In trying to distinguish between acceptable (trace) instability versus physiologically relevant varus, it is often useful to arthroscopically measure the degree to which the lateral compartment opens to varus stress. Opening of greater than 8–10 mm is likely to create undue strain on the PCL reconstruction if the PLC is not addressed. Once the decision to proceed with reconstruction is reached, the lateral side is exposed prior to arthroscopic reconstruction of the central pivot. Dissection is easier prior to imbibition of the tissues with fluid, and the dissected lateral corner allows low-pressure fluid egress, thereby decreasing the risk of compartment syndrome.

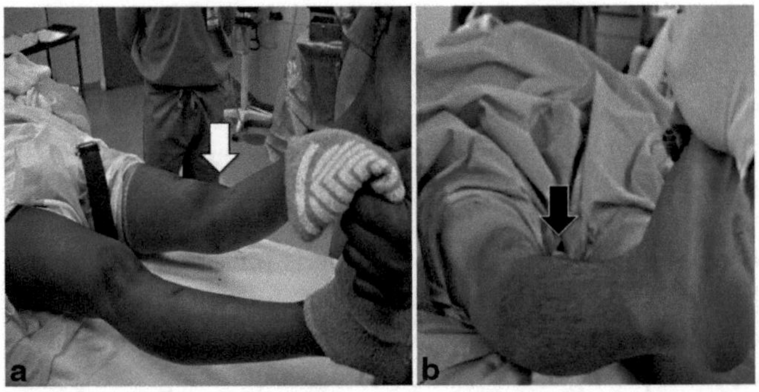

Fig. 16.4 Clinical exam findings of combined PCL and PLC injuries. **a** A markedly positive recurvatum-varus test (*white arrow*) indicates high-grade injury to the PLC, posterolateral ligaments, and posterolateral capsular supporting structures—an ideal indication for repair with a modified LaPrade reconstruction as described in the text. **b** Negative recurvatum-varus test in a patient whose MRI demonstrated injuries to the cruciates and lateral collateral ligament. The relative stability of the knee to rotation and varus makes this knee a potential candidate for a modified Larson sling procedure as described by Rios et al. [67]

Lateral Dissection and Lateral Reconstruction Preparation

The authors advocate augmentation of the PLC even when primary repair is possible, as outcome studies have shown repair with augmentation to be superior to repair alone [48]. In the literature, there are multiple methods of reconstructing the posterolateral corner. Scientific studies have yet to agree on a method of repair that most accurately reconstructs the native ligaments to a state that leads to an optimal clinical result. Good clinical results have been documented with multiple techniques including the Larson technique, anatomic reconstruction described by Arciero, and by anatomic reconstruction described by LaPrade and colleagues [52–54]. Although the merits of each technique can certainly be debated, significant importance should be directed at the effective implementation of a single technique rather than ineffective implementation of multiple techniques.

The severity of injury to the PLC may dictate the best technique for repair (Figs. 16.3 and 16.4). In cases where mild varus and external rotation instability is present in the absence of recurvatum, the authors utilize the Arciero modification of the Larson technique (Fig. 16.5). However, in cases of moderate-to-severe varus and/or external rotation instability, and any time recurvatum is increased, it is preferable to reconstruct the PLC using the technique described by LaPrade [53]. The senior author has modified LaPrade's technique to employ suspensory fixation in the tibia, and

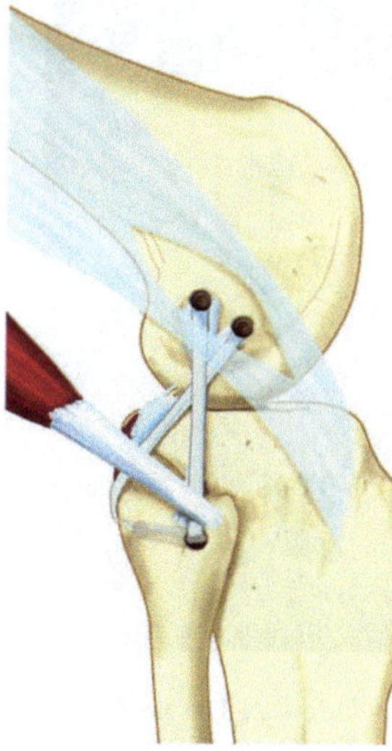

Fig. 16.5 Modified Larson sling PLC reconstruction technique as modified by Arciero (no tibial tunnel). (From [67]. Reprinted with permission from SAGE Publications)

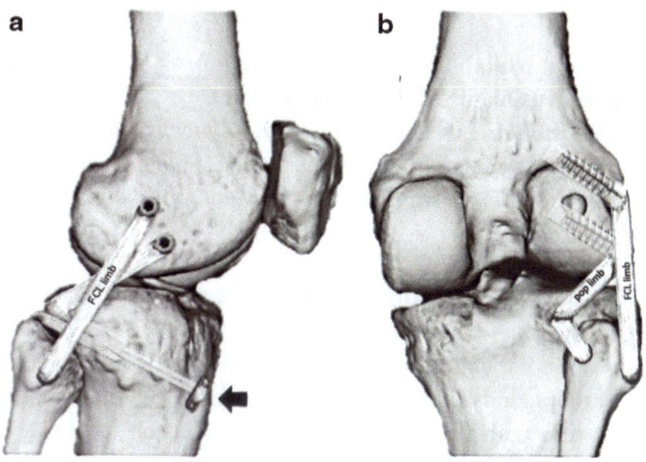

Fig. 16.6 Lateral (**a**) and posterior (**b**) views of the modified LaPrade PLC reconstruction technique using suspensory fixation used by the author. A loop of the soft tissue reconstruction graft is pulled into a posterior tibial tunnel and fixed using suspensory fixation (*black arrow*). One graft limb (pop limb) follows the native popliteus tendon through the popliteal hiatus and is fixed using interference screw fixation at the anatomic insertion of the popliteus on the femur. The second limb (FCL limb) courses from the tibial tunnel into the posteromedial aperture of the fibular tunnel (stabilizing the tibiofibular articulation) and then courses along the path of the native FCL to the lateral epicondyle. Once the ideal (isometric) position of this tunnel is identified, it is tensioned and docked into the tunnel using interference screw fixation

base the FCL femoral tunnel on both isometric and anatomic landmarks (Fig. 16.6). This reconstruction technique theoretically reconstructs key determinants of lateral-sided stability by reconstructing/augmenting the lateral collateral ligament, creates a "static" popliteus limb that also buttresses the posterolateral capsule, and stabilizes the proximal tibiofibular articulation. The use of suspensory fixation allows for a reconstruction using a shorter graft length.

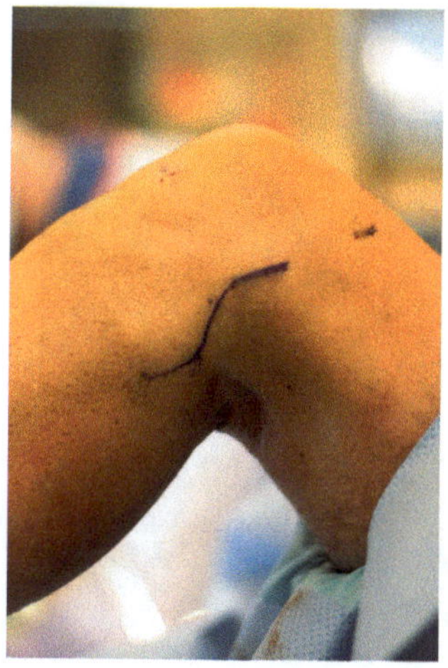

Fig. 16.7 Incision for PLC reconstruction (left knee). A *"lazy-S" incision* starts proximally over the lateral epicondyle and curves gently toward the posterior fibular head, curving along a radius approximately 4.5–5 cm from Gerdy's tubercle

Preferred Surgical Technique

Part 1: Incision, Identification of Anatomic Structures of the PLC, Review of Surgical Windows Incision and Peroneal Nerve

- A "lazy-S" curved incision is made on the lateral side of the knee. The incision starts directly over the lateral epicondyle, and traverses distally toward the posterior aspect of the fibular head, curving gradually anteriorly along a 4.5- to 5-cm radius from Gerdy's tubercle (Fig. 16.7). This incision will allow easy exposure of the peroneal nerve, posterior aspect of the fibula, and a limited exposure of the posteromedial tibiofibular joint.
- The peroneal nerve is typically found deep to a thin fascial layer at the posterior tendinous edge of the biceps femoris, approximately 4–6 cm proximal to the fibular head. *The anatomy may be distorted by scarring or hematoma if injury to the biceps insertion, proximal fibula, or peroneal nerve has occurred.*
- The peroneal nerve is tagged with a short vessel loop and carefully dissected distally to the peroneal fascia (Fig. 16.8).
- In cases of peroneal nerve neurapraxia, a peroneal nerve exploration and neurolysis is performed from proximal to the biceps distally around the fibular neck and into the anterior compartment of the leg.

Window 1: The Proximal Fibula and Posteromedial Tibiofibular Joint

- The fibular collateral ligament normally inserts at the anterolateral aspect of the fibular head. A fibular reconstruction tunnel will be created just distal to this insertion at the widest point of the flare of fibular head. A minimal

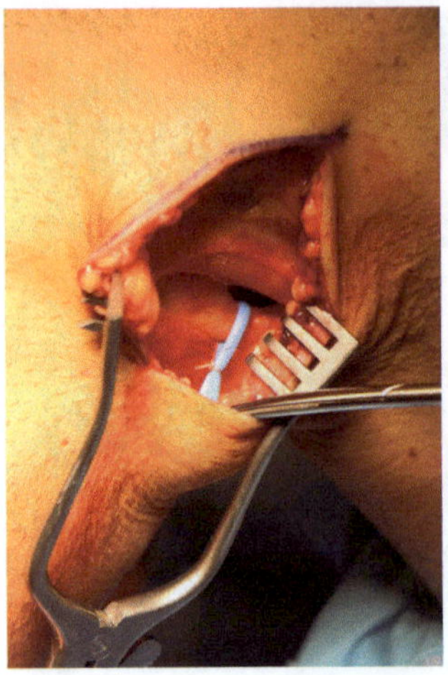

Fig. 16.8 The peroneal nerve is identified subfascially immediately posterior to the posterior border of the biceps femoris tendon. It is tagged with a vessel loop and followed distally toward the fibular neck. A peroneal nerve exploration and neurolysis can be performed if indicated

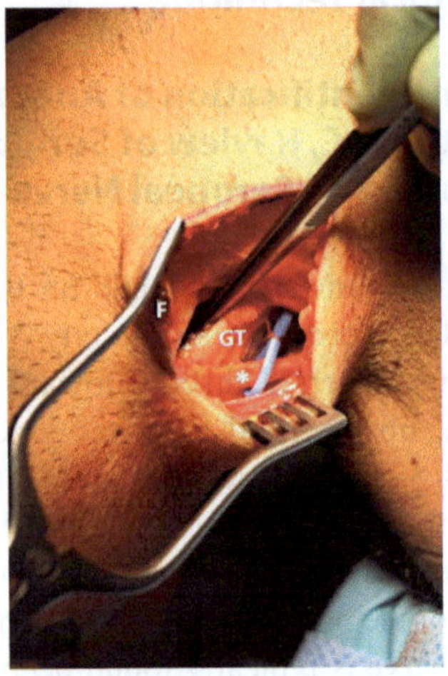

Fig. 16.9 Creation of window 1. A blunt dissection is carried out between the fibular head and proximal peroneal fascia (*F*) anteriorly and the lateral gastrocnemius tendon (*GT*) posteriorly. Care should be taken to free the peroneal nerve distally enough that with 90° knee flexion the posterior tibiofibular joint can be easily approached without undue tension on the nerve

elevation of the periosteal insertion of the biceps femoris can be performed. *Care should be taken not to stray distal to the widest portion of the fibular head, or injury to the peroneal nerve is possible where it courses around the fibular neck.*

- With the common peroneal nerve gently retracted posteriorly, the dissection is carried bluntly posterior to the peroneal muscle origins on the proximal fibula, leaving the soleus and gastrocnemius muscles posterior (window 1, Fig. 16.9). This plane is easily identified with blunt finger dissection across the posterior fibula to the posteromedial tibiofibular joint which is easily palpated. The tendon of the popliteus tendon can be palpated just medial to the

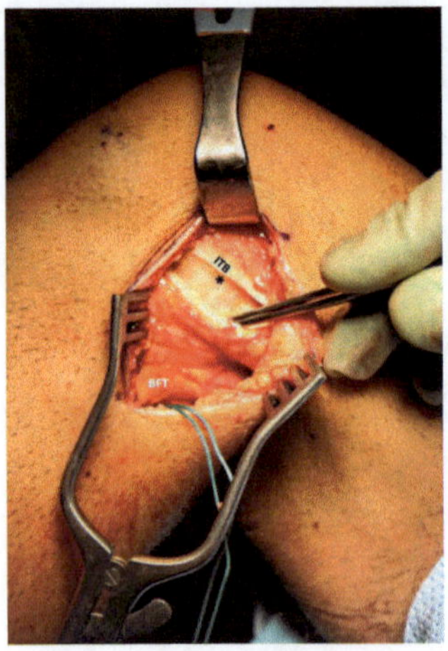

Fig. 16.10 Creation of window 2. The iliotibial band (*ITB*) is incised along its fibers at a point directly overlying the lateral epicondyle (*asterisk*). This fascial incision can be carried distally to the ITB insertion at Gerdy's tubercle, and proximally as far as necessary to allow adequate retraction and visualization of the underlying lateral structures. The surgeon will work intermittently through window 2 and window 1, inferior to the biceps femoris tendon (*BFT*)

posteromedial tibiofibular articulation as it enters the popliteus hiatus from outside the joint.

- *Occasionally, the capsular insertion, biceps femoris, and FCL insertion will avulse en masse from the proximal fibula, with or without a bony avulsion or fracture of the fibula present.*

Window 2: The Iliotibial Band and Lateral Epicondyle

- A split of the iliotibial band is created directly over the lateral epicondyle and carried proximally 4 cm and distally in line with the ITB fibers to the insertion at Gerdy's tubercle (Fig. 16.10). A Weitlaner retractor is placed to open the interval between the ITB and lateral capsule of the knee.
- The origin of the FCL on the lateral epicondyle is located. In cases where the disruption of the FCL is proximal, there may be a bony avulsion off the epicondyle that can be tagged for repair.
- The FCL can be palpated coursing from the lateral epicondyle toward the fibular head.

Window 3: The Lateral Capsule, Popliteus Insertion, and Hiatus

- A limited arthrotomy is carried through the capsule just anterior to the fibular collateral ligament fibers (window 3, Fig. 16.11). Care must be taken to incise only the capsule, as the popliteus tendon insertion is present just anterior and distal to the lateral epicondyle and iatrogenic injury is possible. In addition, the incision can be carried distally to the superior margin of the lateral meniscus, but care should be taken not to cause iatrogenic laceration of the peripheral lateral meniscus.

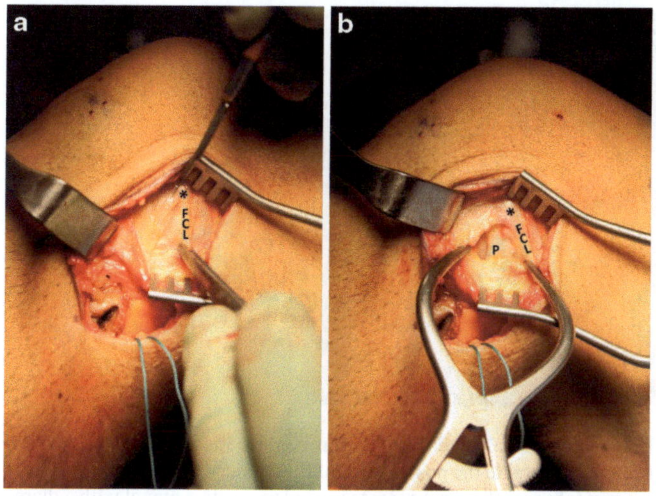

Fig. 16.11 Creation of window 3. **a** A Weitlaner retractor has been placed for retraction of the split iliotibial band. The fibular collateral ligament (*FCL*) can often be palpated if it has not been completely disrupted as it courses from the lateral epicondyle (*asterisk*) toward the proximal fibular head. The lateral capsule should be incised carefully beginning anterodistal to the lateral epicondyle and coursing longitudinally along the anterior border of the FCL. **b** Once the capsular incision has been started, a Gelpi retractor is placed. The capsular incision can be carried distally to the superior border of the meniscus. The popliteus tendon (*P*) insertion on the lateral fibula is identified, and the tendon can be visualized entering the popliteus hiatus of the lateral meniscus

- If the popliteus insertion on the femur is disrupted, the popliteus tendon can usually be identified resting close to the hiatus and tagged for later repair.
- The popliteus hiatus is easily visible just deep and slightly posterior to the FCL fibers. A passing suture can easily be placed from proximal to distal along the popliteus tendon through the hiatus using a curved clamp and retrieved through window 1 at the posterior tibiofibular articulation (Fig. 16.12).

Once all anatomic structures have been identified and tagged for repair, the iliotibial band is closed temporarily to abate excessive arthroscopy fluid outflow while reconstruction of the central pivot (ACL and PCL) is completed. For pearls related to reconstruction of the PCL, please refer to Part 4.

Part 2: Repair and Reconstruction of the Posterolateral Corner (Modified LaPrade Technique)

Repairs with augmentation or reconstruction of the PLC should proceed after all central pivot structures have been stabilized (ACL and/or PCL reconstruction). This is because the author's modification of the LaPrade technique relies on the isometry of the fibular collateral insertion near or at the lateral epicondyle which may be highly abnormal when ACL and/or PCL laxity is present. Anatomic repairs of all injured structures are performed. Avulsions from bone are repaired using suture anchors. It is common with chronic

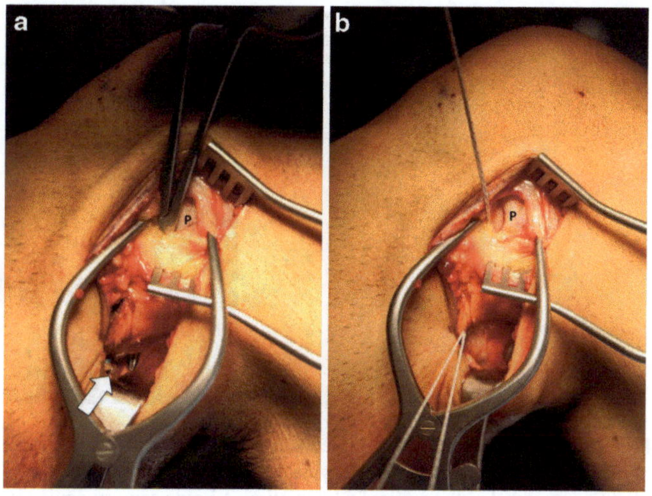

Fig. 16.12 Placing a passing suture for popliteus reconstruction limb. **a** A long Kelly clamp is placed through the popliteus hiatus visible through window 3, passing alongside the popliteus tendon (*P*) to window 1 (*white arrow*). **b** A #2 braided suture is retrieved using the clamp. This suture will be used to shuttle the popliteus reconstruction limb for either the Arciero or modified LaPrade reconstructions

FCL ruptures or midsubstance ruptures that the ligament is too short to be repaired anatomically. In such cases, the torn native remnants can be sewn to the reconstruction grafts using absorbable braided #0 or #1 suture. Also, chronic ruptures of the biceps femoris not infrequently shorten to the extent that they cannot be repaired primarily without undue tension in extension. It is the author's preference to repair the attenuated biceps femoris to a length of allograft tendon (placed through the fibular reconstruction tunnel) alongside the FCL reconstruction limb.

Fibular Tunnel

- A slotted Beath pin will be used to create a tunnel through the fibula with a diameter that matches the single-diameter of the graft (unless a second graft is required to augment an attenuated biceps femoris avulsion). In most cases when using a semitendinosus autograft or tibialis anterior allograft, a 5- to 6-mm tunnel will be sufficient.
- A starting point for a reamer guide pin through a minimal subperiosteal window is created just posterior and inferior to the native FCL insertion at the anterolateral fibula (at the widest point of the flare of the fibular head) (Fig. 16.13a). The pin is directed slightly medially and slightly inferiorly to exit the fibular head at its posteromedial edge, just lateral to the posterior tibiofibular joint. The pin exit can be carefully palpated at the posteromedial fibula prior to over-reaming (Fig. 16.13b). *Care must be taken to make the tunnel along the widest diameter of the fibular head to create an adequate tunnel and avoid iatrogenic fracture of the proximal fibula.*
- The pin is over-reamed to the diameter of the reconstruction graft (Fig. 16.13c).

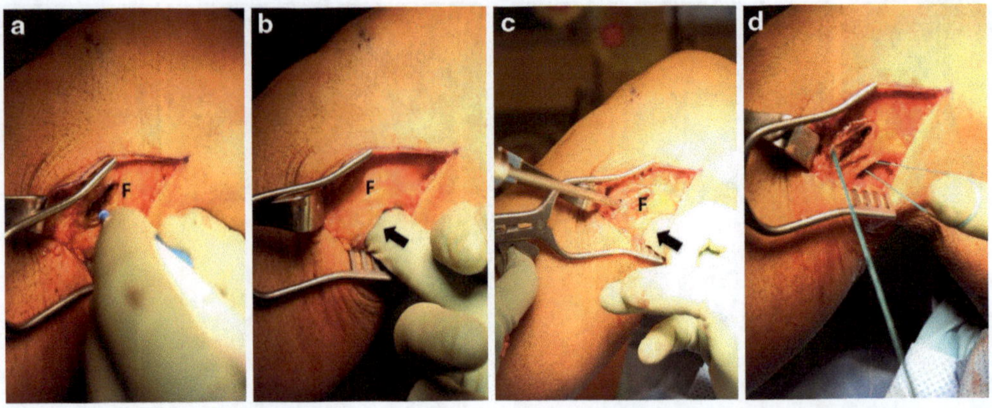

Fig. 16.13 Creation of the FCL reconstruction tunnel. **a** A small subperiosteal approach is made at the widest point of the anterolateral fibula (*F*), just distal to the native FCL insertion. A bovie cautery device is utilized and care is taken not to continue the elevation distally onto the fibular neck to avoid injury to the common peroneal nerve. **b** A finger is placed through window 1 (*black arrow*, interval between the fibula and anterior gastrocnemius/soleus fascia) and the posteromedial tibiofibular joint is palpated. A guide pin is placed along a trajectory from the anterolateral to the posteromedial fibular head, at the widest point of the metaphyseal flare. **c** A reamer is used to create a tunnel with a diameter that matches the reconstruction graft. A finger or retractor should be utilized (*black arrow*) to avoid injury to underlying neurovascular structures. **d** A loop of braided suture is placed to aid in graft passage

- A passing suture can be passed using a HEWSON™ suture passer (Smith & Nephew, Andover, MA) or by passing suture via the slotted end of the Beath pin through the tunnel and retrieving it through window 1 (Fig. 16.13d).

Tibial Tunnel (Modified LaPrade only)

- A curved guide and flexible guide/reamer system is employed (CLANCY™ ANATOMIC CRUCIATE GUIDE, Smith & Nephew Endoscopy, Andover, MA). The guide is placed approximately 1 cm distal to the posterior tibial joint line slightly medial to the proximal tibiofibular articulation, adjacent to the anatomic popliteus tendon. The curved guide should be angled distally to aim the pin/tunnel distal to the tunnels utilized for ACL and/or PCL reconstruction (Fig. 16.14a).
- Drive the flexible guide pin to exit the anterior tibia through a small incision medial to the anterior compartment musculature.
- Overream a 27- to 30-mm socket at the posterior tibia to a diameter that matches the diameter of the looped end of the graft (Fig. 16.14b).
- Ream the anterior cortex of the tibia (either antegrade or retrograde) over the guide pin to 4.5 mm diameter to admit the fixation button (ENDOBUTTON™, Smith & Nephew, Andover, MA) (Fig. 16.14c).
- Pass a passing suture from posterior to anterior through the tibial tunnel.
- Use a depth gauge to measure the total tunnel length. This is done most easily by passing the depth gauge from anterior to posterior through the tunnel and palpating the tip of the pin at the posterior aperture—measure the length at the anterior tibia.
- Select an ENDOBUTTON CL™ with loop length that such that ENDOBUTTON CL™ Length = Total Tunnel Length − 20 mm.

Graft Passage, Popliteus Limb (Modified LaPrade)

- Assemble the graft onto the ENDOBUTTON CL™ with the loop positioned at 1/3 of the total graft length. The popliteus limb with be reconstructed with the shorter (1/3) length of graft, while the FCL will be reconstructed using the longer limb (2/3).
- Pull the ENDOBUTTON CL™/graft complex into the posterior tibial tunnel and deploy the ENDOBUTTON CL™ at the anterior tibial cortex. Leave a minimum of 15–20 mm of graft secured in the tibial tunnel (Fig. 16.15a).
- Using the previously placed "hiatus" passing suture, draw the short limb of the graft from the tibial tunnel exit through the popliteus hiatus from posteroinferior to exit through window 3, at the anatomic insertion of the popliteus on the lateral femur (Fig. 16.15b, c).

Secure the Static Popliteus Limb

- A straight slotted Beath pin is placed at or very near the anatomic insertion of the popliteus tendon insertion on the lateral fibula. *The pin should be aimed proximally and anteriorly to avoid intersection with the ACL and/or PCL femoral tunnels.* Drive the pin through the medial femoral cortex (Fig. 16.16).
- A blind socket is reamed to the diameter of the popliteus limb of the graft for a length of 25 mm (Fig. 16.17a).
- The graft is pulled into the socket using the slotted reamer guide pin (Fig. 16.17b), tensioned (Fig. 16.17c), and secured with an interference screw (Fig. 16.17d).

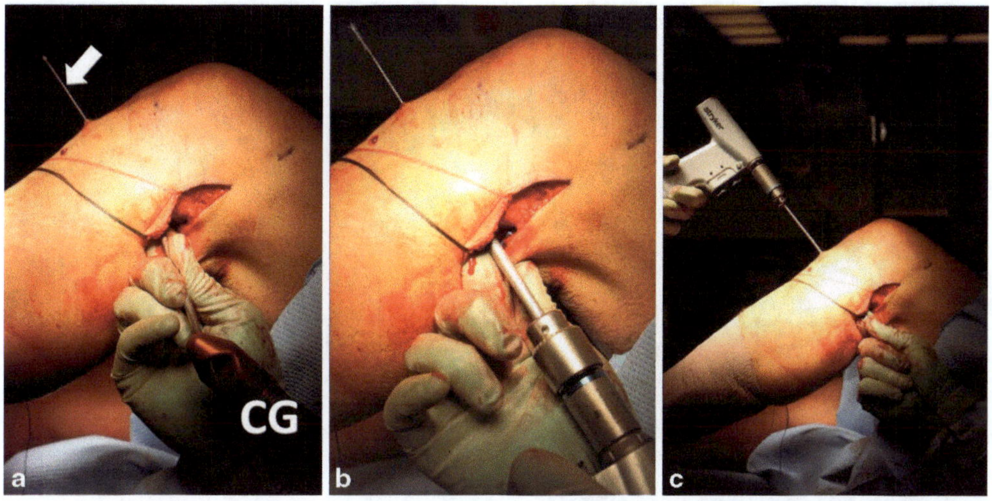

Fig. 16.14 Femoral socket drilling for modified LaPrade PLC reconstruction. **a** A curved flexible ACL guide system (*CG*) is placed on the posterior tibia just medial to the proximal tibiofibular articulation and approximately 1 cm distal to the joint line. The guide can be aimed so that the flexible slotted guide pin will course anteromedially and exit the tibia distal to the location of tibial ACL or PCL tunnels (*white arrow*). **b** A flexible reamer is placed over the pin and used to drill a 25–30-mm socket that matches the diameter of the doubled end of the reconstruction graft. A finger or blunt retractor should be used to maintain a safe distance from neurovascular structures. **c** The anterior tibial cortex is reamed over the flexible guide/passing pin to allow passage of the suspension fixation button. The total tunnel distance can now be measured (anterior tibia to posterior tibia socket aperture). An appropriate size fixation loop is selected to allow docking of at least 20 mm of the looped end of the reconstruction graft in the posterior tibial socket

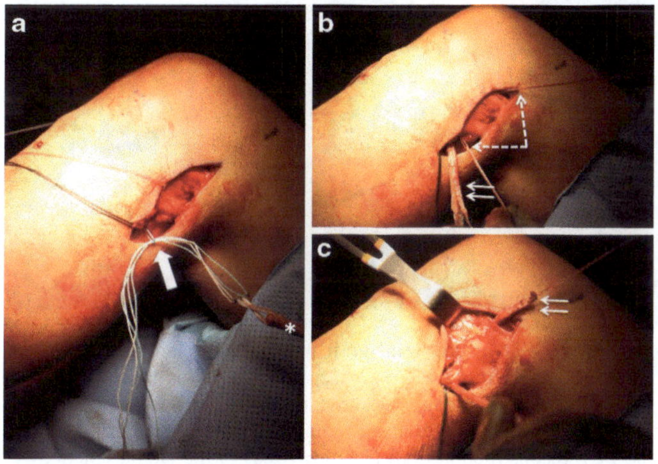

Fig. 16.15 Docking the tibial limb and passage of the static popliteus limb. **a** A passing suture loop (*large white arrow*) is used to draw the closed fixation button, closed loop and graft construct into the tibial tunnel. The fixation button is deployed on the anterior tibial cortex, leaving 20–25 mm of the looped reconstruction graft (*asterisk*) suspended in the tibial socket. **b** The previously placed suture passing loop for the popliteus limb parallels the native popliteus course through the hiatus intraarticularly to the lateral femur (*dashed angled arrow*). This suture loop is used to shuttle the popliteus limb (*double arrow*) from window 1 to window 3 adjacent to the lateral femur and native popliteus insertion. **c** The passed popliteus limb

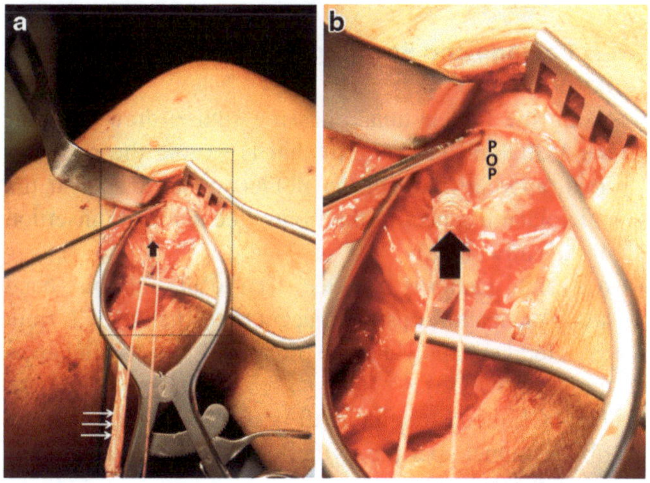

Fig. 16.16 Guide pin placement for the static popliteus femoral tunnel. **a** A Weitlaner retractor exposes window 2 (the split in the iliotibial tract) while a Gelpi retractor is placed through the vertical capsular incision anterior to the fibular collateral ligament (window 3) to expose the native popliteus insertion. A rigid slotted reamer guide pin has been placed at the anatomic insertion of the popliteus tendon on the lateral wall of the femur, drilled on a proximal trajectory to avoid intersection with ACL or PCL femoral tunnels. Note the FCL graft limb (*white arrows*) has not yet been passed, but the popliteus reconstruction limb (*black arrow*) has been passed and is adjacent to the native popliteus tendon. **b** A magnified view of dotted rectangular section of (**a**). The native popliteus limb insertion (*POP*) is visible. The anterior edge of the native FCL is visible to the right of the popliteus (under the arm of the Gelpi retractor) and the lateral edge of the femoral condyle articular surface is visible just distal and posterior to the guide pin where it enters the cortex. The reamer guide pin was placed immediately adjacent to the popliteus insertion. After reaming a socket over the pin, the popliteus reconstruction limb (*large black arrow*) will be docked and fixed

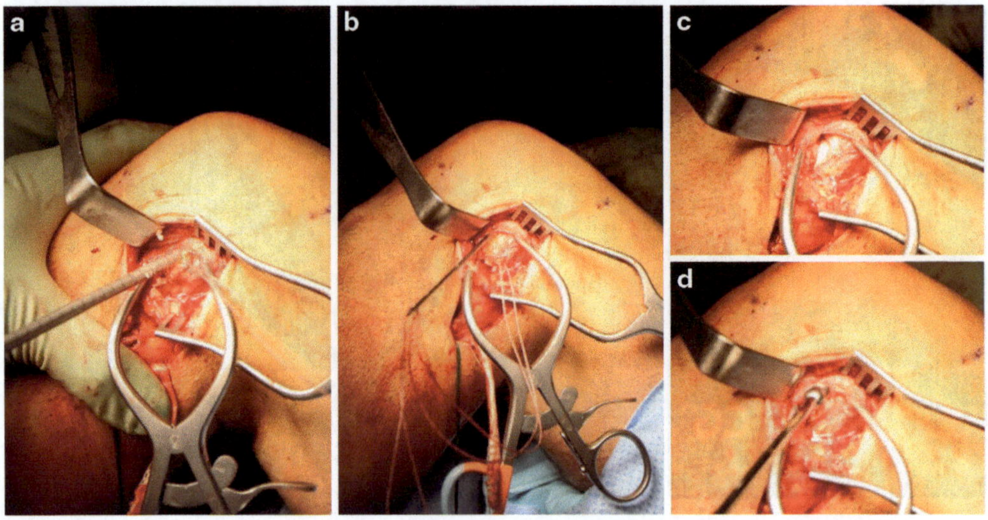

Fig. 16.17 Securing the popliteus limb. **a** A socket is reamed over the guide pin to the diameter of the popliteus reconstruction limb. **b, c** The graft is docked into the tunnel utilizing the slotted guide pin. Note the reconstruction graft immediately adjacent to the native popliteus in **c**. **d** The popliteus limb is secured using interference screw fixation. Window 3 can now be closed with absorbable braided suture, sealing the intraarticular environment

- Window 3 can now be closed using #0 braided absorbable sutures.

Graft Passage and Securing the Isometric Lateral Collateral Limb

- Using the fibular tunnel passing suture, draw the longer FCL limb of the graft that is exiting the posterior tibial aperture through the fibular tunnel to exit at the anterolateral aspect of the fibula (the anatomic insertion of the native FCL)
- A straight clamp is tunneled deep to the iliotibial band along the lateral capsule adjacent to the native FCL from the lateral epicondyle to the proximal fibular tunnel aperture (Fig. 16.18a).
- The FCL reconstruction graft is shuttled from the lateral fibular tunnel aperture to the lateral epicondyle deep to the iliotibial band.
- Using a long slotted reamer guide pin as an isometer, an isometric position is identified at or near the lateral epicondyle, where the FCL reconstruction graft will not change length through a knee ROM from full extension to full flexion. *Typically, the isometric position is very close to the center or slightly anterior on the lateral epicondyle. The pin should be aimed proximally and anteriorly (parallel to the popliteus tunnel) to avoid intersection with the popliteus tunnel and the ACL and/or PCL tunnels* (Fig. 16.18b).
- Once the isometric position for graft placement has been confirmed with the slotted reamer guide pin, the pin is advanced medially across the knee to aid in graft passage and tensioning. A blind socket is reamed to the diameter of the graft with enough length that the graft can be fully docked and tensioned into the tunnel (Fig. 16.19a).
- The graft is secured using an interference screw (Fig. 16.19b).

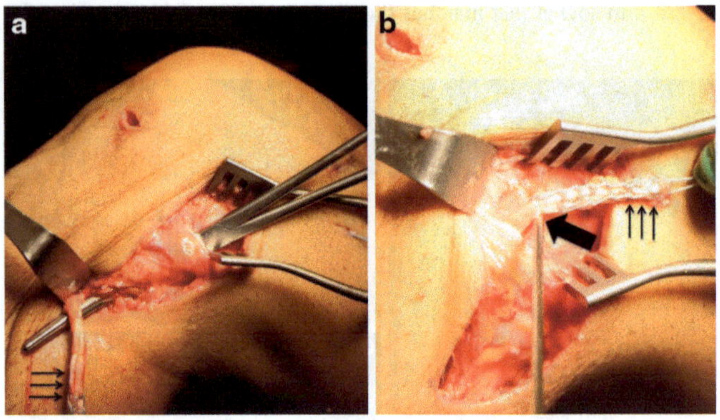

Fig. 16.18 Fibular collateral graft passage and isometry. **a** A blunt clamp is placed from window 2 deep to the iliotibial band adjacent to the lateral capsule along the course of the native FCL to exit at the proximal lateral fibula tunnel aperture. The clamp is used to shuttle the FCL reconstruction graft (*black arrows*) to the lateral epicondyle. **b** A long reamer guide pin (*thick black arrow*) is placed at the lateral epicondyle and introduced into the lateral femoral cortex. The FCL reconstruction graft (*black arrows*) is looped over the pin and the knee is cycled through flexion and extension. If there is excursion of the graft along the pin, the pin placement must be adjusted to identify the isometric position (e.g., if the graft *loosens* in flexion, the pin must be repositioned more anteriorly; if the graft tightens in flexion, the pin must be repositioned posteriorly). When an ideal position is identified, the pin is advanced along a slight proximal/anterior trajectory to exit the medial femoral cortex. Care should be taken to choose a trajectory that will avoid intersection with popliteus, PCL and/or ACL tunnels

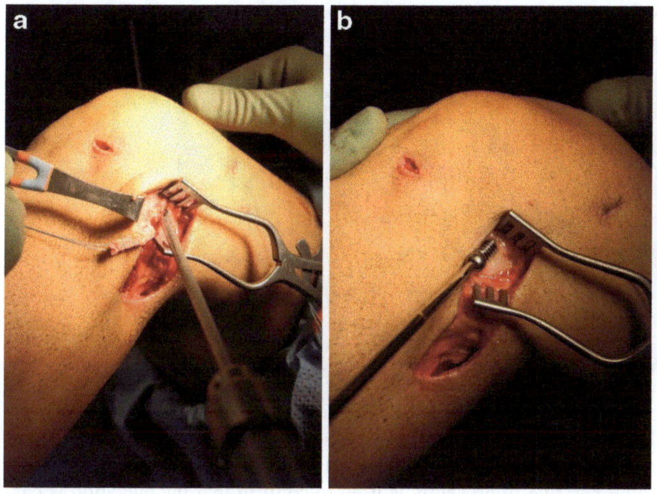

Fig. 16.19 Fibular collateral ligament graft fixation. **a** The slotted reamer guide pin is overreamed to the diameter of the FCL reconstruction graft to a depth that the graft end can be docked into the tunnel under tension. The graft is pulled firmly into the tunnel and cycled multiple times through flexion and extension. **b** The graft is secured using interference screw fixation. The remaining open windows and incisions are closed

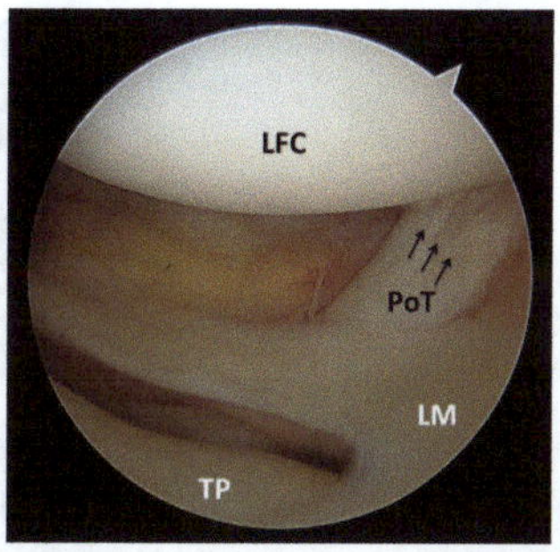

Fig. 16.20 Arthroscopic evaluation of the lateral compartment in a PCL-/PLC-injured knee (KD-2L). Varus stress during arthroscopy demonstrates >1 cm of opening between the tibial plateau (*TP*) and lateral femoral condyle (*LFC*). Note the fraying and attenuation of the popliteus tendon (*PoT*) approaching the femoral insertion (*black arrows*)

Part 3: Repair and Reconstruction of the Posterolateral Corner (Arciero Technique)

In cases of mild varus and external rotation instability and the complete absence of increased recurvatum, it is possible to obtain a satisfactory result without the need for the tibial tunnel (Fig. 16.5). The windows and technique are identical to the modified LaPrade technique except that no tibial tunnel is utilized.

- The reconstruction graft is passed from lateral to posteromedial through the fibular tunnel.
- A passing suture routed from window 3 through the popliteus hiatus to the posteromedial tibia (window 1) is used to pass the "popliteus end" of the graft from the posteromedial fibula, along the native popliteus tendon, to the anatomic insertion distal and anterior to the lateral epicondyle.
- This popliteus limb is docked and secured using an interference screw fixation in an identical fashion to that described for the modified LaPrade technique (Fig. 16.17a–c).
- The "FCL end" of the graft (exiting the lateral fibula tunnel) is tunneled along the native fibular collateral ligament to the lateral epicondyle.
- Identical to the technique described previously, the isometric insertion site is identified using a Beath pin as an isometer, and an appropriately sized tunnel is drilled to a depth to allow docking and tensioning of the graft (Fig. 16.18).
- The FCL limb is secured using interference screw fixation.

Part 4: Diagnostic Arthroscopy and Posterior Cruciate Ligament Reconstruction

Complete a diagnostic arthroscopy to identify and address concomitant intraarticular pathology (meniscal tears, chondral injuries). When repairable, meniscal tears are repaired with an all-inside or inside-out technique, and meniscal root avulsions can be repaired using a transosseous technique. Similarly, osteochondral injuries are either repaired or debrided. If a diagnostic arthroscopy is necessary prior to lateral dissection for confirmation of lateral injury, a lateral drive-through sign should be documented along with lateral joint space widening >8–10 mm with varus stress (Fig. 16.20).

As discussed previously, the PCL has a better propensity for nonsurgical healing, and isolated low-grade PCL injuries are reasonably well tolerated, even by athletes. When the PCL requires reconstruction, there are multiple techniques to accomplish this task including arthroscopic single- or double-bundle reconstruction and open versus arthroscopic tibial inlay single- or double-bundle reconstruction. Although a double-bundle reconstruction may recreate more native knee characteristics biomechanically, the failure to demonstrate significant clinical differences from single-bundle techniques, even in prospective randomized trials, permits surgeons to choose the most optimal technique for PCL reconstruction in their hands [13, 25, 55–61].

The senior author (C.J.W.) prefers a single-bundle PCL reconstruction technique that primarily recreates the anterolateral bundle of the PCL. Any intact remnants of the

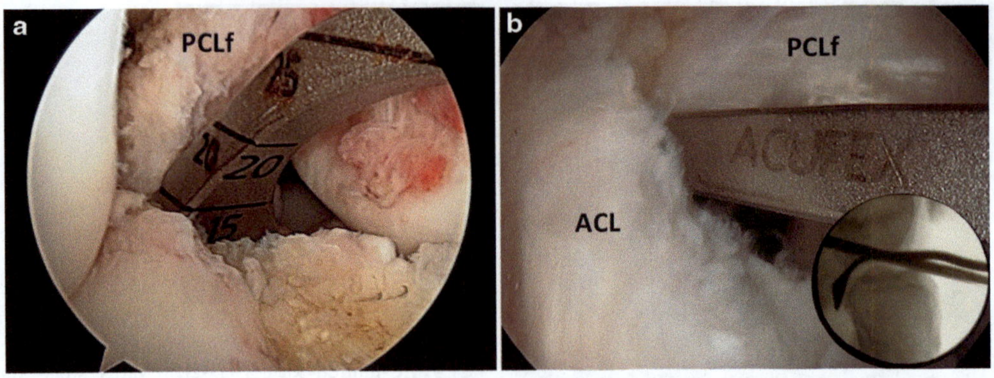

Fig. 16.21 Preparation of the posterior tibial intercondylar facet. **a** A PCL elevator follows any remaining fibers of the native PCL (*PCLf*) to their anterior insertion at the posterior intercondylar facet. Elevation is continued inferiorly at the periosteal insertion of these fibers, leaving the native PCL fibers and posterior capsule interposed between the elevator and the neurovascular structures. **b** When the ACL is intact, visualization of the native PCL fiber insertion is impaired. However, if the elevator is passed between the posterior ACL fibers (*ACL*) and anterior PCL fibers (*PCLf*) the seam can be easily palpated. In all cases, intraoperative fluoroscopy is used to confirm that the elevation is carried out immediately against the bone of the posterior tibia (*inset*)

native PCL (fibers in continuity) are preserved during the reconstruction. While completing the diagnostic scope, the allograft can be prepared. Generally, the preference is to use either Achilles tendon allograft or six-strand hamstring composite autograft with a goal of an 11-mm-diameter graft. Because the reconstruction utilizes interference screw fixation at the femur and tibia, the Achilles allograft bone plug is typically removed, which eases graft passage and is more time efficient. The calcaneal end of the allograft typically becomes the tibial side of the reconstruction. The graft is tapered and tubularized from a long 7-mm tail at one end to leave 8–9 cm of 11 mm graft diameter at the calcaneal end of the graft. The terminal ends, each prepared with nonabsorbable braided #2 sutures, are passed in a Krakow fashion for a length of 3 cm. These sutures aid in graft passage and provide stiffness to the tissue for screw purchase.

Table Set Up and Portals

The operative limb is flexed to 90° and held using an articulated variable leg positioner. A mini- or large C-arm fluoroscopy unit is positioned in a "rainbow" configuration over the limb and a perfect lateral image of the knee is obtained. *A medial parapatellar (working) portal should be made immediately adjacent to the medial edge of the patellar tendon, so that elevation of the PCL in the notch is possible without iatrogenic damage to the medial articular cartilage.* A lateral parapatellar (viewing) portal is created at the level of the distal pole of the patella, so that it may traverse along the roof of the notch (Blumensaat's line) for viewing the PCL tibial insertion. Alternatively, a posteromedial portal can be utilized for viewing of the PCL insertion, though intact fibers of the PCL insertion on the tibia will partially obscure the view to the interval between the anterior PCL and bony insertion. Frayed or torn fibers of the PCL are debrided, leaving any intact fibers in place.

Tibial PCL Tunnel Preparation

- Tibial tunnel preparation begins with a tibial PCL elevator (ACUFEX PCL ELEVATOR™, Smith & Nephew, Andover, MA). A posteromedial portal can be created to aid in visualization of the PCL insertion but is not mandatory.
- If the tibial insertion of the PCL is still intact, a PCL elevator is placed at the seam between the posterior intercondylar eminence and the anterior-most fibers of the PCL insertion. If the ACL is present, this plane can be easily found by following any remaining intact PCL fibers passing posterior to the ACL. A 70° arthroscope can be useful, viewing either through the notch or through an accessory posteromedial portal.
- PCL elevation is performed to dissect fibers from their insertion on the posterior intercondylar facet. *Elevation should always be confirmed under fluoroscopy in the lateral plane. The elevator must remain immediately against the bone of the PCL facet at the posterior tibia as PCL fibers are elevated.* This will leave both PCL fibers as well as the posterior joint capsule between the elevator and the neurovascular structures (Fig. 16.21). *Take care to remain centered on the posterior intercondylar fossa (PCL facet) to avoid injury to the meniscal roots and meniscofemoral ligaments.* The PCL elevation is continued inferiorly and posteriorly until the elevator drops below the level of the posterior tibial metaphyseal flare.

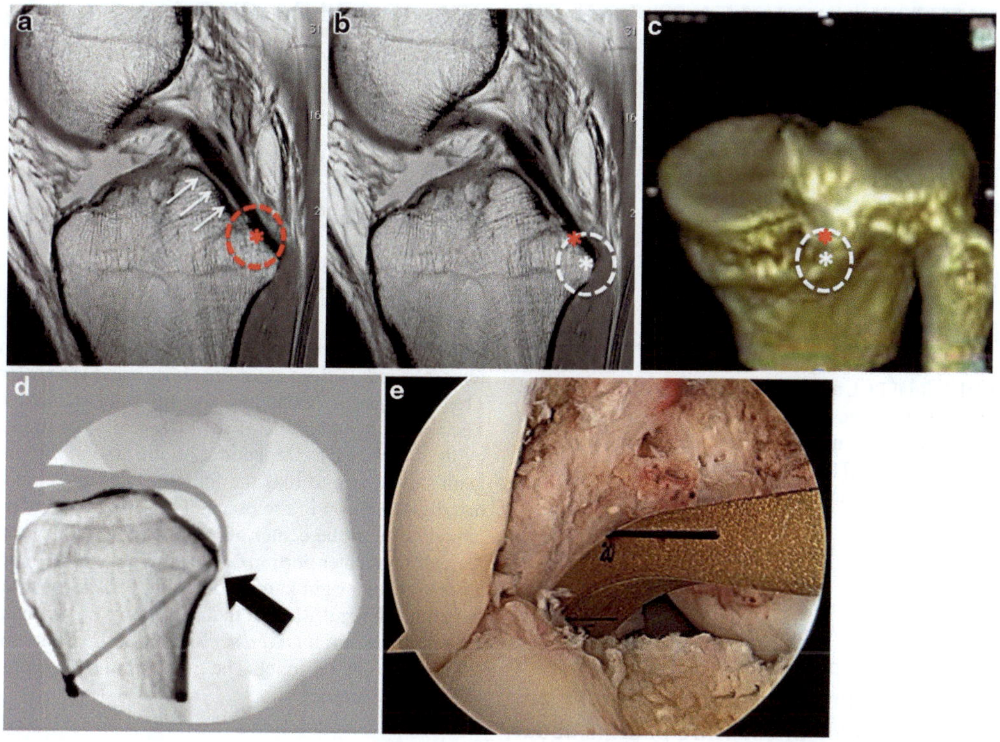

Fig. 16.22 Principles of ideal tibial tunnel placement during PCL reconstruction. **a** A "cam effect" of the posterior tibial eminence (*white arrows*) is critical to providing the normal anterior tibial position maintained by the PCL. Note that the PCL footprint on the tibia is approximately 11 mm and extends to the most posterior aspect of the posterior tibial facet. An 11-mm tunnel centered on the footprint (*red asterisk*) will bring the anterior "working" edge of the tibial tunnel too far anterior and much of the "cam effect" will be lost (diagrammed by the *red dashed circle*). **b** If the center of the tunnel (guide pin) is brought posteriorly to the most inferior segment of the posterior tibial facet (*white asterisk*), the resulting 11-mm tunnel will have its working edge in the center of the PCL footprint (*white dashed circle*). **c** Diagrammatic representation of the ideal center guide pin placement (*white asterisk*) and resulting tibial tunnel aperture (*white dashed circle*) on the posterior tibial eminence. **d** Fusion image demonstrating placement of the PCL guide tip at the far posterior edge of the metaphyseal flare and posterior tibial eminence. Note the relationship of the guide pin to the metaphyseal flare (*thick black arrow*). **e** Intraoperative arthroscopic view of the PCL guide when properly placed. The tip of the pin is 15 mm distal to the anterior edge of the posterior eminence

- A PCL guide (ACUFEX™) is placed at the tibial insertion of the PCL at the intercondylar facet under fluoroscopic guidance. The ideal placement of the guide tip (tunnel) should be approximately one tunnel radius width distal to the center of the anatomic footprint which then places the tunnel approximately 10–15 mm distal to the articular surface. For an 11-mm tunnel, the center of the guide pin will generally exit at the posteriormost point of the facet, placing the anterior (working) edge of the tunnel at the center of the native PCL footprint (Fig. 16.22). *Ideally, the PCL guide should be set to the maximum trajectory that will not obliterate the posterior metaphyseal flare of the tibia, thus preserving the strength of aperture fixation.* Occasionally, a small patient undergoing concomitant ACL and PCL reconstructions may require PCL reaming from the anterolateral tibia, which necessitates elevation of the anterior compartment musculature. Great care should be taken to protect the neurovascular structures at the posterior aspect of the knee during tibial tunnel drilling. In general, the knee should be flexed to 90° to increase the distance between the neurovascular bundle and the posterior capsule. A specialized PCL elevator with a hollow to catch the pin and prevent overpenetration with the reamer can be utilized (ACUFEX PCL ELEVATOR™, Smith & Nephew, Andover, MA). Drilling of the pin and reaming over the pin should be performed under fluoroscopic guidance, and (at the surgeon's discretion) a posteromedial "safety" incision can be utilized (Fig. 16.23).

Femoral PCL Tunnel Preparation

An inside-out or outside-in technique for femoral tunnel drilling can be employed, but it is the author's preference to drill outside-in to avoid an extreme angle as the graft makes the femoral tunnel and also maintain distance from the medial epicondyle (useful in cases where the MCL must also be repaired/augmented).

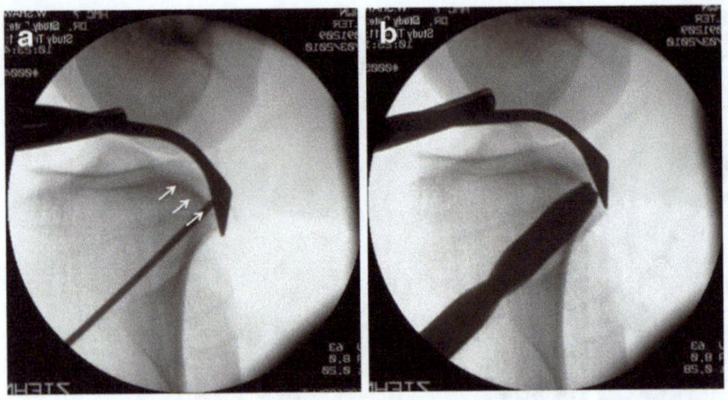

Fig. 16.23 Drilling the tibial PCL tunnel under fluoroscopic guidance. **a** After the PCL guide pin has been placed using the appropriate guide (Fig. 16.22d, e) the pin is captured using a hollowed instrument (ACUFEX™ PCL ELEVATOR/PIN CATCHER, Smith & Nephew, Andover, MA). Note the pin has been placed at the far inferior aspect of the posterior intercondylar facet (*white arrows*). **b** Reaming is performed under fluoroscopic observation. The elevator/pin catcher is helpful to prevent overpenetration by the drill reamer

- A minimal subvastus approach centered between the medial epicondyle and medial articular surface will allow ideal access for tunnel drilling and graft tensioning. The external guide pin starting point is about 1/3 the distance from the medial epicondyle and the articular surface edge. Ideal placement of the femoral tunnel on the notch is critical to proper graft kinematics as this construct recreates primarily the anterolateral fibers of the PCL. Large grafts such as 11 mm or larger grafts can recreate a large portion of the native PCL footprint.
- It is advisable to offset the guide pin (center of the tunnel) distally and anteriorly one tunnel radius width so that the posterior (working) wall of the tunnel will enter the joint at the anatomic center of the origin of the PCL anterolateral bundle footprint (Fig. 16.24). This position is typically described as the "11:00-shallow" (left knee) or "1:00-shallow" (right knee) position, and corresponds to the most anterodistal fibers (anterolateral bundle) of the PCL. For large grafts/tunnels, this may leave only a 1.5- to 2-mm rim of cortical bone between the articular cartilage and the femoral aperture of the PCL tunnel at the distal medial wall of the femoral condyle, but the trajectory of the tunnel should be coursing away from the femoral articular surface.
- The tunnel is drilled outside in to the diameter of the PCL reconstruction graft.

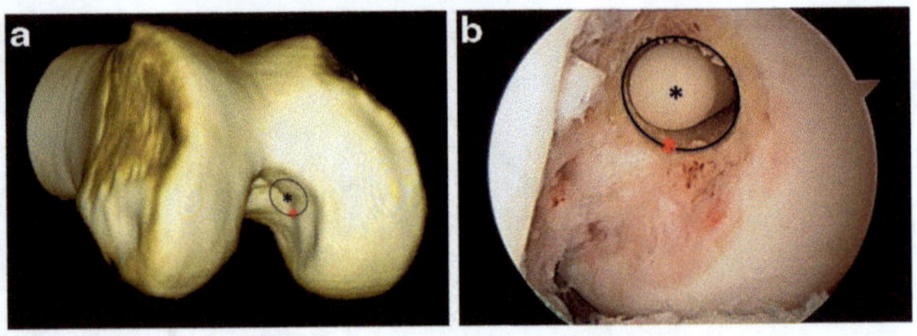

Fig. 16.24 Principles of ideal femoral tunnel placement during PCL reconstruction. **a** Three-dimensional view of the medial side of the intercondylar notch in a right knee. The PCL origin has a broad based fan shape that occupies a large portion of the lateral wall of the medial femoral condyle from anterior (*upper notch*) to posterior (*lower notch*). The *red asterisk* demarcates the approximate center of this footprint. The anterolateral bundle of the PCL originates in the region subtended by the *black circle*. Depending on the size of the graft/tunnel, the surgeon should aim to bias the femoral PCL tunnel anteriorly (*high*) and distally (*shallow*) in the notch. This brings the "working edge" of the tunnel close to the center of the anatomic footprint (*red asterisk*), and recreates a greater portion of the anterolateral PCL bundle. **b** Intraoperative view of a right knee undergoing PCL reconstruction. The femoral tunnel has been drilled so that the approximate anatomic center of the large PCL footprint (*red asterisk*) sits at the posteroproximal "working edge" of the PCL tunnel. The guide pin had been placed in the region of the *black asterisk*

PCL Graft Passage

- A spring-loaded curving suture passer or the coated wire end of a GORE™ SMOOTHER Crucial Tool (Smith & Nephew, Andover, MA) can be used to deliver a passing suture through the tibial tunnel from anterior to the internal aperture at the PCL facet, and into the posterior intercondylar space. There the suture is retrieved through the femoral PCL tunnel and delivered out the subvastus incision.
- A GORE™ SMOOTHER Crucial Tool (Smith & Nephew, Andover, MA) is used to gently chamfer the tunnel apertures as the knee is taken from flexion to extension. *Care should be taken to keep the pull of the smoother parallel to the tunnels, so as not to saw through or enlarge the external apertures.* (Fig. 16.25)
- Next, the PCL graft is passed from tibia through femur until the prepared calcaneal end of the graft lies snug within the tibial tunnel.
- The tibial side is secured using an interference screw driven (under fluoroscopic guidance) to the posterior tibial aperture, shortening the working length of the graft (see Fig. 16.26b).
- The graft is cycled through flexion and extension, and the tibia is held reduced within anterior draw (bringing the anterior tibia ahead of the femoral condyles), neutral to slight internal rotation, and flexed 70–90°.

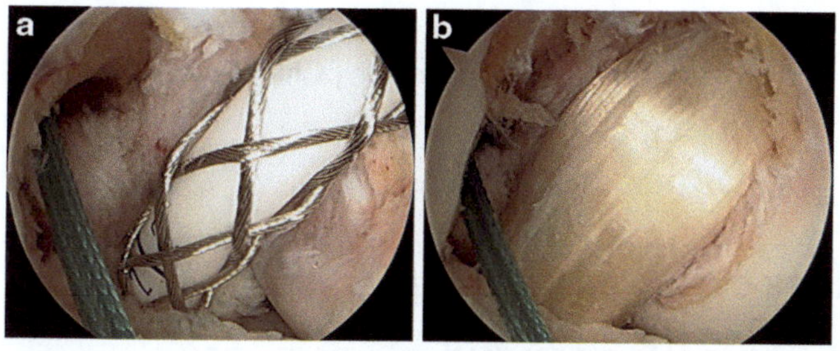

Fig. 16.25 Intraoperative view smoothing PCL tunnels and graft passage. **a** A flexible tunnel smoother (GORE™ SMOOTHER Crucial Tool, Smith & Nephew, Andover, MA) is routed from the tibial tunnel through the joint and femoral tunnel and used to chamfer the tunnel walls. This instrument can also be used to pass the shuttle sutures attached to the femoral side of the PCL graft. **b** The PCL reconstruction graft (Achilles allograft in this case) has been passed through the tibial tunnel, around the posterior tibia, through the joint, and into the femoral tunnel

- The femoral side of the graft is secured with an interference screw placed outside-in to the internal aperture. Once PCL stability has been restored, the remainder of the procedure is performed, first completing the central pivot by reconstructing the ACL (when torn), and moving to the repair and augmentation/reconstruction of the lateral structures (Fig. 16.26).

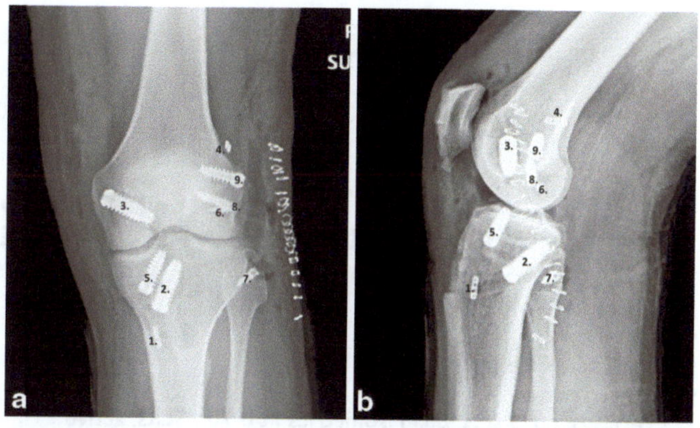

Fig. 16.26 Postoperative AP (**a**) and lateral (**b**) X-rays from an ACL/PCL/PLC reconstruction. The numerals correspond to the order of placement of implants. After exposing the lateral structures and tagging torn tissues for repair: *1* The tibial tunnel for the modified LaPrade PLC reconstruction is created and the graft seated in the posterior tibial socket. *2* Attention is turned to restoration of the central pivot. The PCL (and ACL) tunnels are created and the tibial side of the PCL graft is fixed in the tibial tunnel (note that the interference screw is driven nearly to the posterior tibial aperture to shorten the working length of the graft). *3* The PCL graft is cycled and fixed in the femoral tunnel. *4* The ACL graft is secured in the femoral tunnel. *5* The ACL graft is cycled and fixed in the tibial tunnel (completing the central pivot). *6* The torn proximal popliteus insertion was repaired using a suture anchor. *7* The torn distal fibular collateral ligament insertion was repaired to the proximal fibula using a suture anchor. *8* The popliteus limb of the augmentation graft was passed and secured into the femoral socket. *9* The isometric position for the fibular collateral (FCL) limb of the augmentation graft is identified, and the graft tensioned and secured into the femoral tunnel

Postoperative Rehabilitation

Rehabilitation after a PCL/PLC reconstruction must strike a balance between restoring motion and function of the knee versus maintaining the stability and integrity of graft tissue [62]. To date, there has been only one randomized controlled trial that has posed a question regarding rehabilitation after PCL injury. Yoon et al. in 2013 asked if immobilizing PCL reconstructions in a long leg cast for 5 weeks versus a locked hinged brace resulted in any meaningful difference [63]. They found that the PCL reconstructions immobilized in a cast for 5 weeks demonstrated significantly better results on Telos stress radiographs, but this difference did not bear out to have clinical significance.

Two recent reviews have focused on PCL reconstruction rehabilitation and have found much research remains in optimizing rehabilitation protocols [64, 65]. Most rehabilitation protocols for PCL/PLC injuries focus on delaying full weight bearing for at least 6–8 weeks. Because biomechanical work demonstrated that hamstring contraction increases the posterior shear force on the tibia and stresses the PCL, most protocols allow active knee extension while avoiding active knee flexion until 6 weeks [66]. After 6–8 weeks, motion is encouraged to 90° of flexion. Restoration of normal gait is the goal for 8–12 weeks with restoring full ROM by 12 weeks. Incorporation of resistance and functional sport training occurs gradually with full return to sports or unrestricted activity not expected until 7–10 months [50].

The senior author employs a more aggressive protocol than the recommendations above (Fig. 16.27). The concepts of the protocol are to immobilize at most 2 weeks to allow for uneventful healing of incisions and to allow the acute inflammatory phase to settle. Weeks 3–5 stress recovery with initiation of passive flexion and restoration of terminal symmetrical active extension. Weeks 6–8 bring full weight bearing, continue the progression of motion, and initiate short-crank bicycling/repetition. Weeks 9–11 focus on normalizing gains in gait, step, and proprioception. Active hamstring/flexion strengthening begins at weeks 12–20 along with a progression of functional training. Limited activities are allowed from weeks 21 to 28, and a full return to sport is allowed as early as 29 weeks if the patient has demonstrated adequate strength, flexibility, proprioception, and stability.

Christopher J. Wahl, MD
Associate Clinical Professor | Chief, Sports Medicine

Physical Therapy Prescription
MULTI-LIGANENT KNEE RECONSTRUCTION

PREOPERATIVE:
- Brace fitting
- Cryo-cuff®/ ice
- Crutch training
- Exercises: quad sets, quad isometrics at 0-70°, SLRs, active extension 0-70°, **passive** flexion 0-90°, patellar mobs

HOSPITAL/EARLY HOME: 0-2 Weeks
- Brace locked in full extension, avoiding hyperextension
- NWB with crutches, brace locked in extension
- Cryo-cuff®/ ice
- NO PERIOPERATIVE ACTIVE KNEE FLEXION -- THIS WILL STRESS THE RECONSTRUCTED PCL!

RECOVERY: Weeks 3 - 5
- Active extension 45° - 0° (quad sets, isometrics)
- Progress **passive** flexion target 90° by week 6
- Tandem "mini-squats" with upper extremity assistance (use well leg to bear weight, follow with recon knee)
- TTWB with brace locked in extension
- Quadriceps re-education (e-stim, biofeedback, etc.)
- Hip PRE's
- Patella mobilization
- Continue/advance home exercise program

ROM/STRENGTH PROGRESSION: Weeks 6 – 8
- Progress to FWB with brace unlocked to 0-50° and crutches at all times
- Discontinue crutches at week 8 if normal gait
- Leg press in 90-0° arc
- Multiple angle quadriceps isometrics, 90-0°
- Calf raises
- Bicycle ergometer
- LIDO exercises: isometrics, active extension/passive flexion, concentric/eccentric quad
- Begin quad isotonics 0-70° (distal pad), eccentric first

GAIT/STEP TRAINING: Weeks 9 – 11
- Restore normal gait
- At 10 wks, begin active flex isometrics, isotonics 0-90°, closed chain
- Begin squat/step program
- Proximal muscle PREs
- Begin proprioception program
- Quad isotonics (knee extension) with distal pad in 0-90° arc
- Begin retro program
- LIDO exercises: isotonics, quad eccentrics
- Nordic-track®

FUNCTIOANL TRAINING: Weeks 12 - 20
- Restore full ROM
- Continue proximal muscle PREs
- Quad isotonics (knee extension) in full arc
- Begin functional exercise program
- Progress endurance activities
- Improve lower extremity flexibility
- LIDO exercises: quad isokinetics full arc, quad eccentrics in 0-90° arc
- Stairmaster®, Versaclimber®

LIMITED RETURN TO ACTIVITIES: Weeks 21 - 28
- Full arc PRE's to restore strength, emphasizing quads
- Agility exercises
- Continue functional exercises/grid training
- Begin running program at 6 months (25 weeks) if less than 30% difference in side-to-side hamstring/quad torque on isokinetic testing
- LIDO exercises: full arc quad isokinetics in velocity spectrum
- Return to limited sports (no cutting)

FULL RETURN TO SPORTS: Weeks 29 – 40
- Restore symmetrical strength, function, endurance, agility to lower extremity
- Advance running program
- Functional/grid test assessment
- Symmetrical isokinetic testing
- Return to all activities

Patient: ______________________________ | **Date:**____________

Sessions: _____ x per wk for _____ wks | **Provider:** ______________________________

Fig. 16.27 Physical therapy prescription—multiligament knee reconstruction

Conclusions

Combined PCL and lateral-sided injuries are challenging situations for orthopedic surgeons. Recalling the high association of neurovascular compromise should alert providers to the potential devastating nature of this injury pattern. Furthermore, surgical correction of a PCL injury with failure to recognize and correct even slight lateral-sided laxity leads to worse clinical outcomes than with lateral-sided reconstruction. We recommend PCL reconstruction with an anatomic lateral-sided reconstruction of the LCL, popliteus, and PFL and repair when appropriate. Rehabilitation of these injuries continues to evolve with the goal of restoring normal knee kinematics and stability.

References

1. Freeman RT, Duri ZA, Dowd GS. Combined chronic posterior cruciate and posterolateral corner ligamentous injuries: a comparison of posterior cruciate ligament reconstruction with and without reconstruction of the posterolateral corner. Knee. 2002;9(4):309–12.
2. Kim SJ, Lee SK, Kim SH, Kim SH, Jung M. Clinical outcomes for reconstruction of the posterolateral corner and posterior cruciate ligament in injuries with mild grade 2 or less posterior translation: comparison with isolated posterolateral corner reconstruction. Am J Sports Med. 2013;41(7):1613–20.
3. Fanelli GC, Edson CJ. Posterior cruciate ligament injuries in trauma patients: Part II. Arthroscopy. 1995;11(5):526–9.
4. Fanelli GC. Posterior cruciate ligament injuries in trauma patients. Arthroscopy. 1993;9(3):291–4.
5. Geissler WB, Whipple TL. Intraarticular abnormalities in association with posterior cruciate ligament injuries. Am J Sports Med. 1993;21(6):846–9.
6. Boynton MD, Tietjens BR. Long-term followup of the untreated isolated posterior cruciate ligament-deficient knee. Am J Sports Med. 1996;24(3):306–10.
7. Strobel MJ, Weiler A, Schulz MS, Russe K, Eichhorn HJ. Arthroscopic evaluation of articular cartilage lesions in posterior-cruciate-ligament-deficient knees. Arthroscopy. 2003;19(3):262–8.
8. Voos JE, Mauro CS, Wente T, Warren RF, Wickiewicz TL. Posterior cruciate ligament: Anatomy, biomechanics, and outcomes. Am J Sports Med. 2012;40(1):222–31.
9. Mejia EA, Noyes FR, Grood ES. Posterior cruciate ligament femoral insertion site characteristics. Importance for reconstructive procedures. Am J Sports Med. 2002;30(5):643–51.
10. Gollehon DL, Torzilli PA, Warren RF. The role of the posterolateral and cruciate ligaments in the stability of the human knee. A biomechanical study. J Bone Joint Surg Am. 1987;69(2):233–42.
11. Kennedy NI, Wijdicks CA, Goldsmith MT, et al. Kinematic analysis of the posterior cruciate ligament, part 1: the individual and collective function of the anterolateral and posteromedial bundles. Am J Sports Med. 2013;41(12):2828–38.
12. Mauro CS, Sekiya JK, Stabile KJ, Haemmerle MJ, Harner CD. Double-bundle PCL and posterolateral corner reconstruction components are codominant. Clin Orthop Relat Res. 2008;466(9):2247–54.
13. Wijdicks CA, Kennedy NI, Goldsmith MT, et al. Kinematic analysis of the posterior cruciate ligament, part 2: a comparison of anatomic single- versus double-bundle reconstruction. Am J Sports Med. 2013;41(12):2839–48.
14. Marsh JP, MacDonald PB. Surgical management of ACL, PCL, and lateral-sided injuries: acute and chronic. In: Fanelli GC, editor. The multiple ligament injured knee. New York: Springer; 2013. pp. 267–80.
15. Andrews JR, Baker CL, Curl WW, Gidumal R. Surgical repair of acute and chronic lesions of the lateral capsular ligamentous complex of the knee. New York: Churchill Livingstone; 1988.
16. Seebacher JR, Inglis AE, Marshall JL, Warren RF. The structure of the posterolateral aspect of the knee. J Bone Joint Surg Am. 1982;64(4):536–41.
17. LaPrade RF, Ly TV, Wentorf FA, Engebretsen L. The posterolateral attachments of the knee: a qualitative and quantitative morphologic analysis of the fibular collateral ligament, popliteus tendon, popliteofibular ligament, and lateral gastrocnemius tendon. Am J Sports Med. 2003;31(6):854–60.
18. Staubli HU, Birrer S. The popliteus tendon and its fascicles at the popliteal hiatus: gross anatomy and functional arthroscopic evaluation with and without anterior cruciate ligament deficiency. Arthroscopy. 1990;6(3):209–20.
19. Sanchez AR 2nd, Sugalski MT, LaPrade RF. Anatomy and biomechanics of the lateral side of the knee. Sports Med Arthrosc. 2006;14(1):2–11.
20. Maynard MJ, Deng X, Wickiewicz TL, Warren RF. The popliteofibular ligament. Rediscovery of a key element in posterolateral stability. Am J Sports Med. 1996;24(3):311–6.
21. Schinhan M, Bijak M, Unger E, Nau T. Electromyographic study of the popliteus muscle in the dynamic stabilization of the posterolateral corner structures of the knee. Am J Sports Med. 2011;39(1):173–9.
22. Noyes FR, Stowers SF, Grood ES, Cummings J, VanGinkel LA. Posterior subluxations of the medial and lateral tibiofemoral compartments. An in vitro ligament sectioning study in cadaveric knees. Am J Sports Med. 1993;21(3):407–14.
23. LaPrade RF, Muench C, Wentorf F, Lewis JL. The effect of injury to the posterolateral structures of the knee on force in a posterior cruciate ligament graft: a biomechanical study. Am J Sports Med. 2002;30(2):233–8.
24. Sekiya JK, Haemmerle MJ, Stabile KJ, Vogrin TM, Harner CD. Biomechanical analysis of a combined double-bundle posterior cruciate ligament and posterolateral corner reconstruction. Am J Sports Med. 2005;33(3):360–9.
25. Apsingi S, Nguyen T, Bull AM, Unwin A, Deehan DJ, Amis AA. Control of laxity in knees with combined posterior cruciate ligament and posterolateral corner deficiency: comparison of single-bundle versus double-bundle posterior cruciate ligament reconstruction combined with modified Larson posterolateral corner reconstruction. Am J Sports Med. 2008;36(3):487–94.
26. Howells NR, Brunton LR, Robinson J, Porteus AJ, Eldridge JD, Murray JR. Acute knee dislocation: an evidence based approach to the management of the multiligament injured knee. Injury. 2011;42(11):1198–204.
27. Merritt AL, Wahl C. Initial assessment of the acute and chronic multiple-ligament injured (dislocated) knee. Sports Med Arthrosc. 2011;19(2):93–103.
28. Rihn JA, Groff YJ, Harner CD, Cha PS. The acutely dislocated knee: evaluation and management. J Am Acad Orthop Surg. 2004;12(5):334–46.
29. Stannard JP, Sheils TM, Lopez-Ben RR, McGwin G Jr., Robinson JT, Volgas DA. Vascular injuries in knee dislocations: the role of physical examination in determining the need for arteriography. J Bone Joint Surg Am. 2004;86-A(5):910–5.
30. Johansen K, Lynch K, Paun M, Copass M. Non-invasive vascular tests reliably exclude occult arterial trauma in injured extremities. J Trauma. 1991;31(4):515–9; discussion 519–22.

31. Lynch K, Johansen K. Can Doppler pressure measurement replace "exclusion" arteriography in the diagnosis of occult extremity arterial trauma? Ann Surg. 1991;214(6):737–41.
32. Mills WJ, Barei DP, McNair P. The value of the ankle-brachial index for diagnosing arterial injury after knee dislocation: a prospective study. J Trauma. 2004;56(6):1261–5.
33. Nicandri GT, Chamberlain AM, Wahl CJ. Practical management of knee dislocations: a selective angiography protocol to detect limb-threatening vascular injuries. Clin J Sport Med. 2009;19(2):125–9.
34. Seamon MJ, Smoger D, Torres DM, et al. A prospective validation of a current practice: the detection of extremity vascular injury with CT angiography. J Trauma. 2009;67(2):238–43; discussion 243–34.
35. Abbasi D, May MM, Wall EJ, Chan G, Parikh SN. MRI findings in adolescent patients with acute traumatic knee hemarthrosis. J Pediatr Orthop. 2012;32(8):760–4.
36. Noyes FR, Bassett RW, Grood ES, Butler DL. Arthroscopy in acute traumatic hemarthrosis of the knee. Incidence of anterior cruciate tears and other injuries. J Bone Joint Surg Am. 1980;62(5):687–95, 757.
37. Noyes FR, Paulos L, Mooar LA, Signer B. Knee sprains and acute knee hemarthrosis: misdiagnosis of anterior cruciate ligament tears. Phys Ther. 1980;60(12):1596–601.
38. Malanga GA, Andrus S, Nadler SF, McLean J. Physical examination of the knee: a review of the original test description and scientific validity of common orthopedic tests. Arch Phys Med Rehabil. 2003;84(4):592–603.
39. Petrigliano FA, Lane CG, Suero EM, Allen AA, Pearle AD. Posterior cruciate ligament and posterolateral corner deficiency results in a reverse pivot shift. Clin Orthop Relat Res. 2012;470(3):815–23.
40. Sekiya JK, Whiddon DR, Zehms CT, Miller MD. A clinically relevant assessment of posterior cruciate ligament and posterolateral corner injuries. Evaluation of isolated and combined deficiency. J Bone Joint Surg Am. 2008;90(8):1621–7.
41. Garavaglia G, Lubbeke A, Dubois-Ferriere V, Suva D, Fritschy D, Menetrey J. Accuracy of stress radiography techniques in grading isolated and combined posterior knee injuries: a cadaveric study. Am J Sports Med. 2007;35(12):2051–6.
42. Margheritini F, Mancini L, Mauro CS, Mariani PP. Stress radiography for quantifying posterior cruciate ligament deficiency. Arthroscopy. 2003;19(7):706–11.
43. Petrigliano FA, Suero EM, Voos JE, Pearle AD, Allen AA. The effect of proximal tibial slope on dynamic stability testing of the posterior cruciate ligament- and posterolateral corner-deficient knee. Am J Sports Med. 2012;40(6):1322–8.
44. Savarese E, Bisicchia S, Romeo R, Amendola A. Role of high tibial osteotomy in chronic injuries of posterior cruciate ligament and posterolateral corner. J Orthop Traumatol. 2011;12(1):1–17.
45. Levy BA, Fanelli GC, Whelan DB, et al. Controversies in the treatment of knee dislocations and multiligament reconstruction. J Am Acad Orthop Surg. 2009;17(4):197–206.
46. Levy BA, Dajani KA, Morgan JA, Shah JP, Dahm DL, Stuart MJ. Repair versus reconstruction of the fibular collateral ligament and posterolateral corner in the multiligament-injured knee. Am J Sports Med. 2010;38(4):804–9.
47. Levy BA, Dajani KA, Whelan DB, et al. Decision making in the multiligament-injured knee: an evidence-based systematic review. Arthroscopy. 2009;25(4):430–8.
48. Stannard JP, Brown SL, Farris RC, McGwin G Jr., Volgas DA. The posterolateral corner of the knee: repair versus reconstruction. Am J Sports Med. 2005;33(6):881–8.
49. Stannard JP, Nuelle CW, McGwin G, Volgas DA. Hinged external fixation in the treatment of knee dislocations: a prospective randomized study. J Bone Joint Surg Am. 2014;96(3):184–91.
50. Merritt AL, Wahl CJ. Rationale and treatment of multiple-ligament injured knees: the Seattle perspective. Operat Techn Sports Med. 2011;19(1):51–72.
51. Nicandri GT, Slaney SL, Neradilek MB, Larson RV, Green JR, Wahl CJ. Can magnetic resonance imaging predict posterior drawer laxity at the time of surgery in patients with knee dislocation or multiple-ligament knee injury? Am J Sports Med. 2011;39(5):1053–8.
52. Arciero RA. Anatomic posterolateral corner knee reconstruction. Arthroscopy. 2005;21(9):1147.e1–5.
53. LaPrade RF, Johansen S, Wentorf FA, Engebretsen L, Esterberg JL, Tso A. An analysis of an anatomical posterolateral knee reconstruction: an in vitro biomechanical study and development of a surgical technique. Am J Sports Med. 2004;32(6):1405–14.
54. Larson RV, Sidles JA, Beals CT. Isometry of lateral collateral and popliteofibular ligaments and a technique for reconstruction. Seattle: University of Washington; 1996.
55. May JH, Gillette BP, Morgan JA, Krych AJ, Stuart MJ, Levy BA. Transtibial versus inlay posterior cruciate ligament reconstruction: an evidence-based systematic review. J Knee Surg. 2010;23(2):73–9.
56. Papalia R, Osti L, Del Buono A, Denaro V, Maffulli N. Tibial inlay for posterior cruciate ligament reconstruction: a systematic review. Knee. 2010;17(4):264–9.
57. Markolf KL, Feeley BT, Jackson SR, McAllister DR. Biomechanical studies of double-bundle posterior cruciate ligament reconstructions. J Bone Joint Surg Am. 2006;88(8):1788–94.
58. Kim SJ, Jung M, Moon HK, Kim SG, Chun YM. Anterolateral transtibial posterior cruciate ligament reconstruction combined with anatomical reconstruction of posterolateral corner insufficiency: comparison of single-bundle versus double-bundle posterior cruciate ligament reconstruction over a 2- to 6-year follow-up. Am J Sports Med. 2011;39(3):481–9.
59. Kim SJ, Kim SH, Kim SG, Kung YP. Comparison of the clinical results of three posterior cruciate ligament reconstruction techniques: surgical technique. J Bone Joint Surg Am. 2010;92(Suppl 1 Pt 2):145–57.
60. Kohen RB, Sekiya JK. Single-bundle versus double-bundle posterior cruciate ligament reconstruction. Arthroscopy. 2009;25(12):1470–7.
61. Yoon KH, Bae DK, Song SJ, Cho HJ, Lee JH. A prospective randomized study comparing arthroscopic single-bundle and double-bundle posterior cruciate ligament reconstructions preserving remnant fibers. Am J Sports Med. 2011;39(3):474–80.
62. Edson CJ, Fanelli GC. Postoperative rehabilitation of the multiple ligament injured knee. In: Fanelli GC, editor. The multiple ligament injured knee. New York: Springer; 2013. pp. 437–42.
63. Yoon KH, Park SW, Lee SH, Kim MH, Park SY, Oh H. Does cast immobilization contribute to posterior stability after posterior cruciate ligament reconstruction? Arthroscopy. 2013;29(3):500–6.
64. Kim JG, Lee YS, Yang BS, Oh SJ, Yang SJ. Rehabilitation after posterior cruciate ligament reconstruction: A review of the literature and theoretical support. Arch Orthop Trauma Surg. 2013;133(12):1687–95.
65. Pierce CM, O'Brien L, Griffin LW, Laprade RF. Posterior cruciate ligament tears: functional and postoperative rehabilitation. Knee Surg Sports Traumatol Arthrosc. 2013;21(5):1071–84.
66. Shelburne KB, Pandy MG. Determinants of cruciate-ligament loading during rehabilitation exercise. Clin Biomech. 1998;13(6):403–13 (Bristol, Avon).
67. Rios CG, Leger RR, Cote MP, Yang C, Arciero RA. Posterolateral corner reconstruction of the knee: Evaluation of a technique with clinical outcomes and stress radiography. Am J Sports Med. 2010;38(8):1564–74.
68. Nicandri GT, et al. Are evidence-based protocols which identify vascular injury associated with knee dislocation underutilized? Knee Surg Sports Traumatol Arthrosc. 2010;18(8):1005–12.

Combined Posterior Cruciate Ligament and Posteromedial Reconstruction

17

Adnan Saithna and Peter B. MacDonald

Introduction

Injuries to the posteromedial corner (PMC) have received relatively less attention in the literature than those to the posterolateral corner and as a consequence are often not considered when addressing the posterior cruciate ligament (PCL)-injured knee [1–4]. Unrecognized or inadequately treated associated injuries are reported to have an incidence of 50–90% in the PCL-injured knee and this may explain why some studies have shown unfavorable outcomes at mid-term follow-up [1, 5, 6].

Part of the reason why injuries to the PMC may go unrecognized is due to the fact that the phrase "medial sided injury" has become synonymous with medial collateral ligament (MCL) sprains or tears and therefore it is often assumed that the medial-sided injuries will heal with nonoperative management [7]. However, unlike low-grade MCL tears, injuries to the PMC are a significantly different clinical entity biomechanically and are unlikely to heal particularly in the setting of a multiligament-injured knee. In addition, persistent valgus or posteromedial instability can place additional strain on a reconstructed cruciate ligament and potentially cause late graft failure [7, 8]. Therefore, it is essential to have an appropriate index of suspicion and identify these injuries before cruciate reconstruction so that repair and/or reconstruction of the PMC and MCL can be undertaken at the same time [7].

This chapter seeks to highlight the key features of the anatomy, biomechanics, and surgical management of combined PCL and PMC injuries.

P. B. MacDonald (✉) · A. Saithna
Pan Am Clinic, 75 Poseiden Bay, Winnipeg, Manitoba, R3M 3E4 Canada
e-mail: pmacdonald@panamclinic.com

A. Saithna
e-mail: adnan.saithna@nhs.net

G. C. Fanelli (ed.), *Posterior Cruciate Ligament Injuries*,
DOI 10.1007/978-3-319-12072-0_17,

Anatomy of the Medial Side of the Knee

In their classic article, Warren and Marshall described three layers of the medial side of the knee [9]. Layer I is the superficial fascia that blends with the pes anserinus distally and covers the sartorius and quadriceps proximally and the retinaculum anteriorly. Layer II is the superficial medial collateral ligament (sMCL), with parallel fibers running from the femoral epicondyle to the anteromedial tibial crest, 5–7 cm below the joint line. These fibers blend posteriorly with the oblique fibers of layer III. These oblique fibers attach around the femoral adductor tubercle and pass posterodistally across the tibiofemoral joint line to insert on the rim of the tibial plateau. Hughston and Eilers described these oblique fibers as a distinct structure and named it the posterior oblique ligament (POL). Historically, the literature has been divergent in the description of this structure and there has been a lack of clarity over whether this is a capsular thickening [9, 10], a part of the MCL [11, 12], or a discrete ligament. However, regardless of whether one chooses to recognize the POL as a separate structure or as a thickening of the posteromedial capsule is a matter of semantics. The important distinction to make is that injury to the posteromedial corner has a significant effect on the stability of the knee over and above an isolated MCL injury and failure to recognize and address this can lead to poor outcomes [13].

In any case, more recently, there has been greater consensus as to the anatomy of the POL (Fig. 17.1). Several cadaveric studies have described superficial, central, and proximal branches of the POL and these discrete structures have also been delineated on MRI [4, 12, 14]. These three arms have been described as consisting of fascial attachments extending from the semimembranosus tendon immediately posterior to the sMCL. The origins of the superficial arm fibers blend in with the posterior border of the sMCL anteriorly and course into the other arms of the POL inferiorly and posteriorly. The central arm is considered to be the main component of the POL, arising from the main semimembranosus tendon, reinforcing the deep medial collateral ligament (dMCL) directly

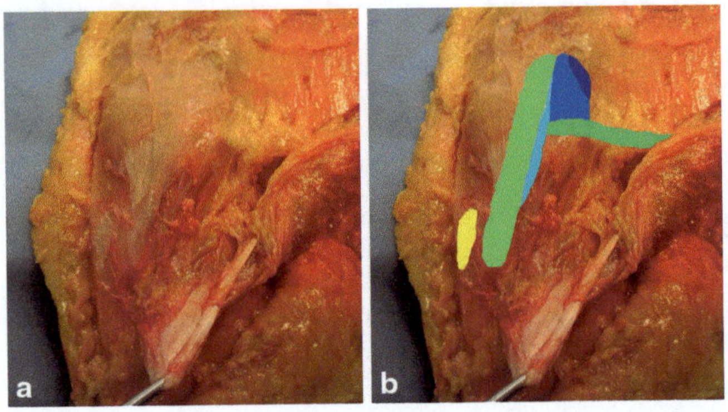

Fig. 17.1 The anatomy of the posterior medial corner including the hamstring tendon attachment (*yellow*), sMCL (*bright green*), fascial arm POL (*light blue*), central arm POL (*mid-blue*), capsular arm POL (*dark blue*), and semimembranosus tendon (*dark Green*). *sMCL* superficial medial collateral ligament, *POL* posterior oblique ligament

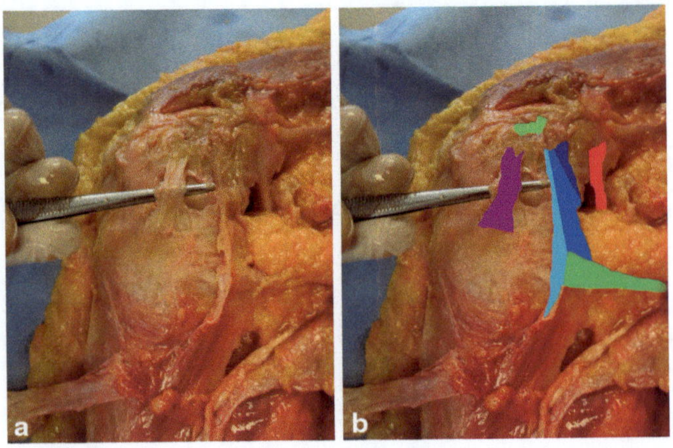

Fig. 17.2 The sMCL reflected to demonstrate the femoral foot print of the sMCL (*bright green*), dMCL (*purple*), fascial arm POL (*light blue*), central arm POL (*mid-blue*), capsular arm POL (*dark blue*), semimembranosus tendon (*dark green*), and the medial gastrocnemius tendon (*red*). *sMCL* superficial medial collateral ligament, *dMCL* deep medial collateral ligament, *POL* posterior oblique ligament

attaching to the posterior joint capsule and posterior meniscus, and blending with the semimembranosus attachment on the tibia. The capsular arm comes off the distal aspect of the semimembranosus tendon, attaching to the meniscofemoral portion of the joint capsule and medial head of the gastrocnemius and over the adductor magnus [4, 7, 12]. On average, the POL attaches on the femur 7.7 mm distal and 6.4 mm posterior to the adductor tubercle and 1.4 mm distal and 2.9 mm anterior to the gastrocnemius tubercle [12].

The anatomy of the medial structures of the knee has also been described from anterior to posterior, extending from the medial border of the patella to the medial edge of the PCL. The anterior third comprises the extensor retinaculum of the quadriceps femoris muscle. The middle third consists of the dMCL and the sMCL. The former is itself made up of meniscofemoral and meniscotibial fibers, and is separated from the sMCL by the MCL bursa (Fig. 17.2). The posterior third represents the posteromedial capsule and again there is some controversy as to what exactly this comprises. However, from previous biomechanical and anatomical studies, those structures that play a functional role include the posterior horn of the medial meniscus, the POL, semimembranosus tendon and insertions, meniscotibial ligaments, the oblique popliteal ligament, and the posteromedial capsule [1, 5, 12–14].

The PMC has been described as a synergistic muscle–ligament–meniscal unit with all of the structures working together to provide stability. The semimembranosus muscle has multiple attachments to the tibia and provides a dynamic component to the PMC. The anterior arm of the semimembranosus attaches to the tibia deep to the proximal attachment of the superficial MCL, whereas the direct arm attaches posterior to the medial tibial crest. In extension, it acts as a restraint to valgus and in flexion it restricts but also tightens the PMC via its attachments to POL and posterior capsule. The resulting posterior retraction of the posterior horn of the medial meniscus serves as a restraint against anterior tibial translation via the "chock block" effect [7].

Superficial Medial Collateral Ligament

The superficial medial collateral ligament consists of one femoral attachment and two tibial attachments. The femoral attachment is on average, 3.2 mm proximal and 4.8 mm posterior to the medial epicondyle. The proximal tibial attachment is primarily to soft tissue over the termination of the anterior arm of the semimembranosus tendon and is located at an average of 12.2 mm distal to the joint line. The distal tibial attachment of the sMCL is located just anterior to the posteromedial crest of the tibia at an average of 61.2 mm distal to the joint line. The two distinct tibial attachments have been reported to result in two distinct functioning divisions of the superficial medial collateral ligament [15].

Deep Medial Collateral Ligament

The deep medial collateral ligament comprises the thickened medial aspect of the joint capsule that is deep to the superficial medial collateral ligament. It is divided into meniscofemoral and meniscotibial components. The meniscofemoral portion has a slightly curved convex attachment, 12.6 mm distal and deep to the femoral attachment of the superficial medial collateral ligament. The meniscotibial portion, which is much shorter and thicker than the meniscofemoral portion, attaches just distal to the edge of the articular cartilage of the medial tibial plateau, 3.2 mm distal to the medial joint line [15].

Biomechanics

The PMC and the POL are biomechanically separate structures from the superficial MCL and play a role in restraint to valgus stress, internal/external rotation, posterior tibial translation (PTT), and anteromedial rotatory instability (AMRI).

Valgus Stress

The PMC is a primary stabilizer of the extended knee providing approximately one third of the restraint to valgus stress. However, with flexion, the PMC slackens, causing the superficial MCL to become the primary stabilizer to valgus stress across the remainder of the flexion–extension arc. At 0°, the PMC resisted 29 % valgus, 14 % at 30° and <5 % at 90° [16].

Internal/External Rotation

The POL is a primary stabilizer for internal rotation at all knee flexion angles although the most load occurs in full extension. In biomechanical studies where the MCL has already been cut, sectioning the POL and capsule causes significant increases in internal and external rotation in all degrees of flexion.

The PMC is not a significant restraint to tibial internal rotation above 30° flexion but is the primary restraint near full extension. The fibers of PMC are slackened by tibial ER and therefore do not contribute to restraining this movement unlike the sMCL and dMCL [16].

Posterior Tibial Translation

The PMC is an important secondary restraint to PTT in the PCL-intact knee. It has been shown to resist 28 % of the posterior tibial load when the tibia was free to rotate, rising to 42 % when the tibia was internally rotated. However, the PMC becomes the primary restraint to PTT in the PCL-deficient knee.

Sectioning of the POL and posteromedial capsule in this setting has been shown to increase posterior tibial translation and this can be helpful for distinguishing between isolated and combined PCL injuries [7].

The effect on PTT is even more pronounced when the knee is in extension because POL fibers slacken with flexion. Weimann et al. reported that the application of valgus rotation with a force of 10 N m causes a significant increase in PTT of the knee with posteromedial instability. This suggests that the POL should be intact if there is no PTT in extension with valgus testing in the PCL-deficient knee. This finding may also be considered as a basis for the observation that isolated PCL injuries may not always cause functional disability and furthermore supports the clinical theory that untreated injuries to the POL may contribute to PCL graft failure [1].

Anteromedial Rotatory Instability

Injury to multiple structures on the medial side of the knee results in the phenomenon of AMRI which is defined as anterior subluxation and external rotation of the medial tibial plateau [7].

Mechanism of Injury

A spectrum of medial-sided injury can occur after the application of a valgus force to the leg. This can range from isolated MCL injury to involvement of the PMC, which is more likely if there is high-velocity trauma or an external rotation component to the forces involved [1, 17–19].

Clinical Examination

The hallmarks of clinical examination are detailed below.

Valgus Stress Testing

For an isolated superficial MCL injury, the greatest joint space opening occurs with the knee in 30° of flexion. Joint space opening with the knee fully extended indicates an injury to the capsule, the POL, or both [20]. Chahal et al. showed that in their series of knee dislocations, all those with grade III medial opening at 0 and 30° had complete tears of the sMCL as well as the POL. No patient with grade I opening had complete tears of POL or sMCL [2].

Posterior Drawer

In combined PCL–PMC injury, a posterior drawer test is performed with the knee flexed at 90° and the foot in neutral rotation and repeated with the foot 10° internally rotated. The PMC acts as a secondary stabilizer with an isolated PCL injury decreasing tibial translation when the foot is held in internal rotation, if intact. With combined PCL–PMC injury, there is increased translation during the posterior drawer when the tibia is internally rotated as these secondary stabilizers are no longer intact [7, 19].

Anterior Drawer and AMRI

AMRI is detected by performing the anterior drawer test while holding the tibia in external rotation. Any evidence of anterior subluxation of the medial tibial plateau during a valgus stress test with the knee in 30° of flexion might also indicate the presence of AMRI [7].

Imaging

Plain Radiographs

All patients should have plain radiographs taken in orthogonal planes to evaluate for fractures, avulsions, or a dislocation [21].

Stress radiographs can be useful to assess the degree of medial opening and PTT. Garavaglia et al. reported that >12 mm of posterior translation at 80° flexion was indicative of a combined PCL–PMC injury [22].

MRI

MRI is the imaging study of choice to evaluate the PMC and can elucidate injuries to SM, the POL, medial meniscocapsular structures, the OPL, and fractures/bone bruising. MRI should be performed prior to fixation of any coexisting periarticular fractures as metal artifact can significantly reduce the quality of imaging [2, 6].

Chahal et al. reported MR findings in 27 consecutive knee dislocations. It is interesting to note that they found evidence of injury to at least one structure in the posteromedial corner in 81 % (22/27) of knees. Of these, 64 % (14/22) had injury to the POL. The semimembranosus and its expansions were injured in 64 % (22/22) and injury to the MT ligament was identified in 50 % (11/22). Of particular note, 9/22 had injuries to the PHMM and of those 100 % had a tear of MT ligament and 67 % had a tear of the POL. They concluded that injuries to the PMC are in fact common with high-grade multiligament knee injuries [2].

A cadaveric study demonstrated that T1-weighted fat-saturated coronal- and coronal-oblique sequences acquired after the injection of intra-articular contrast demonstrated the best visualization of the POL and posteromedial capsule. However, the use of contrast studies is not common practice and noncontrast T1 axial images can provide good visualization of the MCL, POL, and the semimembranosus attachments [21].

It is important to look for evidence of injury to each structure within the PMC as involvement of any of these can disable the functional cascade of the posteromedial capsule [13]. However, Chahal et al. reported that isolated injuries to semimembranosus on MRI did not correlate with clinical medial knee instability [2].

Surgical Management

Immediate Management

The immediate management of knee dislocation is well described elsewhere. In brief, patients should be assessed with respect to standard trauma care principles and life-threatening injuries treated first. The hallmarks of clinical examination of the PCL–PMC injured knee are described above, but in the acute setting a neurological and vascular assessment of the limb is also mandatory. Provided that no emergent management is required (e.g., for open dislocation or vascular injury), the affected limb can be placed into a cricket pad splint while awaiting further imaging, assessment, and definitive management.

Nonoperative Treatment

Nonoperative management is not recommended for combined PCL–PMC injuries. Although low-grade MCL injuries heal predictably with nonsurgical treatment, as stated at the beginning of this chapter, it is important to distinguish these from PMC injuries [23]. This is necessary because PMC injury is associated with AMRI, excessive PTT and medial opening all of which may affect long-term viability of cruciate ligament reconstruction [1, 7, 19, 21, 23]. Furthermore, it is recognized that the nonoperative management of isolated PCL injury also causes a relative change in the kinematics of the medial compartment resulting in a characteristic pattern of arthrosis. It is therefore logical that the increased PTT associated with a PMC injury may exacerbate this progression to degenerative change though there is currently no clinical evidence to support this assumption.

Operative Treatment

There are no series describing the surgical management of PCL and PMC injuries alone but small numbers of cases have been included within larger multiligament knee injury series. A wide variety of surgical techniques have been described. In addition to reconstructing the PCL, these have included repair or reattachment of the posteromedial capsular structures, reconstructing the POL, or both the POL and the MCL [1].

However, Stannard and Fanelli both advocate medial side repair and/or posteromedial capsular shift + autograft/allograft reconstruction of the POL and the evidence and rationale for this is discussed below [19, 23].

Timing of Surgery

Currently, there is no evidence regarding the timing of surgery [20]. However, Tuman et al. recommend surgery within 2 weeks of the injury in order to minimize the formation of scar tissue, maintain tissue planes, and facilitate primary repair. In those patients with chronic injuries (defined as >3 weeks since the injury), primary repair is no longer possible due to abundant scar tissue and the focus of treatment becomes restoration of range of movement prior to elective surgery [24]. When planning the timing of surgery, it is important to note that multiligament injuries repaired acutely have less articular and medial meniscal damage than do those repaired more than 1 year after the injury [7].

PCL Surgery

The surgical technique for PCL repair or reconstruction is described elsewhere in the book. A variety of techniques exist and it is reasonable for surgeons to use the procedure they are most familiar with.

Arthroscopy

In addition to PCL reconstruction, arthroscopy may be used before the open procedure to evaluate intra-articular pathology and perform debridement/meniscal repair as indicated. However, care must be taken to avoid significant fluid extravasation. Other arthroscopic findings may include posterior capsular hemorrhage, pathologic medial "meniscus rise" (meniscus lift off from the tibia during abduction stress testing at 30° flexion) and the "arthroscopic spin sign" (excessive rotation of the tibia beneath the medial meniscus) [3].

Repair Versus Reconstruction of the PMC

There are no clinical studies directly comparing repair versus reconstruction of the PMC and some authors will use both techniques together, particularly in the acute setting. However, Stannard reported failure rates of 4% (PMC reconstruction) and 20% (PMC repair). On the basis of these results, Stannard recommended reconstruction of the MCL/PMC in patients who have sustained a knee dislocation and have medial instability [21, 25].

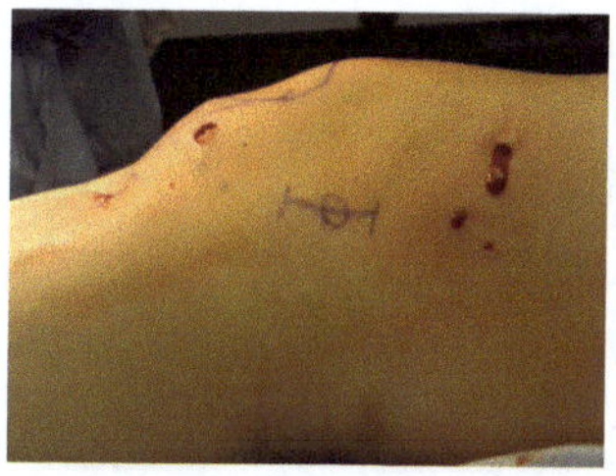

Fig. 17.3 The skin incision for MCL reconstruction described by Marx. *MCL* medial collateral ligament

What Structures to Reconstruct?

Biomechanically, it has been demonstrated that the two arms of the sMCL and the POL all have different functions. Despite this, there are insufficient clinical data in the published literature to determine whether there is any advantage in reconstructing the MCL and POL over an isolated MCL reconstruction in a PCL- injured knee [26]. However, Weimann et al. in a cadaveric biomechanical study demonstrated that reconstruction of the POL with a tendon graft improved PTT in the PCL-reconstructed knee and that supplementary reconstruction of the MCL did not provide significant improvement in knee kinematics [1].

Isolated MCL Reconstruction

Numerous techniques for isolated sMCL reconstruction have been described. As there is little clinical evidence to support one technique over another, it may be preferable to use a simple technique with small incisions. This potentially minimizes the risk of stiffness and reduces operating/tourniquet time, as well as reducing the number of tunnels and fixation devices required when compared to more complex double-bundle reconstructions [26].

Some authors have described the use of semitendinosus autograft but there is a theoretical concern that harvest can further defunction the dynamic stabilizing effect of the pes anserinus complex. If ST autograft is the preferred graft option, an alternative would be to leave the tibial attachment of semitendinosus intact; however,this is then a nonanatomical reconstruction and results in anteriorization of the normal tibial sMCL footprint and risks overtightening in higher flexion angles [26, 27]. Additional arguments for using allograft include reducing morbidity and operating time.

Marx et al. describe the use of Achilles allograft for MCL reconstruction. The graft is prepared creating a 9-mm diameter by 18-mm length bone plug. A 3-cm longitudinal skin incision is made over the medial femoral epicondyle (Fig. 17.3). A guide pin is inserted 3–5 mm proximal and posterior to the medial femoral epicondyle, parallel to the joint line, and in a 15° anterior direction to avoid the

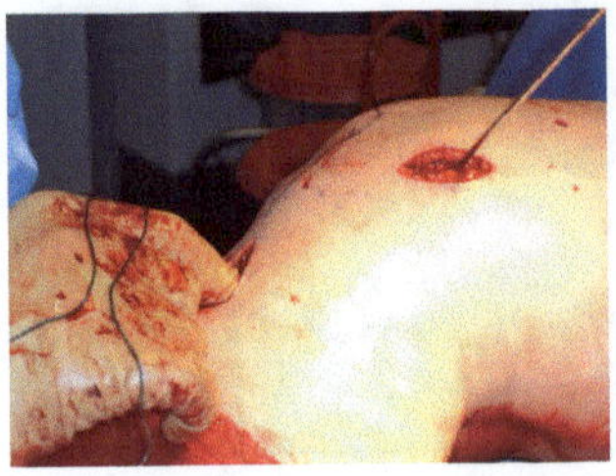

Fig. 17.4 Guidewire placement and testing for isometry by flexing and extending the knee with sutures held at the tibial footprint of the sMCL. *sMCL* superficial medial collateral ligament

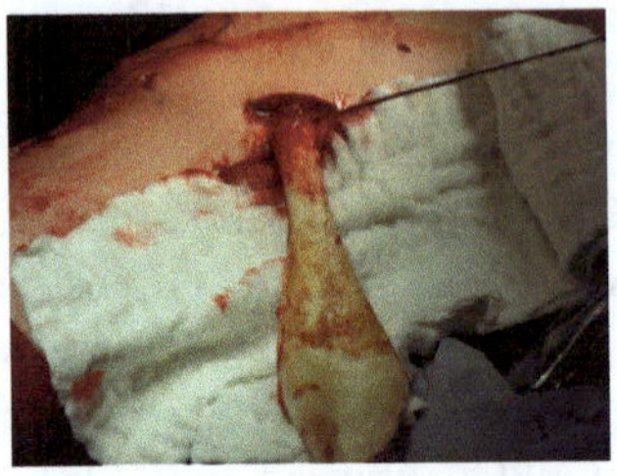

Fig. 17.5 Insertion of Achilles bone plug into femoral tunnel

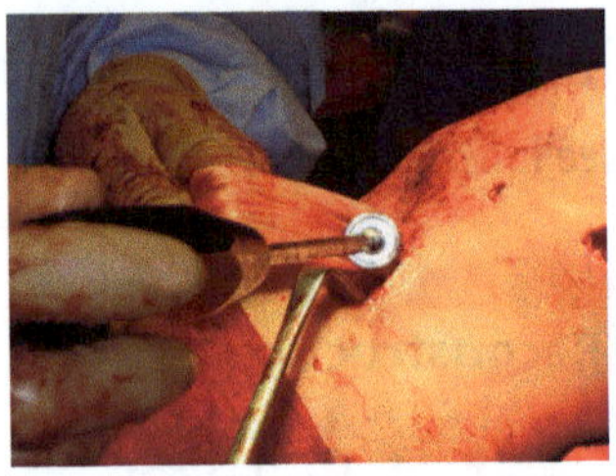

Fig. 17.6 Distal fixation of Achilles graft with screw and washer

intercondylar notch. The skin is undermined to create a tunnel from the femoral guide pin to the sMCL insertion on the tibia. A nonabsorbable suture loop is placed around the guide pin and brought distally through the tunnel and held against the tibia at the estimated anatomic insertion, just posterior to the pes anserinus insertion. Isometricity is tested through knee motion from 0 to 90° (Fig. 17.4). The guide pin is over reamed to a depth of 20 mm. The Achilles bone plug is inserted into the femoral socket and fixed with a metal interference screw (Fig. 17.5). The Achilles tendon tissue is passed through the subcutaneous tunnel and tensioned with the knee at 20° of flexion under varus stress and fixed at the isometric point on the tibia with a 4.5-mm cortical screw and a 17-mm spiked washer (Fig. 17.6). In their series, Marx et al. ($n=11$) reported that at a minimum 2-year follow-up, all reconstructed MCL grafts had a firm endpoint on valgus stress test with no or minimal side-to-side differences [28].

Acute Medial Repair Technique

Bonasia et al. described their preferred technique for repair of medial-sided injuries. This follows a logical progression of repairing from the deepest structure outward using an open technique for the medial meniscus and suture anchors/staples/screws and washers for capsular and ligamentous structures. This technique is performed with the knee held in varus and full extension. Bonasia et al. also reported that it is crucial to attempt to repair the capsular arm of semimembranosus that attaches to the POL so that the dynamic unit stabilizer effect is restored. For this, they recommend that the semimembranosus portion of the POL is sutured to the posterior border of the MCL in a pants-over-vest fashion. Despite advocating this technique, the authors agree that some medial-sided injuries may also require augmentation [20].

Capsular Re-tensioning Procedures

The goal of this technique is to remove the laxity from the injured posteromedial structures by creating increased distance between the origin and insertion. The posteromedial capsule needs to be released from the meniscus and resutured to it in a more advanced position. The proximal and distal attachments of the POL are sequentially advanced forward and slightly proximal and distal, respectively, and sutured to the intact attachments of the MCL. This is followed by mattress stitch imbrication of the mid-portion of the POL to the intact MCL. At this point, the capsular arm of the semimembranosus is identified and palpated for residual laxity. The knee is also tested with gentle valgus stress at 30° and the anteromedial drawer is tested in neutral and external rotation. If there is residual laxity present within the semimembranosus attachment, the capsular arm of the semimembranosus is advanced to the POL [20].

En masse Elevation

This procedure is indicated when a generalized laxity of the posteromedial corner is present rather than injury to an isolated structure. This can be assessed by using simple retraction on the individual structures with a meniscal hook. The structures at the weakest attachment (tibial or femoral) must be released as an entire soft tissue unit which is then re-tensioned, and fixed back to an isometric point on the bone with staples or suture anchors. If the tibial attachments are weaker, then the reattachment point for them should be advanced anteriorly and possibly inferiorly. For the femoral side, the ideal reattachment point would be posteriorly and possibly superiorly. In either case, the tissue should be repaired to a point on the femur or tibia that allows full range of motion with good stability [3, 20].

POL Reconstruction Techniques

A number of techniques have been described and there is some limited clinical outcome and biomechanical data to support them as described below.

POL Reconstruction with Autograft

The Stannard modification of the Kim procedure uses semitendinosus allograft [19, 21, 29]. This is harvested but left intact at the tibial attachment. Fluoroscopy is used to identify the isometric point for the femoral tunnel which is located at the intersection of a line drawn down the anterior aspect of the posterior femoral cortex and Blumensaat's line. The tunnel is directed approximately 30° proximally and 30° anteriorly to avoid interference with tunnels for ACL, PCL, and posterolateral corner reconstructions. A bicortical 4.5-mm screw and an 18-mm spiked ligament washer are placed at this isometric point and inserted approximately three quarters of the way in. Decortication of the femur is performed for a radius of approximately 6 mm under the washer. The semitendinosus graft is then passed around the screw and washer, under the direct head of the semimembranosus tendon, and then back to the intact insertion on the tibia. The graft is then tensioned with the knee in approximately 40° of flexion and a slight varus stress. The screw and washer are then tightened down to the femoral condyle and the graft is sutured back to the insertion of the semitendinosus using a strong permanent suture. The stability of the PMC is then assessed. If it is not as tight as desired, it can be further tightened by suturing the distal two arms of this triangular construct together in a V–Y fashion. Stannard reports good outcomes with only a 3.7 % failure rate with this technique at a minimum follow-up of 2 years [19, 21].

POL Reconstruction with Allograft

Stannard recommends using either one large tibialis anterior tendon split in half or two semitendinosus tendons. The technique is similar to the autograft technique described above. The grafts are fixed in the femoral tunnel using a biotenodesis screw with one limb representing the MCL and the other the POL. A tibial tunnel is drilled at the point of insertion of the conjoined tendon of semitendinosus and gracilis. A 4.5-mm screw with a ligament washer is placed into the drill hole and inserted three quarters of the way into the bone. The knee is then flexed approximately 40° and a slight varus stress is applied. The two grafts are passed around the screw in opposite directions and tensioned, and the 4.5-mm screw and washer are tightened securely to the tibia. Results with this technique have also been good, with only a 4.8 % failure rate in knee dislocation patients with a minimum 2-year follow-up [19, 21].

Combined PCL and MCL with Single Achilles Allograft

Wahl et al. reported a technique for single Achilles allograft MCL and PCL reconstruction. An Achilles tendon allograft is prepared with an 11- to 12-mm bone plug with a gradual taper to 7 mm over approximately 15 cm. A transtibial PCL tunnel is created under fluoroscopic and arthroscopic guidance. The femoral tunnel is prepared in an "outside-in" fashion under direct arthroscopic visualization, originating at the anatomic origin of the MCL on the medial epicondyle and entering the joint at the anatomic origin of the anterolateral bundle of the PCL. The Achilles graft is pulled into the joint through the tibial tunnel and routed into the femoral tunnel so that the soft tissue exits at the medial epicondyle. The bone plug is fluoroscopically guided to the posterior aperture of the tibial tunnel and fixed with a bioabsorbable interference screw. The pretensioned graft is fixed in the femoral tunnel via interference screw fixation with the knee in 90° of flexion. The isometric position of the MCL insertion is identified with a K-wire isometer, and the graft is fixed in place at this point by the use of an interference screw and washer. The use of a single autograft and the need for only one femoral tunnel for both reconstructions is appealing; however, no clinical results have been reported with this technique so far [30].

Combined Anatomical MCL and POL Reconstruction

The LaPrade technique consists of a reconstruction of the sMCL and POL using two separate grafts with four reconstruction tunnels. An anteromedial incision is made along the medial knee and located proximally between the medial border of the patella and the medial epicondyle. The sMCL and POL femoral tunnels are reamed to a depth of 30 mm over eyelet guide pins directed anterolaterally across the femur. A 16-cm semitendinosus graft is passed into the sMCL tunnel and a 12-cm graft is used for the POL and secured with bioabsorbable screws. The tibial fixation tunnels for the distal sMCL and POL anatomical attachment points are reamed to a depth of 30 mm. The distal sMCL tibial tunnel is reamed first. It is important to ensure that the eyelet pin for this tunnel is placed along the posterior edge of the distal sMCL footprint because grafts placed too anterior tend to result in overtightening in higher flexion angles. Next, an eyelet pin is drilled anterolaterally through the center of the tibial attachment of the central arm of the POL, which exits just distal and medial to Gerdy's tubercle. The sMCL graft is then passed laterally through the distal sMCL tunnel, and recessed to a depth of 25 mm. The knee is placed in 30° of flexion, neutral rotation, and a manual varus force is applied to reduce any gapping of the medial compartment. The sMCL reconstruction graft is then tensioned by placing a manual lateral traction force to tighten the graft into the tibial tunnel via a No. 2 nonabsorbable suture, and secured in place with a bioabsorbable screw at the distal aperture of the tunnel. The knee is then placed through a full passive range of motion to verify proper positioning of the sMCL graft. Once proper positioning is verified, the proximal tibial attachment point of the sMCL, which is primarily to soft tissues and located just distal to the joint line is recreated by suturing the sMCL graft to the anterior arm of the semimembranosus muscle. Finally, the POL graft is secured into its tunnels. The POL graft is passed into the tibial tunnel and recessed to a depth of 25 mm. The knee is held in extension and neutral rotation with a varus force applied. The graft is manually tensioned by placing an anterolateral traction force on the No. 2 nonabsorbable suture, and secured into position with a 7-mm bioabsorbable screw placed at the distal aperture of the tunnel. Biomechanical analysis has shown that this reconstruction technique restores native stability. Prospective clinical outcome studies are currently in progress to evaluate the use of this reconstruction technique in vivo [27].

Order of Graft Tensioning and Fixation

It is recommended that the PCL reconstruction is performed first without tensioning or fixation of the graft on one side (e.g., the femoral side if an inlay technique is used), followed by reconstruction of the MCL/PMC again without fixing. Once the PMC graft is in place, the PCL is tensioned and fixed. The final step is fixation of the PMC graft [19, 23].

Postoperative Rehabilitation

There is little consensus on the best way to rehabilitate a knee following PCL and PMC/POL repair or reconstruction. Bonasia et al. recommended that the patient be kept in a hinged knee brace with protected weight bearing for 6 weeks and restriction of motion to between 0 and 90° for 2 weeks [7], whereas Fanelli and Marx both advocate that the knee is braced in full extension and non-weight bearing for a number of weeks followed by progressive range of movement and full weight bearing around 6 weeks postoperatively.

Graft Choice

Both allograft and autograft are acceptable choices but when reconstructing a multiligament-injured knee, it is beneficial to reduce morbidity and thus allograft may be favored. Another advantage of allograft is that it avoids disrupting the pes anserinus complex which has a role as a secondary medial stabilizer of the knee [1, 19, 23].

Areas for Further Study

There is considerable potential for further study. There are no published series reporting comprehensive clinical results or patient-reported outcome measures for combined PCL and PMC injuries. In part, this is due to the rarity of these injuries and the consequently small numbers in single-institution case series. In order to address this deficiency, future studies would benefit from a multicenter design or from the use of ligament registry data. Ligament registries have the added advantages of allowing recognition of trends in practice, helping track new developments, identifying techniques that may have suboptimal outcomes, and providing externally valid outcome data that would enable surgeons to better advise patients on expectations and prognosis.

Conclusions

There appears to be a high incidence of unrecognized injury to the posteromedial corner particularly in the multiligament-injured knee. Failure to address this can result in failure of cruciate ligament reconstruction. Although a number of surgical techniques have been described, the current trend is toward a combined PCL–POL reconstruction. Biomechanical study supports this strategy but clinical outcomes have not been well reported.

References

1. Weimann A, Schatka I, Herbort M, Achtnich A, Zantop T, Raschke M, Petersen W. Reconstruction of the posterior oblique ligament and the posterior cruciate ligament in knees with posteromedial instability. Arthroscopy (J Arthrosc Relat Surg). 2012;28(9):1283–9.
2. Chahal J, Al-Taki M, Pearce D, Leibenberg A, Whelan DB. Injury patterns to the posteromedial corner of the knee in high-grade multiligament knee injuries: a MRI study. Knee Surg Sports Traumatol Arthrosc. 2010;18(8):1098–104.
3. Jackson JB, Ferguson CM, Martin DF. Surgical treatment of chronic posteromedial instability using capsular procedures. Sports Med Arthrosc Rev. 2006;14(2):91–5.
4. Cohen M, Astur DC, Branco RC, de Souza Campos Fernandes R, Kaleka CC, Arliani GG, Jalikjian W, Golano P. An anatomical three-dimensional study of the posteromedial corner of the knee. Knee Surg Sports Traumatol Arthrosc. 2011;19(10):1614–9.
5. Petersen W, Loerch S, Schanz S, Raschke M, Zantop T. The role of the posterior oblique ligament in controlling posterior tibial translation in the posterior cruciate ligament-deficient knee. Am J Sports Med. 2008;36(3):495–501.
6. Geiger D, Chang E, Pathria M, Chung CB. Posterolateral and posteromedial corner injuries of the knee. Radiol Clin North Am. 2013;51(3):413–32.
7. Tibor LM, Marchant MH Jr, Taylor DC, Hardaker WT Jr, Garrett WE Jr, Sekiya JK. Management of medial-sided knee injuries, part 2: posteromedial corner. Am J Sports Med. 2011;39(6):1332–40.
8. Strobel MJ, Schulz MS, Petersen WJ, Eichhorn HJ. Combined anterior cruciate ligament, posterior cruciate ligament, and posterolateral corner reconstruction with autogenous hamstring grafts in chronic instabilities. Arthroscopy. 2006;22(2):182–192.

9. Warren LF, Marshall JL, Girgis F. The prime static stabilizer of the medial side of the knee. J Bone Joint Surg Am. 1974;56:665–74.
10. Robinson JR, Sanchez-Ballester J, Bull AMJ, Thomas RdeW, Amis AA. The posteromedial corner revisited: an anatomic description of the passive restraining structures of the medial aspect of the human knee. J Bone Joint Surg Br. 2004;86:674–81.
11. Brantigan OC, Voshell AF. The tibial collateral ligament: its function, its bursae, and its relation to the medial meniscus. J Bone Joint Surg. 1943;25:121–31.
12. LaPrade RF, Engebretsen AH, Ly TV, Johansen S, Wentorf FA, Engebretsen L. The anatomy of the medial part of the knee. J Bone Joint Surg Am. 2007;89:2000–10.
13. Sims WF, Jacobson KE. The posteromedial corner of the knee: medial-sided injury patterns revisited. Am J Sports Med. 2004;32(2):337–45.
14. House CV, Connell DA, Saifuddin A. Posteromedial corner injuries of the knee. Clin Radiol. 2007;62:539–46.
15. Wijdicks CA, Griffith CJ, Johansen S, Engebretsen L, LaPrade RF. Injuries to the medial collateral ligament and associated medial structures of the knee. J Bone Joint Surg Am. 2010;92:1266–80.
16. Amis AA, Bull AMJ, Gupte CM, Hijazi I, Race A, Robinson JR. Biomechanics of the PCL and related structures: posterolateral, posteromedial and meniscofemoral ligaments. Knee Surg Sports Traumatol Arthrosc. 2003;11:271–81.
17. Fanelli CF. Posterior cruciate ligament injuries in trauma patients. Arthroscopy. 1993;9:291–94.
18. Fanelli GC, Giannotti BF, Edson CJ. Arthroscopically assisted combined posterior cruciate ligament/posterior lateral complex reconstruction. Arthroscopy. 1996;12(5):521–30.
19. Bauer KL, Stannard JP. Surgical approach to the posteromedial corner: indications, technique, outcomes. Curr Rev Musculoskelet Med. 2013;6(2):124–31.
20. Bonasia DE, Bruzzone M, Dettoni F, Marmotti A, Blonna D, Castoldi F, Gasparetto F, D'Elicio D, Collo G, Rossi R. Treatment of medial and posteromedial knee instability: indications, techniques, and review of the results. Iowa Orthop J. 2012;32:173–83.
21. Stannard JP. Medial and posteromedial instability of the knee: evaluation, treatment, and results. Sports Med Arthrosc Rev. 2010;18(4):263–8.
22. Garavaglia G, Lubbeke A, Dubois-Ferriere V, Suva D, Fritschy D, Menetrey J. Accuracy of stress radiography techniques in grading isolated and combined posterior knee injuries: a cadaveric study. Am J Sports Med. 2007;35:2051–6.
23. Fanelli GC, Harris JD. Surgical treatment of acute medial collateral ligament and posteromedial corner injuries of the knee. Sports Med Arthrosc. 2006;14(2):78–83.
24. Tuman JM, Miller MD. Surgical treatment of combined PCL medial side injuries: acute and chronic. In: Fanelli GC, editor. The multiple ligament injured knee. 2nd ed. New York: Springer; 2013. pp. 227–38.
25. Stannard JP, Black BS, Azbell C, Volgas DA. Posteromedial corner injury in knee dislocations. J Knee Surg. 2012;25(5):429–34.
26. Kitamura N, Ogawa M, Kondo E, Kitayama S, Tohyama H, Yasuda K. A novel medial collateral ligament reconstruction procedure using semitendinosus tendon autograft in patients with multiligamentous knee injuries clinical outcomes. Am J Sports Med. 2013;41(6):1274–81.
27. Coobs BR, Wijdicks CA, Armitage BM, Spiridonov SI, Westerhaus BD, Johansen S, Engebretsen L, LaPrade RF. An in vitro analysis of an anatomical medial knee reconstruction. Am J Sports Med. 2010;38(2):339–47.
28. Marx RG, Hestroni I. Surgical technique: medial collateral ligament reconstruction using Achilles allograft for combined knee ligament injury. Clin Orthop Relat Res. 2012;470:798–805.
29. Kim SJ, Lee DH, Kim TE, Choi NH. Concomitant reconstruction of the medial collateral and posterior oblique ligaments for medial instability of the knee. J Bone Joint Surg Br. 2008;90:1323–27.
30. Wahl CJ, Nicandri G. Single–Achilles allograft posterior cruciate ligament and medial collateral ligament reconstruction: a technique to avoid osseous tunnel intersection, improve construct stiffness, and save on allograft utilization. J Arthrosc Relat Surg. 2008;24(4):486–89.

Combined PCL, Posteromedial Corner, and Posterolateral Corner Reconstruction

18

Clayton W. Nuelle and James P. Stannard

Introduction

Knee dislocations are significant orthopedic injuries that result in damage to multiple knee ligaments. The mechanism of injury can be from an athletic injury, but more frequently results from a high-energy blunt trauma, such as motor vehicle collision. In the majority of cases, knee dislocations may be spontaneously reduced prior to presentation to the emergency room, but they still sustain significant injury to the structures within and around the joint [1–3].

Various studies have demonstrated the benefits and pitfalls of repair versus reconstruction of injured ligaments and acute versus delayed operative management after multiple ligament injuries. Multiple studies have shown the benefit of reconstruction of the posteromedial corner (PMC) and posterolateral corner (PLC), in particular, in high-grade ligamentous injuries [4–8]. Multiple patient factors, such as associated injuries to neurovascular structures, the degree of injury to the surrounding skin, and the spectrum of ligament injury, must be taken into account when formulating a treatment plan. Clinical outcomes following these multi-ligament injuries may be poor, with arthrofibrosis, recurrent instability, and persistent pain being common complications [9–12]. Acute versus delayed operative management seeks to achieve early ligamentous stability in an effort to promote early mobilization, with the definition of early mobilization varying from 1 day to approximately 4 weeks after surgery. Many authors prefer early operative treatment and rehabilitation in an effort to achieve early ligamentous stability and joint mobilization [6, 12–14]. An early operative intervention allows early mobilization, which may result in less scar tissue formation and improved final range of motion. A potential risk of acute surgery is a skin envelope that has not had time to completely recover and may have a higher risk for postoperative wound infections.

For active patients who have sustained a knee dislocation with three or four ligament injuries, we recommend a repair or reconstruction within 2–4 weeks to allow early mobilization of the knee. The ideal timing for surgery is not clear in the literature, and may sometimes be dictated by patient comorbidities and associated injuries. Surgeons may choose to repair or reconstruct all torn ligaments at one surgery or may delay the anterior cruciate ligament (ACL) reconstruction after early reconstruction and rehabilitation of the posterior cruciate ligament (PCL), PMC, and PLC. The preferred technique of the senior author incorporates an early reconstruction of the PCL, PMC, and PLC, followed by an ACL reconstruction approximately 6 weeks later. Numerous techniques for each type of reconstruction have been described, but regardless of technique, a successful reconstruction of a combined PCL, PMC, and PLC may be achieved in a single operation.

Surgical Treatment

Preoperative Planning

Appropriate preoperative planning is vital to successful management of a multiligament knee reconstruction. Patients with an abnormal vascular exam or severe soft tissue injury should be delayed from ligament repair or reconstruction and may benefit from a spanning external fixator across the knee until a clean, closed wound and soft tissue envelope can be achieved. An adequate magnetic resonance imaging (MRI) scan should be obtained, if possible, to fully evaluate the degree of ligamentous and soft tissue injury. After these assessments are complete, a plan may be formulated for repair versus reconstruction of ligaments, the timing of surgery, the order in which each ligament may be reconstructed, and an assessment of any further surgeries that may be required.

J. P. Stannard (✉)
Missouri Orthopaedic Institute, Department of Orthopaedic Surgery, University of Missouri, Columbia, MO 65212, USA
e-mail: stannardj@health.missouri.edu

C. W. Nuelle
Orthopaedics, University of Missouri-Columbia, Columbia, MO, USA

G. C. Fanelli (ed.), *Posterior Cruciate Ligament Injuries*,
DOI 10.1007/978-3-319-12072-0_18, © Springer International Publishing Switzerland 2015

Repair versus reconstruction may be dictated by degree of injury and surgeon preference, but for the highly unstable dislocations resulting in Anatomical Classification of Knee Dislocation (KD)-III or IV ligament injuries, studies have shown benefit to multiligament reconstruction rather than repair [15–20]. Autograft or allograft reconstructions may be performed, but primarily allograft is chosen in the multiligament knee to protect as much of the uninjured native anatomy surrounding the knee joint and because of the number of grafts needed to complete reconstruction. Numerous allograft options exist, including Achilles tendon, anterior and posterior tibialis tendons, quadriceps tendon, patellar tendon, and hamstring tendon. Allograft choice should be made based on the number of ligaments being reconstructed and the planned reconstruction techniques. For certain techniques, such as a two-tailed PLC reconstruction, it is vital to obtain a graft that will have plenty of length to complete the reconstruction. For others, such a tibial inlay technique for a PCL reconstruction, an adequate bone block at the end of the tendon is required to complete the procedure. Regardless of the technique chosen, these factors must be taken into account preoperatively to ensure a successful outcome during the operation.

When considering operative treatment of a combined PCL, PMC, and PLC injury, numerous reconstruction techniques exist. For the PCL, these may include an open or arthroscopic tibial inlay technique, an open or arthroscopic transtibial technique, an all-inside arthroscopic technique, a suspensory tension technique, and a single- or double-bundle reconstruction.

For the posteromedial corner, reconstructions utilizing one or two tails with single or multiple fixation tunnels on the femur and tibia exist. The anatomy of the medial side of the knee and an anatomic reconstruction has been described by LaPrade [21–23]. This particular technique incorporates two separate grafts with four separate graft tunnels (two each on the femur and tibia), with one graft reconstructing the superficial medial collateral ligament (MCL) and the second reconstructing the posterior oblique ligament (POL). The preferred technique of the senior author is similar in that it utilizes two separate grafts, but different in that it creates only two separate bone sockets (one on the femur and one on the tibia) for graft fixation. This technique still results in an anatomic reconstruction, but is greatly beneficial in a multiple ligament knee reconstruction as it results in less bone loss from tunnel or socket creation. This is extremely valuable when other tunnels or sockets must be created for multiple ligament reconstructions.

For the PLC, a two-tailed, a figure-of-eight, or a popliteus muscle reconstruction are some of the most commonly described techniques. The indications, benefits, and pitfalls of each of these individual techniques are detailed in other chapters and thus will not be discussed here.

In the setting of a multiple ligament knee reconstruction, knee stability is paramount, but it is also beneficial to begin early range of motion in order to prevent arthrofibrosis and a stiff knee. In this regard, when performing reconstructions of three or four ligaments, particularly in a staged fashion, consideration may be given to placing a compass knee hinge (CKH; Smith and Nephew, Memphis, Tennessee). The CKH is a hinged external fixator that incorporates fixator Schanz pins in multiple planes on both sides of the knee joint, providing excellent stability while allowing sagittal plane motion. This combination results in minimal rotational stress placed on the reconstructed ligaments, allowing the patient to begin early weight bearing and knee range of motion without sacrificing ligament stability. Multiple studies have documented the use of the CKH in the setting of ligament reconstruction after knee dislocation, including a randomized controlled trial that showed decreased ligament reconstruction failures with the use of the hinge versus knee bracing alone [24–28]. The CKH functions as an excellent adjunct to multiple ligament reconstruction and may be especially beneficial in the setting of type IV or type V knee dislocations, fracture dislocation, chronic dislocation, or preoperative flexion deformity of >15°. It should be considered during the preoperative planning of combined ligament reconstructions, particularly in the setting of multiple simultaneous ligament reconstructions or staged operations.

Operative Technique for a Combined PCL, PMC, and PLC Reconstruction

Author's Preferred Technique

For a combined PCL, PMC, and PLC reconstruction in a single procedure, the senior author employs a tibial inlay technique for the PCL, a modified loop reconstruction for the PMC, and modified two-tailed reconstruction for the PLC. In addition to the reconstructions, consideration is frequently given to placement of a CKH as well. An Achilles allograft with a bone block is typically utilized for the PCL, an anterior or posterior tibialis or semitendinosus allograft for the PMC, and an anterior or posterior tibialis allograft for the PLC. It is vital to obtain grafts of adequate length (>27 cm) for the PLC, to ensure the entire reconstruction may be performed and the graft does not end up short. Prior to beginning the open surgical approaches, an examination under anesthesia is performed, followed by a diagnostic knee arthroscopy to assess the overall injury to the joint. Repair or resection of any damaged articular cartilage fragments or menisci may then be subsequently performed. In addition, the remaining ACL and/or PCL stumps may be debrided to visualize the corresponding footprints. The open medial approach to the knee, as described by Burks and Berg, is then utilized as the first step, as open treatment of the PCL and the PMC can be easily accessed via this approach [29, 30]. The PCL is subsequently reconstructed but not tensioned, followed by the PMC (again not yet tensioned) and finally a posterolateral approach to the knee is utilized to reconstruct the posterolateral corner. A key point is that none of the grafts are tensioned, however, until all of the grafts are in position, so as to ensure equal graft tensioning and forces across the knee. The exact techniques utilized for each reconstruction, in particular the ACL and PCL, are not as vital as the operating surgeon being comfortable using their preferred techniques when managing these complex injuries.

Anatomy and Posteromedial Approach to the Knee

The PMC of the knee comprises the structures between the posterior border of the superficial MCL and the medial border of the PCL. This includes the POL, semimembranosus (SM) tendon with its multiple insertions, the oblique popliteal ligament (OPL), and the posterior horn of the medial meniscus, with the medial head of the gastrocnemius also providing support (Fig. 18.1) [31, 32]. A layer system to the approach to PMC has been described using Roman numerals I, II, and III [33]. Layer I is the most superficial layer, with the deeper layers being II and III. Layer I is composed of the patellar retinaculum and sartorius fascia, with the gracilis and semitendinosus tendons located between layers I and II. Layer II is composed of the MCL, SM and POL. Layer III is composed of the deep MCL, joint capsule, and coronary ligament.

For the initial posteromedial approach to the knee, the patient is positioned supine on a flat operating room table. The incision is made along a line from the medial epicondyle to the insertion of the MCL along the posteromedial border of the tibia and the posterior aspect of the MCL. The knee should be flexed to approximately 70° and in the "figure-of-four" position for the deeper portions of the approach. Keeping the knee in this position relaxes the posterior neurovascular bundle and helps to avoid complications. Electrocautery may be used initially, followed by blunt dissection with Metzenbaum scissors to identify individual anatomic structures. The saphenous vein and nerve should be identified and protected if encountered, as injury has can frequently occur (Fig. 18.2). The sartorius fascia is exposed and incised in line with the incision and the pes anserinus tendons are identified and retracted distally. The fascia between the SM and medial head of the gastrocnemius is then identified and incised in line with the incision. The SM has multiple variable insertion points and occasionally requires release at its insertion along the medial aspect of the joint capsule, where it can be tagged for later repair. The medial head of the gastrocnemius should then be identified. This is an important step as the remainder of the approach remains anterior to this muscle, staying right

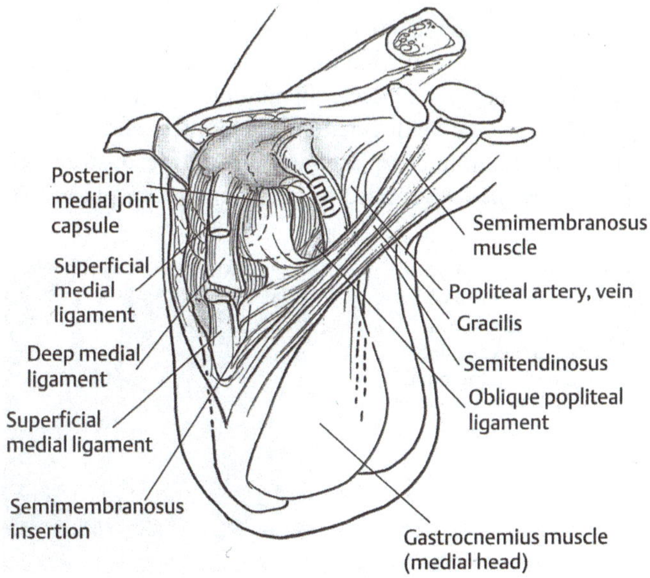

Fig. 18.1 Illustration depicting the anatomy of the posteromedial structures of the knee. (From [43]. Reprinted with permission from Thieme Publishers)

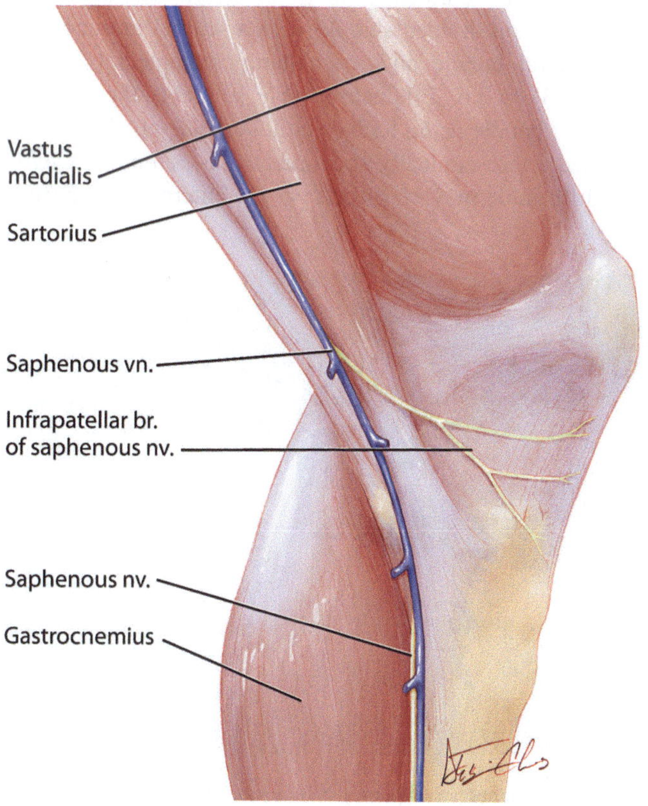

Fig. 18.2 Illustration depicting the anatomy of the saphenous vein and nerve in relation to the posteromedial structures of the knee

on the posterior aspect of the proximal tibia and as close to the medial femoral condyle as possible. The medial head of the gastrocnemius is not typically released and all retractors should remain anterior and anterior to the popliteus muscle which is elevated directly off of the posterior tibia. Staying right on the bone and anterior to popliteus and gastrocnemius allows the surgeon to avoid injury to the posterior neurovascular structures. A Cobb or similar smooth instrument may be utilized to aid the dissection posterior to the joint capsule. The joint line should repeatedly be isolated so as not to dissect too far distally on the posterior tibial condyle. In the setting of a knee dislocation, the capsular structures may be completely disrupted, altering the normal anatomy posterior to the knee but also allowing direct exposure to the joint itself.

PCL Reconstruction

An anatomical PCL reconstruction combines the tibial inlay and two femoral tunnel techniques [34–37]. An Achilles tendon allograft is initially prepared on the back table, trimming the bone block to a length of 20 mm, a width of 15 mm, and a thickness of 10 mm, for a 20 × 15 × 10-mm inlay graft. It is necessary to have an adequate size bone block that is not too thin, as it could fracture when the screw is used to stabilize the bone block in the tibial trough. The tendinous portion is then divided sharply with a scalpel into a larger anterolateral bundle and a smaller posteromedial bundle (Fig. 18.3). A no. 2 nonabsorbable suture is then placed into each bundle using Krakow stitches. The notch is again debrided arthroscopically and, once this is complete, a femoral drill guide may be placed via the anteromedial portal.

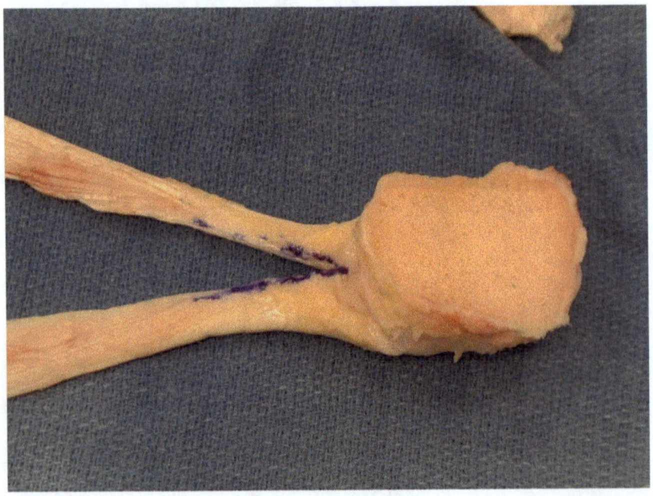

Fig. 18.3 Intraoperative photograph demonstrating the preparation of an Achilles tendon allograft for use in a posterior cruciate ligament reconstruction. (From [43]. Reprinted with permission from Thieme Publishers)

A guidewire is then drilled from outside-in approximately 10 mm from the articular surface as high in the notch as possible to represent the anterolateral tunnel. A second guidewire may then be placed inferior to the first, approximately 8 mm from the articular surface and far enough to allow at least a 4-mm bone bridge between tunnels (Fig. 18.4). Drilling of the anterolateral and posteromedial guidewires should be completed under direct visualization to ensure there is no change in the notch position during drilling. Each tunnel is subsequently reamed to its appropriate size. The tunnel sizes are determined by the size of the Achilles tendon allograft, with a goal of 8–9 mm for the anterolateral tunnel and 6–7 mm for the posteromedial tunnel. A shaver may be placed down the tunnels to remove any bony debris and to debride periosteum at the tunnel openings along the medial condyle to facilitate later screw placement. A nitinol wire is subsequently placed and each tunnel is tapped, respectively. If a 7- or 8-mm tunnel is reamed then either the same size or one size larger tap is utilized, depending on the bone quality.

A trough site similar in size to the bone block is then created in the posterior tibia, extending from approximately a centimeter distal to the posterior joint line and centered over the midline of the posterior tibia at the insertion site of the PCL. The trough may be created using a rongeur or small osteotomes, such as a 0.5-inch osteotome (Fig. 18.5). A blunt retractor, such as a Hohman, may be placed anterior to the popliteus and gastrocnemius across the posterior aspect of the tibia prior to making the trough to help retract the posterior structures. The knee may be flexed to 90° and the ankle externally rotated to aid in visualization of the posterior tibia. A 4.5-mm drill hole is drilled in the center of the bone block in a slightly oblique orientation from posteromedial to anterolateral. The block is subsequently fixed in the trough with a single 4.5-mm cannulated screw and washer (Fig. 18.6). A guidewire is initially utilized to hold the bone block in place and aimed at the tibial tubercle. In multiple ligament injuries, the guidewire may be directed more obliquely and laterally to avoid the tibial tunnel placement for ACL reconstruction. Fluoroscopy may be utilized to check guidewire placement

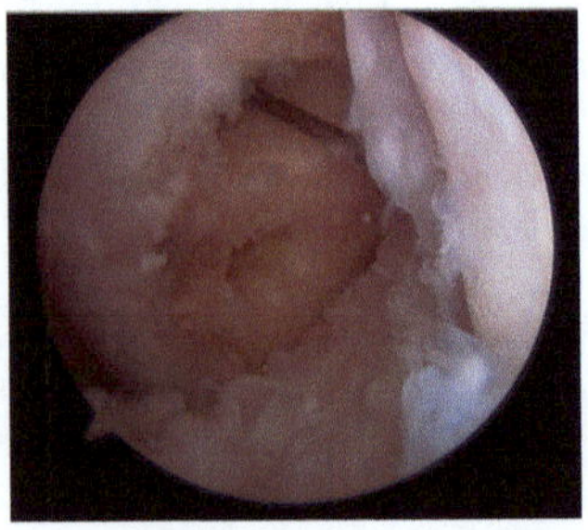

Fig. 18.4 Intraoperative photograph demonstrating the anterolateral and posteromedial tunnels drilled through the medial femoral condyle for a PCL reconstruction. PCL posterior cruciate ligament

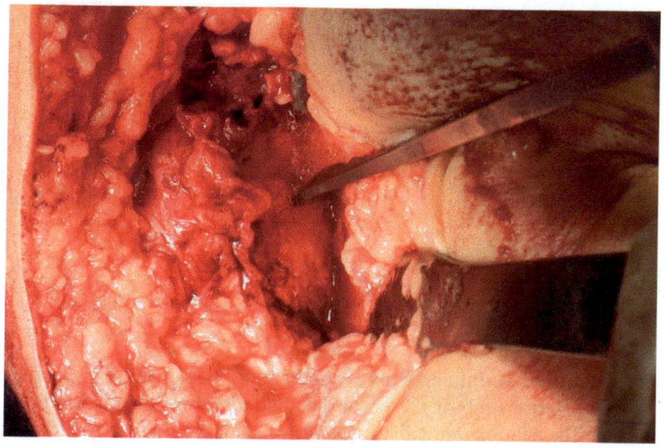

Fig. 18.5 Intraoperative photograph demonstrating preparation of the trough with an osteotome at the posterior aspect of the tibia for an inlay PCL reconstruction. PCL posterior cruciate ligament

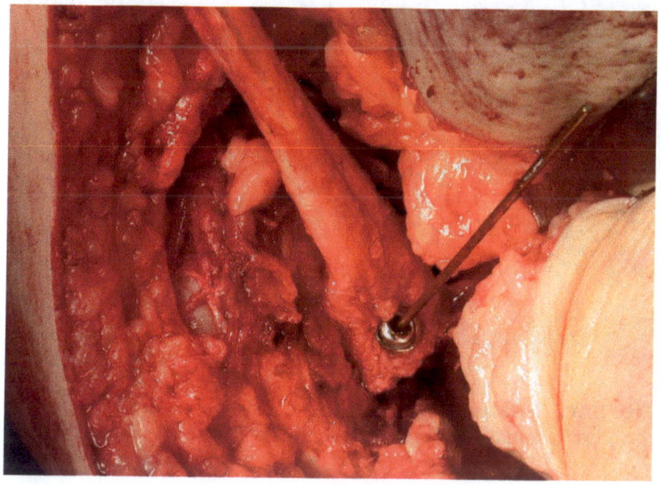

Fig. 18.6 Intraoperative photograph demonstrating cannulated screw fixation of the tibial inlay bone block for a PCL reconstruction. PCL posterior cruciate ligament

and depth. A measurement may be taken directly from the guidewire, taking 8–10 mm off the measured depth for the screw length. The 4.5-mm screw and washer are then placed directly over the guidewire using lag technique (Fig. 18.7). Ideally, the bone block will be flush with the posterior tibia or just slightly proud, but not countersunk. A hole in the posterior capsule may then be made with a Kelly or similar pointed instrument (if posterior capsular damage is not already present from the dislocation) and the two bundles are advanced into the notch. This is accomplished with the aid of a Hewson suture passer, passed in the anteromedial portal, through the notch and out the posterior capsule. Graft passage is then completed under direct arthroscopic visualization. A small arthroscopic grasper is placed retrograde through the femoral tunnels and utilized to pass each graft,

Fig. 18.7 Lateral radiograph demonstrating screw fixation of the tibial bone block for a PCL reconstruction PCL posterior cruciate ligament

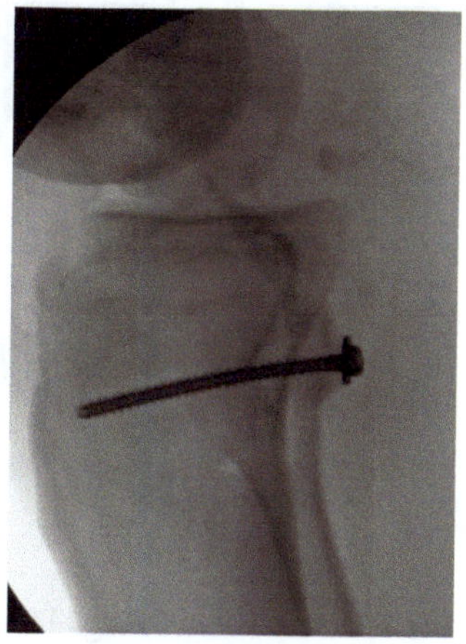

starting with the smaller, posteromedial bundle first. When passing the anterolateral graft, ensure that it remains on the lateral side of the previously passed posteromedial graft. A guidewire is again placed retrograde into each tunnel and the grafts are secured with absorbable interference screws the same size as was previously tapped. The anterolateral bundle should be tensioned at approximately 80° of flexion and the posteromedial tensioned at approximately 10° of flexion when final tensioning is performed.

PMC Reconstruction

The senior author's preferred technique for a PMC reconstruction in the setting of a combined ligament reconstruction utilizes either two semitendinosus grafts or one anterior or posterior tibialis allografts split in half to recreate the triangle of the MCL, POL, and the SM sling. The most preferable technique incorporates two semitendinosus allografts [38]. The grafts may be initially prepared with Krackow (or fiberloop) locking stitches placed at each end of both the grafts. The posteromedial dissection will have already been completed as described above. The isometric point of the knee is then found, either anatomically or radiographically. The radiographic method has been shown to have increased accuracy and is subsequently the method of choice of the senior author [39]. This is accomplished by obtaining a perfect lateral view of the knee using the fluoroscope, lining up the posterior femoral condyles. The isometric point is located where the extension of the posterior femoral cortical line intersects Blumensaat's line (Fig. 18.8). The isometric point is the starting point for guide pin placement in the medial femoral condyle. A threaded guide pin may then be placed from medial to lateral. A cannulated reamer is placed over the guide pin to ream an 8 × 25-mm socket. An 8-mm absorbable biotenodesis screw (Arthrex, Naples, FL) is fixed to one end of each graft, forming two separate limbs, and placed in

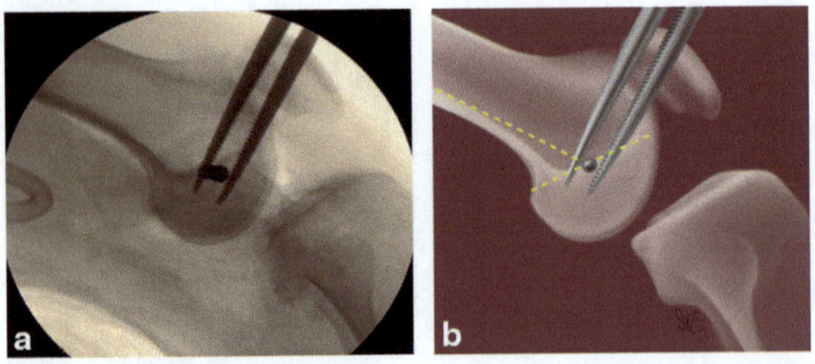

Fig. 18.8 **a** Lateral radiograph and **b** illustration demonstrating the isometric point of the knee

the femoral socket (Fig. 18.9). The tibial insertion site may then be prepared by using a rongeur to debride away the soft tissue just proximal and posterior to the insertion of the semitendinosus, all the way to bone. A 3.2-mm drill bit is utilized to drill a bicortical drill hole across the tibia in preparation for a 4.5-mm screw with a spiked ligament washer. The metal tibial screw and washer are provisionally placed, but not tightened all the way down to bone. A Kelly instrument is then passed deep to the SM from distal to proximal and the free end of the posterior limb of the graft is passed distally to the tibia (Fig. 18.10). The other free end of the graft (the anterior portion) is then passed directly inferior from its femoral insertion distally to the tibial screw in line with the MCL. Each limb of the graft is then passed around the tibial screw, beneath the washer, and a Cobb elevator is subsequently utilized to compress the tibial washer down while the screw is placed the rest of the way down and the graft is appropriately tensioned (Fig. 18.11). The screw is not compressed all the way down, however, until final tensioning is ready to be performed. This procedure reconstructs the superficial MCL (anterior limb of the graft) and the POL (posterior limb) (Fig. 18.12). The graft may tensioned at 30–40°of knee flexion, but again, not until all grafts for all reconstructions are in place. When the graft is finally tensioned, it should be isometric in flexion and extension. The remaining graft ends

Fig. 18.9 Intraoperative photograph demonstrating proximal posteromedial corner graft fixation to the medial femoral condyle with a biotenodesis screw

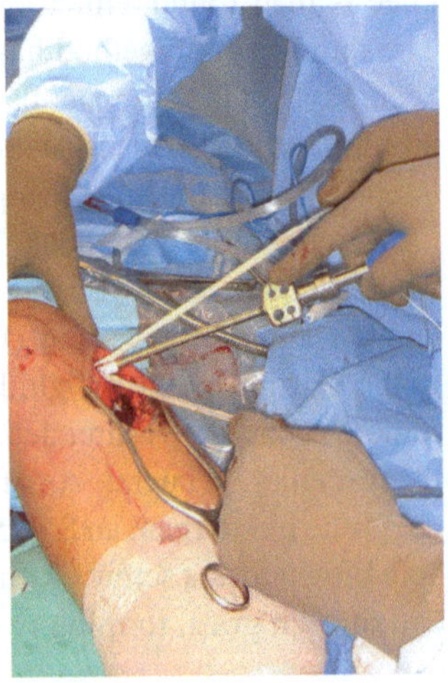

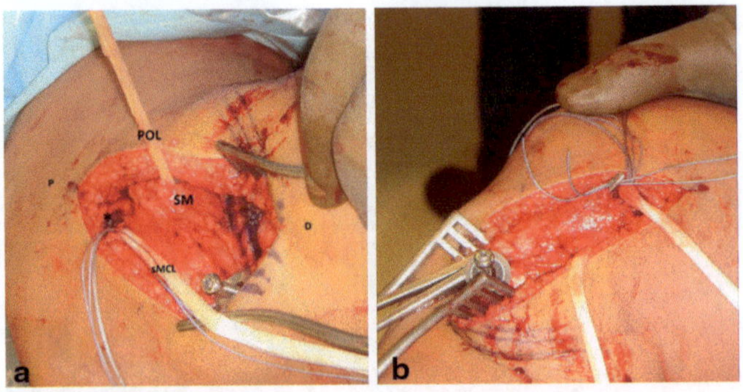

Fig. 18.10 **a**, **b** Intraoperative photographs demonstrating passing of the posterior limb of the posteromedial corner reconstruction graft beneath the semimembranosus. (*asterisk* isometric point, *P* proximal, *D* distal, *sMCL* superficial MCL, *POL* posterior oblique ligament, *SM* semimembranosus)

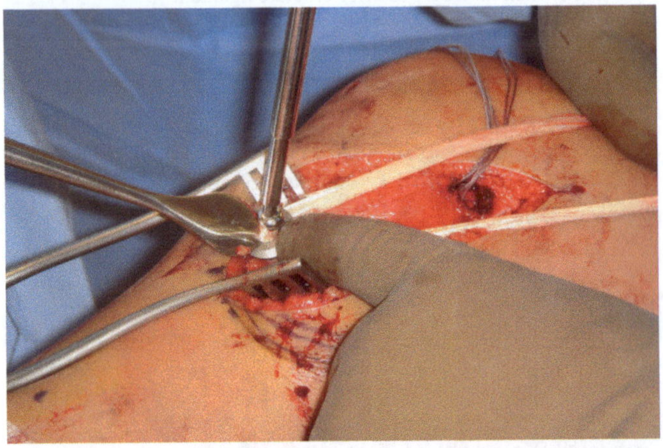

Fig. 18.11 Intraoperative photograph demonstrating distal fixation of the posteromedial corner graft to the tibia with a screw and washer

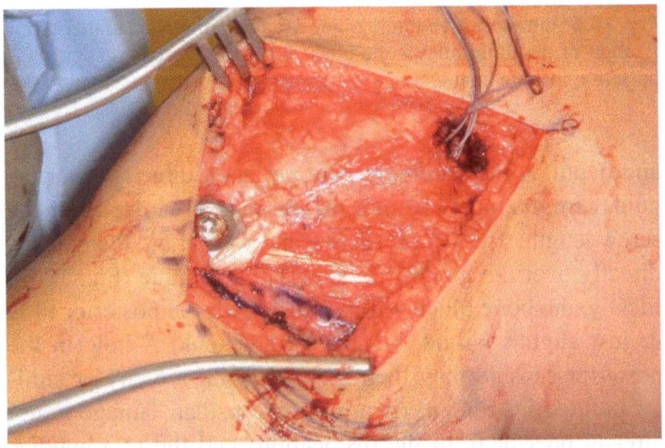

Fig. 18.12 Intraoperative photograph demonstrating the completed posteromedial corner reconstruction

may be sutured together and sutured to the fixed graft using figure of eight stitches and then cut sharply to remove any excess graft material (Fig. 18.12). Attention is subsequently turned to the lateral side of the knee.

Posterolateral Approach and PLC Reconstruction

The PLC is primarily composed of: the fibular (lateral) collateral ligament, the popliteus muscle and tendon, the popliteofibular ligament, the lateral capsule, and variable structures such as the arcuate ligament and the fabellofibular ligament [40, 41]. Similar to the medial side of the knee, the lateral approach has been described in layers: Layer I is composed of the iliotibial tract and the biceps femoris. Layer II is composed of the patellar retinaculum and patellofemoral ligament and layer III is composed of the lateral collateral ligament (LCL), fabellofibular ligament, arcuate ligament, popliteus tendon, popliteofibular ligament, and the joint capsule (Fig. 18.13). It is important to note that the common peroneal nerve typically lies between layers I and II. This nerve must always be isolated prior to deep joint exposure to prevent inadvertent injury. In order to relax and protect the nerve, the approach is best performed with the knee flexed. The incision is placed in line with the fibular head and continues in a straight line proximally. When proximally extended the incision may be carried out between the iliotibial band and biceps femoris tendon. The dissection is taken down to deep fascia with electrocautery, then careful dissection of the peroneal nerve is performed utilizing Metzenbaum scissors. The nerve can typically be palpated and isolated just proximal and posterior to the fibula and then released distally where it curves around the fibula in the soft spot just distal to the fibular head (Fig. 18.14). Once the nerve is identified, it may be protected with a vessel loop or a Penrose drain. The ends of the vessel loop or Penrose drain may be stapled together, but do not clamp or hang any instruments from them, as excessive retraction of the nerve from a hanging instrument can result in a neurapraxia. Blunt dissection is then utilized to establish the plane anterior to the lateral gastrocnemius head. In multiple ligament injuries, this dissection plane may already be formed secondary to the trauma from the injury. When this plane is not formed, however, the lateral gastrocnemius may be slightly more adherent to the posterior capsule, and care should be taken to retract it accordingly. Similar to the medial dissection being anterior to the medial gastrocnemius, no portion of the posterolateral dissection should occur posterior to the lateral gastrocnemius, as it would place the popliteal neurovascular structures at risk (Fig. 18.15). It is important to remember that the popliteal artery normally lies slightly lateral to midline at the level of the knee. Dissection may then be bluntly carried out along the posterior fibula and tibia and a Homann retractor may be carefully placed anterior to the lateral gastrocnemius. Once this dissection is complete, the PLC reconstruction may be performed.

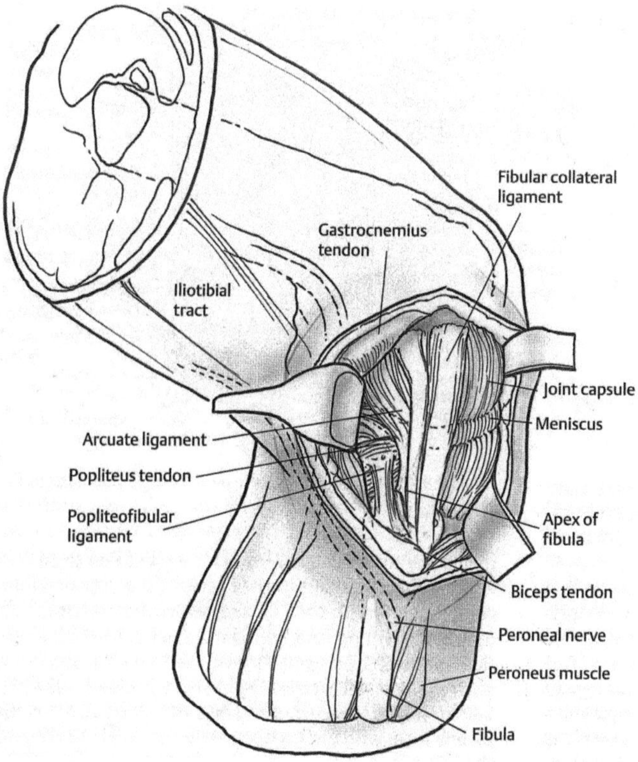

Fig. 18.14 Illustration depicting the superficial anatomy of the posterolateral approach to the knee

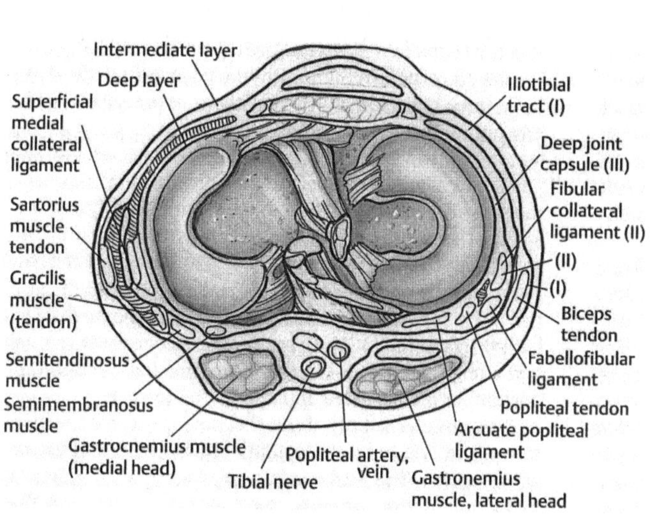

Fig. 18.13 Axial view of the anatomical layers of the knee at the level of the menisci. (From [43]. Reprinted with permission from Thieme Publishers)

In the setting of a combined PCL, PMC, and PLC injury, the preferred technique of the senior author for reconstruction of the PLC is a modified two-tailed reconstruction with either a tibialis anterior or tibialis posterior allograft. These particular types of tendon are preferred because they allow sufficient length of graft (>27 cm) to complete this reconstruction technique. This technique reconstructs the three primary components of the deep layer of the posterolateral corner: the LCL, the popliteus, and popliteofibular ligament. Initial graft preparation requires trimming the graft to

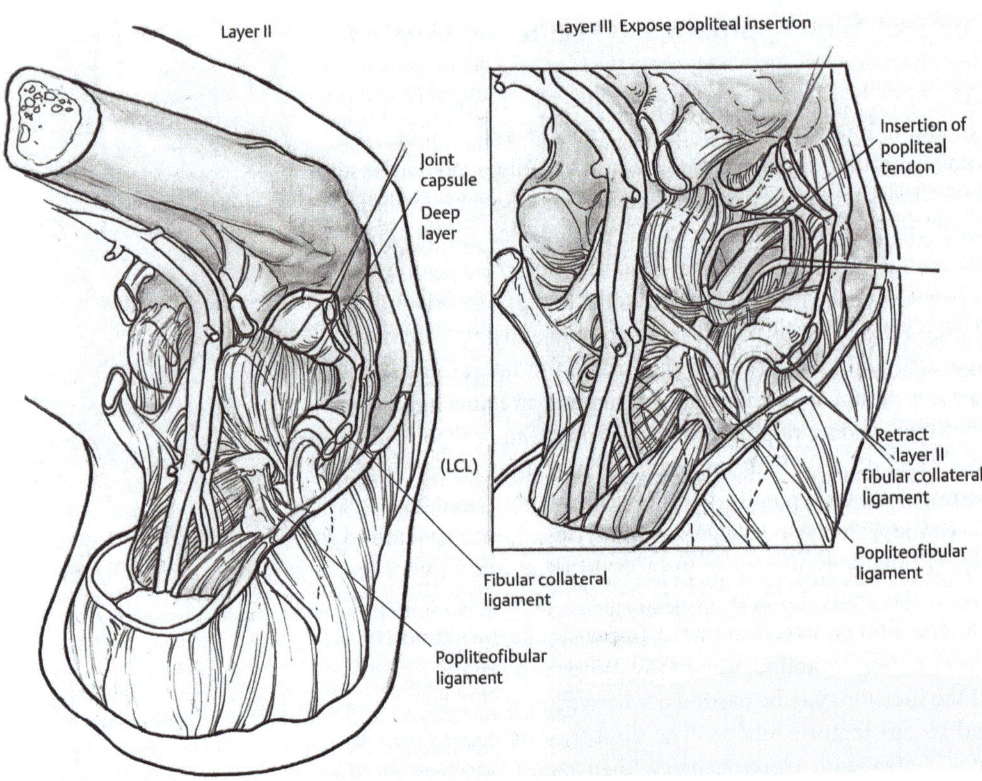

Fig. 18.15 Illustration depicting the deep anatomy of the posterolateral approach to the knee. (From [43]. Reprinted with permission from Thieme Publishers)

approximately 5–6 mm in width, then placing a locking Krackow stitch on one end of the graft with either a #2 nonabsorbable suture or fiberloop. The first step of the technique involves making a small stab incision 3–4 cm inferior to the inferolateral arthroscopy portal. A 5–6-mm drill hole is then placed directly anterior to posterior through the lateral tibia, exiting where the popliteus tendon crosses the posterior aspect of the tibia. A retractor or the surgeon's finger on the non-drilling hand may be placed posterior to the tibia while drilling to prevent drilling out the tibia and damaging the popliteal vessels. A guidewire is then placed in the tunnel and the tunnel is tapped with a 7-mm tap. A suture passer is placed in the tunnel from anterior to posterior and the graft is pulled into the tunnel from posterior to anterior, with just a small amount of graft at the anterior edge of the tibial tunnel. If the length of the graft may not be sufficient for the reconstruction, the graft may be pulled into the tibia so that only approximately 20 mm of graft is in the posterior tibia. The graft is then secured with a bioabsorbable 7-mm screw from anterior to posterior, taking the screw all the way to the posterior cortex. Next, a second 5–6-mm drill hole is placed in the proximal fibula, aiming from anterolateral to posteromedial through the fibular head. The fibula tunnel is not tapped. The isometric point is subsequently located on the lateral femoral condyle as previously described (Fig. 18.6). A 3.2-mm drill bit is placed at the isometric point and is drilled from lateral to medial across the femur, aiming 30° proximally and anteriorly, which will aim away from the possible location of a future ACL reconstruction tunnel. A fully threaded 4.5-mm screw with a washer is then placed within the tunnel but not fully seated. If bone quality is poor, a 6.5-mm screw may be used instead. The bone surrounding the screw may be decorticated to create a bleeding surface for the allograft to heal to the bone. The graft is then passed from the posterior tibia proximally under the biceps femoris and around the screw anteriorly (popliteus limb), then passed under itself back down to the fibular tunnel (popliteofibular limb) (Fig. 18.16). The graft is passed through the fibular tunnel from posterior to anterior and then back to the screw and washer (LCL limb), where it is wrapped around the screw (Fig. 18.17). The graft is typically tensioned with the foot slightly internally rotated and the knee flexed 40°. The final construct recreates the LCL, the popliteus, and the popliteofibular ligament (Fig. 18.18).

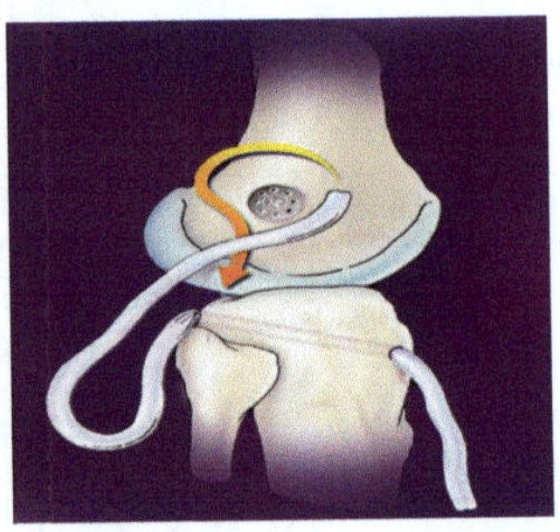

Fig. 18.16 Illustration depicting the initial graft passage for modified two-tailed posterolateral corner reconstruction

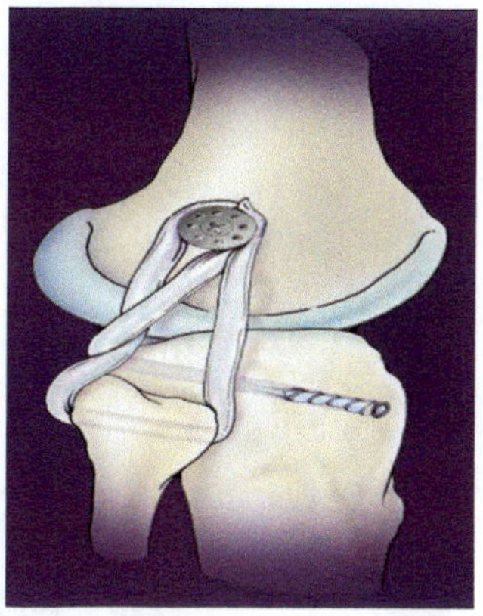

Fig. 18.17 Illustration depicting the final construct for a two-tailed posterolateral corner reconstruction

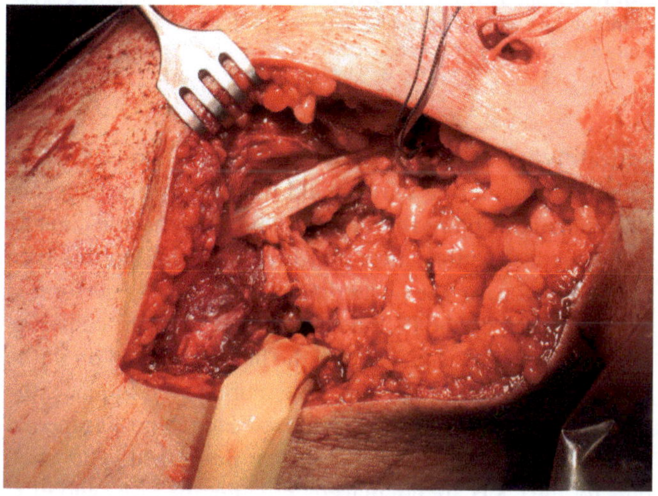

Fig. 18.18 Intraoperative photograph demonstrating a completed two-tailed posterolateral corner reconstruction

Placement of a CKH

The CKH functions as an excellent adjunct to multiple ligament reconstruction, particularly in the setting of type IV or type V dislocation, fracture dislocation, chronic dislocation, or preoperative flexion deformity of >15°. In the setting of a combined PCL, PMC, and PLC reconstruction, the senior author frequently utilizes the CKH to impart added stability to the knee while allowing early range of motion. If an ACL reconstruction is planned for the future, as is most commonly the case, the preferred treatment plan is to keep the hinge in place for 6 weeks and remove it concurrently when the ACL reconstruction is performed. This amount of time allows the soft tissues to recover after the combined reconstructions, allows early ligament healing, and allows the patient to regain knee range of motion prior to the ACL reconstruction. In a randomized, prospective study conducted by the authors, patients who underwent multiple ligament reconstruction after a knee dislocation who were placed in only a conventional hinged knee brace postoperatively had a significantly higher number of ligament failures (21 %) than patients who were treated with a CKH (7 %) [28]. For these reasons, we advocate consideration to placement of the hinge in the setting of these types of combined ligament reconstructions.

Placement of the CKH is placed at the center of rotation of the knee joint based on the same isometric point as previously described. Detailed explanation of the CKH application has been described, but it is relatively straightforward after precise placement of a centering reference wire at the isometric point [42]. The hinge is constructed with two carbon-fiber 5/8 rings bolted to multihole Rancho cubes that connect to 5- or 6-mm external fixator Schanz pins. The proximal and distal rings are subsequently connected by two calibrated hinges that are placed along the medial and lateral sides of the knee. The placement of the hinge is based on a threaded 2.5-mm centering wire that is temporarily placed at the isometric point on the lateral femoral condyle (Fig. 18.19). The wire is checked frequently in both the lateral and anterior–posterior projections to ensure it is properly placed. On the lateral radiograph, the wire should be brought in parallel with the fluoroscope so that it appears as a single dot. It is then drilled across the knee and an anterior–posterior view is checked to ensure that the wire is exactly parallel with the knee joint (Fig. 18.20). If the wire is not parallel, it should be removed and the process should be repeated. After the centering wire is placed, the hinge is created by placing the external fixator pins into the femur and the tibia. Typically, two 6-mm pins are utilized in the femur and three 5-mm pins in the tibia. For the femur, one pin is placed medially and inferiorly off the ring with a one- to three-hole Rancho cube and one pin is placed laterally off the ring with a two-hole Rancho cube, with the cubes facing

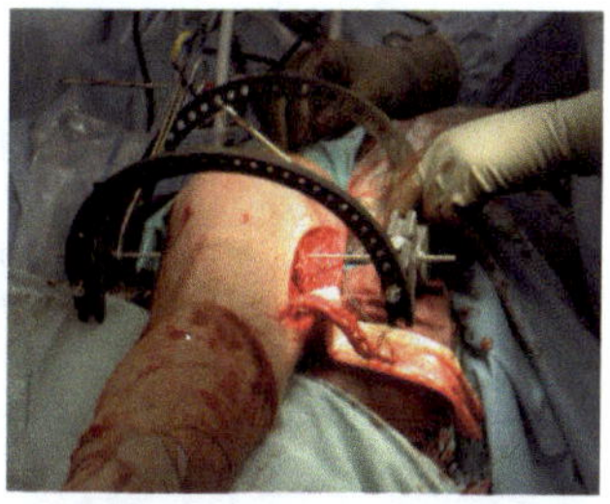

Fig. 18.19 Intraoperative photograph demonstrating placement of the compass knee hinge over a centering wire placed through the isometric point of the knee

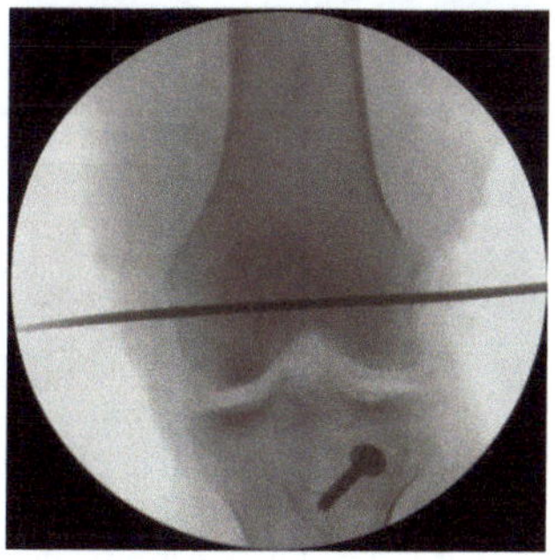

Fig. 18.20 Intraoperative radiograph demonstrating a centering reference wire parallel to the knee joint on an anteroposterior view. (From [43]. Reprinted with permission from Thieme Publishers)

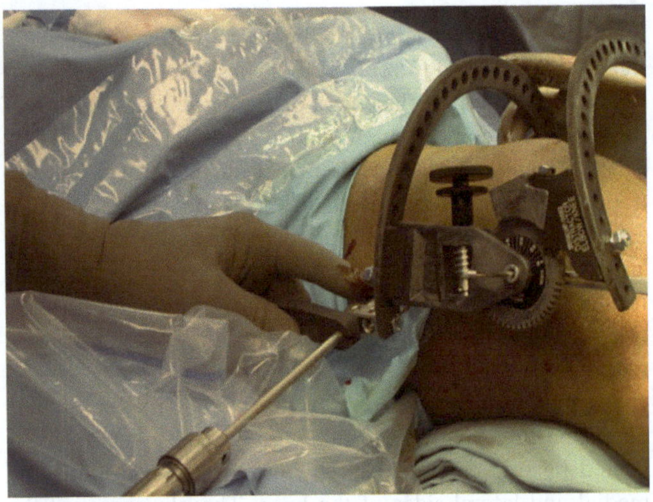

Fig. 18.21 Intraoperative photograph demonstrating placement of a femoral Schanz pin for placement of the compass knee hinge. (From [43]. Reprinted with permission from Thieme Publishers)

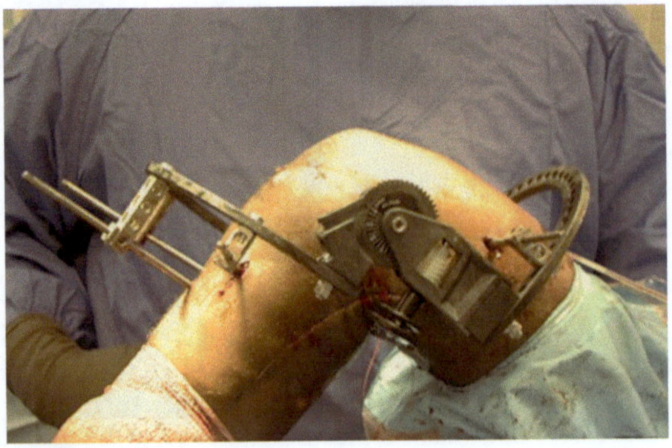

Fig. 18.23 Intraoperative photograph demonstrating completed application of the compass knee hinge. (From [43]. Reprinted with permission from Thieme Publishers)

proximally from the ring (Fig. 18.21). Using different-size Rancho cubes helps to ensure that the pins do not meet in the middle of the femur. The cubes should be placed in the most posterior hole on both the medial and lateral sides of the ring. A Trocar system is included which may be used to guide drilling of the pins. Three 5-mm pins are placed into the tibia through Rancho cubes evenly spaced apart and placed inferiorly from the inferior ring to complete the pin placement (Fig. 18.22). The pins are placed anterior, anteromedial, and lateral, and three-, four-, and five-hole Rancho cubes are utilized to keep the pins at different entry points across the tibia.

When applying the CKH in conjunction with a multiple ligament reconstruction, the timing of the hinge placement is critical. When a combined PMC and PLC is part of the procedure, the centering wire should be placed prior to reconstruction of the injured corners to avoid any potential damage to the reconstructions after they are completed. In this type of combined case, the posteromedial approach is performed first, followed by the PCL reconstruction, then the centering wire for the CKH is placed and the hinge mounted on it, the pins are drilled and placed in the femur and left in place, the hinge and centering wire are removed and the posteromedial and posterolateral reconstruction are performed. The tibial pins for the CKH are not placed until after the PMC and PLC reconstructions, as they can interfere with these procedures. The compass hinge may be kept on the back table during the PMC and PLC reconstructions and then remounted through the same holes in the Rancho cubes on the femoral pins after closure of all wounds. The centering wire does not need to be replaced so long as the femoral pins were placed in precise alignment during initial centering wire placement. The tibial pins are then placed through their respective Rancho cubes to complete the application of the hinge (Fig. 18.23).

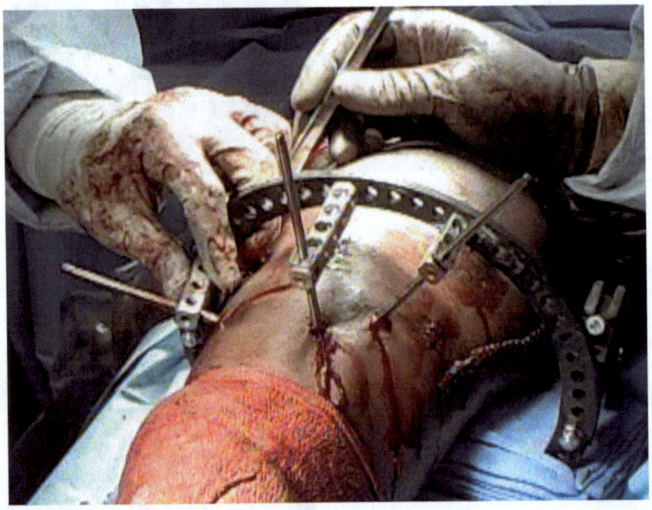

Fig. 18.22 Intraoperative photograph demonstrating completed tibial Schanz pin placement for placement of a compass knee hinge. (From [43]. Reprinted with permission from Thieme Publishers)

Postoperative Management

The balance between early range of motion and protection of knee stability after combined multiple ligament knee reconstructions is important to recognize. When a CKH is placed in conjunction with the combined PCL, PMC, and PLC reconstruction, our protocol dictates an early, progressive attempt to regain range of motion. Patients are allowed to bear weight immediately with the hinge locked in extension. Continuous passive motion machines are utilized when the patient is in bed beginning postoperative day 1. Patients are also asked to lock the hinge in full extension and maximum flexion for at least 1 h each per day. Epidurals, spinal anesthetic blocks, or patient-controlled analgesia is utilized for pain management in the acute postoperative period. Early rehabilitation is incorporated to encourage progressive increases in quadriceps and hamstring strengthening. The CKH is worn for approximately 6 weeks and may be removed at the time of ACL reconstruction, during any other future procedures, or as its own separate procedure. Rehabilitation is then subsequently continued as per the individual surgeon's protocol for multiple ligament knee reconstructions.

Conclusions

Multiple ligament knee reconstructions are complex cases which require adequate preoperative planning and attention to detail. A combined PCL, PMC, and posterolateral reconstruction can be successfully achieved in one operation. Numerous techniques for each reconstruction have been described and are available, but the preferred techniques of the senior author incorporate a tibial inlay for the PCL, a modified loop with two grafts for the PMC, and modified two-tailed technique for the posterolateral corner. These techniques have yielded low failure rates and allowed an aggressive early range of motion rehabilitation protocol. In addition to these techniques, consideration may be given to placement of a CKH for a defined period of time. Patient comorbidities, concomitant injuries, and future expectations must all be taken into account when planning the timing and type of reconstructions performed, but with adequate preparation a successful treatment outcome may be achieved in the treatment of a combined PCL, PMC, and PLC injury.

References

1. Shelbourne KD, Pritchard J, Rettig AC, McCarroll JR, Vanmeter CD. Knee dislocations with intact PCL. Orthop Rev. 1992;21(5):607–8, 610–1.
2. Wascher DC, Dvirnak PC, DeCoster TA. Knee dislocation: initial assessment and implications for treatment. J Orthop Trauma. 1997;11(7):525–9.
3. Peskan, CJ, Levy BA, Fanelli GC, Stannard JP, Stuart MJ, MacDonald PB, Marx RG, Boyd JL, Whelan DB. Diagnosis and management of knee dislocations. Physician Sports Med. 2010;4(38):101–11.
4. Fanelli GC, Edson CJ. Arthroscopically assisted combined anterior and posterior cruciate ligament reconstructions in the multiple ligament injured knee: 2- to 10-year follow-up. Arthroscopy. 2002;18(7):703–14.
5. Bin S-I, Nam T-S. Surgical outcome of 2-stage management of multiple knee ligament injuries after knee dislocation. Arthroscopy. 2007;23(10):1066–72.
6. Levy BA, Dajani KA, Whelan DB, Stannard JP, Fanelli GC, Stuart MJ, Boyd JL, MacDonald PA, Marx RG. Decision making in the multiligament-injured knee: an evidence based systemic review. Arthroscopy. 2009;25(4):430–8.
7. Fanelli GC, Stannard JP, Stuart MJ, MacDonald PB, Marx RG, Whelan DB, Boyd JL, Levy BA. Management of complex knee ligament injuries. J Bone Joint Surg Am. 2010;92(12):2235–46.
8. Mook WR, Ligh CA, Moorman CT, Leversedge FJ. Nerve injury complicating multiligament knee injury: current concepts and treatment algorithm. J Am Acad Orthop Surg. 2013;21:343–54.
9. Noyes FR, Barber-Westin SD. Reconstruction of the anterior cruciate and posterior cruciate ligaments after knee dislocation: Use of early protected postoperative motion to decrease anrthrofibrosis. Am J Sports Med. 1997;25:769–778.
10. Sisto DJ, Warren RF. Complete knee dislocation: A follow-up study of operative treatment. Clin Orthop Relat Res. 1985;198:94–101.
11. Cole BJ, Harner CD. Complex topics in knee surgery: The multiple ligament injured knee. Clin Sports Med. 1999;18(1):241–62.
12. Yeh WL, Tu YK, Su JY, Hsu RW. Knee dislocation: Treatment of high-velocity knee dislocation. J Trauma. 1999;46(4):693–701.
13. Shelbourne KD, Porter DA, Clingman JA, McCarroll JR, Rettig AC. Low-velocity knee dislocation. Orthop Rev. 1991;20(11):995–1004.
14. Howells NR, Brunton LR, Robinson J, Porteus AJ, Eldridge JD, Murray JR. Acute knee dislocation: An evidenced based approach to the multiligament injured knee. Injury. 2011;42:1198–204.
15. Wascher DC, Becker JR, Dexter JG, Blevins FT. Reconstruction of the anterior and posterior cruciate ligaments after knee dislocation. Am J Sports Med. 1999;27(2):189–96.
16. Schenck RC Jr. The dislocated knee. Instr Course Lect. 1994;43:127–36.
17. Stannard JP, Brown SL, Farris RC, McGwin G, Volgas DV. The posterolateral corner of the knee: repair versus reconstruction. Am J Sports Med. 2005;33(6):881–8.
18. Engebretsen L, Risberg MA, Robertson B, Ludvigsen TC, Johansen S. Outcome after knee dislocations at 2-9 years follow-up of 85 consecutive patients. Knee Surg Sports Tramatol Arthrosc. 2009;1:1013–26.
19. Strobel MJ, Martin SS, Wolf JP, Eichhorn HJ. Combined anterior cruciate ligament, posterior cruciate ligament, and posterolateral corner reconstruction with autogenous hamstring grafts in chronic instabilities. Arthroscopy. 2006;22(2):182–92
20. Stannard JS, Black BS, Axbell C, Volgas DA. Posteromedial corner injury in knee dislocations. J Knee Surg. 2012;25:429–34.
21. Laprade RF, Engebretsen AH, Ly TV, Johansen S, Wentorf FA, Engebretsen L. The anatomy of the medial part of the knee. J Bone Joint Surg Am. 2007;89:2000–10.
22. Laprade RF, Wijdicks CA. The management of injuries to the medial side of the knee. J Orthop Sports Phys Therapy. 2012;42(3):221–33.
23. Coobs BR, Wijdicks CA, Armitage BM. An in vitro analysis of an anatomical medial knee reconstruction. Am J Sports Med. 2010;38:339–47.
24. Richter M, Lobenhoffer P. Chronic posterior knee dislocation: treatment with anthrolysis, posterior cruciate ligament reconstruction and hinged external fixation device. Injury. 1998;29(7):546–9.
25. Simonian PT, Wickiewicz TL, Hotchkiss RN, Warren RF. Chronic knee dislocation: reduction, reconstruction, and application of a skeletally fixed hinge. A report of two cases. Am J Sports Med. 1998;26(4):591–6.
26. Stannard JP, Sheils TM, McGwin G, Volgas DA, Alonso JE. Use of a hinged external knee fixator after surgery for knee dislocation. Arthroscopy. 2003;19(6):626–31
27. Fitzpatrick DC, Sommers MB, Kam BC, Marsh JL, Bottlang M. Knee stability after articulated external fixation. Am J Sports Med. 2005;33(11):1735–41.
28. Stannard JP, Nuelle CW, McGwin G, Volgas DA. Hinged external fixation in the treatment of knee dislocations: A prospective randomized study. J Bone Joint Surg Am. 2014;96(3):184–91.
29. Berg EE. Positive cruciate ligament tibial inlay reconstruction. Arthroscopy. 1995;11:69–76.
30. Walker D, Rogers W, Schenck RC. Immediate vascular and ligamentous repair in a closed knee dislocation: A case report. J Trauma. 1994;36:898–900.

31. Sims WF, Jacobson KE. The posteromedial corner of the knee, medial-sided injury patterns revisited. Am J Sports Med. 2004;32(2):337–45.
32. Tibor LM, Marchant MH Jr, Taylor DC, Hardaker WT, Garrett WE, Sekiya JK. Management of medial-sided knee injuries, Part 2, posteromedial corner. Am J Sports Med. 2011;39:1332–40.
33. Warren RF, Marshall JL. The supporting structures and layers on the medial side of the knee: An anatomical analysis. J Bone Joint Surg. 1979;61A:56–62.
34. Miller MD, Gordon WT. Posterior cruciate ligament reconstruction: Tibial inlay technique-principles and procedure. Oper Tech Sports Med. 1999;7:127–33.
35. St. Pierre P, Miller MD. Posterior cruciate ligament injuries. Clin Sports Med. 1999;18:199–221.
36. Clancy WG Jr, Bisson LJ. Double tunnel technique for reconstruction of the posterior cruciate ligament. Oper Tech Sports Med. 1999;7:110–7.
37. Petrie RS, Harner CD. Double bundle posterior cruciate ligament reconstruction technique: University of Pittsburgh approach. Oper Tech Sports Med. 1999:118–36.
38. Stannard JP, Bauer KL. Current concepts in knee dislocations: PCL, ACL, and medial sided injuries. J Knee Surg. 2012;25:287–94.
39. Stannard JP, Hammond A, Tunmire D, Clayton M, Johnson C, Moura C. Determining the isometric point of the knee. J Knee Surg. 2012;25:71–4.
40. LaPrade RF, Ly TV, Wentorf FA, Engebretsen L. The posterolateral attachments of the knee: A qualitative and quantitative morphologic analysis of the fibular collateral ligament, popliteus tendon, popliteofibular ligament, and lateral gastrocnemius tendon. Am J Sports Med. 2003;31:854.
41. Medvecky MJ, Noyes FR. Surgical approaches to the posteromedial and posterolateral aspects of the knee. J Am Acad Orthop Surg. 2005;13(2):121–8.
42. Nuelle CW, Stannard JP. Application of a compass knee hinge: surgical technique. JBJS Essent Surg Tech. 2014;4(1):e 2 1–6.
43. Stannard JP, Schmidt AH, Kregor PJ, editors. Surgical treatment of orthopaedic trauma. New York: Thieme; 2007.

Posterior Cruciate Ligament Reconstruction in Patients 18 Years of Age and Younger

19

Gregory C. Fanelli and David G. Fanelli

Introduction

The purpose of this chapter is to present the senior author's Gregory C. Fanelli (GCF) experience in treating posterior cruciate ligament (PCL) injuries and PCL-based multiple ligament knee injuries in patients who are 18 years of age and younger. This chapter discusses patient age at the time of surgery, mechanisms of injury, surgical techniques, considerations in patients with open growth plates, a review of the literature, and the author's surgical outcomes in PCL and PCL-based multiple knee ligament reconstructions in patients 18 years of age and younger.

Patient Population

PCL reconstructions in patients 18 years of age and younger represent approximately 14 % of our total PCL reconstruction experience at a rural tertiary care medical center. This 14 % consists of 58 patients in the combined PCL-collateral ligament group, and 25 patients in the combined PCL–anterior cruciate ligament (ACL)-collateral ligament group for a total of 83 patients. Mechanisms of injury in the PCL-collateral ligament group are sports related in 72 %, motor vehicle accident related in 25 %, and trampoline accidents in 3 %. Mechanisms of injury in the PCL–ACL-collateral ligament group are sports related in 39 %, motor vehicle accident related in 57 %, and trampoline-related accidents in 4%.

The diagnosis of the PCL-based multiple ligament knee injuries in this patient population of 18 years of age and under broken down by percentages are: PCL-lateral side 39 %, PCL-medial side 1 %, PCL-medial–lateral sides 28 %, PCL–ACL-lateral side 17 %, PCL–ACL-medial side 12 %, and PCL–ACL-medial–lateral sides 3 %. Ninety-seven percent of the PCL-collateral group was chronic injuries, while 3 % were acute injuries. In contrast, 57 % of the PCL–ACL-collateral ligament-injured knees were chronic, while 43% of these knee injuries were acute. Forty-nine percent of the PCL-collateral ligament reconstruction group was right knees, and 51 % were left knees. Fifty-eight percent of the PCL–ACL-collateral ligament reconstruction group was right knees, and 42 % were left knees.

The mean age at the time of surgery in the PCL-collateral ligament reconstruction group was 16.3 years (range 6–18 years). Three percent of the patients in this group were less than 10 years old, 9 % were 10–14 years old, and 88 % were 15–18 years old. Sixty-seven percent of the PCL-collateral ligament reconstruction group was boys, and 33 % of this group was girls. The age groups of the boys who were less than 10 years old were 0 %, 10–14 years old 8 %, and 15–18 years old 92 %. The age groups of the girls who were less than 10 years old were 11 %, 10–14 years old 11 %, and 15–18 years old 78 %.

The mean age at the time of surgery in the PCL–ACL-collateral ligament reconstruction group was 16.7 years (range 13–18 years). Zero percent of the patients in this group were less than 10 years old, 4 % were 10–14 years old, and 96 % were 15–18 years old. Seventy-six percent of the PCL–ACL-collateral ligament reconstruction group was boys, and 24 % of this group was girls. The age groups of the boys who were less than 10 years old were 0 %, 10–14 years old 0 %, and 15–18 years old 100 %. The age groups of the girls who were less than 10 years old were 0 %, 10–14 years old 17 %, and 15–18 years old 83 %.

Preoperative Planning: Special Considerations

The concern in the pediatric and adolescent patient population with open growth plates is the potential for growth arrest and resultant angular deformity about the knee after

G. C. Fanelli (✉) · D. G. Fanelli
303 Kaseville Road, Danville, PA 17821, USA
e-mail: gregorycfanelli@gmail.com

D. G. Fanelli
email: fanellidavid@gmail.com

G. C. Fanelli (ed.), *Posterior Cruciate Ligament Injuries*,
DOI 10.1007/978-3-319-12072-0_19, © Springer International Publishing Switzerland 2015

surgical intervention. This risk can be decreased by insuring that no fixation devices or bone blocks cross or damage the physis during ligament reconstruction. Growth remaining and physiologic stage of development of the patient is very important, and is considered in the preoperative planning for the treatment of these complex knee ligament injuries [1, 2]. Adults with PCL injuries will often have mid-substance disruptions of the PCL, while children may have an increased incidence of PCL avulsion-type injuries, both cartilaginous and bony in nature leading to the consideration of primary repair, primary repair with augmentation, and reconstruction of the injured ligaments [3]. Additionally, an understanding of the relationships of the PCL and collateral ligaments to the physis is important when planning the surgical procedure [4].

Surgical Techniques and Outcomes in the Literature

Many surgeons have described successful surgical techniques to treat PCL and multiple knee ligament injuries in patients' with open growth plates. These studies are presented for a broad view of the treatment of these complex knee ligament injuries. Kocher et al. reviewed two separate patient groups with adolescent and pediatric PCL injuries: those managed nonoperatively and those treated surgically with ligament reconstruction or direct repair [3]. The group reviewed 26 PCL (1 bilateral) injuries in patients under age 18 over a 16-year period with a mean follow-up time of 27.8 months. Fourteen patients (15 knees) were treated operatively, and the other 11 patients had nonoperative treatment. All patients were evaluated using Tegner, Lysholm, and Pediatric International Knee Documentation Committee (Pedi-IKDC) scores. The group determined that patient outcomes for nonoperative treatment of nondisplaced avulsion injuries or partial PCL tears are viable in pediatric populations. They also concluded that PCL reconstruction or repair is a suitable treatment option for young patients with multiligament injuries or isolated PCL injuries who fail conservative treatment.

Warme and Mickelson present a case report of a 10-year-old boy who sustained an avulsion of the PCL from the insertion site on the tibia [5]. The boy required a PCL reconstruction after failing conservative treatment and a primary repair attempt. The team completed physeal sparing reconstruction using a modified femoral tunnel placement method combined with tibial inlay technique. The presented method prevented transphyseal drilling and also attained favorable anatomic graft placement. This technique also avoided the "killer" turn often associated with a transtibial approach. The boy had complete return to the pre-injury level of activity.

Solayar and Kapoor present a case report of a pediatric patient with a PCL avulsion off the insertion site of the tibia with an accompanying posterior horn medial meniscal tear from the posterior capsule [6]. The boy was treated with an open reduction and internal fixation of the detached fragment and suture repair for the meniscal tear. Solayar and Kapoor stress the importance of managing associated intra-articular injuries when treating pediatric PCL tibial avulsions.

Kwon et al. present a case of a 13-year-old girl with tibial detachment of the PCL that was surgically treated with arthroscopic reduction and pullout suture [7]. The procedure left the epiphyseal plate intact by using a posterior transseptal portal. The Kwon group suggests that this alternative treatment to PCL detachment injuries in pediatric patients will avoid injury to the physeal and maintain ligament tension during healing. However, this is yet to be proven in terms of biomechanical benefit.

The Anderson group reports the case of a pediatric patient with posterolateral knee and posterior instability [8]. The patient failed nonoperative treatment and was successfully treated with physeal-saving intra-articular PCL reconstruction and extra-articular posterolateral structure reconstruction.

The Bovid group presents the case of an 11-year-old boy with a high-grade intrasubstance PCL injury [9]. The injury was operatively treated and reconstructed using the all-arthroscopic tibial inlay technique with a modification to minimize physeal injury risk. The patient returned to pre-injury level of activity by 17 months follow-up with no posterior sag and a grade 1 posterior drawer. Radiographs did not indicate degenerative changes. Both the distal femoral and proximal tibial physes were widely patent and showed no angular deformity. The operative limb was longer following surgery with a 1-cm leg-length discrepancy.

Accadbled et al. present a case report of an 11-year-old boy with a PCL rupture [10]. He was operatively treated with an arthroscopic PCL reconstruction employing a single-bundle four-strand hamstring autograft. At 24 months follow-up, the patient had resumed the pre-injury level of activity with no growth disturbance indicators and a normal clinical examination.

Stadelmaier et al. studied the inhibitive effects of soft tissue grafts on the formation of a bony bridge within drill tunnels across open tibial and femoral growth plates for a canine model [11]. A fascia lata autograft was positioned in tunnels drilled across the proximal tibial and distal femoral physes in four skeletally immature canines. A control group of four additional canines had a similar procedure, but all drill holes were left unfilled. All growth plates were evaluated at either 2 weeks or 4 months following the procedure with high-resolution radiography and histologic study. This study indicates that a soft tissue graft of fascia lata inserted in drill holes across an open growth plate prevents bony bridge formation. These findings support other clinical studies that report no apparent changes to growth plate function following pediatric intra-articular ACL reconstruction.

MacDonald et al. present a case report of a 6-year-old boy with a partial radial tear of the medial meniscus and a chronic PCL tear [12]. He was treated nonoperatively and at 5 years post injury presented with a looseness sensation in the knee and occasional anterior knee pain. The group concluded that additional follow-up will be necessary to determine whether instability will develop into arthritic changes.

Shen et al. present a case report of a 5-year-old boy with posterolateral rotatory instability and PCL injury [13]. The patient was surgically treated and returned to the pre-injury level of activity by 4-year follow-up. The findings of the Shen group suggest that operative treatment of acute PCL/PLC injuries can be successful in this patient population.

Author's Surgical Technique

Graft Selection

Our preferred graft for the PCL reconstruction is the Achilles tendon allograft without bone plug for single-bundle PCL reconstructions and Achilles tendon allograft without bone plug and tibialis anterior allografts for double-bundle PCL reconstructions. Achilles tendon allograft without bone plug or other all soft tissue allograft are the preferred grafts for the ACL reconstruction when combined PCL–ACL reconstruction is indicated. The preferred graft material for the lateral posterolateral reconstruction is all soft tissue (no bone plugs) allograft tissue combined with a primary repair, and posterolateral capsular shift procedure. Our preferred method for medial-side injuries is a primary repair of all injured structures combined with posteromedial capsular shift and all soft tissue allograft (no bone plugs) supplementation–augmentation as needed. All soft tissue grafts adhere to the principles of Stadelmaier [11].

General Concepts

The principles of reconstruction in the PCL-injured knee and the multiple-ligament-injured knee are to identify and treat all pathology, accurate tunnel placement, anatomic graft insertion sites, utilize strong graft material, mechanical graft tensioning, secure graft fixation, and a deliberate postoperative rehabilitation program [14–26]. The concern in the patient population of 18 years of age and younger with open growth plates is the potential for growth arrest and resultant angular deformity about the knee after surgical intervention. This risk can be decreased by insuring that no fixation devices or bone blocks cross or damage the physis during ligament reconstruction. Therefore, in patients with open physes, soft tissue allografts without the bone plugs are used, and no fixation devices cross the physis. Patients with closed or nearly closed growth plates may be treated with the same surgical techniques as adults. Our preference is to perform single-bundle PCL reconstruction in patients with open growth plates, while single- or double-bundle PCL reconstruction have both been successful in patients with closed or nearly closed growth plates. We have had no patients with growth arrest and resultant angular deformity about the knee after surgical intervention.

PCL Reconstruction

The patient is placed on the operating room table in the supine position, and after satisfactory induction of anesthesia, the operative and nonoperative lower extremities are carefully examined [23–26]. A tourniquet is applied to the upper thigh of the operative extremity, and that extremity is prepped and draped in a sterile fashion. The well leg is supported by the fully extended operating room table which also supports the surgical leg during medial- and lateral-side surgery. A lateral post is used to control the surgical extremity. An arthroscopic leg holder is not used. Preoperative and postoperative antibiotics are given, and antibiotics are routinely used to help prevent infection in these time-consuming, difficult, and complex cases. Allograft tissue is prepared prior to bringing the patient into the operating room to minimize general anesthesia time for the patient, and to facilitate the flow of the surgical procedure. The reader is referred to Chaps. 9 and 15 for additional information regarding the principles and techniques of surgical reconstruction in the PCL-injured knee and the multiple-ligament-injured knee.

The arthroscopic instruments are inserted with the gravity inflow through the superolateral patellar portal. Arthroscopic fluid pumps are not used. Instrumentation and visualization are positioned through inferomedial and inferolateral patellar portals, and can be interchanged as necessary. Additional portals are established as needed. Exploration of the joint consists of an evaluation of the patellofemoral joint, the medial and lateral compartments, medial and lateral menisci, and the intercondylar notch. The residual stumps of the PCL are debrided; however, the PCL anatomic insertion sites are preserved to serve as tunnel reference points. When a combined PCL–ACL reconstruction is performed, the same principles apply to preparing for the ACL reconstruction, and the notchplasty for the anterior cruciate ligament portion of the procedure is performed at this time. Care is taken throughout the procedure to protect the proximal tibial and distal femoral growth plates.

An extracapsular extra-articular posteromedial safety incision is made by creating an incision approximately 1.5–2 cm long starting at the posteromedial border of the tibia approximately 1 in. below the level of the joint line and extending distally. Dissection is carried down to the crural fascia, which is incised longitudinally. An interval is developed between the medial head of the gastrocnemius muscle and the nerves and vessels posterior to the surgeon's finger, and the capsule of the knee joint anterior to the surgeon's finger. The posteromedial safety incision enables the surgeon to protect the neurovascular structures, confirm the accuracy of the PCL tibial tunnel, and to facilitate the flow of the surgical procedure. There is no subperiosteal stripping or elevation from the proximal tibia or distal femur.

The curved over-the-top PCL instruments (Biomet Sports Medicine, Warsaw, IN, USA) are used to sequentially lyse adhesions in the posterior aspect of the knee, and elevate the capsule from the posterior tibial ridge. This will allow accurate placement of the PCL/ACL drill guide, and correct placement of the tibial tunnel. Care is taken to gently elevate the posterior capsule only, and not to strip or elevate the periosteum or damage the posterior proximal tibial growth plate.

The arm of the PCL/ACL guide (Biomet Sports Medicine, Warsaw, IN, USA) is inserted through the inferior medial patellar portal. The tip of the guide is positioned at the inferior lateral aspect of the PCL anatomic insertion site. This is below the tibial ridge posterior and in the lateral aspect of the PCL anatomic insertion site. The bullet portion of the guide contacts the anteromedial surface of the proximal tibia at a point midway between the posteromedial border of the tibia, and the tibial crest anterior at or just below the level of the tibial tubercle away from the proximal tibial physis. This will provide an angle of graft orientation such that the graft will turn two very smooth 45° angles on the posterior aspect of the tibia. The tip of the drill guide, in the posterior aspect of the tibia is confirmed with the surgeon's finger through the extracapsular extra-articular posteromedial safety incision. Intraoperative anteroposterior (AP) and lateral X-ray may also be used; however, I do not routinely use intraoperative X-ray. When the PCL/ACL guide is positioned in the desired area, a blunt spade-tipped guide wire is drilled from anterior to posterior below the level of the proximal tibial physis. The surgeon's finger confirms the position of the guide wire through the posterior medial safety incision.

The appropriately sized standard cannulated reamer is used to create the tibial tunnel. The surgeon's finger through the extracapsular extra-articular posteromedial incision monitors the position of the guide wire. When the drill is engaged in bone, the guide wire is reversed, blunt end pointing posterior, for additional patient safety. The drill is advanced until it comes to the posterior cortex of the tibia. The chuck is disengaged from the drill, and completion of the tibial tunnel is performed by hand.

Our preference is to perform single-bundle PCL reconstruction in patients with open growth plates in order to protect the distal femoral growth plate, while single- or double-bundle PCL reconstruction have both been successful in patients with closed or nearly closed growth plates. This is a decision the surgeon will need to make on each case based on the anatomy at the time of surgery, the patient's development, and expected potential growth remaining. The PCL single- or double-bundle femoral tunnels are made from inside out using the double-bundle aimers, or an endoscopic reamer can be used as an aiming device (Biomet Sports Medicine, Warsaw, IN, USA). The appropriately sized double-bundle aimer or endoscopic reamer is inserted through a low anterior lateral patellar arthroscopic portal to create the PCL anterior lateral bundle femoral tunnel. The double-bundle aimer or endoscopic reamer is positioned directly on the footprint of the femoral anterior lateral bundle PCL insertion site. The appropriately sized guide wire is drilled through the aimer or endoscopic reamer, through the bone, and out a small skin incision. Care is taken to prevent any compromise of the articular surface. The double-bundle aimer is removed, and the endoscopic reamer is used to drill the anterior lateral PCL femoral tunnel from inside to outside.

When the surgeon chooses to perform a double-bundle double-femoral tunnel PCL reconstruction, the same process is repeated for the posterior medial bundle of the PCL. Care must be taken to ensure that there will be an adequate bone bridge (approximately 5 mm) between the two femoral tunnels prior to drilling. This is accomplished using the calibrated probe, and direct arthroscopic visualization of the PCL femoral anatomic insertion sites. Once again, care is taken throughout the procedure to protect the proximal tibial and distal femoral growth plates.

The surgical technique of PCL femoral tunnel creation from inside to outside is preferred for two reasons. First, there is a greater distance and margin of safety between the PCL femoral tunnel or tunnels and the medial femoral condyle articular surface using the inside-to-outside method. Second, a more accurate placement of the PCL femoral tunnels is possible, in the senior author's opinion, because the double-bundle aimer or endoscopic reamer can be placed on the anatomic footprint of the anterior lateral or posterior medial PCL insertion site under direct visualization.

A Magellan suture retriever (Biomet Sports Medicine, Warsaw, IN, USA) is introduced through the tibial tunnel into the joint, and retrieved through the femoral tunnel. The traction sutures of the graft material are attached to the loop of the Magellan suture retriever, and the graft is pulled into position. The graft material is secured on the femoral side using a bioabsorbable interference screw for primary aperture-opening fixation, and a polyethylene ligament fixation button for backup fixation.

The cyclic dynamic method of graft tensioning using the Biomet graft-tensioning boot (Biomet Sports Medicine, Warsaw, IN, USA) is used to tension the posterior and anterior cruciate ligament grafts [24]. This tensioning method is discussed in Chap. 21 of this book. Tension is placed on the PCL graft distally using the Biomet graft-tensioning boot (Biomet Sports Medicine, Warsaw, IN, USA). Tension is gradually applied with the knee in 0° of flexion (full extension) reducing the tibia on the femur. This restores the anatomic tibial step-off. The knee is cycled through a full range of motion multiple times to allow pretensioning and settling of the graft. The process is repeated until there is no further change in the torque setting on the graft tensioner. The knee is placed in 70–90° of flexion, and fixation is achieved on the tibial side of the PCL graft with a bioabsorbable interference screw placed just inside the cortex of the tibia, and backup fixation with a bicortical screw and spiked ligament washer or polyethylene ligament fixation button. No fixation devices or bone plugs cross or violate the growth plates.

Anterior Cruciate Ligament Reconstruction

When combined posterior and anterior cruciate ligament reconstructions are performed, the PCL reconstruction is performed first followed by the ACL reconstruction. With the knee in approximately 90° of flexion, the anterior cruciate ligament tibial tunnel is created using a drill guide. The senior author's preferred method of anterior cruciate ligament reconstruction is the transtibial femoral tunnel endoscopic surgical technique. The arm of the drill guide enters the knee joint through the inferior medial patellar portal. The bullet of the drill guide contacts the anterior medial proximal tibia externally at a point midway between the posterior medial border of the tibia, and the anterior tibial crest just above the level of the tibial tubercle away from the proximal tibial physis. An approximate 1-cm bone bridge exists between the PCL and ACL tibial tunnel starting points on the proximal tibia. The guide wire is drilled through the guide and positioned so that after creating the anterior cruciate ligament tibial tunnel, the graft will approximate the tibial anatomic insertion site of the anterior cruciate ligament. A standard cannulated reamer is used to create the tibial tunnel.

With the knee in approximately 90–100° of flexion, an over-the-top femoral aimer is introduced through the tibial tunnel, and used to position a guide wire on the medial wall of the lateral femoral condyle to create a femoral tunnel approximating the anatomic insertion site of the anterior cruciate ligament. The anterior cruciate ligament graft is positioned, and fixation achieved on the femoral side using cortical suspensory fixation with a polyethylene ligament fixation button. No fixation devices or bone plugs cross or violate the growth plates.

The cyclic dynamic method of tensioning of the anterior cruciate ligament graft is performed using the Biomet graft-tensioning boot [24] (Biomet Sports Medicine, Warsaw, IN, USA). Traction is placed on the anterior cruciate ligament graft sutures with the knee in 0° of flexion, and tension is gradually applied reducing the tibia on the femur. The knee is then cycled through multiple full flexion and extension cycles to allow settling of the graft. The process is repeated until there is no further change in the torque setting on the graft tensioner, and the Lachman and pivot shift tests are negative. The knee is placed in approximately 30° of flexion, and fixation is achieved on the tibial side of the anterior cruciate ligament graft with a bioabsorbable interference screw placed just inside the cortex of the tibia, and backup fixation with a polyethylene ligament fixation button. No fixation devices or bone plugs cross or violate the growth plates.

Posterolateral Reconstruction

Our most commonly utilized surgical technique for posterolateral reconstruction is the fibular-head-based figure-of-eight free-graft technique utilizing semitendinosus allograft, or other soft tissue allograft material. This procedure requires an intact proximal tibiofibular joint, and the absence of a severe hyperextension external rotation recurvatum deformity. This technique combined with capsular repair and posterolateral capsular shift procedures mimics the function of the popliteofibular ligament and lateral collateral ligament, tightens the posterolateral capsule, and provides a post of strong allograft tissue to reinforce the posterolateral corner. When there is a disrupted proximal tibiofibular joint, or severe hyperextension external rotation recurvatum deformity, a two-tailed (fibular head, proximal tibia) posterior lateral reconstruction is performed in addition to the posterolateral capsular shift procedure, once again protecting the proximal tibial and distal femoral growth plates.

In acute cases, primary repair of all lateral-side-injured structures is performed with suture anchors, and permanent sutures through drill holes as indicated. The primary repair is then augmented with an allograft tissue reconstruction. No fixation devices or bone plugs cross or violate the growth plates. Posterolateral reconstruction with the free-graft figure-of-eight technique utilizes semitendinosus or other soft tissue allograft. A lateral curvilinear incision is made. Dissection is carried down to the layer 1 fascia level. The peroneal nerve is identified, peroneal nerve neurolysis is performed, and the peroneal nerve is protected throughout the entire procedure. When the distal femoral growth plates are open, no hardware or drill holes are made on the lateral aspect of the knee. The common biceps tendon at its insertion into the fibular head is identified. A semitendinosus or other all soft tissue allograft is looped around the common biceps tendon insertion at the head of the fibula, and sewn with number 2 permanent braided sutures where the common biceps tendon inserts into the fibular head. Care is taken to not damage the fibular physis.

The iliotibial band is incised in line with its fibers. Dissection is carried down to the anatomic insertion site of the fibular collateral ligament and the popliteus tendon. A longitudinal incision is made posterior and parallel to the fibular collateral ligament. This incision provides access to the posterolateral compartment of the knee to assess capsular insertion sites for primary repair, and to enable the posterolateral capsular shift. Primary repair is performed as indicated. Posterolateral capsular shift is performed with permanent number 2 ethibond suture.

The semitendinosus allograft limb positioned lateral to the common biceps femoris tendon is passed medial to the iliotibial band and parallel to the fibular collateral ligament. This represents the fibular collateral ligament arm of the fibular head-common biceps femoris-tendon-based figure-of-eight posterolateral reconstruction. The semitendinosus allograft limb positioned medial to the common biceps femoris tendon is passed medial to the iliotibial band and medial to the fibular collateral ligament, and parallel to the popliteus tendon. This limb represents the force vector of the popliteus tendon and popliteal fibular ligament. The two limbs of the semitendinosus allograft are crossed in a figure-of-eight fashion, and sewn into the respective anatomic insertion sites of the fibular collateral ligament and popliteus tendon on the distal lateral aspect of the femur using number 2 permanent braided suture. The posterolateral capsule that had been previously incised is then shifted and sewn into the strut of figure-of-eight graft tissue material using number 2 ethibond permanent braided suture. The allograft tissue used for the posterolateral reconstruction is also sewn into the underlying fibular collateral ligament, popliteus tendon, and popliteofibular ligament also using number 2 permanent braided suture. Throughout the procedure, there is protection of both the fibula and the distal femoral physes, and the peroneal nerve. At the completion of the lateral-side procedure, the wound is thoroughly irrigated and closed in layers. When the growth plates of the proximal tibia and distal femur are functionally closed, the posterolateral reconstruction is carried out as described in Chap. 15.

When there is a disrupted proximal tibiofibular joint, or hyperextension external rotation recurvatum deformity, a two-tailed (fibular head, proximal tibia) posterior lateral reconstruction is utilized combined with a posterolateral capsular shift. A 7- or 8-mm drill hole is made over a guide wire approximately 2 cm below the lateral tibial plateau and below the proximal tibial physis. A tibialis anterior or other soft tissue allograft is passed through this tibial drill hole and follows the course of the popliteus tendon to its anatomic insertion site on the lateral femoral epicondylar region. Nerves and blood vessels are protected. The tibialis anterior or other soft tissue allograft is secured with a suture anchor, and multiple number 2 braided nonabsorbable ethibond sutures at the popliteus tendon anatomic femoral insertion site, and there is no violation of the distal femoral physis. The knee is cycled through multiple sets of full flexion and extension cycles, placed in 90° of flexion, the tibia slightly internally rotated, slight valgus force applied to the knee, and the graft tensioned, and secured in the tibial tunnel with a bioabsorbable interference screw that does not violate the growth plate, and polyethylene ligament fixation button. The fibular-head-based reconstruction and posterolateral capsular shift procedures are then carried out as described above. Number 2 permanent braided ethibond suture is used to sew the allograft to the deep capsular layers for additional reinforcement. When the growth plates of the proximal tibia and distal femur are functionally closed, the posterolateral reconstruction is carried out as described in Chap. 15.

Posteromedial Reconstruction

The surgical leg positioned on the extended operating room table in a supported flexed knee position. Posteromedial and medial reconstructions are performed through a medial curved incision taking care to maintain adequate skin bridges between incisions. In acute cases, primary repair of all medial-side-injured structures is performed with suture anchors and permanent sutures as indicated. The primary repair is then augmented with an allograft tissue reconstruction. Care is taken to make sure that there is no compromise or violation of the proximal tibia or distal femoral growth plates.

In chronic cases of posteromedial reconstruction, the Sartorius fascia is incised and retracted exposing the superficial medial collateral ligament and the posterior medial capsule. Nerves, blood vessels, and the growth plates are protected throughout the procedure. A longitudinal incision is made just posterior to the posterior border of the superficial medial collateral ligament. Care is taken not to damage the medial meniscus during the capsular incision. Avulsed capsular structures are primarily repaired using suture anchors and number 2 permanent braided sutures. The interval between the posteromedial capsule and medial meniscus is developed. The posteromedial capsule is shifted in an anterior and superior direction. The medial meniscus is repaired to the new capsular position, and the shifted capsule is sewn into the medial collateral ligament using three number 2 ethibond permanent braided sutures in a horizontal mattress fashion, and that suture line is reinforced using a running number 2 ethibond permanent braided suture.

When superficial medial collateral ligament reconstruction is indicated, this is performed using allograft tissue after completion of the primary capsular repair, and posteromedial capsular shift procedures are performed as outlined above. This graft material is attached at the anatomic insertion sites of the superficial medial collateral ligament on the tibia using a screw and spiked ligament washer, or suture anchors. Care is taken to make sure that there is no compromise or violation of the proximal tibia or distal femoral growth plates. The graft is looped around the adductor magnus tendon, tensioned, and sewn back to itself using number 2 ethibond permanent braided sutures. The final graft-tensioning position is approximately 30–40° of knee flexion. It is my preference to secure the tibial insertion site first, and to perform the final tensioning and fixation of the allograft tissue on the femoral side. Number 2 ethibond permanent braided sutures are used to sew the allograft to the deep capsular layers for additional reinforcement. In patients with closed growth plates, screw and washer fixation may be used if desired on both the tibia and femur to secure the allograft tissue.

Postoperative Rehabilitation Program

The knee is maintained in full extension for 3–5 weeks non-weight bearing. Progressive range of motion begins during postoperative week 3–5. Progressive weight bearing occurs at the beginning of postoperative weeks 3 through 5. Progressive closed kinetic chain strength training, proprioceptive training, and continued motion exercises are initiated very slowly beginning at postoperative week 12. The long leg range of motion brace is discontinued after the 10th week. Return to sports and heavy labor occurs after the 9th to 12th postoperative month when sufficient strength, range of motion, and proprioceptive skills have returned [27–30]. It is very important to carefully observe these complex knee ligament injury patients, and get a feel for the "personality of the knee." The surgeon may need to make adjustments and individualize the postoperative rehabilitation program as necessary. Careful and gentle range of motion under general anesthesia is a very useful tool in the treatment of these complex cases, and is utilized as necessary. Our postoperative rehabilitation program is discussed in more detail in Chap. 25 of this book.

Authors' Results

We present the senior author's results of PCL reconstructions in patients 18 years of age and younger representing approximately 14 % of our total PCL reconstruction experience at a rural tertiary care medical center. This 14 % consists of 58 patients in the combined PCL-collateral ligament group, and 25 patients in the combined PCL–ACL-collateral ligament group for a total of 83 patients. Mechanisms of injury in the PCL-collateral ligament group are sports related in 72 %, motor vehicle accident related in 25 %, and trampoline accidents in 3%. Mechanisms of injury in the PCL–ACL-collateral ligament group are sports related in 39 %, motor vehicle accident related in 57%, and trampoline-related accidents in 4%.

The diagnosis of the PCL-based multiple ligament knee injuries in this patient population of 18 years of age and under broken down by percentages are PCL-lateral side 39 %, PCL-medial side 1 %, PCL-medial–lateral sides 28 %, PCL–ACL-lateral side 17 %, PCL–ACL-medial side 12 %, and PCL–ACL-medial–lateral sides 3 %. Ninety-seven percent of the PCL-collateral group was chronic injuries, while 3% were acute injuries. In contrast, 57 % of the PCL–ACL-collateral ligament-injured knees were chronic, while 43 % of these knee injuries were acute. Forty-nine percent of the PCL-collateral ligament reconstruction group was right knees, and 51 % were left knees. Fifty-eight percent of the PCL–ACL-collateral ligament reconstruction group was right knees, and 42 % was left knees.

The mean age at the time of surgery in the PCL-collateral ligament reconstruction group was 16.3 years (range 6–18 years). Three percent of the patients in this group were less than 10 years old, 9 % were 10–14 years old, and 88 % were 15–18 years old. Sixty-seven percent of the PCL-collateral ligament reconstruction group was boys, and 33 % of this group was girls. The age groups of the boys who were less than 10 years old were 0 %, 10–14 years old 8 %, and 15–18 years old 92 %. The age groups of the girls who were less than 10 years old were 11 %, 10–14 years old 11 %, and 15–18 years old 78 %.

The mean age at the time of surgery in the PCL–ACL-collateral ligament reconstruction group was 16.7 years (range 13–18 years). Zero percent of the patients in this group were less than 10 years old, 4 % were 10–14 years old, and 96 % were 15–18 years old. Seventy-six percent of the PCL–ACL-collateral ligament reconstruction group was boys, and 24 % of this group was girls. The age groups of the boys who were less than 10 years old were 0 %, 10–14 years old 0%, and 15–18 years old 100 %. The age groups of the girls who were less than 10 years old were 0 %, 10–14 years old 17 %, and 15–18 years old 83 %. All patients in this series received the surgical techniques they required as described in this chapter.

It is very important for the reader to understand that the majority of patients in our series were in the 15–18-year-old age group, and that our surgical technique was adjusted to accommodate to stage of development of the growth plate at the time of surgery as described in the surgical technique section of this chapter. The concern in the patient population of 18 years of age and younger with open growth plates is the potential for growth arrest and resultant angular deformity about the knee after surgical intervention. This risk can be decreased by insuring that no fixation devices or bone blocks cross or damage the physis during ligament reconstruction.

Therefore, in patients with open physes, soft tissue allografts without the bone plugs are used, and no fixation devices cross the physis. Patients with closed or nearly closed growth plates may be treated with the same surgical techniques as adults. Our preference is to perform single-bundle PCL reconstruction in patients with open growth plates; however, single- and double-bundle PCL reconstruction have both been successful in patients with closed or nearly closed growth plates. Thus far, we have had no patients with growth arrest and resultant angular deformity about the knee after surgical intervention in any age group.

Postoperatively, the patients were evaluated with the range of knee motion, KT 1000 arthrometer, 90° knee flexion stress radiography, Lysholm, Tegner, and Hospital for Special Surgery knee ligament rating scales, X-ray, and physical examination [31–33]. Each evaluation criterion compared the postoperative surgical knee to the uninjured nonsurgical normal knee.

PCL + Collateral Ligament Group

The results of our combined PCL and collateral ligament reconstruction group (PCL + collateral ligament) are presented first. Fifty-one percent of the patients in this group (29/57) had single-bundle PCL reconstruction, while 49% (28/57) of the PCL-collateral ligament group received a double-bundle PCL reconstruction. The mean follow-up for this group of 58 patients was 3.5 years with a range of 1–17 years. The postoperative mean range of motion difference between the surgical knee and the nonsurgical normal knee was a 9.6° loss of terminal flexion with a range of 0–32° of terminal flexion loss. There were no flexion contractures in this series of patients.

Tibiofemoral displacement measurements were performed using the KT 1000 knee arthrometer (Medmetric Corporation, San Diego, CA, USA) and the Telos stress radiography device (Austin Associates, Baltimore, MD, USA). Postoperative mean KT 1000 side-to-side difference measurements in millimeters (mm) for the PCL screen, corrected posterior, and corrected anterior were 2.5 mm (range −0.5 to 6.0 mm), 3.3 mm (range −1.0 to 7.0 mm), and 0.1 mm (range −1.5 to 3.0 mm), respectively. The KT 1000 arthrometer 30-pound anterior displacement side-to-side difference measurement at 30° of knee flexion was 1.6 mm (range −2.0 to 5.0 mm). Ninety-degree knee flexion stress radiography with a posterior directed force applied to the proximal tibia using the Telos device side-to-side difference measurement was 2.5 mm (range −0.4 to 18.1 mm).

Lysholm, Hospital for Special Surgery, and Tegner knee ligament rating scales were used to evaluate the patient outcomes postoperatively. The Lysholm, Hospital for Special Surgery, and Tegner mean postoperative values were 93/100 (range 83–100), 90/100 (range 75–100), and 6/10 (range 3–9), respectively. Sixty-seven percent (32/48) of patients returned to their pre-injury Tegner level of function, while 15% (7/48), 6% (3/48), 4% (2/48), and 8% (4/48) of the patients were 1, 2, 3, and 4 Tegner levels below their pre-injury Tegner level of function, respectively.

Physical examination tests used to evaluate the postoperative outcomes of the combined PCL collateral ligament group included the posterior drawer, Lachman, pivot shift, varus stress, valgus stress, and the axial rotation dial tests. All physical examination tests compared the postoperative surgical knee to the normal uninjured nonsurgical knee. The posterior drawer test was normal in 63% (34/54), grade 1/2 laxity in 9% (5/54), grade 1 laxity in 26% (14/54), and grade 3 laxity in 2% (2/54). The Lachman and pivot shift tests were 100% normal in this intact anterior cruciate ligament group of patients as expected. The varus stress test at 0° and 30° of knee flexion were symmetrical to the normal knee in all patients tested (54/54). The valgus stress test at 0° and 30° of knee flexion were symmetrical to the normal knee in 98% (53/54) and grade 1 laxity in 2% (1/54). The axial rotation dial test at 30° and 90° of knee flexion was symmetrical to the contralateral normal knee in 87% (47/54) of patients, and less external rotation than the contralateral normal knee in 13% (7/54). There were no patients with growth arrest and resultant angular deformity about the knee after surgical intervention in any age group.

PCL + ACL + Collateral Ligament Group

The results of our combined PCL, anterior cruciate ligament, and collateral ligament (PCL + ACL + collateral ligament) reconstruction group are presented here. Fifty-nine percent of the patients in this group (13/22) had single-bundle PCL reconstruction, while 41% (9/22) of the PCL-collateral ligament group received a double-bundle PCL reconstruction. The mean follow-up for this group of 22 patients was 4.5 years with a range of 1–10 years. The postoperative mean range of motion difference between the surgical knee and the nonsurgical normal knee was an 11.3° loss of terminal flexion with a range of 0–43° of terminal flexion loss. There were no flexion contractures in this series of patients.

Tibiofemoral displacement measurements were performed using the KT 1000 knee arthrometer (Medmetric Corporation, San Diego, CA, USA) and the Telos stress radiography device (Austin Associates, Baltimore, MD, USA). Postoperative mean KT 1000 side-to-side difference measurements in millimeters (mm) for the PCL screen, corrected posterior, and corrected anterior were 1.7 mm (range 0.0–3.0 mm), 2.0 mm (range −1.0 to 5.0 mm), and 0.6 mm (range −1.5 to 4.0 mm), respectively. The KT 1000 arthrometer 30-pound anterior displacement side-to-side difference measurement at 30° of knee flexion was 2.2 mm (range −1.0 to 5.0 mm). Ninety-degree knee flexion stress radiography with a posterior directed force applied to the proximal tibia using the Telos device side-to-side difference measurement was 2.9 mm (range 0.0–12.7 mm).

Lysholm, Hospital for Special Surgery, and Tegner knee ligament rating scales were used to evaluate the patient outcomes postoperatively. The Lysholm, Hospital for Special Surgery, and Tegner mean postoperative values were 93/100 (range 69–100), 89/100 (range 76–96), and 5/10 (range 3–9), respectively. Fifty-five percent (11/20) of patients returned to their pre-injury Tegner level of function, while 20 % (4/20), 10 % (2/20), and 15 % (3/20) of the patients were 1, 2, and 3 Tegner levels below their pre-injury Tegner level of function, respectively.

Physical examination tests used to evaluate the postoperative outcomes of the combined PCL-collateral ligament group included the posterior drawer, Lachman, pivot shift, varus stress, valgus stress, and the axial rotation dial tests. All physical examination tests compared the postoperative surgical knee to the normal uninjured nonsurgical knee. The posterior drawer test was normal in 65 % (13/20), grade 1 laxity in 30 % (6/20), and grade 2 laxity in 5 % (1/20). The Lachman and pivot shift tests were symmetrical to the normal knee in 95 % (19/20), and grade 1 laxity in 5% (1/20). The varus stress test at 0° and 30° of knee flexion was symmetrical to the normal knee in all patients tested (20/20). The valgus stress test at 0° and 30° of knee flexion was symmetrical to the normal knee in all patients tested (20/20). The axial rotation dial test at 30° and 90° of knee flexion was symmetrical to the contralateral normal knee in 100 % (20/20) of patients in the PCL + ACL + collateral ligament group. There were no patients with growth arrest and resultant angular deformity about the knee after surgical intervention in any age group.

Case Presentation

The patient is a 12-year-old boy referred to me 3 weeks after a right knee injury sustained playing baseball. The patient slid into base and collided with another player and the fixed base with his knee in 90° of flexion. Initial evaluation by another physician revealed a bloody effusion upon aspiration, posterior tibial translation at 90° of flexion, and a magnetic resonance imaging (MRI) study of the right knee demonstrating a PCL tear. The patient was referred to me for evaluation and treatment.

Physical examination comparing the injured right knee to the uninvolved left knee revealed the skin and neurovascular status to be intact. Range of knee motion was symmetrical to the uninvolved left knee. There was no pain or restriction of motion at the hip or ankle on the involved or normal side. The tibial step-offs were decreased, and the posterior drawer test was positive. There were positive posterolateral and posteromedial drawer tests, and the dial test was positive at both 30° and 90° of knee flexion. The knee was stable to valgus stress at 0° and 30° of knee flexion, and there was varus laxity at both 0° and 90° of knee flexion with a soft end point. The hyperextension external rotation recurvatum test was negative, and the heel liftoff test was symmetrical on the injured and noninjured side. The Lachman test and pivot shift tests were both negative.

Initial radiographs taken in the orthopedic clinic demonstrated open growth plates on the distal femur and the proximal tibia with no fractures (Fig. 19.1). There was no physeal injury noted on stress radiography, or MRI imaging. MRI showed a tear of the PCL, and bone marrow edema without fracture in the anterior tibial epiphysis in the midline. There were no articular cartilage injuries or meniscus tears.

KT 1000 arthrometer testing revealed the following side-to-side difference measurements: PCL screen at 90° of knee flexion 6 mm, corrected posterior measurement at 70° of knee flexion 6 mm, corrected anterior measurement at 70° of knee flexion 4 mm, and the 30-pound anterior displacement measurement at 30° of knee flexion was 1 mm. Side-to-side difference on stress radiography at 90° of knee flexion with a posterior displacement force applied to the tibial tubercle area of the proximal tibia using the Telos device comparing the involved to the normal knee was 10 mm (Fig. 19.2).

Preoperative testing with three knee ligament rating scales revealed the following: Hospital for Special Surgery score was 42/100, Lysholm score was 44/100, and the Tegner activity score was 3 (pre-injury, the patient was level 7).

The diagnosis in this patient is a right knee subacute PCL-based multiple-ligament-injured knee with PCL tear, posteromedial instability type A, and posterolateral instability type B in a patient with open growth plates. The decision was made to proceed with arthroscopic single-bundle transtibial PCL reconstruction using fresh-frozen Achilles tendon allograft without bone plug combined with a fibular-head-based figure-of-eight posterolateral reconstruction using fresh-frozen semitendinosus allograft. The PCL reconstruction femoral tunnel crossed the distal femoral physis, and the PCL tibial tunnel was positioned distal to the tibial physis. Cortical suspensory fixation with two stacked polyethylene ligament fixation buttons were used on the femoral side, and a bioabsorbable interference screw and bicortical screw and spiked ligament washer were used on the tibial side fixation. No fixation device crossed the growth plates, and there were no bone plugs on the Achilles tendon allograft tissue, so no bone plug crossed the growth plate (Fig. 19.3).

The posterolateral reconstruction was a fibular-head-based figure-of-eight reconstruction using a fresh-frozen semitendinosus allograft. The allograft was looped around the common biceps tendon at the fibular head and sewn there

Fig. 19.1 Preoperative radiographs in a 12-year-old boy. The diagnosis in this patient is a right knee posterior-cruciate-ligament-based multiple-ligament-injured knee with posterior cruciate ligament tear, posteromedial instability type A, and posterolateral instability type B in a patient with open growth plates

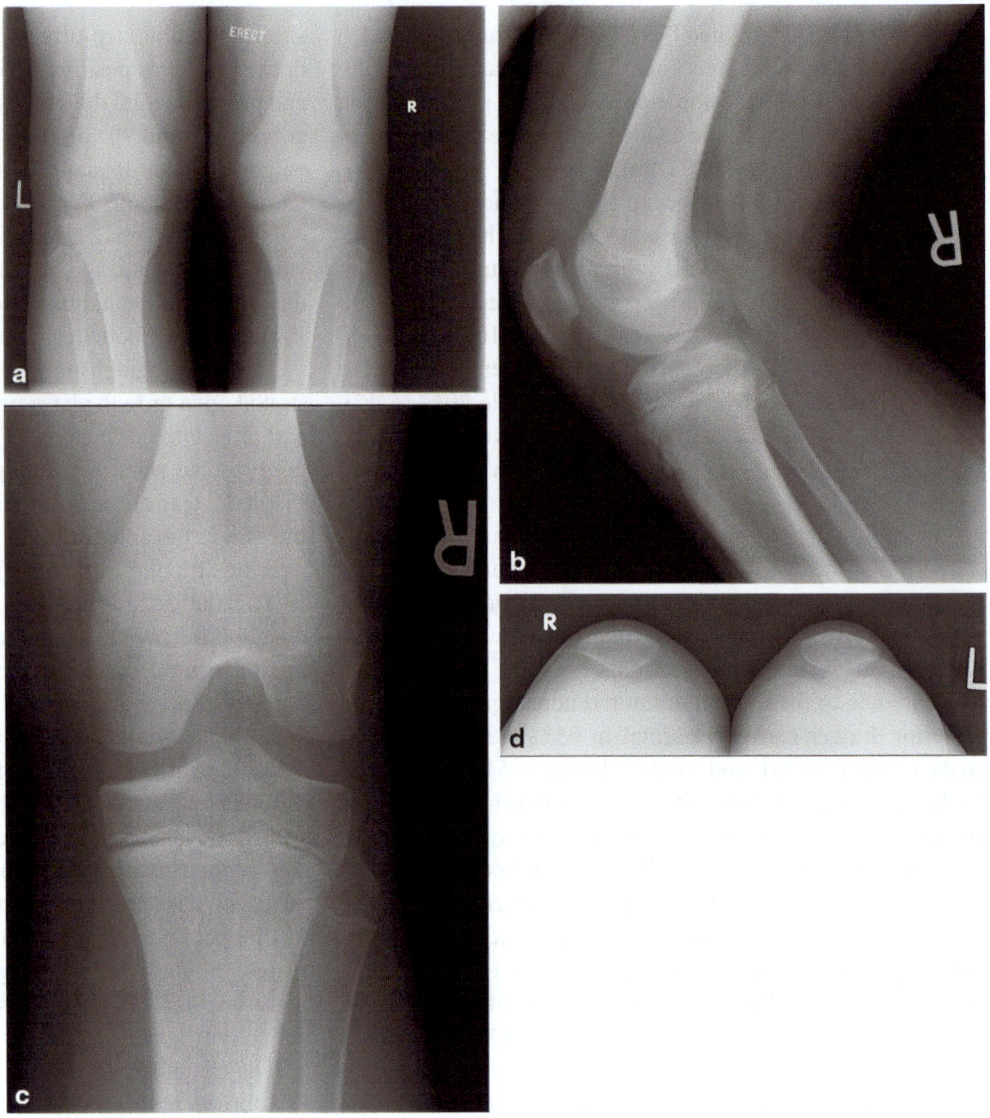

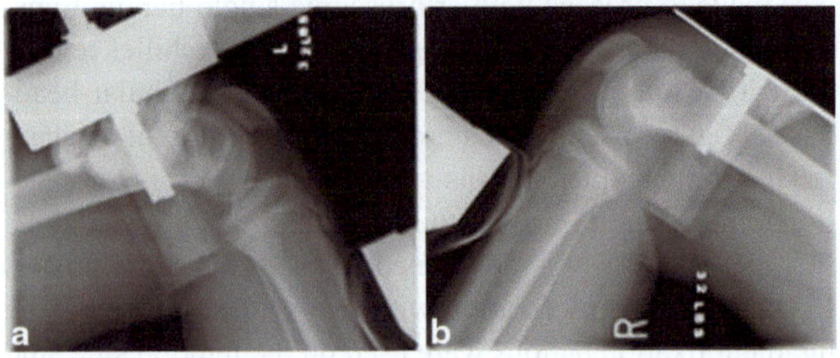

Fig. 19.2 Preoperative stress radiography with a posterior directed force applied to the proximal tibia of the normal uninjured knee (**a**) and the PCL, posterolateral, posteromedial injured knee (**b**). These stress radiographs demonstrate increased posterior translation at approximately 90° of knee flexion in the injured knee compared to the normal knee. Side-to-side difference on stress radiography at 90° of knee flexion with a posterior displacement force applied to the tibial tubercle area of the proximal tibia using the Telos device comparing the involved to the normal knee was 10 mm increased posterior tibial translation compared to the normal knee. PCL posterior cruciate ligament

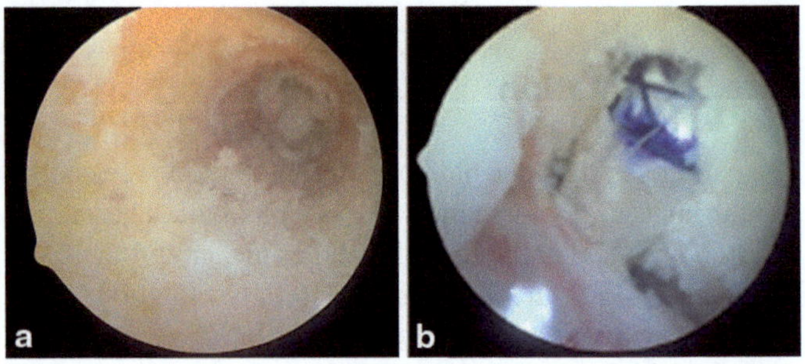

Fig. 19.3 The posterior cruciate ligament reconstruction femoral tunnel crossed the distal femoral physis (**a**), and the PCL tibial tunnel was positioned distal to the tibial physis. Cortical suspensory fixation with two stacked polyethylene ligament fixation buttons were used on the femoral side, and a bioabsorbable interference screw and bicortical screw and spiked ligament washer were used on the tibial side fixation. No fixation device crossed the growth plates, and there were no bone plugs on the Achilles tendon allograft tissue, so no bone plug crossed the growth plate (**b**). PCL posterior cruciate ligament

using permanent braided suture. The fibular collateral ligament component was passed medial to the iliotibial band, and the popliteofibular popliteus tendon component passed medial to the common biceps tendon and the iliotibial band. The allograft limbs were crossed in a figure-of-eight fashion with the fibular collateral component being lateral to the popliteus tendon component. The graft limbs were sewn into their respective anatomic femoral insertion sites with number 2 braided permanent sutures with a slight valgus applied to the knee to close the lateral compartment with the knee in approximately 90° of flexion. The allograft was then sewn to the deep capsular layers for additional reinforcement, and a posterolateral capsular shift was also performed. There were no drill holes through or around the lateral-side growth plates (Fig. 19.4).

The posteromedial reconstruction was performed using the posteromedial capsular shift technique (Fig. 19.5). This was an all suture posteromedial capsular advancement procedure performed with the knee in approximately 45° of flexion as described in Chap. 15. The PCL reconstruction, the posterolateral reconstruction, and the posteromedial reconstruction procedures were all protective of the growth plates. Postoperatively, the surgical knee was immobilized in a long leg brace locked in full extension, and was non-weight bearing with crutches. Prophylactic preoperative and postoperative antibiotics were utilized. Progressive weight bearing and the range of knee motion were gradually initiated according to our postoperative rehabilitation program detailed in Chap. 25.

Six-year follow-up postoperative examination of the patient at the age of 19 reveals equal leg lengths, normal and symmetrical carrying angles, and normal gait during ambulation. Radiographs reveal closed distal femoral and proximal tibial physes that are symmetrical to the normal knee with no malalignment, no evidence of growth arrest, and no degenerative changes (Fig. 19.6). Physical examination of the surgical right knee compared to the normal left knee reveals the posterior drawer is negative, posteromedial and posterolateral drawer tests are negative, and the dial test is symmetrical at 30° and 90° of knee flexion. The Lachman test is negative, the pivot shift test is negative, and the surgical knee is stable to varus and valgus stress throughout the flexion extension arc. The hyperextension external rotation recurvatum and heel liftoff tests are symmetrical compared to the normal knee.

Three-year postoperative KT 1000, stress radiography, and knee ligament rating scale measurements reveal the following. Range of motion is 0–125° on the surgical right knee, and 0–130° on the uninvolved left knee. Side-to-side difference on KT 1000 measurements on the PCL screen, corrected posterior, and corrected anterior measurements are 2.0, 2.5, and −2.0 mm respectively. Side-to-side difference on the KT 1000 anterior displacement measurement at 30° of knee flexion is 2.0 mm. Stress X-rays at 90° of knee flexion using the Telos device comparing the surgical to the knee normal knee reveal a 1.8 mm side-to-side difference (Fig. 19.7). The Hospital for Special Surgery, Lysholm, and Tegner knee ligament rating scale scores are 98/100, 99/100, and 7. The patient's pre-injury Tegner score was 7 indicating a return to pre injury level of function.

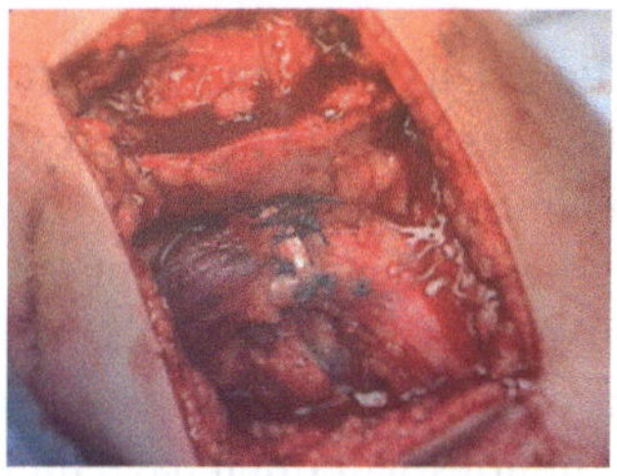

Fig. 19.4 The posterolateral reconstruction was a fibular-head-based figure-of-eight reconstruction using a fresh-frozen semitendinosus allograft. The allograft was looped around the common biceps tendon at the fibular head and sewn there using permanent braided suture. The fibular collateral ligament component was passed medial to the iliotibial band, and the popliteofibular popliteus tendon component passed medial to the common biceps tendon and the iliotibial band. The allograft limbs were crossed in a figure-of-eight fashion with the fibular collateral component being lateral to the popliteus tendon component. The graft limbs were sewn into their respective anatomic femoral insertion sites with number 2 braided permanent sutures with a slight valgus applied to the knee to close the lateral compartment with the knee in approximately 90° of flexion. The allograft was then sewn to the deep capsular layers for additional reinforcement, and a posterolateral capsular shift was also performed. There were no drill holes through or around the lateral-side growth plates

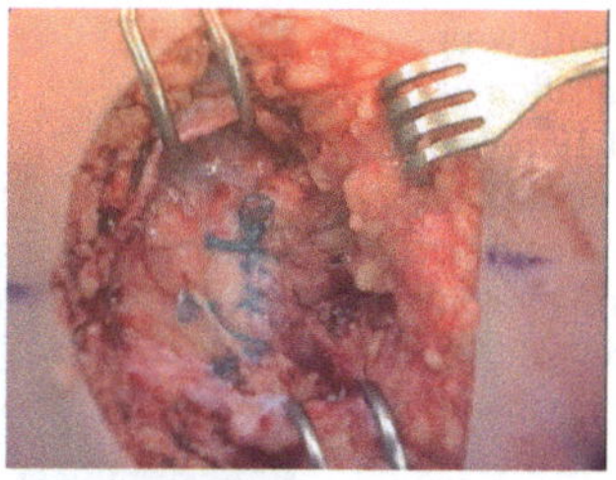

Fig. 19.5 The posteromedial reconstruction was performed using the posteromedial capsular shift technique. This was an all suture posteromedial capsular advancement procedure performed with the knee in approximately 45° of flexion. A longitudinal incision is made just posterior to the posterior border of the superficial medial collateral ligament. Care is taken not to damage the medial meniscus during the capsular incision. Avulsed capsular structures are primarily repaired using suture anchors and number 2 permanent braided sutures. The interval between the posteromedial capsule and medial meniscus is developed. The posteromedial capsule is shifted in an anterior and superior direction. The medial meniscus is repaired to the new capsular position, and the shifted capsule is sewn into the medial collateral ligament using three number 2 ethibond permanent braided sutures in horizontal mattress fashion, and that suture line is reinforced using a running number 2 ethibond permanent braided suture

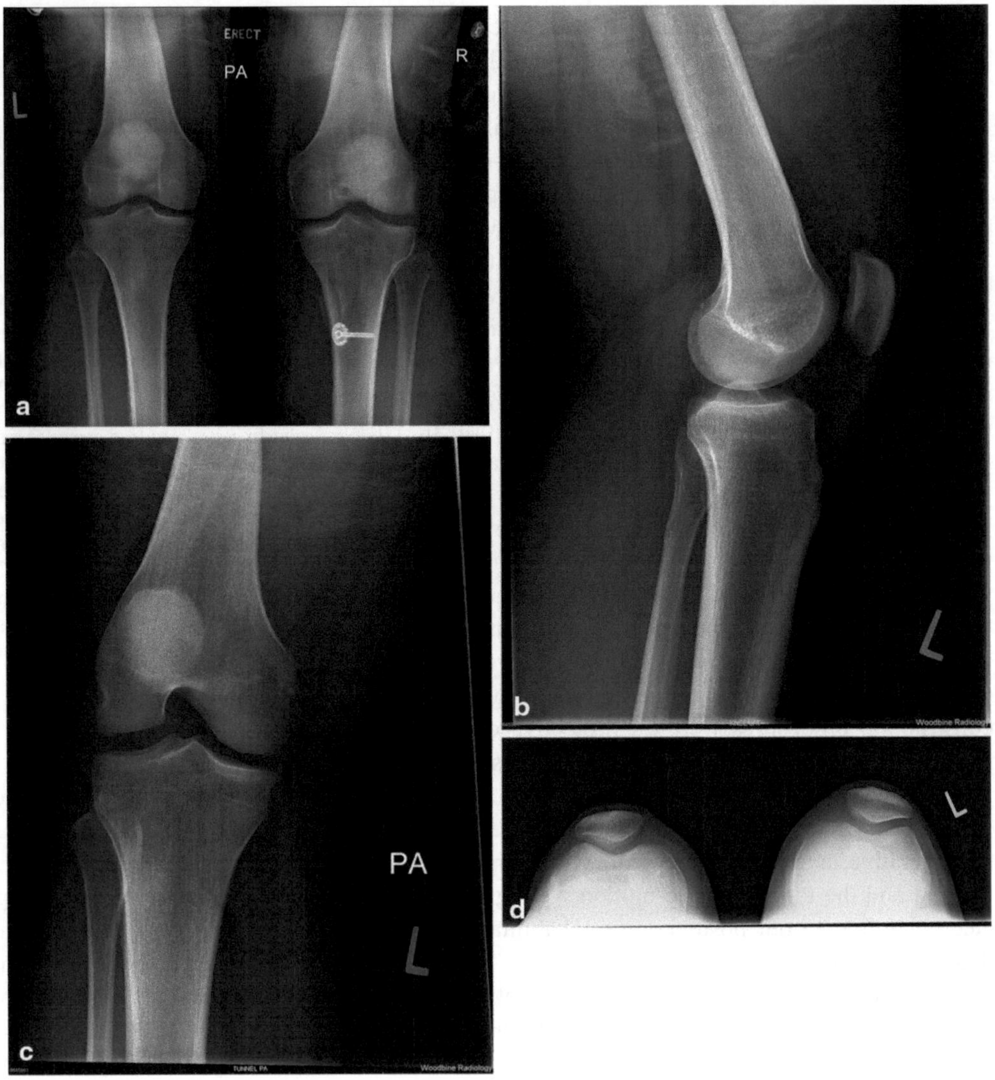

Fig. 19.6 Six-year follow-up postoperative examination of the patient at the age of 19 reveals equal leg lengths, normal and symmetrical carrying angles, and normal gait during ambulation. Radiographs reveal closed distal femoral and proximal tibial physes that are symmetrical to the normal knee with no malalignment, no evidence of growth arrest, and no degenerative changes

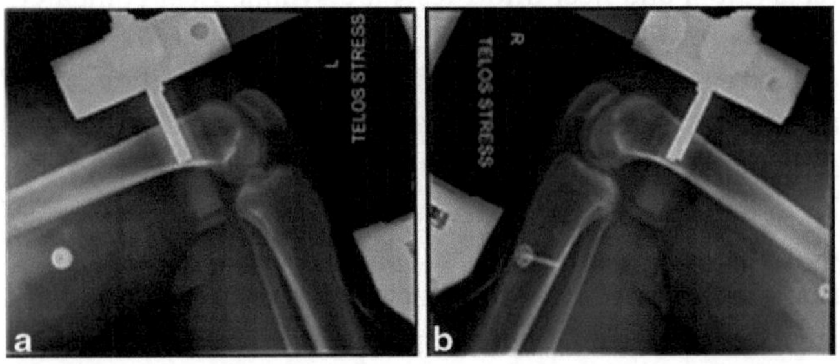

Fig. 19.7 Six -year postoperative stress X-rays at 90° of knee flexion using the Telos device comparing the normal knee (**a**) to the surgical knee (**b**) reveal a 1.8 mm side-to-side difference

Summary

The concern in the pediatric and adolescent patient population with open growth plates is the potential for growth arrest and resultant angular deformity about the knee after surgical intervention. This risk can be decreased by insuring that no fixation devices or bone blocks cross or damage the physis during ligament reconstruction. Growth remaining and physiologic stage of development of the patient is very important, and is considered in the preoperative planning for the treatment of these complex knee ligament injuries. Adults with PCL injuries will often have mid-substance disruptions of the PCL, while children may have an increased incidence of PCL avulsion-type injuries, both cartilaginous and bony in nature, leading to the consideration of primary repair, primary repair with augmentation, and reconstruction of the injured ligaments. Additionally, an understanding of the relationships of the PCL and collateral ligaments to the physis is important when planning the surgical procedure.

The majority of patients in our experience are in the 15–18-year-old age group, and our surgical technique was adjusted to accommodate to the stage of development of the growth plate at the time of surgery as described in the surgical technique section of this chapter. Many surgeons have described successful surgical techniques to treat PCL and multiple knee ligament injuries in patients' with open growth plates, and these concepts should be incorporated into the surgical planning in patients with open growth plates. Patients with closed or nearly closed growth plates may be treated with the same surgical techniques as adults, while skeletally immature patients require modified surgical techniques outlined in this chapter. Our preference is to perform single-bundle PCL reconstruction in patients with open growth plates, while single- or double-bundle PCL reconstruction have both been successful in patients with growth plates that are closed or nearly closed. Anterior cruciate ligament and collateral ligament surgery must also respect the stage of development of the physis. Thus far, in the senior author's experience, there have been no patients with growth arrest and resultant angular deformity about the knee after surgical intervention in any age group.

References

1. Greulich WW, Pyle SI. Radiographic atlas of skeletal development of the hand and wrist. Stanford: Stanford University Press; 1959.
2. Tanner JM, Whitehouse RH. Clinical longitudinal standards for height, weight, height velocity, weight velocity, and stages of puberty. Arch Dis Child. 1976;51:170–179.
3. Kocher MS, Shore B, Nasreddine AY, Heyworth BE. Treatment of posterior cruciate ligament injuries in pediatric and adolescent patients. J Pediatr Orthop. 2012;32(6):553–60.
4. Shea KG, Polousky JD, Jacobs JC, Ganley TJ. Anatomical dissection and CT imaging of the posterior cruciate and lateral collateral ligaments in skeletally immature cadaver knees. J Bone Joint Surg Am. 2014;96:753–9.
5. Warme WJ, Mickelson D. All-epiphyseal semitendinosus PCL reconstruction in a 10-year-old child. J Pediatr Orthop. 2010;30(5):465–8.
6. Solayar GN, Kapoor H. PCL tibial avulsion with an associated medial meniscal tear in a child: a case report on diagnosis and management. J Pediatr Orthop B. 2012;21(4):356–8.
7. Kwon OS, Park MJ, Kelly JD 4th. Arthroscopic treatment of a PCL avulsion fracture in a skeletally immature patient. Orthopedics. 2011;34(2):137.
8 Anderson AF, Anderson CN. Posterior cruciate and posterolateral ligament reconstruction in an adolescent with open physes. A case report. J Bone Joint Surg Am. 2007;89(7):1598–604.
9. Bovid KM, Salata MJ, Vander Have KL, Sekiya JK. Arthroscopic posterior cruciate ligament reconstruction in a skeletally immature patient: a new technique with case report. Arthroscopy. 2010;26(4):563–70.
10. Accadbled F, Knörr J, Sales de Gauzy J. All inside transtibial arthroscopic posterior cruciate ligament reconstruction in skeletally immature: surgical technique and a case report. Orthop Traumatol Surg Res. 2013;99(3):361–5.
11. Stadelmaier DM, Arnoczky SP, Dodds J, Ross H. The effect of drilling and soft tissue grafting across open growth plates. A histologic study. Am J Sports Med. 1995;23(4):431–5.
12. MacDonald PB, Black B, Old J, Dyck M, Davidson M. Posterior cruciate ligament injury and posterolateral instability in a 6-year-old child. A case report. Am J Sports Med. 2003;31(1)135–136.
13. Shen HC, MD, Yang JJ, MD, Chang JH, MD, Wang SJ, MD. Surgical treatment of injury of the posterior cruciate ligament and posterolateral instability in the knee of a 5-year-old child. A case report. Am J Sports Med. 2007;35(5)831–834.
14. Fanelli GC, Feldmann DD. Arthroscopically assisted combined anterior cruciate ligament/posterior cruciate ligament reconstruction. A practical guide to management. In: Fanelli GC, editor. Posterior cruciate ligament injuries. New York: Springer; 2001. pp. 215–236.
15. Fanelli GC. Arthroscopic PCL reconstruction: transtibial technique. A guide to practical management. In: Fanelli GC, editor. Posterior cruciate ligament injuries. New York: Springer; 2001. pp. 141–156.
16. Fanelli GC. Combined ACL PCL medial lateral side injuries of the knee. A practical guide to management. In: Fanelli GC, editor. The multiple ligament injured knee. New York: Springer; 2004. pp. 111–131.
17. Fanelli GC, Edson CJ, Reinheimer KN. Evaluation and treatment of the multiple ligament injured knee. Instr Course Lect. 2009;58:389–395.
18. Levy B, Dajani KA, Whalen DB, Stannard JP, Fanelli GC, Stuart MJ, Boyd JL, MacDonald PA, Marx RG. Decision making in the multiple ligament injured knee: an evidence based systematic review. Arthroscopy. 2009;25(4):430–438.
19. Levy B, Fanelli GC, Whalen D, Stannard J, MacDonald P, Boyd J, Marx R, Stuart M. Modern perspectives for the treatment of knee dislocations and multiligament reconstruction. J Am Acad Orthop Surg. 2009;17(4):197–206.
20. Fanelli GC, Stannard JP, Stuart MJ, MacDonald PB, Marx RG, Whelan DB, Boyd JL, Levy BA. Management of complex knee ligament injuries. J Bone Joint Surg Am. 2010;92-A(12):2235–2246.
21. Fanelli GC, Beck JD, Edson CJ. Double bundle posterior cruciate ligament reconstruction. Surgical technique and results. Sports Med Arthrosc. 2010;18(4):242–248.
22. Fanelli GC, Beck JD, Edson CJ. Combined PCL ACL lateral and medial side injuries: treatment and results. Sports Med Arthrosc. 2011;19(2):120–130.
23. Fanelli GC. Rationale and surgical technique for PCL and multiple knee ligament reconstruction. 3rd Edn. Warsaw: Biomet Sports Medicine; 2012.
24. Fanelli GC. Mechanical graft tensioning in multiple ligament knee surgery. A practical guide to management. 2nd Edn. In: Fanelli GC, editor. The multiple ligament injured knee. New York: Springer; 2013. pp. 323–330.
25. Fanelli GC. The multiple ligament injured knee: what I have learned. A practical guide to management. 2nd Edn. In: Fanelli GC, editor. The multiple ligament injured knee. New York: Springer; 2013. pp. 3–14.
26. Fanelli GC. Surgical treatment of combined PCL ACL medial and lateral side injuries (global laxity): acute and chronic. A practical guide to management. 2nd Edn. In: Fanelli GC, editor. The multiple ligament injured knee. New York: Springer; 2013. pp. 281–301.
27. Fanelli GC. Posterior cruciate ligament rehabilitation: how slow should we go? Arthroscopy. 2008;24(2):234–235.
28. Edson CJ, Fanelli GC, Beck JD. Rehabilitation after multiple ligament reconstruction of the knee. Sports Med Arthrosc. 2011;19(2):162–166.
29. Edson CJ, Fanelli GC, Beck JD. Postoperative rehabilitation of the posterior cruciate ligament. Sports Med Arthrosc. 2010;18(4):275–279.
30. Edson CJ, Fanelli GC. Postoperative rehabilitation of the multiple ligament injured knee. A practical guide to management. 2nd Edn. In: Fanelli GC, editor. The multiple ligament injured knee. New York: Springer; 2013. pp. 437–442.
31. Daniel DM, Akeson W, O'Conner J, editors. Knee ligaments-structure, function, injury, and repair. New York: Raven; 1990. pp. 421–447.
32. Tegner Y, Lysholm J. Rating system in the evaluation of knee ligament injuries. Clin Orthop. 1985;198:43–49.
33. Windsor RE, Insall JN, Warren RF, Wickiewicz TL. The hospital for special surgery knee ligament rating form. Am J Knee Surg. 1988;1:140–145.

Revision Surgery in Posterior Cruciate Ligament Reconstruction

20

Kevin N. Jiang, Scott R. Kling, Timothy L. Miller and Christopher D. Harner

Overview and Historical Treatment Techniques

The treatment of posterior cruciate and multiple ligament knee injuries (MLI) has evolved since the late nineteenth century. In the first half of the twentieth century, cast immobilization was the treatment of choice for the multiple-ligament-injured knee with most patients experiencing decreased function, decreased strength, recurrent instability, or severe stiffness. Beginning with the work of O'Donoghue in the 1950s [1], surgical treatment with primary ligamentous repair became recognized as a more reliable treatment option than conservative management [2, 3]. However, due to the limited potential of cruciate ligaments to heal primarily, ligamentous reconstruction has been recognized as the treatment of choice for high-grade posterior cruciate ligament (PCL) and multiple ligament knee injuries since the 1980s [4–8].

In the twenty-first century, the goal of revision PCL and multiple knee ligament surgery is to optimize patient functional outcomes. This is accomplished with the use of anatomic reconstruction and repair of all associated soft tissue injuries [9–14]. Combined correction of abnormalities of the bony architecture may also be necessary to support ligament reconstruction. Revision surgery includes arthroscopically assisted cruciate ligament reconstruction, collateral ligament repair or reconstruction, posterolateral corner (PLC) reconstruction or repair, and meniscus repair or partial excision. Secondary procedures often necessary for revision reconstruction include staged procedures, bone grafting of suboptimal bone tunnels, and proximal tibial osteotomy.

The failed PCL and multiple-ligament-injured knee reconstruction is a difficult problem that necessitates concise evaluation and treatment by an experienced knee surgeon [15]. This chapter is meant to present up-to-date treatment principles on injury classification, surgical treatment strategy and techniques, and prevention of complications associated with revision surgery for the PCL and MLI knee. These recommended treatment principles are based on current literature and the 25-year clinical experience of the senior author.

General Treatment Principles

The first step in revision knee ligament surgery is appropriate classification of the injury. This is done based on the cause of surgical failure, timing of the injury, ligaments injured, and associated injuries. All factors are intimately related to one another, but in the revision situation establishing the cause of failure for the primary surgery is most important [16–18]. Cause of failure for primary PCL and multiple knee ligament reconstructions can most often be divided into one of three categories: iatrogenic, biologic, or traumatic. One of the most common causes for failure of primary surgery in the senior author's practice is a missed PLC injury. Other common causes are listed in Table 20.1.

Determining the timing of the failure as acute or chronic is important not only for understanding the etiology of failure but also for determining the viability of primary repair of structures versus reconstruction [19–24]. Chronicity of the treatment failure hints to the possibility of further internal derangement to the meniscus and articular surfaces. In the case of the posterolateral structures, chronicity may make revision repair impossible due to healing and excess scar formation [16–18].

K. N. Jiang (✉)
Orthopaedic Sports, Department of Orthopaedic Surgery, University of Pittsburgh Medical Center, Pittsburgh, PA, USA
e-mail: Jiang.kev@gmail.com

S. R. Kling
UPMC Center for Sports Medicine, Department of Orthopaedic Surgery, University of Pittsburgh, Pittsburgh, PA, USA
e-mail: klingsr@upmc.edu

T. L. Miller
Orthopaedic Surgery, Sports Medicine Division, The Ohio State University Wexner Medical Center, Granville, OH, USA
e-mail: timothy.miller@osumc.edu

C. D. Harner
Department of Orthopaedic Surgery, University of Pittsburgh Medical Center, Pittsburgh, PA, USA
e-mail: harnercd@msx.upmc.edu; harnercd@upmc.edu

G. C. Fanelli (ed.), *Posterior Cruciate Ligament Injuries*,
DOI 10.1007/978-3-319-12072-0_20, © Springer International Publishing Switzerland 2015

Further classification of knee ligamentous injury includes precise diagnosis of which ligaments are insufficient and what associated injuries are present. This requires assessment of the cruciate ligaments, collateral ligaments, posterolateral structures, the meniscus, and articular cartilage. The two most common combined injury patterns after knee dislocations include the anterior cruciate ligament (ACL), PCL, and medial collateral ligament (MCL), and the ACL, PCL, lateral collateral ligament (LCL), and PLC [8, 16–18, 25].

Associated injuries include damage to the patellar tendon, the iliotibial (IT) band, popliteal vascular structures and the common peroneal nerve, as well as bony avulsion fractures [26, 27]. As with all knee injuries, appropriate diagnosis and classification is based on an accurate history, thorough physical examination, and appropriate timely imaging studies [28–32].

Preoperative Evaluation

Patient History and Review of Previous Records

The preoperative evaluation for failed PCL and multiple ligament surgery begins with a thorough history. Though the history is obtained from the patient and family members, a review of the patient's old records is essential for determining what original procedure was performed. Often patients are unreliable sources of objective information and, therefore, operative reports, clinic notes, arthroscopic photographs, and physical therapy reports all provide the revision surgeon with vital information for preoperative planning. Key information to glean from old records includes the timing of surgery, results of the examination under anesthesia, what structures were repaired or reconstructed, grafts used, the status of intraarticular structures, and the type of fixation used [16–18].

Information to be obtained directly from the patient pertains more to current symptoms, the mechanism of injury or reinjury, and the circumstances of the surgical failure [16–18, 33].The surgeon must be able to discern from the patient whether the chief complaint is knee pain or recurrent instability. This distinction alone often determines the course of treatment, with instability more often requiring surgical treatment and pain alone indicating conservative management. Finally, smoking history and the level of patient compliance should be addressed in order to understand the factors related to treatment failure. While the patient is often the best source for describing the circumstances of injury, postoperative level of compliance may be best sought from clinic notes and physical therapy reports.

Table 20.1 Etiology of failure of primary PCL and multiple knee ligament reconstruction

Iatrogenic
Untreated combined instabilities
Missed posterolateral corner injury
Nonanatomic tunnel placement
Incorrect graft tensioning/inadequate fixation
Untreated or unrecognized meniscal or articular pathology
Biologic
Failure of graft incorporation (especially with allograft)
Soft tissue graft elongation
Traumatic
"Aggressive" early rehab before adequate biological healing
Major trauma/reinjury
Combined etiologies

PCL posterior cruciate ligament

Physical Examination

Once the patient's chief complaint and the circumstances of treatment failure have been established from history and review of records, a thorough physical examination of both lower extremities in their entirety should be performed [16–18]. Examination findings are often time dependent. Key physical examination findings to evaluate are listed in Table 20.2. In the initial portion of the evaluation, the

Table 20.2 Key physical examination tests for the failed PCL and multiple ligament reconstructed knee

Global
Gait pattern
Varus thrust
Quadriceps atrophy
Soft tissue injury
Previous incisions
Neurovascular status
Active straight leg raise
Active and passive range of motion
Patellofemoral joint
Medial and lateral patellar glide
Passive patellar tilt
Crepitation with range of motion
Medial and lateral facet tenderness
Lateral patellar apprehension
Meniscus
Joint line tenderness
McMurray's test
Ligamentous laxity examination
Lachman
Anterior drawer (internal, neutral, and external rotation)
Posterior drawer (internal, neutral, and external rotation)
Pivot shift (reverse and internal)
Posterolateral rotatory instability (30° and 90° of flexion)
Varus and valgus stress (0° and 30° of flexion)

PCL posterior cruciate ligament

examiner should pay close attention to gait pattern, varus thrust, the soft tissue envelope, atrophy of the quadriceps musculature, the presence or absence of an effusion, ability to perform an active straight leg raise, neurovascular status, and active and passive range of motion [16–18, 27, 34–38]. More focused evaluation of the knee joint should include a detailed assessment of the patellofemoral joint for crepitation, tenderness to palpation, and the integrity of the medial patellofemoral ligament. Not uncommonly an associated patellofemoral subluxation or dislocation may occur with a tibiofemoral dislocation. Medial and lateral patellar glide as well of patellar tilt and lateral apprehension testing helps to determine the status of the medial checkrein structures [16–18].

Joint line tenderness as well as the flexion McMurray's test is utilized to assess the status of the meniscus medially and laterally. Ligamentous laxity patterns are then evaluated using the Lachman, anterior and posterior drawer, pivot shift, quadriceps active, varus and valgus stress, and posterolateral rotator instability tests [16–18, 39, 40]. Anterior and posterior drawer tests should be performed in internal rotation, neutral, and external rotation. Varus and valgus stress tests should be performed in 0° and 30° of flexion, and posterolateral rotatory instability (PLRI) tests in 30° and 90° of flexion. Keep in mind that there are two laxity patterns involved with a PLC injury: varus (LCL) and rotation (PLC). They may occur separately or in combination [41]. These tests should be meticulously performed and graded, then compared to the uninjured limb to determine asymmetry.

Preoperative Imaging: Radiographs, MRI, and Vascular Studies

Complete and appropriate imaging studies serve as a road map for revision PCL and multiple ligament knee surgery. In addition to the bones and soft tissue structures, imaging should also be used to evaluate arterial and venous structures prior to revision surgery [16–18].

Radiographs

For all failed knee ligament reconstruction patients, standard knee series X-rays should be obtained and ideally compared with the patient's original preoperative X-rays. In the senior author's practice, all patients receive a standing bilateral 45° posterior-anterior (PA) flexion X-ray, a bilateral 30° merchant view X-ray, bilateral lateral views, and a standing bilateral long cassette image. Important information to be ascertained from this imaging series includes: (1) patella height, (2) tunnel position and size, (3) degree of tibiofemoral subluxation, (4) mechanical and anatomic axes, (5) position of retained hardware, and (6) associated fractures and osteopenia. Stress radiographs may also be helpful to determine the presence of fixed subluxation. Figure 20.1 shows the preoperative bilateral AP radiographs after a failed PCL reconstruction.

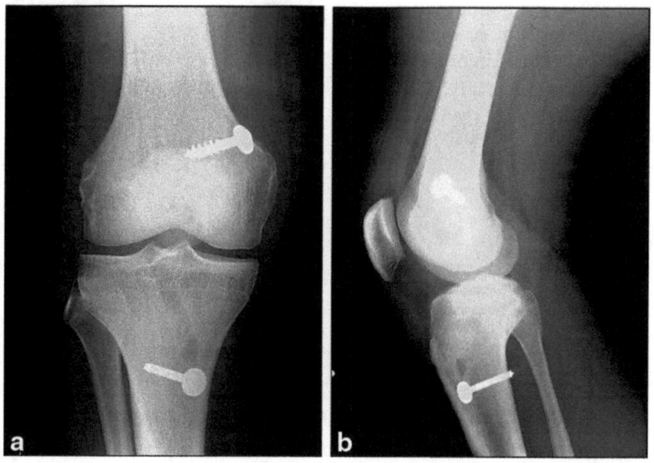

Fig. 20.1 AP and lateral X-rays of a 31-year-old female soccer player with recurrent instability after failed PCL reconstruction. PCL posterior cruciate ligament (With permission from Ref. [62], Fig. 21.1)

MRI

A recent magnetic resonance imaging (MRI) should be obtained to evaluate the soft tissue structures prior to revision surgery. It should be born in mind, however, that postsurgical changes may confuse the injury pattern picture. All imaging series should be scrutinized by the surgeon and an experienced musculoskeletal radiologist to determine new injury from postsurgical changes. Care should be taken to evaluate all ligamentous structures, the patellar tendon, medial and lateral menisci, the articular cartilage, and posterolateral structures [16, 18, 19, 42, 43].

MRI can also be used to evaluate the arterial anatomy at the posterior knee. Revision surgery is significantly more risky with proximity of the popliteal artery due to scarring or variant anatomy of the vasculature. An aberrant anterior tibial artery which runs anterior to the popliteus muscle and adjacent to the posterior capsule and tibial cortex occurs in 2.1 % of extremities [44]. Recognition of the presence of this anatomical variant is important to decrease the risk of injury during tibial tunnel drilling and proximal tibial osteotomy when necessary.

Arteriogram/CT Angiogram

Though often more pertinent in the acute setting after knee dislocation and prior to primary reconstruction, an arteriogram or a computed tomography (CT) angiogram of the lower extremity should be obtained in any patient with suspected vascular injury [16–18, 27, 45]. Spasm, intimal injury, or complete tear may all alter vascular status to the injured limb and must be thoroughly evaluated prior to revision surgery [46–50]. It is strongly recommended that when there is

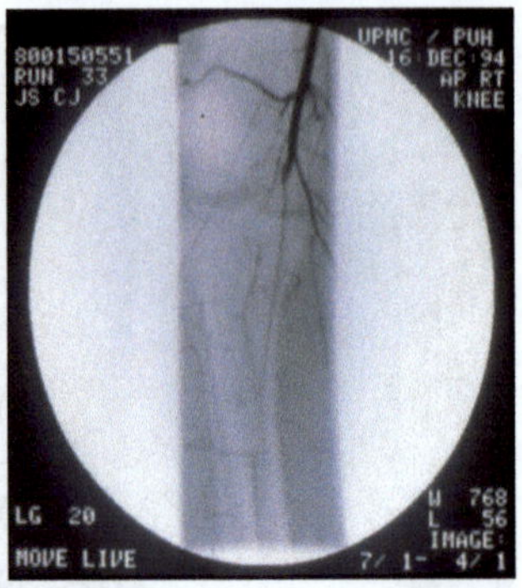

Fig. 20.2 Preoperative arteriogram demonstrating a popliteal arterial injury. (With permission from Ref. [62], Fig 21.2)

any doubt regarding the vascular status of the extremity, a preoperative arteriogram should be obtained [16–18, 50–52]. Figure 20.2 demonstrates a preoperative arteriogram in a patient with popliteal artery occlusion after a knee dislocation.

Venous Duplex Doppler Ultrasound

All patients with combined ligamentous injuries and failed reconstructions should undergo a venous duplex Doppler ultrasound to rule out deep vein thrombosis (DVT). Given the decreased ambulatory status and limited range of motion of the traumatized knee, patients with MLI are predisposed to clot formation [16–18]. It is recommended that bilateral Doppler ultrasounds be obtained after the initial office visit and 1 day prior to revision surgery.

Patient Counseling

Discussions with patients prior to revision posterior cruciate and multiple ligament reconstructions should stress the importance of realistic expectations. Functional needs for activities of daily living and occupational requirements should take precedence over return to sporting activities. The lengthy recovery time, rehab commitment, and increased risk of complications after revision knee ligament surgery should be thoroughly understood by the patient and family members before proceeding to surgery. Degenerative changes to the joint are likely no matter how great the technical ability of the surgeon. It should be further stressed that the use of tobacco products may further delay or inhibit the patient's healing ability postoperatively, and efforts should be made to discontinue tobacco use.

Revision PCL and Multiple Knee Ligament Surgery

Indications and Contraindications

Indications for revision PCL or multiple ligament reconstructions include a patient with a previous failed PCL or MLI reconstruction and continued symptoms of instability with or without pain. As previously noted, a thorough preoperative assessment of combined instabilities and associated injuries should be performed. Concomitant injuries should be addressed along with the revision reconstruction [53]. Contraindications to revision reconstruction include severe loss of range of motion, fixed posterior subluxation, advanced osteoarthritis, and active infection.

Preoperative Planning

Timing of Surgery

The appropriate timing of revision PCL and multiple knee ligament surgery is dependent on multiple factors. Key elements in determining ideal timing of surgery include patient-related factors, equipment availability, and qualified personnel. Patient-related factors affecting surgical timing pertain to the general health of the patient, availability of patient assistance after hospital discharge, and the presence of active infection. Available equipment must include desired allografts, necessary fixation devices, and intraoperative fluoroscopy [16–18, 26, 40]. Qualified personnel necessary for successful revision reconstruction includes an experienced knee surgeon, familiar operating room staff, and occasionally a vascular surgeon on standby. The procedure should be performed as the first and/or only case of the day when the reconstructive surgeon is well rested. Plans should be in place for the patient to be admitted to an inpatient orthopedic ward or ICU for the first 24 h postoperatively.

Graft Selection

Graft selection is dependent on autograft or allograft availability, previously used graft type, surgeon experience, and surgeon preference. In the revision situation, it is prudent to consider allograft reconstruction particularly for MLI cases. This is done in order to limit the amount of soft tissue disruption inflicted on an already traumatized soft tissue envelope. If autograft reconstruction is chosen, it is crucial to be aware of the type of any previously used autograft to assure intraoperative availability of the graft. Review of previous operative notes is essential for assuring graft availability and operative efficiency.

Autograft tissue may be harvested from the ipsilateral or contralateral extremity and has the advantage of better graft incorporation and remodeling [16–18]. At our institution, Achilles tendon and Tibialias Anterior allografts have been traditionally favored for revision reconstructions [1]. In recent years, quadriceps tendon autograft with a patellar bone plug has gained favor for younger patients. The advantages of using allograft tissue include: decreased operative time and no donor site morbidity [16–18, 54, 55].

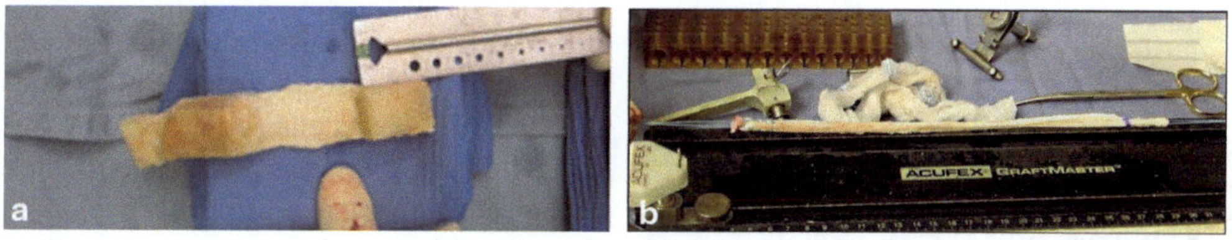

Fig. 20.3 Two commonly used allograft options for MLI reconstructions. (*From top to bottom*) **a** Bone-patellar tendon-bone and **b** anterior tibialis allografts. MLI multiple ligament injuries (With permission from Ref. [62], Fig. 21.3)

Risks of allograft usage include an increase in cost, delay in incorporation, elongation of the soft tissue portion, and potential disease transmission [55]. Figure 20.3 illustrates commonly used allograft options.

Previous Skin Incisions

Prior to undertaking revision knee ligament surgery, all previously used skin incisions should be known and marked with an indelible marker. When practical, previous incisions should be utilized to avoid further disruption to the soft tissue envelope. Patients should be aware, however, that previous incision may need to be extended for adequate visualization and separate incisions may be necessary. Ideally, a discussion of incisions should be carried out with the patient in the clinic and expected incisions should be drawn and demonstrated to the patient.

Diagnostic Arthroscopy and Staged Procedures

In the case of malpositioned or overly dilated bone tunnels, bone grafting and staging of revision reconstruction may be necessary [16–18]. Most modern digital imaging programs include a ruler tool allowing for more accurate measurement of tunnel width. Preoperative radiographs should be scrutinized and tunnel widths noted. These results should then be compared with operative notes from the primary surgery to determine the presence of tunnel dilation. Preparations should be made for harvesting bone graft or inserting prepackaged allograft bone dowels if poor bone stock or malpositioned tunnels are present. Regardless of the results of preoperative X-rays, a diagnostic arthroscopy should be performed to determine the need for staged revision prior to proceeding with graft harvest. If excessive tunnel widening or reabsorption is encountered, previous fixation hardware should be removed, the tunnels grafted, and adequate time allowed for healing and incorporation (usually 6 months) [16–18].

Intraoperative Fluoroscopy

Intraoperative fluoroscopy has become an invaluable tool in primary as well as revision knee ligament reconstruction. The utility of readily available fluoroscopy lies in the ability to place precise anatomic tunnels in the femur and tibia and prevent the potential complication of tunnel convergence. Not only is fluoroscopy useful for guide pin and tunnel placement but also it helps the surgeon to perform a more accurate preoperative examination under anesthesia [16–18]. With fluoroscopic examination under anesthesia, real-time evaluation can be made of ligamentous laxity. This is especially useful in evaluating fixed posterior tibial translation with PCL injuries [16–18]. Figure 20.4 shows an intraoperative lateral fluoroscopic knee X-ray with a PCL tibial tunnel guide positioned for guide pin placement.

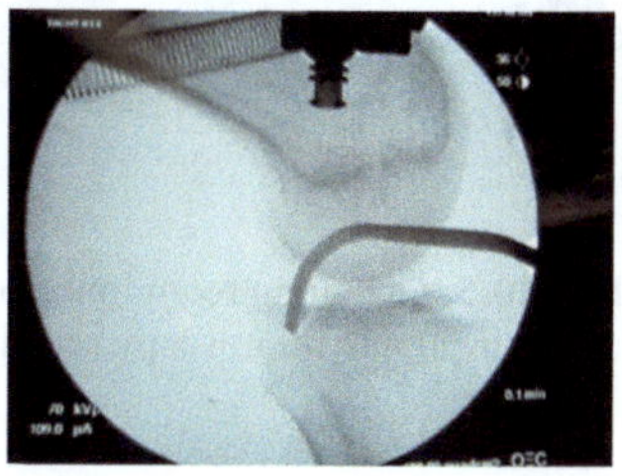

Fig. 20.4 Intraoperative fluoroscopic image showing positioning of PCL tibial tunnel guide. PCL posterior cruciate ligament (With permission from Ref. [62], Fig. 21.4)

Surgical Technique (Section Adapted and Modified from Ref. [63], Chaps. 47 and 49)

Anesthesia

The choice of anesthesia is made in conjunction with the surgeon, the anesthesiologist, and the patient. The anesthesia team typically chooses between a general anesthesia or an epidural anesthetic with intravenous sedation. If the anesthesiologist is at all concerned regarding airway management, general anesthesia is performed. At our institution, preoperative femoral and sciatic nerve blocks are routinely used. The nerve blocks not only provide anesthesia for the surgical procedure but also provide up to 12 h of postoperative pain relief. A Foley catheter is placed for monitoring fluid status, and a vascular surgeon is on call in case a vascular injury occurs during the procedure.

Patient Positioning

The patient is placed in the supine position on a flat top table with the patient's heels at the end of the operative table. No well-leg holder, or tourniquet, is used for the procedure. A foot post is secured to the operative table to maintain the knee in a 90° flexed position. A side post is secured to the table at the level of the lesser trochanter, and a soft bump

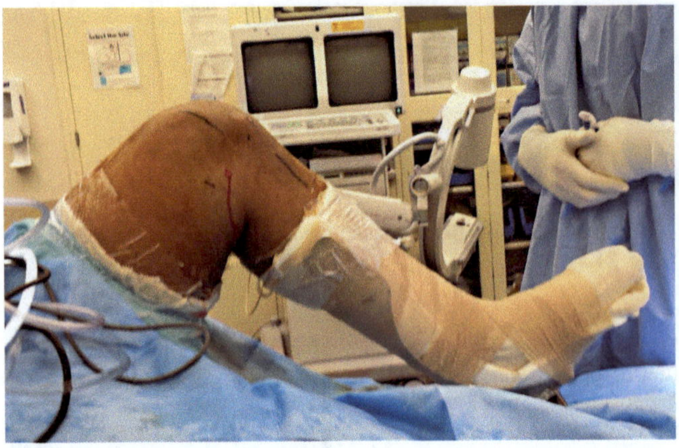

Fig. 20.5 Operating room limb positioning with arthroscopic leg holder and available fluoroscopy seen in the background

is placed under the hip of the injured limb. Alternatively, a well-padded arthroscopic leg holder can be used to hold the leg. Figure 20.5 demonstrates the senior author's operative setup for limb positioning and available fluoroscopic imaging. All limbs are well padded for the procedure, particularly the uninjured lower extremity.

Examination under Anesthesia

After successful induction of anesthesia in the operating room, a thorough examination under anesthesia is performed and correlated with clinical assessment and imaging findings. It is of utmost importance to examine the uninjured extremity and use it as a reference. Passive range of motion is first tested noting any deficits or asymmetry to the uninjured limb. The anterior drawer, Lachman, and pivot shift tests are then performed to evaluate the ACL.

Posterior tibial sag and translation with posterior drawer testing are then used to evaluate the PCL. The knee is then placed into the figure-four position, and the LCL is palpated with a bowstring test. Varus and valgus stress is then applied to the knee in 0° and 30° of flexion to evaluate the LCL and MCL, respectively. PLC structures are then evaluated by applying an external rotation force to the proximal tibia and fibula at 30° and 90° of flexion with the proximal tibia held in a reduced position. Degree of external rotation is then referenced with the uninjured limb. Greater than a 15° increase in external rotation is an indication of PLC injury.

Surface Landmarks and Skin Incisions

An indelible marker is used to identify the surface anatomy and the incisions that will be utilized during the procedure. The osseous landmarks including the inferior pole of the patella, the tibial tubercle, Gerdy's tubercle, and the fibular head are identified and marked. The peroneal nerve is then palpated and marked superficial to the fibular neck. The medial and lateral joint lines are then identified. All previous and potential skin incisions are then marked. The anterolateral arthroscopy portal is placed adjacent to the lateral border of the patella above the joint line. The anteromedial arthroscopy portal is placed approximately 1 cm medial to the patellar tendon at the same level. A superolateral outflow portal is placed 1 cm proximal to the superior pole of the patella and posterior to the quadriceps tendon.

A longitudinal 3-cm incision originating 2 cm distal to the joint line and 2 cm medial to the tibial tubercle is drawn on the anteromedial proximal tibia for the ACL and PCL tibial tunnels. A 2-cm incision is placed just medial to the medial trochlea articular surface and along the subvastus interval for the PCL femoral tunnel. The incision for the lateral and posterolateral structures is a curvilinear 12-cm incision that is drawn midway between Gerdy's tubercle and the fibular head. It is traced proximal to the lateral femoral epicondyle while the knee is in 90° of flexion [16–18]. If a medial injury is present, the distal incision for the tibial tunnels is traced proximally to the medial epicondyle in a curvilinear fashion.

Diagnostic Arthroscopy/Intra-Articular Evaluation

An arthroscopic approach is advocated to assist in the planning of potential skin incisions needed for the procedure based on the pattern of injury. Gravity inflow or dry arthroscopy is recommended for the prevention of iatrogenic compartment syndrome. If inflow is used, the posterior leg musculature should be palpated intermittently to assess for developing compartment syndrome. If excess fluid extravasation is noted, then the arthroscopic technique should be abandoned in favor of an open approach.

All compartments within the knee are assessed. The MCL and the meniscal attachment to the deep MCL are assessed to determine if tibial-sided injury is present. In the lateral compartment, the popliteus tendon is visualized and probed to discern if its function has been compromised. Both cruciate ligaments should be evaluated at their femoral and tibial insertion sites along with both menisci and the articular cartilage. If intra-articular pathology is present, any concomitant articular cartilage or meniscal injury must be addressed. Every effort should be made to preserve as much meniscus tissue as possible. Peripheral meniscus tears are repaired with an inside-out technique while irreparable tears may be debrided. If inside-out repair is performed, the sutures should be tied directly onto the joint capsule at 30° of flexion.

The necessary debridement of the joint is performed with a 4.5-mm arthroscopic shaver and basket forceps. This includes debridement of the notch while preserving any remaining intact PCL tissue. The tibial insertion site of the PCL is removed by inserting a shaver or a curette through a posteromedial portal and developing a plane between the PCL and the posterior capsule. Every attempt is made to debride the tibial insertion of the PCL to help with eventual placement of the guide wire for the tibial tunnel. In the senior author's practice, a limited notchplasty is performed. The fat pad should be preserved if at all possible to prevent patellar fat pad entrapment syndrome.

Biplanar Opening Wedge High Tibial Osteotomy

When performing a high tibial osteotomy, preoperative templating using standing long cassette radiographs is essential. The planned osteotomy should be drawn, and an estimate of the proximal tibial width and necessary plate size should be made. The width of the opening wedge osteotomy on the tibia is determined by the degree of desired correction.

The patient is placed in the supine position as described above. An incision is made midway between the tibial tubercle and the posterior border of the tibia. This incision begins 1 cm inferior to the joint line and extends approximately 5 cm distally. Exposure is made down to the superficial fibers of the MCL. Subcutaneous flaps are created to allow exposure of the patellar tendon and the tibial tubercle. The patellar tendon is retracted laterally. An incision is then made in the sartorius fascia just superior to the gracilis tendon, and a subperiosteal dissection is carried out superiorly to release the superficial fibers of the MCL off of bone. Care must be taken to prevent violating the fibers of the MCL.

A tibial guide wire is placed from an anteromedial to a posterolateral direction angled 15° cephalad along the proposed osteotomy, and its position is confirmed with fluoroscopy. The line of osteotomy should be just superior to the tibial tubercle. The width of the proximal tibia should then be confirmed using a free Kirschner (K)-wire to confirm that the actual tibial width at the osteotomy site matches the template tibial width on preoperative radiographs. This allows confirmation of an adequate tibial osteotomy correction. A 1-in. osteotome is used to begin the osteotomy, using the K-wire as the directional guide. Once the osteotomy plane is established, the K-wire may be removed and the osteotomy completed with an oscillating saw or osteotome. Care must be taken to protect the lateral hinge of cortical bone. To safely complete the osteotomy across the posterior tibial cortex and protect the neurovascular structures, the osteotome must be angled to avoid excess perforation of the posterior cortex.

An opening wedge osteotomy system with a wedge device is then inserted into the osteotomy site to create the desired angle of correction. The appropriate plate is then selected and placed in the anteromedial aspect to the osteotomy for a biplanar effect. The alignment of the leg is again checked using the Bovie cord and fluoroscopy with the cord recreating the mechanical axis of the knee joint. The axis should cross lateral to the tibial spine. The plate is then secured in place with two cancellous screws proximally that are directed parallel to the joint line. The plate is fixed distally with 4.5 mm screws with purchase into the lateral tibial cortex. Wedge cuts of bone graft are then inserted into the osteotomy site. The superficial MCL is then repaired to the medial proximal tibial metaphysis with suture anchors. Figure 20.6 shows the AP and lateral X-rays after a biplanar osteotomy and plate fixation with PCL reconstruction.

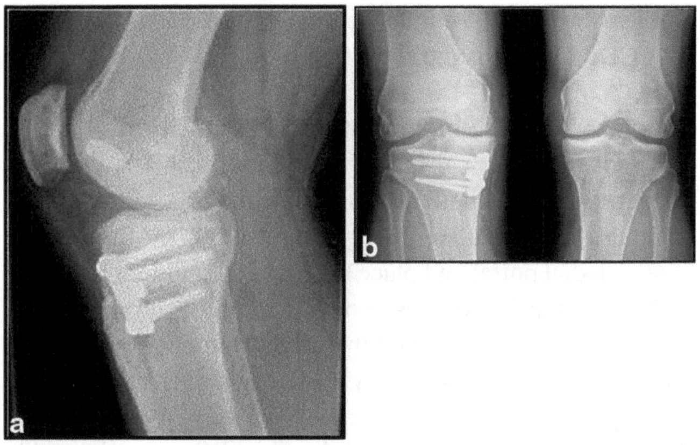

Fig. 20.6 Postoperative lateral and AP X-rays after a biplanar osteotomy and plate fixation with PCL reconstruction. PCL posterior cruciate ligament (With permission from Ref. [62], Fig. 21.6)

Graft Preparation

ACL A bone-patellar tendon-bone allograft is preferred for our ACL revision reconstructions. We prefer 10-mm by 18-mm cylindrical bone plugs with a 10-mm tendon width. Two #5 nonabsorbable sutures are passed through drill holes placed in both bone plugs.

PCL An Achilles tendon allograft is preferred for revision PCL reconstructions. This graft choice provides adequate length, a significant cross-sectional area, and a large calcaneal bone block. For the measurement of graft length needed, a suture may be passed retrograde into the tibial PCL tunnel. The end of the suture is placed at the entrance to the femoral PCL tunnel and the suture is marked at the opening of the distal tibial PCL tunnel; 20 mm is added to this length to account for the length of graft in the femoral PCL tunnel. Precise measurement of graft length needed will ensure the bone plug portion of the graft is flush or slightly recessed at the distal tibial PCL tunnel. The graft is cut to proper length and the central portion of the bone block is fashioned to a 10-mm by 18-mm bone plug. Two #2 nonabsorbable sutures are passed through the bone plug, and the tendon is tubularized with a double-armed #5 nonabsorbable suture. Alternatively, a quadriceps tendon allograft with an 18-mm by 10-mm bone plug is harvested, and two #2 nonabsorbable sutures are passed through the bone plug. The proximal 20 mm of the tendinous portion is then baseball stitched with #5 nonabsorbable suture.

LCL A tibialis anterior tendon allograft is used for the LCL. The graft is tubularized with #2 sutures at each end to allow passage through 6–7-mm bone tunnel fibular head and femoral LCL attachment site.

Cruciate Tunnel Placement and Preparation

The PCL tibial tunnel is addressed first as this is the most dangerous and challenging portion of the procedure. We introduce a 15-mm offset PCL guide set at 50–55° through the anteromedial portal and place the tip of the guide at the distal and lateral third of the insertion site of the PCL on the tibia. The 3- to 4-cm medial proximal tibial skin incision is made, and the periosteum is sharply dissected from the bone. The starting point of the K-wire is approximately 3–4 cm distal to the joint line. The trajectory of the tibial PCL tunnel roughly parallels the angle of the proximal tibiofibular joint. We then pass a 3/32-mm K-wire into the desired position and perforate the far cortex of the tibia at the PCL insertion; this is done under direct arthroscopic visualization. Caution must be taken when passing the guide wire through the cortex of the tibial insertion of the PCL because of the close proximity of the neurovascular structures. Oftentimes, the PCL tibial insertion site has a cancellous feel when the far cortex is breeched and no hard cortex can be felt while the K-wire is advanced. The location of this pin placement is then confirmed with the mini C-arm fluoroscopy machine on the true lateral projection of the knee. Occasionally, the wire is too proximal of the PCL tibial insertion site and a 3- to 5-mm parallel pin guide will be used to obtain the ideal placement of the PCL tibial tunnel. The K-wire for the PCL tibial tunnel is left in place and attention is paid to the ACL tibial tunnel. The tibial guide set at 47.5° is introduced into the anteromedial portal and a 3/32-mm guide wire placed in the center of the ACL tibial footprint. This position should rest approximately 7 mm anterior to the PCL and should coincide with the posterior extent of the anterior horn of the lateral meniscus. The location of the ACL tibial tunnel is also confirmed on the full extension lateral projection with the mini C-arm machine. The guide wire should rest posterior to the Blumenstaat line on the full extension lateral projection to ensure proper placement of the ACL tibial tunnel. The ACL tibial tunnel is proximal and anterior to the PCL tibial tunnel (Fig. 20.7).

After acceptable placement of the ACL and PCL tibial tunnel guide wires is confirmed, the PCL tunnel is drilled. A curette is placed directly on top of the guide wire over the area of the drill site. The 10-mm compaction drill bit is passed under direct arthroscopic visualization with a 30° arthroscope that is introduced through the posteromedial portal. This is initially passed through the tibia on power to the posterior tibial cortex then completed by hand. The PCL tibial tunnel is then expanded to a diameter of 10–11 mm (the size of the graft) using dilators in 0.5-mm increments. The ACL tibial tunnel is then drilled in a similar manner with a 9-mm compaction drill. The ACL tibial tunnel is expanded to a diameter of 10 mm using the dilators in 0.5-mm increments. We prefer at least a 1–2-cm bone bridge between the ACL and PCL tibial tunnels.

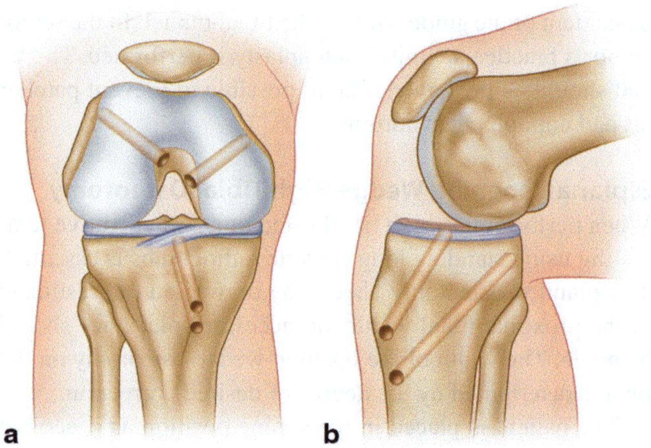

Fig. 20.7 Diagram of tibial and femoral tunnel positions for ACL and PCL reconstruction. ACL anterior cruciate ligament, PCL posterior cruciate ligament (With permission from Ref. [62], Fig. 21.7)

The femoral tunnels for the ACL and PCL are now established. For a single-bundle PCL reconstruction, the insertion for the PCL on the intercondylar notch is identified and the K-wire is placed from the anterolateral portal to a point approximately 7–10 mm from the articular margin within the anterior portion of the PCL femoral footprint. This is then overdrilled with a 10-mm compaction drill to a depth of approximately 24–35 mm. The tunnel is then dilated to the size of the graft by 0.5-mm increments. Next, the ACL femoral tunnel is established approximately 6 mm anterior to the back wall or over the top position of the femur and "northwest" or "northeast" position for right and left knees, respectively. We prefer the medial portal technique to the traditional transtibial technique due to the ability to place a more anatomically positioned insertion site on the femur. The K-wire is overdrilled with the 9-mm compaction drill to a depth of 25–35 mm. This tunnel is then expanded as before to a diameter of 10 mm with the dilators in 0.5-mm increments.

Graft Passage

In the case of multiple ligament reconstruction, the graft for the PCL is passed first. A looped #2 suture is passed retrograde into the PCL tibial tunnel and retrieved out through the anterolateral arthroscopy portal with an arthroscopic grasper. A separate looped #2 suture on a Beath pin is passed through the femoral PCL tunnel and out through the anteromedial femur through the anterolateral portal. Both tibial and femoral tunnel loops sutures are retrieved out the anteromedial portal. The nonabsorbable suture that has secured the tendon portion of the graft is shuttled with the looped tibial tunnel suture retrograde up the PCL tibial tunnel into the joint and out the anteromedial portal. This graft suture is then pulled through the femoral PCL tunnel out the anteromedial thigh with the previously placed looped shuttling suture. First the graft is pulled into the joint with the assistance of a looped towel clamp or right angle clamp around the turn from tibial PCL tunnel into the notch. Once 20–25 mm of the tendon portion of the graft has been pulled past the femoral PCL tunnel, then the sutures to the graft are shuttled out to the anteromedial thigh with the previous looped suture. The graft is now pulled into the femoral PCL tunnel with the help of a probe. The bone plug of the PCL graft should now be slightly recessed or flush with the tibial cortex.

The ACL is passed in the usual fashion using the medial portal technique. The Beath pin with a #5 suture attached eyelet is passed through the femoral tunnel via the medial portal. An arthroscopic suture retriever device is passed retrograde through the tibial tunnel and the #5 suture is retrieved. The graft is then passed from the tibial tunnel into the femoral tunnel with arthroscopic assistance. A heavy right angle clamp is again used to aid in positioning the bone plug for femoral tunnel passage. The femoral fixation of the cruciate grafts is done at this time using a suspensory implant secured on the femoral cortex. Fluoroscopic imaging is used to assure that the suspensory device is seated properly on the femoral cortex. The grafts are not tensioned, however, until the end of the case.

LCL Reconstruction

An anatomical LCL reconstruction is performed with a 7 mm tibialis anterior allograft as previous described by LaPrade et al. [56]. A lateral hockey stick incision is made extending from the posterolateral thigh to the anterolateral tibia over Gerdy's tubercle using previous incision if possible. Dissection is carried down to the IT band and long and short heads of the biceps. Common peroneal exposure is performed and the nerve is protected during the reconstruction. The LCL femoral attachment site is identified just posterior to the lateral epicondyle and a guide pin is placed exiting at the anteromedial aspect of the thigh. A 6-mm bone tunnel is drilled and then dilated to 7 mm. The LCL fibular attachment is then identified at the lateral aspect of the fibular head. The posteromedial aspect of the fibular head is dissected with care to protect the common peroneal nerve. A guide pin is placed from the LCL attachment site laterally to the posteromedial aspect of the fibular head. A 6-mm bone tunnel is then reamed and dilated to 7 mm. The graft is passed from posteromedial to lateral on the fibular head. The proximal graft end is then passed under the IT band and into the femoral tunnel with a shuttling suture exiting the anteromedial thigh. Bioabsorbable interference screws are used for fixation at both the femoral and fibular tunnels. Alternatively, the graft can be routed around the fibular head laterally and sutured to itself for fixation.

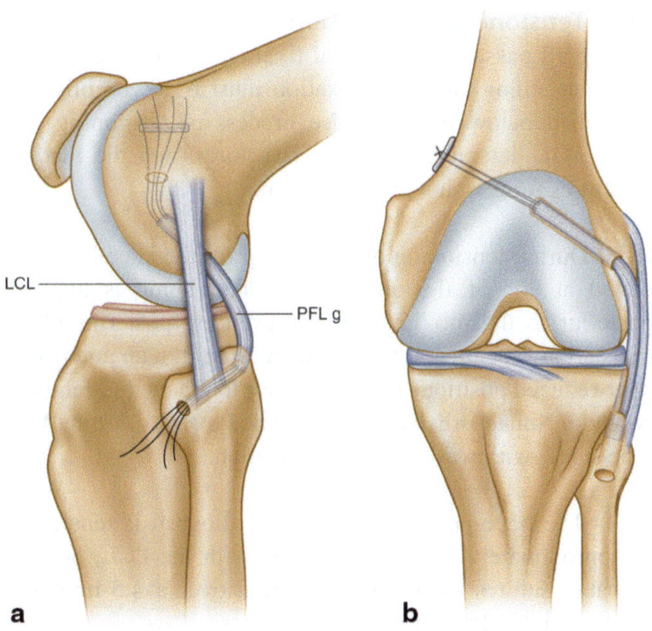

Fig. 20.8 Popliteofibular ligament reconstruction. (With permission from Ref. [62], Fig. 21.8)

Popliteofibular Ligament Reconstruction

The goal of reconstruction is reconstitution of the static portion of the PLC complex. The preferred grafts for this reconstruction include hamstring autograft or anterior tibialis allograft. The lateral epicondyle of the femur is exposed and the popliteus tendon is subperiosteally dissected off of its anatomic insertion. A whipstitch is placed in the popliteus tendon with a #2 nonabsorbable suture. A 6-mm femoral drill tunnel is then placed at the lateral epicondyle to a depth of 25–30 mm and the tunnel is expanded to 7 mm in diameter with the serial dilators. The posterior border of the fibula at the insertion of the PFL is exposed by incising horizontally just below the biceps insertion and proximal to the peroneal nerve. The anterior border of the fibula is also exposed from the anterior tibial musculature. A guide wire is then passed from anterior to posterior across the fibular head. Care must be taken not to violate the LCL tunnel if one has been previously drilled. The PFL tunnel is then drilled over the guide wire medially in the fibular head and then dilated to a diameter of 7 mm. The graft is passed from posterior to anterior through the tunnel using a Hewson suture passer. The proximal end of the graft is then passed medial to the LCL and into the previously drilled femoral tunnel at the popliteus insertion site. Both the graft and the dissected popliteus tendon and pulled into the tunnel. Approximately 25 mm of graft and 10 mm of popliteus tendon are pulled into the femoral tunnel and secured with an AO screw post or a suspensory device. A diagram of the popliteofibular ligament reconstruction is shown in Fig. 20.8.

Graft Tensioning and Fixation

Once graft passage and femoral fixation are complete, final graft tensioning and distal fixation must be accomplished. Described below is a stepwise process of tensioning the PCL, ACL, lateral ligamentous structures, and the medial structures for revision reconstruction.

PCL During tensioning of the PCL graft, the knee is maintained at 90° of flexion and a padded bump is applied posterior to the proximal tibia, preventing posterior tibial translation. The medial tibial plateau is held in an anteriorly over-reduced position, 10 mm anterior to the medial femoral condyle. Nonabsorbable sutures are tied over a 4.5-mm AO-type screw with washer for tibial fixation.

ACL The bone-patellar tendon-bone allograft is tensioned in approximately 15° of flexion. As with the PCL, nonabsorbable sutures of the graft are tied over a 4.5-mm AO screw with washer which serves as a post.

LCL and PLC The LCL and popliteofibular ligament are tensioned in 30° of flexion and the posterolateral corner (when timing of the revision reconstruction allows) with an internal rotation force on the tibia and fibula. The LCL graft is then fixed either in the fibular head with an interference screw or with bone tunnel passage and suture technique. The popliteofibular graft is passed through a bone tunnel in the proximal fibula and fixed either with an interference screw or suspensory device.

Medial Structures The MCL is fixed at 30° of flexion, while the posterior oblique ligament is stabilized near full extension, preventing over-constraint of the knee. The repaired or reconstructed ligamentous complex is then fixed using either suture anchors or nonabsorbable sutures tied over an AO screw post.

Closure and Dressings

Prior to closure, it is pertinent to obtain an intraoperative X-ray imaging to establish that the joint is reduced in the AP and lateral planes and all hardware is in the appropriate position. After thorough irrigation of all wounds with antibiotic saline solution, deep fascia and periosteal layers are closed in a mattress fashion with #2 silky poly-dec nonabsorbable sutures. The subcutaneous tissues are then closed with 2-0 absorbable suture and the skin is re-approximated with either staples or 4-0 Caprosyn suture in a subcuticular fashion. Arthroscopic portals are then closed using 3-0 nylon suture.

Prior to application of dressings, a vascular examination using either direct palpation or Doppler ultrasound is performed to ensure the presence of a dorsalis pedis and posterior tibial pulse. The calf musculature is then palpated to assure that iatrogenic compartment syndrome has not occurred. Dressings consisting of Adaptic, sterile 4×4 gauze, ABDs, Webril, and an ACE wrap are applied to the extremity. Finally, a hinged knee brace locked in full extension is applied to the knee (Fig. 20.9). Tight, constrictive braces and dressings should be avoided to prevent increased risk for compartment syndrome and peroneal nerve injury.

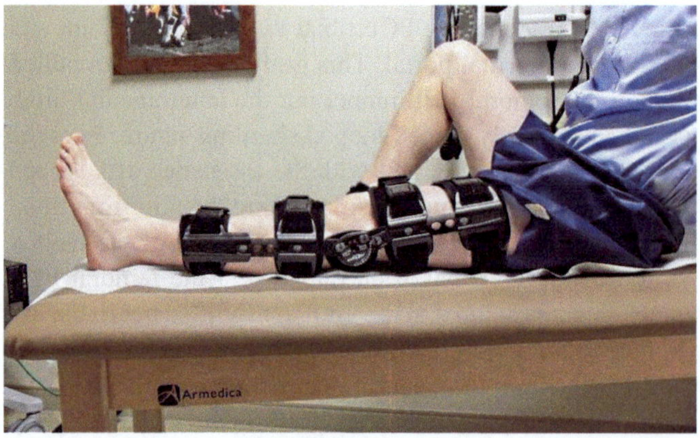

Fig. 20.9 A hinged knee brace locked in extension is applied immediately post-op and discontinued when quadriceps function returns. (With permission from Ref. [62], Fig. 21.9)

Immediate Postoperative Care

Given the need for general anesthesia, extended surgical time, and the risk of compartment syndrome, patients should be admitted for the first postoperative night. Give appropriate preoperative and postoperative antibiotics. Prophylactic anticoagulation with subcutaneous enoxaparin should be used in all high-risk patients. Aspirin is indicated in low-risk patients. In the senior author's practice, smoking and the use of oral contraceptive pills are considered to be risk factors for thrombosis.

Particularly in the first 4 weeks postoperatively, the surgeon should anticipate potential problems and complications. It is recommended that patients be seen and evaluated in follow-up three times during the first month postoperatively. A high index of suspicion for infection and venous thrombosis should be maintained during the first 4 weeks post-op. Venous duplex Doppler ultrasound studies should be used liberally during this timeframe to rule out DVT.

Rehabilitation Protocol

An appropriate and individualized postoperative rehabilitation program is integral to optimizing patient outcomes after revision surgery [37]. Immediately post-op, the limb is placed into a hinged knee brace locked in extension. A footdrop splint may be used for patients with peroneal nerve injury. Initial postoperative rehabilitation is very conservative. The patient is braced in full extension for the first 4 weeks post-op. Weightbearing as tolerated is allowed except in cases with LCL reconstruction where they are made non-weightbearing. The patients do quad sets, straight-leg raises, and calf pumps. Continuous passive motion machines are not recommended in this situation.

At 1 month post-op, closed chain activities are started by unlocking the brace and doing mini squats. They are weight-bearing as tolerated (WBAT) with crutches until 2 months post-op. Passive- and active-assisted range of motion exercises are then initiated to increase knee flexion beyond 90° with the goal of reaching symmetric motion to the uninjured knee by 12 weeks. [57] In the senior author's practice approximately 10–20 % of patients require manipulation under anesthesia between 8 and 12 weeks to reach 90° of flexion.

Patients performing sedentary occupations and light duty may often return to work after 2–4 weeks. Heavy laborers should not expect to return to work for 6–9 months. Return to sports activity should not be expected until 1 year post-revision surgery, if ever. Of note, maintaining close contact with the patient's physical therapist throughout the recovery period from revision knee ligament reconstruction can be vital for preventing reinjury or surgical failure due to overly aggressive rehab. Furthermore, knowing the patient's expected level of compliance and keeping the first 4 weeks of rehabilitation as simple as possible will help to prevent reinjury of the reconstructed knee. A team approach between surgeon, patient, family members, and physical therapists is vital for treatment success.

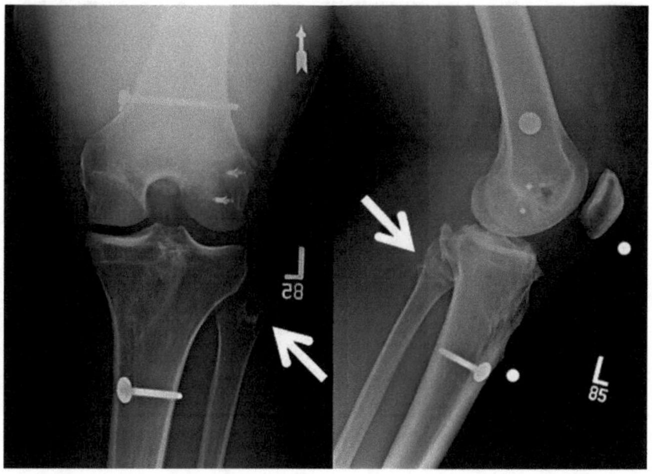

Fig. 20.10 L knee X-ray showing previous screw and washer posts along with metal suture anchors. No significant bone loss is present in the femur, tibia, and fibular head. Note transverse tunnel in fibular head from previous LCL reconstruction (*arrows*). LCL lateral collateral ligament

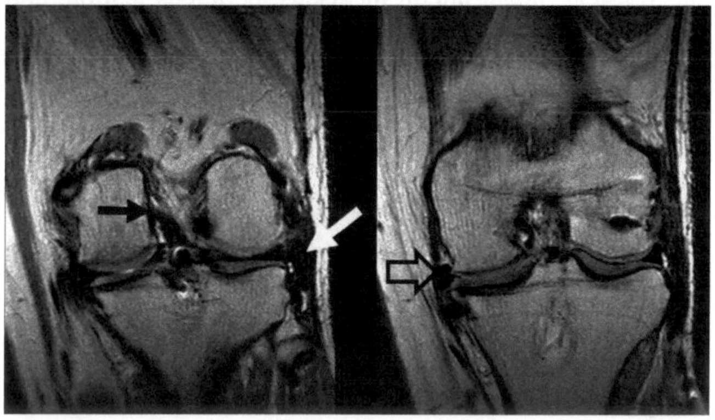

Fig. 20.11 MRI images showing attenuated PCL graft (*black arrow*), LCL reconstruction scarring (*white arrow*), and medial meniscus extrusion (*open arrow*). PCL posterior cruciate ligament, LCL lateral collateral ligament

Case Example

We present a case here to help illustrate the important principles of management in failed PCL reconstruction and associated pathologies. This is a 25-year-old male who was a collegiate soccer player presenting to the office 6 years status post left knee injury and surgical management by an outside orthopedist. Initially, he sustained two injuries, a hyperextension injury during a soccer game followed by an awkward landing onto his knee from a fall off a 3-foot incline. Initial work up revealed high-grade PCL, LCL, and PLC injuries as well as associated meniscal tears. He subsequently underwent arthroscopic PCL reconstruction with Achilles tendon allograft, and PLC reconstruction (LCL augmentation, biceps and popliteus tendon repair).

Postoperatively, he was not compliant with rehabilitation and progressed quickly to try to return to sport. He was not able to return to soccer due to significant pain and instability with increased activity level although his knee was not symptomatic with activities of daily living. He now presents with lateral-sided pain with activities of daily living and instability especially with walking down stairs.

On examination, he had a normal gait with no varus thrust. With stairs, he had instability especially with going down where he feels his knee shift. Range of motion was symmetric from −5° to 120°. He had 10 % quadriceps atrophy and no effusion. Ligament examination revealed 3+ posterior drawer, 2+ varus laxity at 30°, 1+ in full extension, no posterolateral rotatory laxity, 1A Lachman, and 1+ valgus stress. Radiographs showed symmetric bilateral 6° varus knee alignment, no joint space narrowing, and no significant widening of femoral, tibial, or anterior–posterior fibular tunnels (Fig. 20.10). MRI showed extrusion of the medial meniscus and a medial meniscus root tear. There was significant scarring of the LCL reconstruction and an attenuated PCL graft. His PLC structures appeared intact (Fig. 20.11).

An examination under anesthesia and diagnostic arthroscopy was performed to better evaluate knee stability, bone

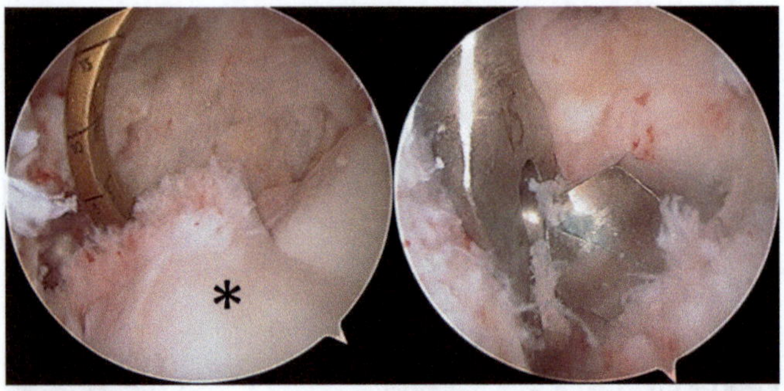

Fig. 20.12 View: Posteromedial portal. *Left*: PCL guide placed at tibial insertion site. Medial meniscal root tear can be seen (*). *Right*: reamer finished by hand and protected by PCL wire catcher. PCL posterior cruciate ligament

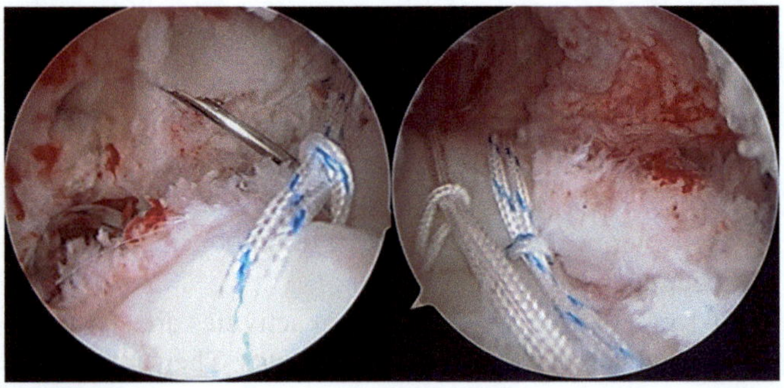

Fig. 20.13 *Left*: Posteromedial view showing looped suture through medial meniscus root. Suture passes through root repair tunnel and dilator through PCL tunnel is seen in background. *Right*: Anterior view (from anterolateral portal) of medial meniscus root repair suture. PCL posterior cruciate ligament

loss, tunnel position, menisci, and cartilage. Examination under anesthesia (EUA) confirms the office examination with 3+ posterior drawer, 3+ varus laxity at 30°, and symmetric posterolateral rotatory laxity. Diagnostic arthroscopy revealed a low femoral PCL tunnel, complete medial meniscal root tear, intact lateral meniscus, popliteus tendon, and well-preserved cartilage with few grade I changes in all three compartments.

The patient was seen back to discuss the definitive surgical management. The risks, benefits, complications, techniques, and expectations of treatment of the diagnosis, chronic failed PCL and LCL reconstruction with medial meniscal root tear were discussed with the patient at length. Surgical management included revision PCL reconstruction with Achilles tendon allograft, LCL reconstruction with tibialis anterior allograft, and medial meniscal root repair. A new femoral PCL tunnel adjacent to the previous low femoral tunnel was planned. No significant bone loss was present in the tibia, therefore, anatomic PCL tibial and meniscal root suture tunnels can be used. The previous LCL reconstruction fibular tunnel measured 6 mm and was placed in the AP direction with significant bone stock left over for an anatomic LCL reconstruction with a lateral-posteromedial directed tunnel. No proximal tibial osteotomy was planned due to symmetric limb alignment, lack of varus thrust and normal posterior tibial slope.

The patient was taken to the operating room 5 months later. EUA again confirmed the diagnosis. The previous PCL graft was debrided and the tibial insertion site identified. A 10-mm tibial tunnel was carefully created first by placing the PCL guide and guide pin, then by reaming to the posterior tibial cortex and finishing by hand (Fig. 20.12). This tunnel was dilated to 11.5 mm. The medial meniscal root tear was repaired with two looped sutures using a suture shuttling device, a bone tunnel placed with an ACL guide, and a suture passer (Fig. 20.13). The tibial PCL tunnel and meniscal root repair tunnels were created at the anteromedial tibial cortex. Fluroscopy was used to confirm anatomic tunnel placement (Fig. 20.14). An anatomic AL PCL femoral tunnel was created with a 10-mm reamer and then dilated to 11.5 mm (Fig. 20.15). An 11-mm Achilles tendon allograft was prepped with a baseball stitch and passed retrograde through the tibial tunnel into the joint and the femoral tunnel (Fig. 20.16).

Fig. 20.14 Intraoperative fluoroscopy confirming anatomic PCL tunnel placement (tunnel dilator) and nonconvergence of meniscal root repair tunnel (3/32 K-wire). PCL posterior cruciate ligament

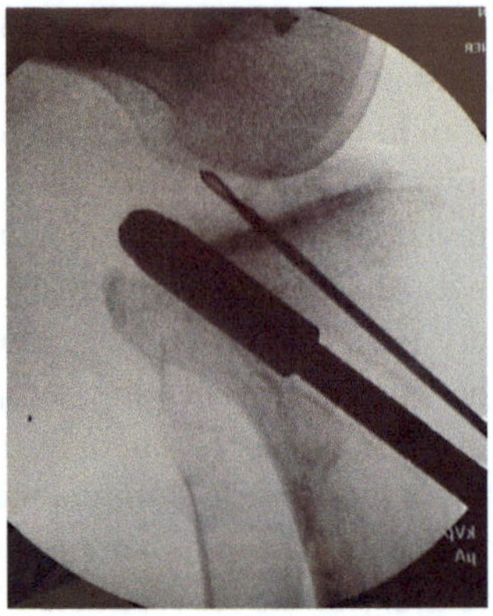

The previous lateral hockey stick incision was used to perform the anatomic LCL reconstruction. The common peroneal nerve was identified and protected. The lateral epicondyle was exposed and after debridement of the previous graft, a 7-mm tunnel at the LCL insertion site was created. The posteromedial aspect of the fibular head was exposed and a 7-mm lateral to posteromedial tunnel was created. A 7-mm tibialis anterior allograft was passed from posteromedial to lateral through the fibular tunnel and then tunnel under the biceps fascia and IT band to the femoral tunnel (Fig. 20.17). The LCL graft was secured with interference screws at the femoral and fibular tunnels with a valgus stress at 30° knee flexion. The PCL graft was secured with an exchanged screw and washer post at the anteromedial femur. The graft was then secured with an exchanged screw and washer post at the anteromedial tibia with an anterior drawer at 90° knee flexion. Meniscal root repair suture was tied to the same tibia post.

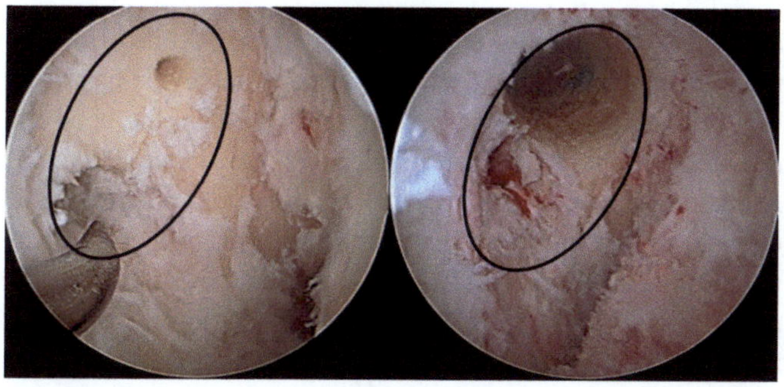

Fig. 20.15 Anterior view (anterolateral portal) *Left*: PCL femoral insertion. Approximate PCL footprint outlined. Steadman awl marks previous femoral tunnel and pilot hole marks new tunnel position. *Right*: New tunnel is in anterolateral footprint and does not overlap with previous tunnel. PCL posterior cruciate ligament

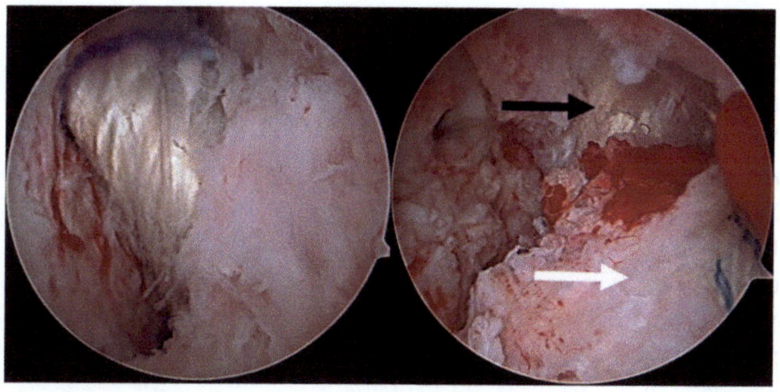

Fig. 20.16 *Left*: PCL graft viewed from anterolateral portal. *Right*: PCL graft (*black arrow*) and meniscal root repair (*white arrow*) viewed from posteromedial portal. PCL posterior cruciate ligament

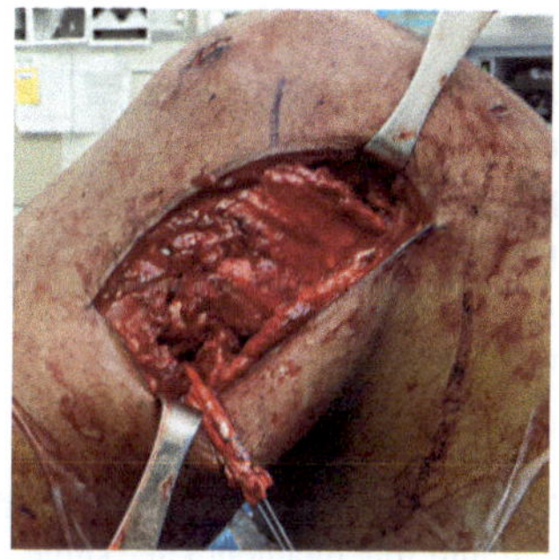

Fig. 20.17 LCL graft passed under IT band and biceps fascia from fibular head to lateral epicondyle (*black arrow*). LCL lateral collateral ligament

Postoperatively, the patient was placed in a hinged knee brace locked in extension and made nonweightbearing with crutches for 6 weeks. Passive motion was progressed during this time with knee flexion limited to 90° due to the meniscal root repair. Weightbearing and range of motion was then progressed along with strengthening after this period. The patient progressed well through the rehabilitation protocol previously described and returned to activities of daily living without significant instability.

Results

Patients have significant improvements in pain and function after revision PCL reconstruction although results are inferior to that of primary surgery. Noyes and Barber-Westin reported on their case series of 15 knees undergoing revision PCL reconstruction with quadriceps tendon patellar bone autograft with a mean follow-up of 44 months [58]. Patients' pain and function scores improved significantly although only 53 % of patients were able to participate in light recreational activities without symptoms. Stress radiographs showed significantly improved posterior tibial translation from 11.7°mm preoperatively to 5.1°mm at follow-up.

Lee et al. reported on results of 22 revision PCL reconstructions with a modified tibial-inlay double-bundle technique using Achilles tendon allograft with at least 24-month follow-up [59]. Stress radiography showed improved side-to-side difference from 9.9 mm preoperatively to 2.8 mm at last follow-up. Mean subjective IKDC score improved significantly from 39.1 to 60.4 while 77 % of patients were able to resume normal activities of daily living.

Complications

Complications of revision PCL and MLI reconstruction can be divided into three categories based on timing: preoperative, intraoperative, and postoperative. Most preoperative complications involve the neurovascular structures, including the popliteal artery and vein and the common peroneal nerve [9, 16–18, 60]. Intraoperative complications are typically related to technique, case setup, and poor preoperative planning. Finally, postoperative complications involve patient compliance, improper rehabilitation protocols, soft tissue management, infection, and thromboembolic events.

As with all revision procedures, the risk of complications of revision knee ligament reconstruction is significantly increased over primary reconstruction. When performing these procedures, the surgeon must be aware and prepared to treat these problems. The most common complications for revision PCL and MLI reconstruction procedures are listed in Table 20.3. The key to treatment of these complications is prevention, which involves detailed preoperative planning, proper surgical technique, and a specific postoperative rehabilitation program. Table 20.4 illustrates the senior author's top ten key points for prevention of complications with revision PCL and MLI knee reconstruction.

Table 20.3 Common and severe complications of revision PCL and multiple knee ligament reconstruction

Preoperative
Vasculature
Arterial
Spasm
Intimal injury
Complete tear
Venous (DVT)
Nerve (sensory, motor, complete)
Intraoperative
Intraoperative vascular injury
Iatrogenic compartment syndrome
Intraoperative mortality
Postoperative
Arthrofibrosis wound breakdown/skin slough
Infection
DVT/PE
Recurrent instability
Peroneal nerve neuropraxia
Pain syndromes

PCL posterior cruciate ligament, *DVT* deep vein thrombosis, *PE* pulmonary embolism

Table 20.4. Top ten tips for avoiding complications of revision PCL and multiple ligament knee surgery

(1) Thorough history and physical examination
(2) Detailed preoperative planning (timing, equipment, graft choice, assistants, vascular backup)
(3) Adequate imaging studies (X-rays, MRI, arteriogram/CT angiogram, venous duplex Doppler)
(4) Pad all extremities well and place a Foley catheter
(5) Examination under anesthesia
(6) Intraoperative fluoroscopy
(7) Perform MLI reconstruction cases as first or only case of the day and when well rested
(8) Always admit the patient overnight
(9) DVT/PE prophylaxis
10) Patient-specific rehab protocol and familiar physical therapists

PCL posterior cruciate ligament, *MLI* multiple ligament injuries, *DVT* deep vein thrombosis, *PE* pulmonary embolism, *CT* computed tomography

Conclusions

Failed PCL and multiple knee ligament reconstructions are a difficult problem for the knee surgeon. In order to effectively treat this problem, it is essential to classify the extent of the injury and determine the cause of the failure of the index procedure. Revision reconstruction for PCL and MLI knee injuries is fraught with complications, and clinical results are much less predictable for revision reconstruction than for primary reconstruction [16, 58, 59, 61].

With the treatment principles described in this chapter, the majority of our patients have been able to return to activities of daily living without difficulty. Ability to participate in sports after revision surgery, however, has been less predictable. To optimize patient outcomes, the need for detailed preoperative planning cannot be overemphasized. A thorough history and physical examination, adequate and optimal preoperative workup with imaging, proper surgical technique, careful soft tissue management, and an individualized postoperative rehab program are essential for treatment success and prevention of complications.

References

1. O'Donoghue DH. An analysis of end results of surgical treatment of major injuries to the ligaments of the knee. J Bone Joint Surg Am. 1955;37-A(1):1–13 (passim).
2. Quinlan AG, Sharrard WJ. Postero-lateral dislocation of the knee with capsular interposition. J Bone Joint Surg Br. 1958;40-B(4):660–3.
3. Quinlan AG. Irreducible posterolateral dislocation of the knee with button-holing of the medial femoral condyle. J Bone Joint Surg Am. 1966;48(8):1619–21.
4. Kennedy JC. Complete dislocation of the knee joint. J Bone Joint Surg Am. 1963;45:889–904.
5. Meyers MH, Harvey JP Jr. Traumatic dislocation of the knee joint. A study of eighteen cases. J Bone Joint Surg Am. 1971;53(1):16–29.
6. Roman PD, Hopson CN, Zenni EJ Jr. Traumatic dislocation of the knee: a report of 30 cases and literature review. Orthop Rev. 1987;16(12):917–24.
7. Shields L, Mital M, Cave EF. Complete dislocation of the knee: experience at the Massachusetts General Hospital. J Trauma. 1969;9(3):192–215.
8. Sisto DJ, Warren RF. Complete knee dislocation. A follow-up study of operative treatment. Clin Orthop Relat Res. 1985;(198):94–101.
9. Harner CD, et al. Surgical management of knee dislocations. J Bone Joint Surg Am. 2004;86-A(2):262–73.
10. Noyes FR, Barber-Weston S, Grood E. Newer concepts in the treatment of posterior cruciate ligament ruptures. In: Scott WN, editor. Surgery of the knee. New York: Churchill Livingstone; 2001. p. 841–78.
11. Noyes FR, Barber-Westin SD. Reconstruction of the anterior and posterior cruciate ligaments after knee dislocation. Use of early protected postoperative motion to decrease arthrofibrosis. Am J Sports Med. 1997;25(6):769–78.
12. Owens BD, et al. Primary repair of knee dislocations: results in 25 patients (28 knees) at a mean follow-up of four years. J Orthop Trauma. 2007;21(2):92–6.
13. Sekiya JK, et al. A clinically relevant assessment of posterior cruciate ligament and posterolateral corner injuries. Evaluation of isolated and combined deficiency. J Bone Joint Surg Am. 2008;90(8):1621–7.
14. Wascher DC, et al. Reconstruction of the anterior and posterior cruciate ligaments after knee dislocation. Results using fresh-frozen nonirradiated allografts. Am J Sports Med. 1999;27(2):189–96.
15. Muller W. The knee: Form, function and ligament reconstruction. Berlin: Springer; 1982.
16. Almekinders LC, Logan TC. Results following treatment of traumatic dislocations of the knee joint. Clin Orthop Relat Res. 1992;284:203–7.

17. Cole BJ, Harner CD. The multiple ligament injured knee. Clin Sports Med. 1999;18(1):241–62
18. Cooper DE, et al. Complete knee dislocation without posterior cruciate ligament disruption. A report of four cases and review of the literature. Clin Orthop Relat Res. 1992;284:228–33
19. Donaldson WF 3rd, Warren RF, Wickiewicz T. A comparison of acute anterior cruciate ligament examinations. Initial versus examination under anesthesia. Am J Sports Med. 1985;13(1):5–10.
20. Fanelli GC, et al. Treatment of combined anterior cruciate-posterior cruciate ligament-medial-lateral side knee injuries. J Knee Surg. 2005;18(3):240–8
21. Fanelli GC, Giannotti BF, Edson CJ. Arthroscopically assisted combined anterior and posterior cruciate ligament reconstruction. Arthroscopy. 1996;12(1):5–14
22. Fanelli GC, Harris JD. Late MCL (medial collateral ligament) reconstruction. Tech Knee Surg. 2007;6(2):99–105.
23. Fanelli GC, Harris JD. Surgical treatment of acute medial collateral ligament and posteromedial corner injuries of the knee. Sports Med Arthrosc. 2006;14(2):78–83.
24. Fanelli GC. Treatment of combined anterior cruciate ligament-posterior cruciate ligament-lateral side injuries of the knee. Clin Sports Med. 2000;19(3):493–502.
25. Bratt HD, Newman AP. Complete dislocation of the knee without disruption of both cruciate ligaments. J Trauma. 1993;34(3):383–9.
26. Khanna G, Herrera DA, Wolters BW, Dajani KA, Levy BA. Staged protocol for high energy knee dislocation: Initial spanning external fixation versus hinged knee brace. Presented as an e-poster at the 27th Annual Meeting of the Arthroscopy Association of North America, 24–27 Apr 2008; Washington, DC.
27. Welling RE, Kakkasseril J, Cranley JJ. Complete dislocations of the knee with popliteal vascular injury. J Trauma. 1981;21(6):450–3.
28. Schenck RC Jr, et al. Knee dislocations. Instr Course Lect. 1999;48:515–22.
29. Schenck RC Jr. The dislocated knee. Instr Course Lect. 1994;43:127–36.
30. Spindler K, Walker RN. General approach to ligament surgery. In: Fu FH, Harner CD, Vince KP, editors. Knee surgery. Baltimore: Williams & Wilkins; 1994. p. 643–65.
31. Taylor AR, Arden GP, Rainey HA. Traumatic dislocation of the knee. A report of forty-three cases with special reference to conservative treatment. J Bone Joint Surg Br. 1972;54(1):96–102.
32. Tzurbakis M, et al. Surgical treatment of multiple knee ligament injuries in 44 patients: 2–8 years follow-up results. Knee Surg Sports Traumatol Arthrosc. 2006;14(8):739–49
33. Bergfeld JA, et al. A biomechanical comparison of posterior cruciate ligament reconstruction techniques. Am J Sports Med. 2001;29(2):129–36.
34. Fanelli GC, Orcutt DR, Edson CJ. The multiple-ligament injured knee: evaluation, treatment, and results. Arthroscopy. 2005;21(4):471–86.
35. Frassica FJ, et al. Dislocation of the knee. Clin Orthop Relat Res. 1991;263:200–5.
36. Good L, Johnson RJ. The dislocated knee. J Am Acad Orthop Surg. 1995;3(5):284–92.
37. Medvecky MJ, Zazulak BT, Hewett TE. A multidisciplinary approach to the evaluation, reconstruction and rehabilitation of the multi-ligament injured athlete. Sports Med. 2007;37(2):169–87.
38. Ranawat A, et al. Posterolateral corner injury of the knee: evaluation and management. J Am Acad Orthop Surg. 2008;16(9):506–18.
39. Hughston JC, Jacobson KE. Chronic posterolateral rotatory instability of the knee. J Bone Joint Surg Am. 1985;67(3):351–9.
40. Levy BA, Dahm DL, Herrera DA, MacDonald PB, Dajani KA, Stuart MJ. Acute repair of posteromedial and posterolateral corners in multiligament knee injury is not indicated. Presented at the 27th Annual Meeting of the Arthroscopy Association of North America, 24–27 Apr 2008; Washington, DC.
41. Rihn JA, et al. The acutely dislocated knee: evaluation and management. J Am Acad Orthop Surg. 2004;12(5):334–46.
42. Harner CD, et al. Quantitative analysis of human cruciate ligament insertions. Arthroscopy. 1999;15(7):741–9.
43. Harner CD, et al. Anterior cruciate ligament reconstruction: endoscopic versus two-incision technique. Arthroscopy. 1994;10(5):502–12.
44. Klecker RJ, et al. The aberrant anterior tibial artery: Magnetic resonance appearance, prevalence, and surgical implications. Am J Sports Med. 2008;36(4):720–7.
45. Varnell RM, et al. Arterial injury complicating knee disruption. Third place winner: Conrad Jobst award. Am Surg. 1989;55(12):699–704.
46. Chapman JA. Popliteal artery damage in closed injuries of the knee. J Bone Joint Surg Br. 1985;67(3):420–3.
47. Green NE, Allen BL. Vascular injuries associated with dislocation of the knee. J Bone Joint Surg Am. 1977:59(2):236–9
48. Hoover NW. Injuries of the popliteal artery associated with fractures and dislocations. Surg Clin North Am. 1961;41:1099–112.
49. Jones RE, Smith EC, Bone GE. Vascular and orthopedic complications of knee dislocation. Surg Gynecol Obstet. 1979;149(4):554–8.
50. Levy BA, et al. Screening for extermity arterial injury with the arterial pressure index. Am J Emerg Med. 2005;23(5):689–95.
51. Hollis JD, Daley BJ. 10-year review of knee dislocations: is arteriography always necessary? J Trauma. 2005;59(3):672–5 (discussion 675–6).
52. Levy BA, et al. Controversies in the treatment of knee dislocations and multiligament reconstruction. J Am Acad Orthop Surg. 2009;17(4):197–206.
53. Richter M, et al. Comparison of surgical repair or reconstruction of the cruciate ligaments versus nonsurgical treatment in patients with traumatic knee dislocations. Am J Sports Med. 2002;30(5):718–27.
54. Olson EJ, et al. Clinical use of fresh, frozen soft tissue allografts. Orthopedics. 1992;15(10):1225–32.
55. Shapiro MS, Freedman EL. Allograft reconstruction of the anterior and posterior cruciate ligaments after traumatic knee dislocation. Am J Sports Med. 1995;23(5):580–7.
56. LaPrade RF, et al. Fibular collateral ligament anatomical reconstructions: a prospective outcomes study. Am J Sports Med. 2010;38(10):2005–11.
57. Irrgang JJ, Fitzgerald GK. Rehabilitation of the multiple-ligament-injured knee. Clin Sports Med. 2000;19(3):545–71.
58. Noyes FR, Barber-Westin SD. Posterior cruciate ligament revision reconstruction, part 2: results of revision using a 2-strand quadriceps tendon-patellar bone autograft. Am J Sports Med. 2005; 33(5):655–65.
59. Lee SH, et al. Revision posterior cruciate ligament reconstruction using a modified tibial-inlay double-bundle technique. J Bone Joint Surg Am. 2012;94(6):516–22.
60. Reckling FW, Peltier LF. Acute knee dislocations and their complications. J Trauma. 1969;9(3):181–91.
61. Almekinders LC, Dedmond BT. Outcomes of the operatively treated knee dislocation. Clin Sports Med. 2000;19(3):503–18.
62. Harner C, et al. The multiple ligament injured knee: a practical guide to management, revision surgery in the posterior cruciate ligament and multiple ligament injured knee. 2nd ed. New York: Springer Science+Business Media; 2013. p. 303–19.
63. El Attrache N, Harner C, et al. Surgical techniques in sports medicine. Philadelphia, PA: Lippincott Williams & Wilkins; 2007.

Part VI
Other Considerations

Mechanical Graft Tensioning in Posterior Cruciate Ligament Reconstruction

21

Gregory C. Fanelli

Introduction

The principles of reconstruction in the multiple-ligament-injured knee are to identify and treat all pathology, accurate tunnel placement, anatomic graft insertion sites, utilize strong graft material, mechanical graft tensioning, secure graft fixation, and a deliberate postoperative rehabilitation program [1]. This chapter concentrates on my experience using a mechanical graft-tensioning boot, the Biomet graft-tensioning boot (Biomet Sports Medicine, Warsaw, Indiana), during posterior cruciate ligament (PCL) reconstruction and anterior cruciate ligament (ACL) reconstruction, in the case of the multiple-ligament-injured knee. The tensioning boot, the PCL and ACL reconstruction surgical techniques, the cyclic dynamic method of graft tensioning, and the comparative results using the graft-tensioning boot are presented in this chapter.

The Mechanical Graft-Tensioning Device

The graft-tensioning boot (Biomet Sports Medicine, Warsaw, Indiana) is a device used to tension posterior and ACL grafts after graft preparation, and prior to final fixation during the PCL and/or ACL reconstruction surgical procedure. The graft-tensioning boot consists of a frame that has a ratcheted torque wrench attached to the frame (Fig. 21.1). After completion of graft preparation, the allograft or autograft tissue is placed on the tensioning boot, and tension is gradually applied to pretension the graft tissue prior to implantation. The graft is wrapped in a damp sponge, and the tensioning boot graft assembly is protected on the back table until it is time to implant the allograft or autograft tissue (Fig. 21.2). During the surgical procedure, the sterile tensioning boot is fitted over the surgical extremity foot and shin areas, and attached to the surgical leg with a sterile bandage (Fig. 21.3). The cyclic dynamic method of graft tensioning is the intraoperative process that is used, and this method is described in detail in the surgical technique section below.

Combined PCL ACL Reconstruction Surgical Technique Using Mechanical Graft Tensioning

My surgical technique for PCL reconstruction, and combined PCL ACL medial and lateral side reconstruction is presented in Chaps. 9 and 15 of this textbook. This chapter specifically addresses the surgical technique for posterior and ACL reconstruction using the Biomet graft-tensioning boot.

The patient is placed on the operating room table in the supine position, and after satisfactory induction of anesthesia, the operative and nonoperative lower extremities are carefully examined [1–11]. A tourniquet is applied to the upper thigh of the operative extremity, and that extremity is prepped and draped in a sterile fashion. The well leg is supported by the fully extended operating room table that also supports the surgical leg during medial and lateral side surgery. A lateral post is used to control the surgical extremity. An arthroscopic leg holder is not used. Pre- and postoperative antibiotics are given, and antibiotics are routinely used to help prevent infection in these time consuming, difficult, and complex cases. Allograft tissue is prepared prior to bringing the patient into the operating room. Autograft tissue is harvested prior to beginning the arthroscopic portion of the procedure.

The arthroscopic instruments are inserted with the inflow through the superolateral patellar portal. Instrumentation and visualization are positioned through inferomedial and inferolateral patellar portals, and can be interchanged as necessary. Additional portals are established as necessary. Exploration of the joint consists of evaluation of the patellofemoral joint, the medial and lateral compartments, medial and lateral menisci, and the intercondylar notch. The residual stumps of both the anterior and PCL are debrided; however,

G. C. Fanelli (✉)
303 Kaseville Road, Danville, PA 17821, USA
e-mail: gregorycfanelli@gmail.com

G. C. Fanelli (ed.), *Posterior Cruciate Ligament Injuries*,
DOI 10.1007/978-3-319-12072-0_21,

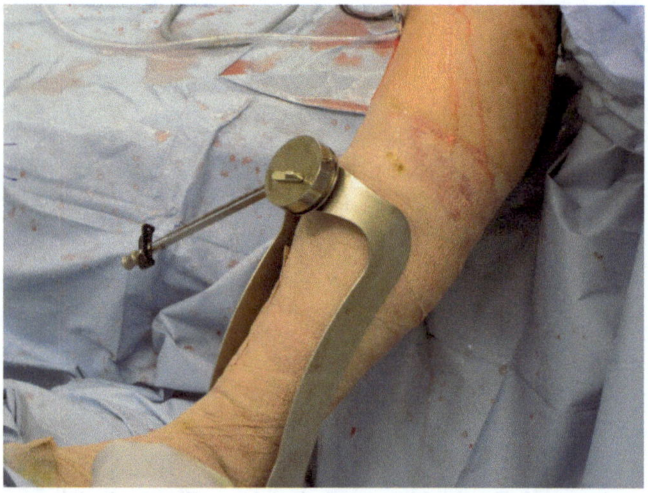

Fig. 21.1 The graft-tensioning boot consists of a frame that has a ratcheted torque wrench attached to the frame. The device fits over the surgical foot and leg. (From Fanelli 2013 [1]. Reprinted with permission)

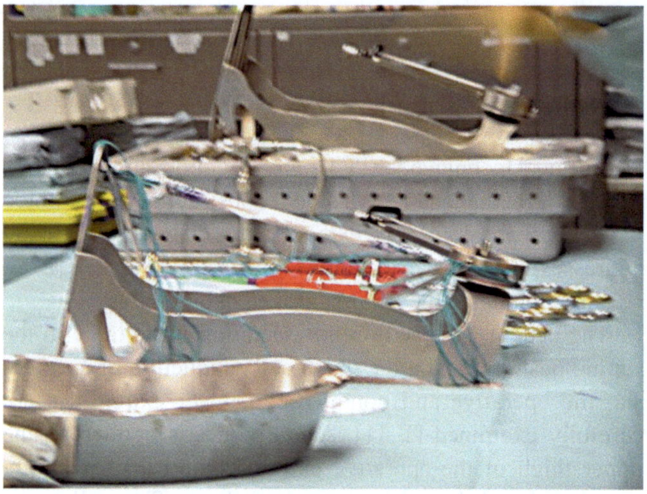

Fig. 21.2 The graft-tensioning device is used to pretension the prepared allograft or autograft tissue prior to implantation. After completion of graft preparation, the allograft or autograft tissue is placed on the tensioning boot, and tension is gradually applied to pretension the graft tissue prior to implantation. The graft is wrapped in a damp sponge, and the tensioning boot graft assembly is protected on the back table until it is time to implant the allograft or autograft tissue. (From Fanelli 2013 [1]. Reprinted with permission)

the posterior and ACL anatomic insertion sites are preserved to serve as tunnel reference points. The notchplasty for the ACL portion of the procedure is performed at this time.

An extra capsular extra-articular posteromedial safety incision is made by creating an incision approximately 1.5–2 cm long starting at the posteromedial border of the tibia approximately 1 in. below the level of the joint line and extending distally. Dissection is carried down to the crural fascia, which is incised longitudinally. An interval is developed between the medial head of the gastrocnemius muscle

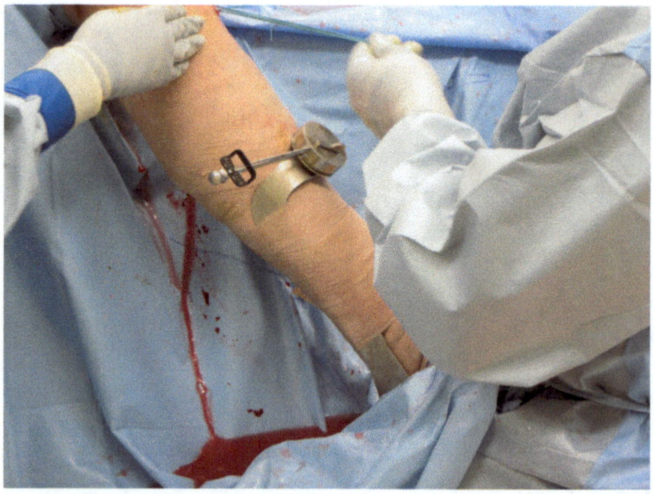

Fig. 21.3 During the surgical procedure, the sterile tensioning boot is fitted over the surgical extremity foot and shin areas, and attached to the surgical leg with a sterile bandage. (From Fanelli 2013 [1]. Reprinted with permission)

and the nerves and vessels posterior to the surgeon's finger, and the capsule of the knee joint anterior to the surgeon's finger. The posteromedial safety incision enables the surgeon to protect the neurovascular structures, confirm the accuracy of the PCL tibial tunnel, and to facilitate the flow of the surgical procedure.

The curved over-the-top PCL instruments (Biomet Sports Medicine, Warsaw, Indiana) are used to sequentially lyse adhesions in the posterior aspect of the knee, and elevate the capsule from the posterior tibial ridge. This allows the accurate placement of the PCL/ACL drill guide, and correct placement of the tibial tunnel.

The arm of the PCL/ACL guide (Biomet Sports Medicine, Warsaw, Indiana) is inserted through the inferior medial patellar portal. The tip of the guide is positioned at the inferior lateral aspect of the PCL anatomic insertion site. This is below the tibial ridge posterior and in the lateral aspect of the PCL anatomic insertion site. The bullet portion of the guide contacts the anteromedial surface of the proximal tibia at a point midway between the posteromedial border of the tibia, and the tibial crest anterior at or just below the level of the tibial tubercle. This will provide an angle of graft orientation such that the graft will turn two very smooth 45° angles on the posterior aspect of the tibia. The tip of the guide in the posterior aspect of the tibia is confirmed with the surgeon's finger through the extra capsular extra-articular posteromedial safety incision. Intraoperative anteroposterior (AP) and lateral X-ray may also be used; however, I do not routinely use intraoperative X-ray. When the PCL/ACL guide is positioned in the desired area, a blunt spade-tipped guide wire is drilled from anterior to posterior. The surgeon's finger confirms the position of the guide wire through the posterior medial safety incision.

The appropriately sized standard cannulated reamer is used to create the tibial tunnel. The surgeon's finger through the extra capsular extra-articular posteromedial incision is monitoring the position of the guide wire. When the drill is engaged in bone, the guide wire is reversed, blunt end pointing posterior, for additional patient safety. The drill is advanced until it comes to the posterior cortex of the tibia. The chuck is disengaged from the drill, and completion of the tibial tunnel is performed by hand.

The PCL single- or double-bundle femoral tunnels are made from inside out using the double-bundle aimers, or an endoscopic reamer can be used as an aiming device (Biomet Sports Medicine, Warsaw, Indiana). The appropriately sized double-bundle aimer or endoscopic reamer is inserted through a low anterior lateral patellar arthroscopic portal to create the PCL anterior lateral bundle femoral tunnel. The double-bundle aimer or endoscopic reamer is positioned directly on the footprint of the femoral anterior lateral bundle PCL insertion site. The appropriately sized guide wire is drilled through the aimer or endoscopic reamer, through the bone, and out a small skin incision. Care is taken to prevent any compromise of the articular surface. The double-bundle aimer is removed, and the endoscopic reamer is used to drill the anterior lateral PCL femoral tunnel from inside to outside. When the surgeon chooses to perform a double-bundle double-femoral tunnel PCL reconstruction, the same process is repeated for the posterior medial bundle of the PCL. Care must be taken to ensure that there will be an adequate bone bridge (approximately 5 mm) between the two femoral tunnels prior to drilling. This is accomplished using the calibrated probe, and direct arthroscopic visualization of the PCL femoral anatomic insertion sites.

My preferred surgical technique of PCL femoral tunnel creation from inside to outside is for two reasons. There is a greater distance and margin of safety between the PCL femoral tunnels and the medial femoral condyle articular surface using the inside-to-outside method. In addition, a more accurate placement of the PCL femoral tunnels is possible, in my opinion, because I can place the double-bundle aimer or endoscopic reamer on the anatomic footprint of the anterior lateral or posterior medial PCL insertion site under direct visualization.

A Magellan suture retriever (Biomet Sports Medicine, Warsaw, Indiana) is introduced through the tibial tunnel into the joint, and retrieved through the femoral tunnel. The traction sutures of the graft material are attached to the loop of the Magellan suture retriever, and the graft is pulled into position. The graft material is secured on the femoral side using a bioabsorbable interference screw for primary aperture opening fixation, and a polyethylene ligament fixation button for backup fixation.

With the knee in approximately 90° of flexion, the ACL tibial tunnel is created using a drill guide. My preferred method of ACL reconstruction is the transtibial femoral tunnel endoscopic surgical technique. The arm of the drill guide enters the knee joint through the inferior medial patellar portal. The bullet of the drill guide contacts the anterior medial proximal tibia externally at a point midway between the posterior medial border of the tibia, and the anterior tibial crest just above the level of the tibial tubercle. A 1-cm or greater bone bridge exists between the PCL and ACL tibial tunnels. The guide wire is drilled through the guide and positioned so that after creating the ACL tibial tunnel, the graft will approximate the tibial anatomic insertion site of the ACL. A standard cannulated reamer is used to create the tibial tunnel.

With the knee in approximately 90–100° of flexion, an over-the-top femoral aimer is introduced through the tibial tunnel, and used to position a guide wire on the medial wall of the lateral femoral condyle to create a femoral tunnel approximating the anatomic insertion site of the anterior cruciate ligament. The ACL graft is positioned and fixation is achieved on the femoral side using a bioabsorbable interference screw, and cortical suspensory backup fixation with a polyethylene ligament fixation button. Additional drawings and photographs of this surgical technique are presented in Chap. 20 [9].

The Cyclic Dynamic Method of Cruciate Graft Tensioning

The cyclic dynamic method of graft tensioning using the Biomet graft-tensioning boot is used to tension the posterior and ACL grafts. During this surgical technique, the PCL and/or ACL grafts are secured on the femoral side first with the surgeon's preferred fixation method. The technique described is a tibial-sided tensioning method. I routinely use polyethylene ligament fixation buttons for cortical suspensory fixation, and aperture interference fixation with bioabsorbable interference screws for femoral side PCL and ACL fixation. In combined PCL ACL reconstructions, the PCL graft is tensioned first, followed by final PCL graft(s) tibial fixation. The ACL graft tensioning and fixation follows that of the PCL.

With the tensioning boot applied to the foot and leg of the surgical extremity, tension is placed on the PCL graft(s) distally using the Biomet graft-tensioning boot (Biomet Sports Medicine, Warsaw, Indiana) (Fig. 21.4). Tension is gradually applied with the knee in 0° of flexion (full extension) reducing the tibia on the femur. This restores the anatomic tibial step-off. Although there are numbers on the torque wrench dial, these numbers are not used to set the tension. The numbers on the torque wrench serve as a reference point during the cycling process, and readjustment process, and are not indicators of final tension in the graft. The tension is determined by reduction of the tibia on the femur in 0°

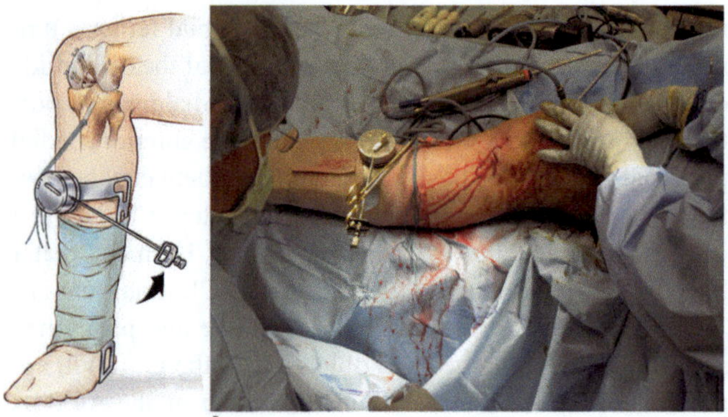

a b

Fig. 21.4 **a** The graft-tensioning boot is applied to the traction sutures of the PCL graft. (From Fanelli 2012 [2]. Reprinted with permission). **b** Tension is gradually applied with the knee in 0° of flexion (full extension) reducing the tibia on the femur. This restores the anatomic tibial step-off. Although there are numbers on the torque wrench dial, these numbers are not used to set the tension. The numbers on the torque wrench serve as a reference point during the cycling process, and readjustment process, and are not indicators of final tension in the graft. The tension is determined by reduction of the tibia on the femur in 0° of knee flexion (full extension), the restoration of the anatomic tibial step-offs, a negative posterior drawer on intraoperative examination of the knee, and full range of motion of the knee. (From Fanelli 2013 [1]. Reprinted with permission)

of knee flexion (full extension), the restoration of the anatomic tibial step-offs, a negative posterior drawer on intraoperative examination of the knee, and full range of motion of the knee. The knee is cycled through a full range of motion multiple times to allow pretensioning and settling of the graft. The process is repeated until there is no further change on the torque setting on the graft tensioner with the knee at 0° of flexion (full extension). When there are no further changes or adjustments necessary in the tension applied to the graft, the knee is placed in 70–90° of flexion, and fixation is achieved on the tibial side of the PCL graft with a bioabsorbable interference screw for interference fit fixation, and backup cortical suspensory fixation with a bicortical screw and spiked ligament washer or polyethylene ligament fixation button (Fig. 21.5).

The cyclic dynamic method of tensioning the ACL graft is performed using the Biomet graft-tensioning boot (Biomet Sports Medicine, Warsaw, Indiana) after tensioning and final fixation of the PCL graft(s) has been performed (Fig. 21.6). Traction is placed on the ACL graft sutures with the knee in 0° of flexion (full extension), and tension is gradually applied reducing the tibia on the femur. The knee is then cycled through multiple full flexion and extension cycles to allow settling of the graft. The Lachman and pivot shift tests are performed. The process is repeated until there is no further change in the torque setting on the graft tensioner at full extension (0° of knee flexion), and the Lachman and pivot shift tests are negative. Although there are numbers on the torque wrench dial, these numbers are not used to set the tension. The numbers on the torque wrench

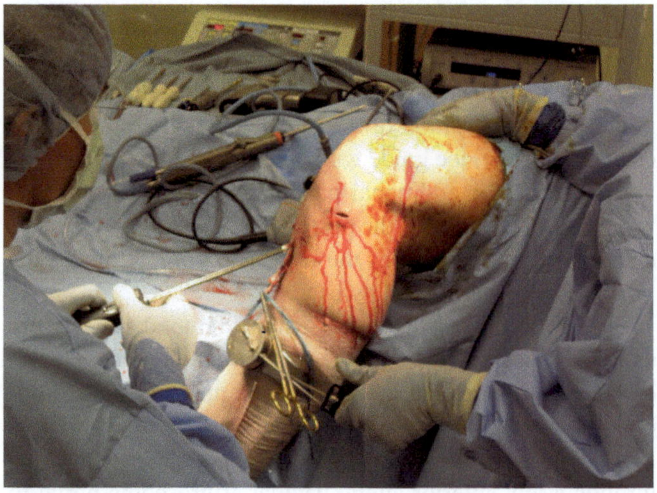

Fig. 21.5 When the tensioning sequence described in the chapter text is complete, the knee is placed in 70–90° of flexion, and fixation is achieved on the tibial side of the PCL graft with a bioabsorbable interference screw for interference fit fixation, and backup cortical suspensory fixation with a bicortical screw and spiked ligament washer or polyethylene ligament fixation button. (From Fanelli 2013 [1]. Reprinted with permission)

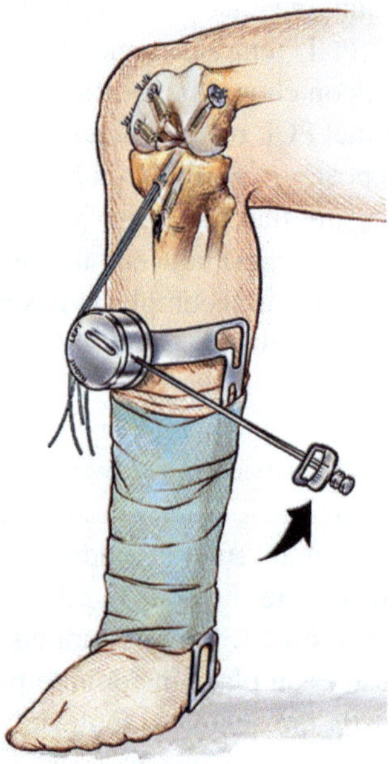

Fig. 21.6 This drawing depicts the graft-tensioning boot applied to the traction sutures of the ACL graft. (From Fanelli 2012 [2]. Reprinted with permission)

serve as a reference point during the cycling process, and readjustment process, and are not indicators of final tension in the graft. Final ACL graft tension is determined by the Lachman and pivot shifts becoming negative, and achieving full range of motion of the knee. The knee is placed in approximately 30° of flexion, and fixation is achieved on the tibial side of the ACL graft with a bioabsorbable interference screw, and backup fixation with a polyethylene ligament fixation button (Fig. 21.7).

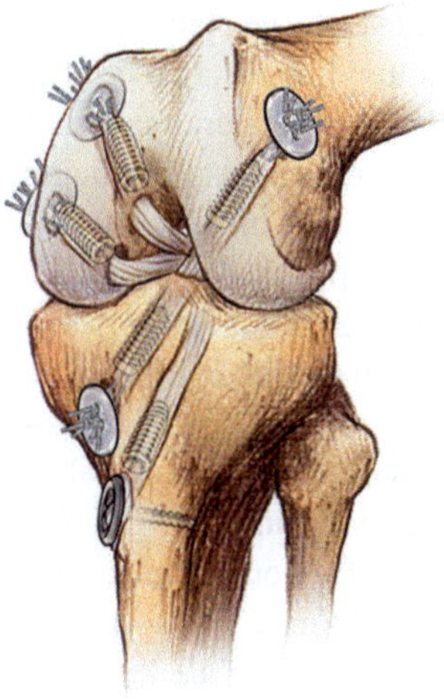

Fig. 21.7 This figure shows final fixation of the posterior and ACL grafts. (From Fanelli 2012 [2]. Reprinted with permission)

Results

Fanelli and Edson in 2004 published the 2–10-year (24–120 month) results of 41 chronic arthroscopically assisted combined PCL/posterolateral reconstructions evaluated pre- and postoperatively using Lysholm, Tegner, and Hospital for Special Surgery (HSS) knee ligament rating scales, KT-1000 arthrometer testing, stress radiography, and physical examination [12, 13]. PCL reconstructions were performed using the arthroscopically assisted single femoral tunnel–single-bundle transtibial tunnel PCL reconstruction technique using fresh frozen Achilles tendon allografts in all 41 cases. In all 41 cases, posterolateral instability reconstruction was performed with combined biceps femoris tendon tenodesis, and posterolateral capsular shift procedures. Postoperative physical examination revealed normal posterior drawer/tibial step-off for the overall study group in 29/41 (70 %) of knees. Normal posterior drawer and tibial step-offs were achieved in 91.7 % of the knees tensioned with the Biomet Sports Medicine mechanical graft tensioner. Posterolateral stability was restored to normal in 11/41 (27 %) of knees, and tighter than the normal knee in 29/41 (71 %) of knees evaluated with the external rotation thigh foot angle test. Thirty-degree varus stress testing was normal in 40/41 (97%) of knees, and grade 1 laxity in 1/41 (3 %) of knees. Postoperative KT-1000 arthrometer testing mean side-to-side difference measurements were 1.80 mm (PCL screen), 2.11 mm (corrected posterior), and 0.63 mm (corrected anterior) measurements. This is a statistically significant improvement from preoperative status for the PCL screen and the corrected posterior measurements ($p=0.001$). The postoperative stress radiographic mean side-to-side difference measurement measured at 90° of knee flexion, and 32 lb. of posterior directed force applied to the proximal tibia using the Telos device was 2.26 mm. This is a statistically significant improvement from preoperative measurements ($p=0.001$). Postoperative Lysholm, Tegner, and HSS knee ligament rating scale mean values were 91.7, 4.92, and 88.7, respectively, demonstrating a statistically significant improvement from preoperative status ($p=0.001$). The authors concluded that chronic combined PCL/posterolateral instabilities can be successfully treated with arthroscopic PCL reconstruction using fresh-frozen Achilles tendon allograft combined with posterolateral corner (PLC) reconstruction using biceps tendon tenodesis combined with posterolateral capsular shift procedure. Statistically significant improvement is noted ($p=0.001$) from the preoperative condition at 2–10-year follow-up using objective parameters of knee ligament rating scales, arthrometer testing, stress radiography, and physical examination.

About 2–10-year results of combined ACL–PCL reconstructions without the Biomet Sports Medicine Graft-Tensioning Boot have been published by Fanelli and Edson in 2002 [14]. This study presented the 2–10-year (24–120 month) results of 35 arthroscopically assisted combined ACL/PCL reconstructions evaluated pre- and postoperatively using Lysholm, Tegner, and HSS knee ligament rating scales, KT-1000 arthrometer testing, stress radiography, and physical examination.

This study population included 26 males, 9 females, 19 acute, and 16 chronic knee injuries. Ligament injuries included 19 ACL/PCL/posterolateral instabilities, 9 ACL/PCL/MCL instabilities, 6 ACL/PCL/posterolateral/MCL instabilities, and 1 ACL/PCL instability. All knees had grade III preoperative ACL/PCL laxity, and were assessed pre- and postoperatively with arthrometer testing, three different knee ligament rating scales, stress radiography, and physical examination. Arthroscopically assisted combined ACL/PCL reconstructions were performed using the single-incision endoscopic ACL technique, and the single femoral tunnel-single bundle transtibial tunnel PCL technique. PCLs were reconstructed with allograft Achilles tendon (26 knees), autograft BTB (7 knees), and autograft semitendinosus/gracilis (2 knees). ACLs were reconstructed with autograft BTB (16 knees), allograft BTB (12 knees), Achilles tendon allograft (6 knees), and autograft semitendinosus/gracilis (1 knee). Medial collateral ligament (MCL) injuries were treated with bracing or open reconstruction. Posterolateral instability was treated with biceps femoris tendon transfer, with or without primary repair, and posterolateral capsular shift procedures as indicated. No Biomet graft-tensioning boot was used in this series of patients.

Postoperative physical examination results revealed normal posterior drawer/tibial step-off in 16/35 (46 %) of knees, and normal Lachman and pivot-shift tests in 33/35 (94 %) of knees. Posterolateral stability was restored to normal in 6/25 (24 %) of knees, and tighter than the normal knee in 19/25 (76 %) of knees evaluated with the external rotation thigh foot angle test. Thirty-degree varus stress testing was normal in 22/25 (88 %) of knees, and grade 1 laxity in 3/25 (12 %) of knees. Thirty-degree valgus stress testing was normal in 7/7 (100 %) of surgically treated MCL tears, and normal in 7/8 (87.5 %) of brace treated knees. Postoperative KT-1000 arthrometer testing mean side-to-side difference measurements were 2.7 mm (PCL screen), 2.6 mm (corrected posterior), and 1.0 mm (corrected anterior) measurements, a statistically significant improvement from preoperative status ($p=0.001$). Postoperative stress radiographic side-to-side difference measurements measured at 90° of knee flexion, and 32 pounds of posteriorly directed proximal force were 0–3 mm in 11/21 (52.3 %), 4–5 mm in 5/21 (23.8 %), and 6–10 mm in 4/21 (19 %) of knees. Postoperative Lysholm, Tegner, and HSS knee ligament rating scale mean values were 91.2, 5.3, and 86.8, respectively, demonstrating a statistically significant improvement from preoperative status ($p=0.001$). No Biomet graft-tensioning boot was used in this series of patients.

The conclusions drawn from the study were that combined ACL/PCL instabilities could be successfully treated with arthroscopic reconstruction and the appropriate collateral ligament surgery. Statistically significant improvement was noted from the preoperative condition at 2–10-year follow-up using objective parameters of knee ligament rating scales, arthrometer testing, stress radiography, and physical examination. Postoperatively, these knees are not normal, but they are functionally stable. Continuing technical improvements would most likely improve future results.

The results of allograft multiple ligament knee reconstructions using the Biomet Sports Medicine (Warsaw, IN) mechanical graft-tensioning device were published by Fanelli et al. in 2005 [13]. The data present the 2-year follow-up results of 15 arthroscopic assisted ACL/PCL allograft reconstructions using the Biomet Sports Medicine graft-tensioning boot. This study group consists of 11 chronic and 4 acute injuries. These injury patterns included six ACL PCL PLC injuries, four ACL PCL MCL injuries, and five ACL PCL PLC MCL injuries. The Biomet Sports Medicine tensioning boot was used during the procedures as in the surgical technique described above. All knees had grade III preoperative ACL/PCL laxity, and were assessed pre- and postoperatively using Lysholm, Tegner, and HSS knee ligament rating scales, KT-1000 arthrometer testing, stress radiography, and physical examination.

Arthroscopically assisted combined ACL/PCL reconstructions were performed using the single-incision endoscopic ACL technique, and the single femoral tunnel–single- bundle transtibial tunnel PCL technique. PCLs were reconstructed with allograft Achilles tendon in all 15 knees. ACLs were reconstructed with Achilles tendon allograft in all 15 knees. MCL injuries were treated surgically using primary repair, posteromedial capsular shift, and allograft augmentation as indicated. Posterolateral instability was treated with allograft semitendinosus free graft, with or without primary repair, and posterolateral capsular shift procedures as indicated. The Biomet Sports Medicine graft-tensioning boot was used in this series of patients.

Post-reconstruction physical examination results revealed normal posterior drawer/tibial step-off in 13/15 (86.6 %) of knees. Normal Lachman test in 13/15 (86.6 %) knees, and normal pivot shift tests in 14/15 (93.3 %) knees. Posterolateral stability was restored to normal in all knees. When evaluated with the external rotation thigh– foot angle test, nine knees were equal to the normal knee and two knees were tighter than the normal knee. Thirty-degree varus stress testing was restored to normal in all 11 knees with posterolateral lateral instability. Thirty- and zero-degree valgus stress testing was restored to normal in all nine knees with medial side laxity. Postoperative KT-1000 arthrometer testing mean side-to-side difference measurements were 1.6 mm (range 3–7 mm) for the PCL screen, 1.6 mm (range 4.5–9 mm) for the corrected posterior, and 0.5 mm (range 2.5–6 mm) for the corrected anterior measurements, a significant improvement from preoperative status. Postoperative stress radiographic side-to-side difference measurements measured at 90° of knee flexion, and 32 pounds of posteriorly directed proximal force using the Telos stress radiography device were 0–3 mm in 10/15 knees (66.7 %), 4 mm in 4/15 knees (26.7 %), and 7 mm in 1/15 knees (6.67 %). Postoperative Lysholm, Tegner, and HSS knee ligament rating scale mean values were 86.7 (range 69–95), 4.5 (range 2–7), and 85.3 (range 65–93), respectively, demonstrating a significant improvement from preoperative status.

The authors concluded that the study group demonstrates the efficacy and success of using allograft tissue and a mechanical graft-tensioning device (Biomet Sports Medicine graft-tensioning boot) in single-bundle single-femoral tunnel arthroscopic PCL reconstruction in the multiple-ligament-injured knee. Without the tensioning boot there were 46 % normal posterior drawer and tibial step-off examinations, and with the graft-tensioning boot the normal tibial step-offs and posterior drawer examinations improved to 86.6 % of the PCL reconstructions in the study group.

Summary and Conclusions

The principles of reconstruction in the multiple-ligament-injured knee are to identify and treat all pathology, accurate tunnel placement, anatomic graft insertion sites, utilize strong graft material, mechanical graft tensioning, secure graft fixation, and a deliberate postoperative rehabilitation program. This chapter has presented my experience using a mechanical graft-tensioning boot during PCL and ACL reconstruction in the multiple-ligament-injured knee. The cyclic dynamic method of posterior and ACL graft-tensioning pretensions the grafts, allows graft settling, and confirms knee range of motion and knee stability before final fixation of posterior and ACL reconstruction. Our results demonstrate the efficacy and success of using allograft tissue and a mechanical graft-tensioning device (Biomet Sports Medicine graft-tensioning boot) in single-bundle single-femoral tunnel arthroscopic PCL reconstruction in the multiple-ligament-injured knee. We have also found the graft-tensioning boot to be equally effective in double-bundle PCL reconstructions in the multiple-ligament-injured knee, and with up to 18-year postoperative follow-up [2, 3, 15, 16].

References

1. Fanelli GC. Mechanical graft tensioning in multiple ligament knee surgery. A practical guide to management. 2nd ed. In: Fanelli GC, editor. The multiple ligament injured knee. New York: Springer; 2013. pp. 323–30.
2. Fanelli GC. Rationale and surgical technique for PCL and multiple knee ligament reconstruction. 3rd ed. Warsaw: Biomet Sports Medicine; 2012.
3. Fanelli GC, Beck JD, Edson CJ. Double bundle posterior cruciate ligament reconstruction. Surgical technique and results. Sports Med Arthrosc Rev. 2010;18(4):242–48.
4. Fanelli GC, Beck JD, Edson CJ. Combined PCL ACL lateral and medial side injuries: treatment and results. Sports Med Arthrosc Rev. 2011;19(2):120–30.
5. Fanelli GC, Boyd J. How I manage PCL injuries. Op Techniques Sports Med. 2009;17(3):175–93.
6. Fanelli GC, Beck JD, Edson CJ. How I manage the multiple ligament injured (dislocated) knee. Op Techniques Sports Med. 2010;18(4):198–210.
7. Levy B, Dajani KA, Whalen DB, Stannard JP, Fanelli GC, Stuart MJ, Boyd JL, MacDonald PA, Marx RG. Decision making in the multiple ligament injured knee: an evidence based systematic review. Arthroscopy. 2009;25(4):430–38.
8. Fanelli GC, Stannard JP, Stuart MJ, MacDonald PB, Marx RG, Whelan DB, Boyd JL, Levy BA. Management of complex knee ligament injuries. J Bone Joint Surg. 2010;92-A(12):2235–46.
9. Levy B, Fanelli GC, Whalen D, Stannard J, MacDonald P, Boyd J, Marx R, Stuart M. Modern perspectives for the treatment of knee dislocations and multiligament reconstruction. J Am Academy Orthopaedic Surgeons. 2009;17(4):197–206.
10. Fanelli GC. Surgical treatment of combined PCL ACL medial and lateral side injuries (global laxity): acute and chronic. A practical guide to management. 2nd ed. In: Fanelli GC, editor. The multiple ligament injured knee. Chapter 20 (currently in production).
11. Fanelli GC, Beck JD, Edson CJ. Arthroscopic trans tibial double bundle PCL reconstruction. J Knee Surg. 2010;23(2):89–94.
12. Fanelli GC, Edson CJ. Combined posterior cruciate ligament–posterolateral reconstruction with achilles tendon allograft and biceps femoris tendon tenodesis: 2–10 year follow-up. Arthroscopy. 2004;20(4):339–45.
13. Fanelli GC, Edson CJ, Orcutt DR, Harris JD, Zijerdi D. Treatment of combined ACL PCL medial lateral side injuries of the knee. J Knee Surg. 2005;28(3):240–48.
14. Fanelli GC, Edson CJ. Arthroscopically assisted combined ACL/PCL reconstruction. 2–10 year follow-up. Arthroscopy. 2002;18(7):703–14.
15. Fanelli GC, Beck JD, Edson CJ. Single compared to double bundle PCL reconstruction using allograft tissue. J Knee Surg. 2011;24(4) (currently in production).
16. Fanelli GC, Edson CJ. Surgical treatment of combined PCL, ACL, medial, and lateral side injuries (global laxity): surgical technique and 2 to 18 year results. J Knee Surg. 2012;25(4):307–16.

22 The Role of Osteotomy in the Treatment of Posterior Cruciate Ligament (PCL) Injuries

Jonathan A. Godin, Kathryne J. Stabile and Claude T. Moorman, III

Introduction

Isolated grade I-II posterior cruciate ligament (PCL) injuries are often not addressed surgically. However, after PCL injury, patellofemoral joint pressure increases. This is due to an increase in internal femoral rotation and increased posterior tibial translation resulting in increased tension on the patellar tendon. The change in knee kinematics and joint contact pressure in the PCL-deficient knee leads to degenerative cartilaginous changes in the knee, most commonly osteoarthritic degeneration in the medial compartment of the knee along with the lateral facet and inferior pole of the patella [1–6].

The chronic PCL-deficient knee can be organized in the three main groups: (1) Isolated PCL in which reconstruction may or may not be considered; (2) varus deformity (rarely valgus); and (3) combined ligament injury requiring ligament reconstruction. Patients who may benefit from a high tibial osteotomy (HTO) are those who have a PCL-deficient knee with varus deformity with medial tibiofemoral narrowing symptoms. The group of chronic PCL-deficient patients who have arthrosis so advanced that reconstruction is no longer recommended but they may be too young or too active for knee arthroplasty. An HTO can provide an option to relieve symptoms.

The ideal candidate for an osteotomy is a young, thin, active patient with full knee range of motion and without patellofemoral symptoms. Considering the patient's expectations and desired activity level is an important part of the preoperative discussion. Patient selection is an important factor when considering an osteotomy for a chronic PCL-deficient patient. Patients who have had prior medial and lateral meniscectomy as well as obese individuals who exceed ideal body weight by 1.3 times have consistently worse outcomes [7–9].

History and Physical Examination

A thorough history is a crucial aspect in the evaluation of patients with PCL injuries. Many patients, even those with complete PCL tears, present with relatively benign, often vague, symptoms. Provocative and palliative measures should be noted, as well as any prior treatment. The surgeon should always note the duration of symptoms and any etiological factors. The most common mechanism is a posteriorly directed force to the proximal tibia of the flexed knee [10]. This mechanism is frequently encountered when a patient's knee strikes the dashboard in a motor vehicle collision, when the leg is struck during sporting events, or during a fall onto a flexed knee, particularly with a plantarflexed ankle. Indirect mechanisms of injury include cutting, twisting, or hyperextension during athletic competition [10]. The posterior force can be combined with a varus/valgus or rotational force, thereby leading to concomitant medial, lateral, posteromedial, or posterolateral injury. For example, patients with a posterolateral corner (PLC) injury usually report an impact to the anteromedial aspect of the knee, contact or noncontact hyperextension, and a varus noncontact force. Because common peroneal nerve injury occurs in 15–40% of multiple ligament injured knees, it is vital to ask the patient about numbness, paresthesias, or weakness, especially with ankle dorsiflexion or great toe extension [11, 12]. As with any patient encounter, the clinician should guide expectation management and provide counseling on a case-by-case basis, especially when treating athletes with return to sport ambitions.

J. A. Godin (✉)
Department of Orthopaedic Surgery, Duke University Hospital, 2000 Trent Drive, Box 3000, Room 5309, Orange Zone, Durham, NC 27710, USA
e-mail: jonathan.godin@dm.duke.edu

K. J. Stabile · C. T. Moorman, III
129 Turvey Court, Chapel Hill, NC 27514, USA
e-mail: kathryne.stabile@dm.duke.edu

C. T. Moorman, III
e-mail: t.moorman@dm.duke.edu

G. C. Fanelli (ed.), *Posterior Cruciate Ligament Injuries*,
DOI 10.1007/978-3-319-12072-0_22, © Springer International Publishing Switzerland 2015

Physical examination should include the following:

- Inspection: Open wounds, overlying skin changes, erythema, knee swelling, limb alignment, and posterior sag.
- Palpation: Assess for joint line tenderness, patellar grind, cysts, or masses.
- Range of motion: Both active and passive.
- Neurovascular: A thorough examination should be performed in all patients.
- Gait: Patients with PLC instability often present with hyperextension varus thrust gait. Several reports note that patients with varus thrust gait have poorer outcomes than patients without a gait abnormality [13, 14]. The clinician should also note the presence of a varus recurvatum alignment with stance or gait.

In addition, the following special tests assess for PCL and PLC injury:

- Posterior sag sign: While the patient lies supine with both hips and knees flexed 90°, the examiner holds patient's heels and assesses posterior tibial translation from a lateral view.
- Posterior drawer test: While the patient lies supine with both hips and knees flexed 90°, the examiner sits on the patient's feet and applies a posterior force to the proximal tibia and compares translation to the contralateral side.
- Posterolateral drawer test: The patient lies supine with the knee flexed to 90° and the foot externally rotated 15° while the examiner applies a posterior force to the proximal tibia. Increased translation compared to the contralateral side suggests a popliteus tendon or popliteofibular ligament injury.
- Quadriceps contraction test: While lying supine and starting with the hip and knee flexed to 90°, the patient slowly extends his/her knee. In doing so, the tibia translates anteriorly if a PCL injury is present.
- Dial test: The patient lies prone, and an assistant stabilizes the thighs with the knees flexed to 30°. The examiner externally rotates the legs and compares the sides. The test is positive for PLC injury if there is 30° of absolute rotation or 15° more external rotation than the unaffected side. The same test is then performed at 90° of knee flexion. If there is further discrepancy compared to the contralateral side, then a PCL injury is present.
- External rotation recurvatum test: The patient lies supine with knees extended while the examiner lifts the great toes. A positive examination elicits knee hyperextension, external rotation, and varus deformity.
- Varus/valgus stress test: The patient lies supine and the knee is flexed to 30° of flexion, and the examiner grasps the thigh of the patient with one hand and the foot or the lower leg with the other hand and applies a varus or valgus force to the knee. The amount of lateral or medial compartment opening indicates the grade of the lateral or medial collateral lesion: grade I (0–5 mm), grade II (6–10 mm), and grade III (>10 mm). Increased tibial internal or external rotation should also be documented.
- Reverse pivot shift test: With the patient lying supine and the knee flexed to 70–80° and the foot externally rotated, posterior tibial subluxation suggests PLC injury. This subluxation reduces with knee extension to ~20° of flexion. It is important to test the uninjured side to assess for a falsely positive normal knee.
- McMurray test: With the patient lying supine, the knee is deeply flexed and externally and internally rotated while extending the knee to assess for medial and lateral meniscus tears, respectively. Several studies note the rate of concomitant meniscal injury with acute PCL injury between 16 and 28 % [15, 16].

It is important to note physical examination findings consistent with severe arthrosis, as these patients will not benefit from PCL reconstruction.

Imaging

Preoperative imaging is necessary to ensure careful and thorough planning to avoid under- or overcorrection. In 1992, Dugdale et al. were the first to mathematically analyze the effects of varus deformity on the weight-bearing axis of the extremity and its implications for HTO planning [17]. Since then, a number of other reports have been published as imaging modalities have evolved. We recommend obtaining the following imaging studies to appropriately evaluate and plan HTO in the PCL/PLC-deficient patient.

Standing Full-Length Bilateral A-P Radiograph

A standing full-length bilateral A-P X-ray (Fig. 22.1) is essential to evaluate overall tibiofemoral alignment [18]. An A-P X-ray is taken from the hips to the ankles with the patient standing and the patellae facing anterior. This view is the main view to evaluate varus alignment by evaluating mechanical axis as shown in Fig. 22.2. Mechanical axis is drawn from the center of the femoral head to the center of the ankle joint (not plafond). In a valgus knee, the mechanical axis passes through the knee joint lateral to the center of the knee. In a varus knee, the mechanical axis passes medial to the center of the knee. This can lead to overloading of the medial compartment and articular cartilage degeneration. *Primary varus* includes osseous alignment including the added varus due to loss of meniscus and articular cartilage (Fig. 22.3). *Double varus* is the varus tibiofemoral osseous alignment combined with separation of the lateral compartment due to lateral soft tissues stretching out. *Triple varus*

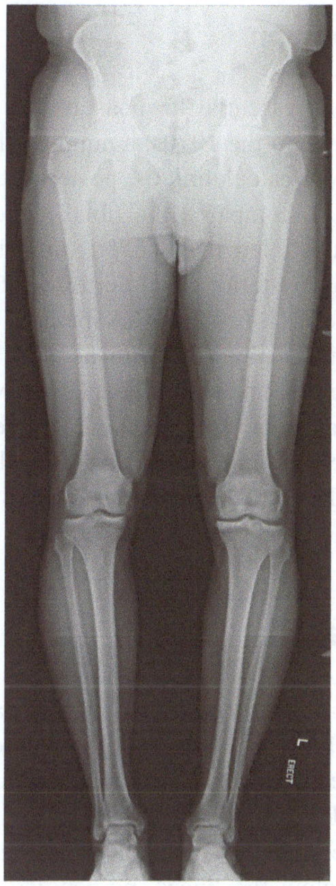

Fig. 22.1 Illustrates standing full-length radiographs. This allows for assessment of varus and determination of mechanical axis

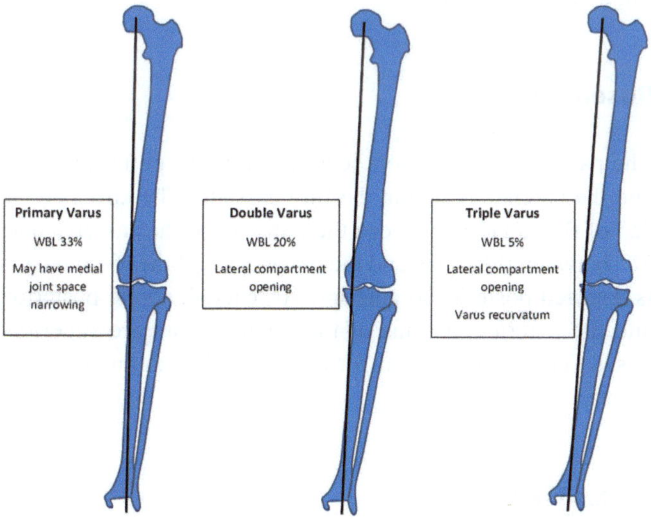

Fig. 22.2 Demonstrates the difference between primary, double, and triple varus

includes tibiofemoral osseous alignment, soft-tissue stretching, and chronic abnormalities resulting in recurvatum and external tibial rotation [19].

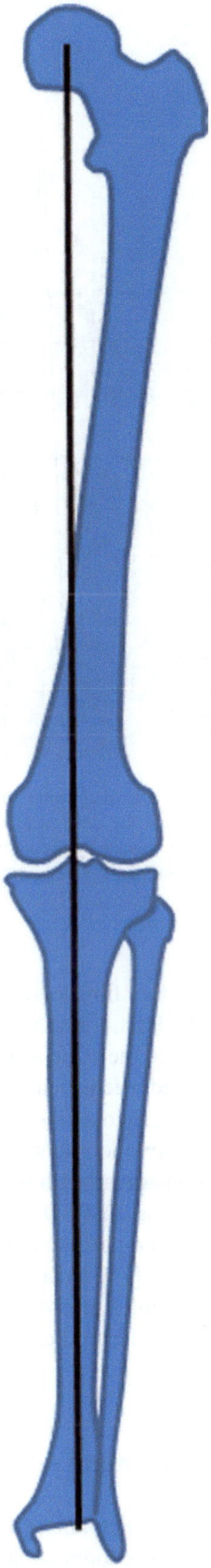

Fig. 22.3 Mechanical axis shown in this figure is drawn from the center of the femoral head to the center of the ankle joint (not plafond)

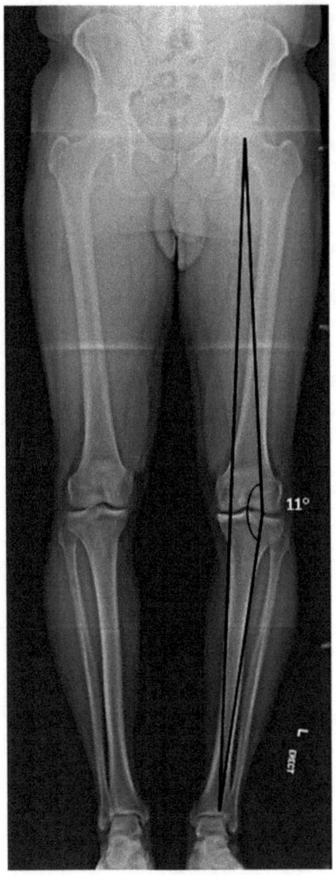

Fig. 22.4 Demonstrates how to determine mechanical axis correction. The point through which the desired mechanical axis will pass is first identified. The angle created by the intersection of the femoral and tibial mechanical axis and the desired point is the amount of correction needed

Dugdale et al. used this film to identify the amount of correction needed [17]. First, a line is drawn from the center of the femoral head to the point along the tibial plateau through which the desired mechanical axis will pass. Next, a line from the center of the tibiotalar joint to this point is draw [17]. The angle created by the intersection of these lines is the amount of correction needed with HTO to achieve the desired mechanical axis (Fig. 22.4). Dugdale et al. also stated that every 1° of varus is proportional to a 1-mm increase in lateral joint line widening [17]. In addition, the A-P view of the knee can be very helpful to observe Segond and arcuate avulsion fractures of the lateral capsule and fibular head, respectively.

Supine Full-Length Bilateral A-P Radiograph

Supine radiographs are important to obtain because they eliminate the added varus brought about by insufficiency to the lateral and posterolateral soft-tissue structures. This allows the surgeon to measure the true amount of correction needed.

Lateral Radiograph

A lateral X-ray is essential to measure the posterior tibial slope. Dating back to the 1970s, a number of methods have been suggested for calculating the posterior tibial slope [20, 21]. Brazier et al. compared the tibial slope measurement methods and concluded that the proximal tibial anatomic axis (PTAA) and posterior tibial cortex (PTC) methods are the most reliable [21]. In the PTAA method, a line is drawn along the proximal tibial anatomical axis and another is drawn along the tibial plateau. The angle between these two lines is the tibial slope [20]. In the PTC method, a line is drawn along the PTC and another is drawn along the medial tibial plateau. The angle between these two lines is the tibial slope [21].

Merchant's View

This radiograph is obtained by having the patient lie in the supine position with the knees at 45° of flexion over the end of the table. The knees are held to maintain the femora parallel to the floor. The beam is directed proximal to distal, forming a 30° angle with the table. The film cassette is placed about 30 cm below the knees, perpendicular to the tibial shaft. This view is helpful for looking at the patellofemoral joint. Specifically, in this patient group, Merchant's view helps assess patellofemoral degenerative changes, patellar tilt, and maltracking.

Rosenberg's View

The patient stands on both legs with thumbs pointing ahead and the patellae touching the film cassette. The knees are at 45° of flexion (25° between the femora and the cassette, and 20° between the tibiae and the cassette), and the X-ray beam is directed posterior to anterior, 10° caudal, so the posterior and the anterior margins of the tibial plateau are superimposed. This view is ideal for assessing the lateral compartment.

Stress View

A number of methods have been described for obtaining a stress view of the knee. Jacobsen first described a method for obtaining a lateral stress radiograph of the knee in 1976 [22]. This description calls for the patient to lie in the lateral decubitus position with the knee flexed to 90°. The heel is fixed to a stand, and the arm of the Telos GA II (Telos, Weterstadt, Germany) applies a posterior force to the tibia [22]. A lateral X-ray is then taken in this position. A radiograph is then taken with the knee in 25° of flexion. This method is very important in chronic PCL-deficient knees to evaluate both anterior and posterior tibial translation with regard to the femur, and it is useful to detect fixed posterior tibial subluxation. The lateral stress view using the kneeling method asks the patient to kneel on a flat, elevated surface with the knee flexed to 90° while a lateral X-ray is taken [23]. Meanwhile, the hamstring contraction method has the patient lie in the lateral decubitus position or in a seated position with the knee at 90° of flexion and the heel fixed to a stand. A lateral X-ray is taken while the patient contracts his/her hamstring [24]. The gravity method asks the patient to lie supine with the hip and knee flexed to 90°, supported by an assistant, with the leg in neutral rotation. In this position, a lateral X-ray is taken [25]. Lastly, Puddu et al. described an axial stress test in 2000 [26]. The patient lies in supine position with both knees at 70° of flexion, feet in moderate plantar flexion, and the tibia in neutral rotation. The X-ray beam is directed parallel to the longitudinal patellar axis, from distal to proximal, and the distance between the anterior tibial profile and the center of the femoral groove is measured [26]. The side-to-side difference is the amount of posterior instability.

Jung et al. compared all five of these methods, focusing on posterior translation, side-to-side difference, condyle rotation, time to perform the test, and pain during the test. Considering all these factors, they stated that the most effective methods are Telos view at 90° of knee flexion and the kneeling method, even if they are painful and time-consuming [24]. Despite being the most expensive method, the Telos method is the most reliable in detecting posterior tibial subluxation [24].

MRI

Magnetic resonance imaging (MRI) is useful in evaluating the PCL-deficient knee, especially associated soft-tissue injuries and subchondral bony edema. Gross et al. introduced a classification system for PCL tears and noted 100% sensitivity and specificity for diagnosing a PCL tear using T1-weighted MRI [27]. Bellelli et al. incorporated T2-weighted spin echo (SE) and short-tau inversion recovery (STIR) scans to augment the classification system established by Gross et al [28]. In the new classification scheme, the two bundles of the PCL were treated independently. Type I lesions involve high-intensity signal within the ligament with low intensity along the borders of the ligament. Type II lesions are partial and involve the dorsal edge of the ligament (posteromedial bundle). Type III lesions are partial and involve the ventral edge of the ligament (anterolateral bundle). Type IV lesions represent a complete tear with both the dorsal and ventral edges involved [28].

MRI is also helpful for evaluating the PLC. LaPrade et al. recommend using at least a 1.5-T scanner with dedicated PLC sectioning using thin-sliced (2 mm) proton density coronal oblique images, which include the entire fibular head and styloid [5]. Doing so affords evaluation of the iliotibial band, long head of the biceps femoris, short head of the biceps femoris, fibular collateral ligament, popliteus complex, and the fabellofibular ligament.

Indications

In general, indications for HTO in the setting of PCL deficiency include the following:

- Young, healthy patients in whom arthroplasty would fail due to excessive wear
- Good vascular status
- Pain and/or disability interfering with daily living
- Compliant patient who will abide by postoperative protocols

Contraindications

Contraindications to HTO include the following:

- Severe osteoporosis
- Inflammatory disease
- Infection
- Severe tricompartmental OA
- Prior lateral meniscectomy
- Knee flexion < 90°

Relative contraindications include the following:

- Morbid obesity
- Age greater than 65 years
- Patellofemoral OA
- Tobacco use

Preoperative Planning

Careful preoperative planning is essential prior to performing an HTO. PCL and PLC lesions are often associated with malalignment of the knee, and they should be addressed in a staged fashion 6–8 months after HTO if the knee is still unstable. Poor results are common after soft-tissue procedures alone in the setting of the malaligned knee. This is due to the forces on these structures, which do not decrease if the underlying malalignment is not corrected, as the bony deformity overstresses them. Instead, HTO reduces these forces and improves the stability and biomechanics of the knee [5, 13, 19, 29–31].

If medial compartment OA with joint-space narrowing is present, then the new weight bearing axis should be positioned to intersect at 62–66 % of the tibial plateau (where 0 % indicates the medial margin of the tibial plateau and 100 % the lateral margin), as this alignment increases the pressure on the lateral compartment of the knee [17, 19]. This slight overcorrection has been shown to prevent progression of medial compartment OA and early recurrence of varus [19]. If degenerative narrowing of the medial compartment is not present, the new mechanical axis should split the tibial plateau in half [19]. Medial opening wedge HTO improves symptoms of patellofemoral OA because the anterior translation of the tibia reduces the tension on the patellar tendon, thereby reducing stress on the lateral facet [3]. Because of this, patellofemoral pain is not a contraindication to HTO.

The type of osteotomy performed to correct the deformity alters the posterior tibial slope in a fairly predictable manner. Lateral closing wedge and dome HTOs have been shown to decrease posterior tibial slope [32]. Although decreasing slope may be beneficial in the anterior cruciate ligament (ACL)-deficient knee, it may exacerbate instability in a PCL-deficient knee. Conversely, medial opening HTO tends to increase posterior tibial slope [33]. Noyes et al. determined that the height of the anterior osteotomy gap at the tibial tubercle must be one half the height of the posteromedial gap to maintain normal sagittal alignment [34]. Furthermore, the authors showed that a gap error of a single millimeter will result in approximately 2° of change in the posterior tibial slope [34].

If meniscal lesions are associated, they should be addressed at the same time as. HTO. A preoperative rehabilitation protocol consisting of strengthening and gait training has been suggested in the literature as a measure to avoid recurrence of hyperextension varus thrust gait after surgery [19]. In the patient with a chronic PCL-deficient knee associated with double or triple varus, HTO should be performed before soft-tissue procedures. The patient should be evaluated 6–8 months later, and soft-tissue reconstruction can subsequently be undertaken if the knee remains unstable.

Operative Technique

The patient is placed on the operating room table in a supine position. A thigh tourniquet can be used on the operative leg. However, this may occlude possible vascular injury that may need to be addressed after the tourniquet is let down. Some authors prefer to use iliac crest bone autograft harvested from the ipsilateral side. In this case, the iliac crest is also prepped and draped along with the surgical limb.

The initial incision is medially based over the pes anserine vertically oriented halfway between the tibial tubercle and the PTC. The sartorius fascia is sharply incised parallel to the underlying hamstring tendons. Care should be taken to preserve the sartorius fascia so that it can be repaired upon closure of the wound. In the case of concurrent ligament reconstruction of the ACL or PCL, the hamstring may be harvested at this time. The superficial medial collateral ligament (MCL) is then exposed by retracting the hamstrings (if still in place) medially. The superior portion of the MCL attachment is released with an elevator to expose the posteromedial border of the tibia. On the anterior aspect of the tibia, the fascia is dissected at the level of the patellar tendon insertion. Visualization and exposure are key and blunt retractors are placed under the MCL and patellar tendon.

After exposure is obtained, a guide wire is placed in a medial-to-lateral fashion across the proximal tibia. The guide is placed 4 cm distal to the medial joint line at the level of the superior aspect of the tibial tubercle. The guide is oriented in an oblique fashion to end 1 cm below the joint line on the lateral cortex. The tip of the fibular head is used as a reference point. Fluoroscopy is used throughout this portion of the procedure. The guide wire is used to guide the oscillating saw that is placed on the underside of the wire to minimize the risk of intra-articular fracture. The osteotomy is made starting from the medial and posteromedial cortex. Thin osteotomes are used to complete the osteotomy which should end 1 cm short of the lateral tibial cortex. Once anterior and posterior cortices are penetrated and the osteotomy is completed, a predetermined-sized osteotomy wedge is used medially to open the osteotomy. Care should be taken during this step to prevent fracture propagation.

Once the desired osteotomy opening has been made based on fluoroscopic evaluation of mechanical axis and tibial slope, the osteotomy plate is placed. There are two systems typically used: the Puddu plate (Arthrex, Inc, Naples, FL) or the Tomofix plate (Synthes, West Chester, PA). The plate is placed with the leg in extension and using two 4.5 mm cortical screws distally with two 6.5 mm cancellous screws proximally, as shown in Fig. 22.5. Bone grafting is commonly performed to ensure bony union. The author's preference is autograft combined with allograft cancellous chips or synthetic bone matrix with the addition of platelet-rich plasma. The wound is then irrigated and closed with care to repair the Sartorius.

Patients are placed in a hinged knee brace with nonweight bearing for 4 weeks initially. They are then advanced to touch down weight bearing for 4 weeks followed by an additional 4 weeks of 50 % weight bearing. Radiographs are used to evaluate union and guide weight bearing status.

Clinical Results

The main body of published literature focuses on outcomes following HTO in the setting of the ACL-deficient knee. HTO associated with ACL reconstruction has shown promising results in young patients with varus malalignment and

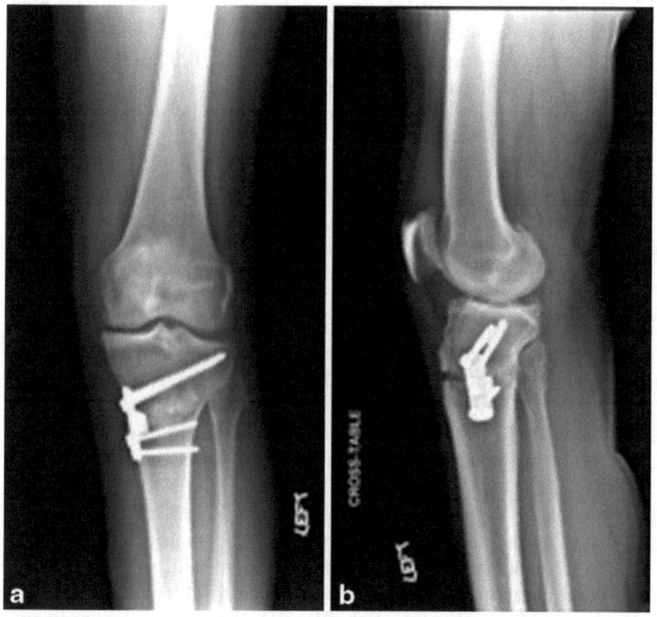

Fig. 22.5 a and b Representative postoperative radiographs of a high tibial osteotomy with an 11° correction using plate fixation. The anteriorposterior and lateral radiographs are shown

ACL deficiency. Zaffagnini et al. recently reported outcomes of thirty-two patients who underwent closing wedge HTO and ACL reconstruction simultaneously for varus malalignment and ACL deficiency [35]. Subjective and objective International Knee Documentation Committee (IKDC), Tegner, and EQ-5D scores significantly improved from preoperative status to final follow-up, while KT-1000 evaluation showed a mean side-to-side difference of 2.2 ± 1.0 mm [35]. The mean correction of the limb alignment was 5.6° ± 2.8°, and posterior tibial slope decreased at a mean of 1.2° ± 0.9° [35]. No patients underwent revision surgery [35].

Noyes et al. reported on a total of 41 knees (23 double varus, 18 triple varus) treated with proximal tibial closing wedge osteotomy and ACL reconstruction [19]. In addition, all triple-varus knees underwent reconstruction of the posterolateral structures [19]. At a mean of 4.5 years follow-up, reduction in pain was found in 71 % (29 knees); elimination of giving way in 85 % (35 knees); and resumption of light recreational activities in 66 % (27 knees) [19]. Subjective patient-reported outcome was normal or very good in 37 % (15 knees) and good in 34 % (14 knees) [19]. The mean Cincinnati Knee Rating Score significantly improved from 63 to 82 points (24). Correction of varus alignment was maintained in 33 knees (80 %) [19]. Two patients required revision osteotomy, while another four underwent revision ACL reconstruction for graft rupture [19].

Similarly, Badhe et al. treated 14 patients with varus alignment and knee instability [36]. Five patients with double varus were treated with single-stage closing wedge tibial osteotomy and ACL reconstruction [36]. The remaining nine patients had varying amount of posterior cruciate and PLC ligament injuries with varus angulation (triple varus) [36]. Six of these patients had a ligament reconstruction, while the remaining three had a tibial osteotomy without ligament reconstruction [36]. Four of the nine patients with triple varus had an opening wedge tibial osteotomy, and the remaining five had a closing wedge tibial osteotomy [36]. At a mean follow-up of 2.8 years after tibial osteotomy, 12 knees (86 %) were stable [36]. Thirteen (93 %) of the patients were able to participate in light recreational activities. None of these patients could return to competitive sports [36]. Five (35 %) continued to have pain of varying degree. The mean Cincinnati Knee Score improved from a mean preoperative of 53 to a mean postoperative of 74, thereby yielding two poor, four fair and eight good results [36]. In-patients with triple-varus alignment, opening wedge tibial osteotomy resulted in better scores than those with closing wedge osteotomy [36].

Lerat et al. reported the results of 28 patients with an average follow-up of over 4 years who underwent closing or opening wedge proximal tibial osteotomy in conjunction with ACL reconstruction using a bone-patellar tendon-bone autograft [37]. Forty-three percent of patients were able to return to sport, while eight patients suffered an ACL graft rupture [37]. Meanwhile, Lattermann et al. compared three groups of patients treated for varus alignment and chronic anterior knee instability: HTO alone, simultaneous HTO and ACL reconstruction, and staged HTO and subsequent ACL reconstruction [38]. Pain and positive pivot-shift test was present in all groups, though to the greatest proportion in the simultaneous HTO and anterior cruciate ligament reconstruction (ACLR) group [38]. Nevertheless, the overall IKDC score improved in 23/27 patients and 25/27 patients noted that they would undergo the same procedure again [38]. Neuschwander et al. reported the outcomes of five patients treated with simultaneous HTO and ACLR [39]. Postoperatively, the medial compartment pain improved, instability episodes were eliminated, there were no complications, and functional levels were improved in all patients [39].

Naudie et al. assessed the functional outcome of opening wedge HTO in a young, active group of 16 patients (17 knees) with instability [40]. At a mean of 56 months follow-up, all patients had an increase in their activity score postoperatively. Nine patients rated their symptoms as significantly better and seven as somewhat better [40]. Femorotibial axis coronal alignment was changed to a mean of 6° valgus, while posterior tibial slope was increased a mean of 8° [40].

Conclusions/Discussion

The chronically deficient PCL patient is at risk for increased medial compartment wear and patellofemoral wear. An HTO remains a viable option for patients who have a full range of motion, are too young for knee arthroplasty and prefer to maintain a high level of activity. It is essential to evaluate the mechanical axis in each patient prior to considering an osteotomy. Evaluation of the deformity in the coronal and sagittal planes is particularly important in patients who are PCL deficient due to the effect of tibial slope on knee kinematics. Correct bone alignment in both the coronal and sagittal planes should be obtained before performing any type soft-tissue surgery. HTO offers patients a chance to get relief of symptoms and continue activity while avoiding or delaying arthroplasty and its associated limitations.

References

1. Skyhar MJ, Warren RF, Ortiz GJ, Schwartz E, Otis JC. The effects of sectioning of the posterior cruciate ligament and the posterolateral complex on the articular contact pressures within the knee. J Bone Joint Surg Am. 1993;75(5):694–9.
2. Ramaniraka NA, Terrier A, Theumann N, Siegrist O. Effects of the posterior cruciate ligament reconstruction on the biomechanics of the knee joint: a finite element analysis. Clin Biomech. 2005;20(4):434–42.
3. Li G, Gill TJ, DeFrate LE, Zayontz S, Glatt V, Zarins B. Biomechanical consequences of PCL deficiency in the knee under simulated muscle loads–an in vitro experimental study. J Orthop Res. 2002;20(4):887–92.
4. Lephart SM, Pincivero DM, Rozzi SL. Proprioception of the ankle and knee. Sports Med. 1998;25(3):149–55.
5. LaPrade RF, Wentorf F. Diagnosis and treatment of posterolateral knee injuries. Clin Orthop Relat Res. 2002;9(402):110–21.
6. Kumagai M, Mizuno Y, Mattessich SM, Elias JJ, Cosgarea AJ, Chao EY. Posterior cruciate ligament rupture alters in vitro knee kinematics. Clin Orthop Relat Res. 2002;2(395):241–48.
7. Slawski DP. High tibial osteotomy in the treatment of adult osteochondritis dissecans. Clin Orthop Relat Res. 1997;8(341):155–61.
8. Morrey BF. Upper tibial osteotomy for secondary osteoarthritis of the knee. J Bone Joint Surg Br. 1989;71(4):554–9.
9. Coventry MB, Ilstrup DM, Wallrichs SL. Proximal tibial osteotomy. A critical long-term study of eighty-seven cases. J Bone Joint Surg Am. 1993;75(2):196–201.
10. Cosgarea AJ, Jay PR. Posterior cruciate ligament injuries: evaluation and management. J Am Acad Orthop Surg. 2001;9(5): 297–307.
11. Mook WR, Ligh CA, Moorman CT, 3rd, Leversedge FJ. Nerve injury complicating multiligament knee injury: current concepts and treatment algorithm. J Am Acad Orthop Surg. 2013;21(6):343–54.
12. Savarese E, Bisicchia S, Romeo R, Amendola A. Role of high tibial osteotomy in chronic injuries of posterior cruciate ligament and posterolateral corner. J Orthop Traumatol. 2011;12(1):1–17.
13. Miller MD, Cooper DE, Fanelli GC, Harner CD, LaPrade RF. Posterior cruciate ligament: current concepts. Instr Course Lect. 2002;51:347–51.
14. Noyes FR, Dunworth LA, Andriacchi TP, Andrews M, Hewett TE. Knee hyperextension gait abnormalities in unstable knees. Recognition and preoperative gait retraining. Am J Sports Med. 1996;24(1):35–45.
15. Hamada M, Shino K, Mitsuoka T, Toritsuka Y, Natsu-Ume T, Horibe S. Chondral injury associated with acute isolated posterior cruciate ligament injury. Arthroscopy 2000;16(1):59–63.
16. Fowler PJ, Messieh SS. Isolated posterior cruciate ligament injuries in athletes. Am J Sports Med. 1987;15(6):553–7.
17. Dugdale TW, Noyes FR, Styer D. Preoperative planning for high tibial osteotomy. The effect of lateral tibiofemoral separation and tibiofemoral length. Clin Orthop Relat Res. 1992;1(274):248–64.
18. Moreland JR, Bassett LW, Hanker GJ. Radiographic analysis of the axial alignment of the lower extremity. J Bone Joint Surg Am. 1987;69(5):745–9.
19. Noyes FR, Barber-Westin SD, Hewett TE. High tibial osteotomy and ligament reconstruction for varus angulated anterior cruciate ligament-deficient knees. Am J Sports Med. 2000;28(3):282–96.
20. Dejour H, Bonnin M. Tibial translation after anterior cruciate ligament rupture. Two radiological tests compared. J Bone Joint Surg Br. 1994;76(5):745–9.
21. Brazier J, Migaud H, Gougeon F, Cotten A, Fontaine C, Duquennoy A. [Evaluation of methods for radiographic measurement of the tibial slope. A study of 83 healthy knees]. Rev Chir Orthop Reparatrice Appar Mot. 1996;82(3):195–200.
22. Jacobsen K. Stress radiographical measurement of the anteroposterior, medial and lateral stability of the knee joint. Acta Orthop Scand. 1976;47(3):335–4.
23. Louisia S, Siebold R, Canty J, Bartlett RJ. Assessment of posterior stability in total knee replacement by stress radiographs: prospective comparison of two different types of mobile bearing implants. Knee Surg Sports Traumatol Arthrosc. 2005;13(6):476–82.
24. Jung TM, Reinhardt C, Scheffler SU, Weiler A. Stress radiography to measure posterior cruciate ligament insufficiency: a comparison of five different techniques. Knee Surg Sports Traumatol Arthrosc. 2006;14(11):1116–21.
25. Staubli HU, Jakob RP. Posterior instability of the knee near extension. A clinical and stress radiographic analysis of acute injuries of the posterior cruciate ligament. J Bone Joint Surg Br. 1990;72(2):225–30.
26. Puddu G, Gianni E, Chambat P, De Paulis F. The axial view in evaluating tibial translation in cases of insufficiency of the posterior cruciate ligament. Arthroscopy 2000;16(2):217–20.
27. Gross ML, Grover JS, Bassett LW, Seeger LL, Finerman GA. Magnetic resonance imaging of the posterior cruciate ligament. Clinical use to improve diagnostic accuracy. Am J Sports Med. 1992;20(6):732–37.
28. Bellelli A, Mancini P, Polito M, David V, Mariani PP. Magnetic resonance imaging of posterior cruciate ligament injuries: a new classification of traumatic tears. Radiol Med. 2006;111(6):828–35.
29. McNamara I, Birmingham TB, Fowler PJ, Giffin JR. High tibial osteotomy: evolution of research and clinical applications–a Canadian experience. Knee Surg Sports Traumatol Arthrosc. 2013;21(1):23–31.
30. Giffin JR, Shannon FJ. The role of the high tibial osteotomy in the unstable knee. Sports Med Arthrosc. 2007;15(1):23–31.
31. Andrews JR, Edwards JC, Satterwhite YE. Isolated posterior cruciate ligament injuries. History, mechanism of injury, physical findings, and ancillary tests. Clin Sports Med. 1994;13(3):519–30.
32. Hohmann E, Bryant A, Imhoff AB. The effect of closed wedge high tibial osteotomy on tibial slope: a radiographic study. Knee Surg Sports Traumatol Arthrosc. 2006;14(5):454–9.
33. Bombaci H, Canbora K, Onur G, Gorgec M. [The effect of open wedge osteotomy on the posterior tibial slope]. Acta Orthop Traumatol Turc. 2005;39(5):404–10.
34. Noyes FR, Goebel SX, West J. Opening wedge tibial osteotomy: the 3-triangle method to correct axial alignment and tibial slope. Am J Sports Med. 2005;33(3):378–87.
35. Zaffagnini S, Bonanzinga T, Grassi A, et al. Combined ACL reconstruction and closing-wedge HTO for varus angulated ACL-deficient knees. Knee Surg Sports Traumatol Arthrosc. 2013;21(4):934–41.
36. Badhe NP, Forster IW. High tibial osteotomy in knee instability: the rationale of treatment and early results. Knee Surg Sports Traumatol Arthrosc. 2002;10(1):38–43.

37. Lerat JL, Moyen B, Garin C, Mandrino A, Besse JL, Brunet-Guedj E. [Anterior laxity and internal arthritis of the knee. Results of the reconstruction of the anterior cruciate ligament associated with tibial osteotomy]. Rev Chir Orthop Reparatrice Appar Mot. 1993;79(5):365–74.
38. Lattermann C, Jakob RP. High tibial osteotomy alone or combined with ligament reconstruction in anterior cruciate ligament-deficient knees. Knee Surg Sports Traumatol Arthrosc. 1996;4(1):32–8.
39. Neuschwander DC, Drez D Jr, Paine RM. Simultaneous high tibial osteotomy and ACL reconstruction for combined genu varum and symptomatic ACL tear. Orthopedics. 1993;16(6):679–84.
40. Naudie DD, Amendola A, Fowler PJ. Opening wedge high tibial osteotomy for symptomatic hyperextension-varus thrust. Am J Sports Med. 2004;32(1):60–70.

Articular Cartilage Restoration in the PCL-Injured Knee

23

Clay G. Nelson and Kevin F. Bonner

Introduction

Posterior cruciate ligament (PCL) injuries represent a heterogeneous patient population, which includes both low- and high-energy mechanisms. Higher-energy mechanism injuries, with motor vehicle accidents being the most common, often have concomitant ligamentous, meniscal, chondral, or osteochondral lesions [1, 2]. Lower-energy injuries, as a general rule, are more likely to be relatively isolated and lower grade, although that is certainly not always the case [3]. The PCL literature justifiably tends to focus on the management and outcomes of the isolated or multiligamentous injury reconstruction options to restore joint stability [4–11]. Relatively few studies comment on the incidence of chondral lesions in the setting of an acute PCL disruption with or without multiligament involvement. Some studies reveal articular damage to be present in 12–52 % of cases overall, although multiligament, higher-grade injuries tend to be associated with a higher likelihood of significant acute chondral injury (Fig. 23.1) [12–18]. Most authors, however, do not discuss articular cartilage injury let alone their acute or chronic management in this setting [4–9, 15].

PCL insufficiency has known detrimental effects on joint mechanics of the knee, and the kinematics can be altered dramatically depending on the individual's activities [19]. Sectioning of the PCL increases both patellofemoral and medial compartment contact pressures [20, 21]. The magnitude and location of peak articular cartilage contact pressures during knee flexion are altered with PCL deficiency, both increasing absolute peak loads and shifting contact pressures to a more anterior and medial location within the medial compartment [22]. These altered kinematics help to explain the more typical locations of the resulting symptoms and degenerative changes that may result with PCL insufficiency over time, with the medial femoral condyle being the most likely (31–78 %) affected region followed by the patellofemoral compartment (23–47 %) [14, 23].

Following a severe multiligament injury, the development of progressive degenerative changes is often ubiquitous with time [15–18]. This degenerative course is felt to be multifactorial, and despite the high rate of articular degeneration that occurs following these injuries, there is no current evidence to suggest that a focal, acute chondral injury will become symptomatic or be the primary cause of progressive joint degeneration [24]. Degenerative changes following ligamentous knee injury are influenced by many factors including altered joint kinematics, persistent instability, meniscus integrity, weight, body mass index, as well as macroscopic- and cellular level articular cartilage damage [18, 25–30]. Many of these patients may ultimately require an arthroplasty to address their advanced posttraumatic arthritis [31].

With chronic isolated PCL instability, patients often also go on to develop articular degeneration with time, although progression rate may be variable [23, 32–34]. Similar to the multiligament situation, factors leading to the degenerative course are likely multifactorial and it is currently often unknown the contribution an acute chondral lesion will make to this degenerative progression. The natural history of most acute chondral injuries is poorly understood, and it is often unknown whether the treatment will even alter the natural history, especially in a joint with abnormal kinematics. Many chondral lesions will remain asymptomatic for a period of time without any treatment. Others may be quite debilitating and progress with time. Determining which course an acute lesion will take in the setting of an acute PCL or multiligamentous injury is realistically impossible at this time.

With limited evidence that procedures addressing the articular damage will necessarily alter the overall natural history of the joint, it is important to evaluate the lesion, joint, and patient characteristics to determine optimal treatment.

K. F. Bonner (✉)
Jordan-Young Institute, 5716 Cleveland St, Suite 200, Virginia Beach, VA 23462, USA
e-mail: kfbonner@cox.net

C. G. Nelson
Eastern Virginia Medical School, Norfolk, VA, USA
e-mail: nelsoncg@evms.edu

G. C. Fanelli (ed.), *Posterior Cruciate Ligament Injuries*,
DOI 10.1007/978-3-319-12072-0_23, © Springer International Publishing Switzerland 2015

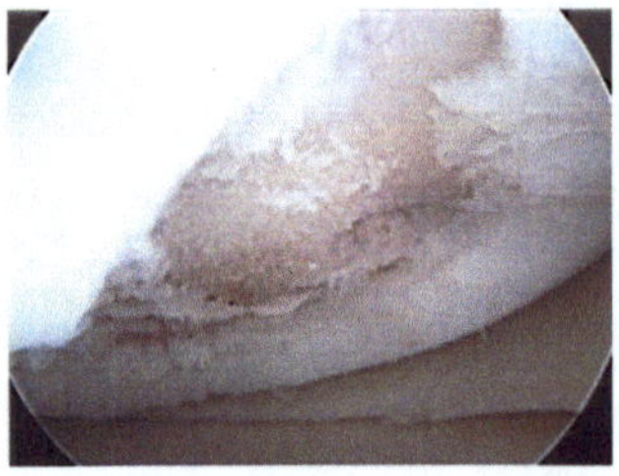

Fig. 23.1 Traumatic full-thickness chondral lesion of the medial femoral condyle

Given the spectrum of cartilage lesions that may be encountered, different treatment options can be considered to address a specific lesion. Inherent to the discussion of articular cartilage surgery is the reality that optimal treatment is often unknown and controversial, thus individual surgeon preferences and personal algorithms often play a significant role in treatment.

Cartilage restorative options are more limited in the acute multiligament injury setting since surgical intervention is often recommended within 3 weeks of the injury [35]. It is reasonable to treat the majority of high-grade lesions with low-morbidity, expeditious, available interventions in the acute setting [28]. For the subset of lesions that cause persistent symptoms despite primary acute treatment, secondary articular-cartilage resurfacing procedures are performed according to accepted algorithms. Many lesions may never require further treatment; however, degenerative changes often occur in patients over time. When contemplating treatment of a more chronic articular-cartilage lesion, it is important to appreciate the potential contributing factors to the development of the lesion. Some of these issues may be able to be addressed, while others may not. Realizing despite our best efforts, this can be a very challenging patient population. The goal of the articular cartilage surgeon is to address symptomatic lesions in order to improve pain and function, with the hope of delaying the need for future arthroplasty. Realistically, however, with time many patients with isolated PCL injury and most with severe multiligamentous injury will eventually require arthroplasty to address degenerative changes that often progress with time.

Treatment of Acute Articular-Cartilage Lesions Associated with PCL Injury

With limited evidence to support definitive recommendations for addressing articular defects occurring with a concomitant ligamentous injury in the acute setting, there is considerable debate among orthopedists regarding the most appropriate surgical treatment for an incidental and potentially asymptomatic lesion versus what may be a potentially symptomatic defect [24, 36–38]. In the acute setting, it may be impossible to determine if a chondral lesion is or will remain symptomatic. While many patients with PCL insufficiency will go on to develop chronic degenerative changes over time, it is truly unknown the specific contribution an acute defect will make, versus other factors, to this frequent ultimate outcome [4, 15, 23–26, 32, 36, 39]. When considering data on acute anterior cruciate ligament (ACL) injury, patients with an acute high-grade articular cartilage defect left untreated were shown to only have slightly inferior outcomes compared to patients without chondral lesions 15 years following ACL reconstruction [24, 36]. Other studies, however, report that these focal lesions can cause significant morbidity [29, 38, 40]. At this time, we feel that it is reasonable to treat a high-grade lesion in the acute setting in a patient who is undergoing surgery for another primary indication. However, the authors favor expeditious, less-invasive techniques, which minimize morbidity when treating chondral lesions in this acute treatment group.

Perhaps in the future, we will be able to better determine if "more invasive" cartilage procedures or even acute treatment at all will change the natural history of the single or multiligament-injured knee. Currently, there are no trials that investigate the effect of treatment versus no treatment. Additionally, there are not many comparison studies among treatments in not only the PCL or multiligament-injury group but also in the much larger isolated ACL reconstruction population. Several investigators have published case series of combined ACL reconstruction and osteochondral autograft transfer, microfracture, or autologous chondrocyte implantation (ACI) with reasonable short-term outcomes [11, 29]. One recent study did show higher subjective outcome scores with osteochondral autograft transfer when compared to microfracture in an ACL reconstruction population at 3-year follow-up [41]. Other studies, which have focused more on symptomatic lesions, have more variable results. Some show superiority or perhaps greater durability of more invasive procedures like osteochondral autologous transfer system (OATS) or ACI, while others do not [41–43]. There does seem to be a trend towards inferiority of microfracture relative to hyaline-resurfacing options in terms of durability with time; however, this is still a topic of debate [44–46].

Although it makes sense to try and resurface a high-grade defect based on our experience with treating symptomatic defects, the results of any cartilage restoration procedure for an acute traumatic or incidental lesion may have optimal results relative to other cohorts. However, since certainly some patients with higher-grade lesions do go on to become symptomatic in our and others' experience, treatment over nontreatment is reasonable in this setting [11, 29, 40]. An acute treatment algorithm is proposed based on available options yet attempting to minimize morbidity when treating full-thickness defects in an often young individual (Fig. 23.2). The senior author (KFB) acknowledges that this is based on

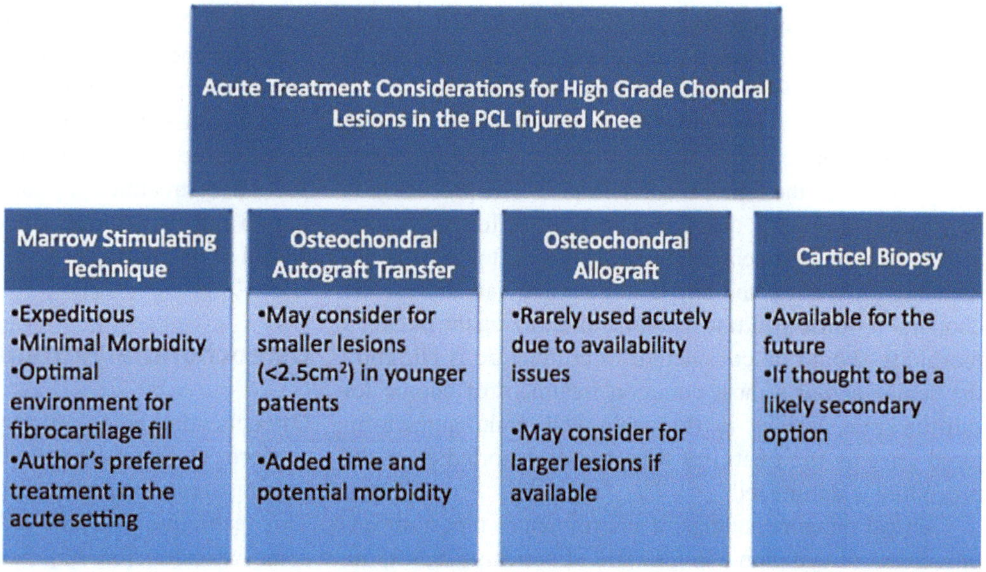

Fig. 23.2 Acute treatment algorithm for a high-grade chondral lesion in the PCL or multiligament-injured knee. *PCL* posterior cruciate ligament. (With kind permission from Springer Science+Business Media: The Multiple Ligament Injured Knee [31])

anecdotal experience, and there is no good evidence to support one treatment method over another in an acute and potentially asymptomatic lesion [11, 40].

Debridement/Chondroplasty

Arthroscopic chondroplasty is the treatment of choice whenever a partial-thickness (ICRS Grade 2) articular cartilage lesion is present with unstable edges or fragments. The senior author routinely will use this simple procedure for higher-grade (ICRS 3a) lesions if there is still a layer of articular cartilage present over the calcified cartilage layer. If this layer has been violated and calcified cartilage is visible (ICRS Grade 3b or Outerbridge Grade 4), other treatment options are preferred, especially in younger, more active populations.

Chondroplasty is used to help alleviate mechanical symptoms that may be caused by loose, unstable fragments of cartilage. Removing only the unstable cartilage gives the surgeon a quick, low-morbidity treatment option to address a chondral lesion when reconstructing the PCL or multiligament knee in the acute setting. Having an expeditious treatment option is beneficial as the reconstruction itself can be a time-consuming procedure. Debridement of the cartilage is done with either a mechanical shaver or a more modern radiofrequency-type device, and there is some debate over which is the better option. Cell death from thermal injury has been cited as a concern with radiofrequency devices although this is controversial [29, 47].

Microfracture

Marrow-stimulating techniques, such as microfracture, are often used in an attempt to induce the formation of primarily fibrocartilage repair tissue within a high-grade to full-thickness defect. Lesion edges are debrided to a stable rim followed by penetration of the subchondral plate by either an awl-type impaction device by drilling utilizing a small bit. These small subchondral access holes, which should be separated by 3–5 mm, serve as a conduit for blood components into the defect site (Fig. 23.3). The goal is to create a stable fibrin clot within the defect, which will remain to support the formation of repair tissue. Marrow-derived fibrin clot contains mesenchymal stem cells, which can differentiate into fibrochondrocytes. These cells produce a fibrocartilage repair tissue that contains type I and type II collagen [48, 49]. Microfracture has been shown to produce variable fibrocartilage defect fill, based off of short-term magnetic resonance imaging (MRI) data [50–52]. While this repair tissue has inferior biomechanical properties and wear characteristics

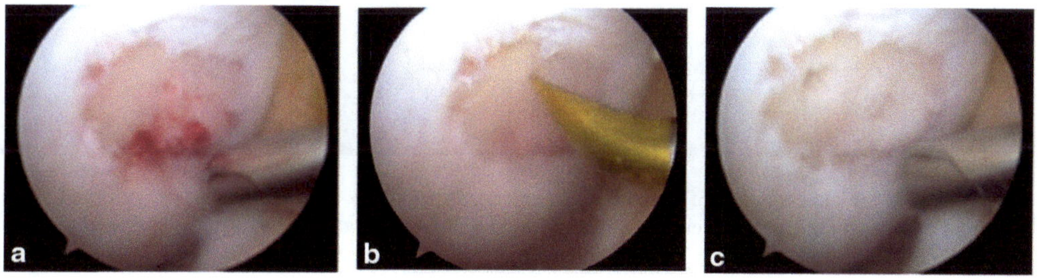

Fig. 23.3 **a** Traumatic full-thickness chondral lesion of the femoral condyle sustained during a knee dislocation. **b** and **c** Microfracture of the relatively small lesion performed during acute reconstruction

compared to hyaline cartilage, there is a correlation, at least in the short term, between the amount of fibrocartilage repair tissue found on MRI and patient outcomes [49–53].

Microfracture is generally considered a good first-line treatment option for many acute full-thickness lesions, especially lesions of the femoral condyle [54]. The procedure is fairly straightforward, quick, and very cost-effective. Again, a PCL or multiligament reconstruction is often a time-demanding procedure, and any treatment that can address the chondral lesion expeditiously while minimizing the patient's morbidity should be considered. Microfracture is currently the senior author's most common treatment of choice for full-thickness lesions in the acute PCL/multiligament-injured knee as the treatment time and the morbidity of the procedure is minimized.

Clinical outcome studies of microfracture report an improvement of symptoms in 50–90% of patients [29, 49, 50, 55–58]. These results vary, however, based on the characteristics of the lesion as well as the patient's demographics, activity level, and duration of symptoms [55–59]. Patients tend to do worse with lesions > 2 cm^2, age > 35 years, higher body mass index, patellofemoral lesions (particularly patella lesions), and symptomatology > 1 year [50, 55, 56, 59]. While microfracture has been shown to improve patients' function in the short term, limited data is available on the long-term results following the procedures [55]. Available long-term data show that microfracture improves International Knee Documentation Committee (IKDC), Lysholm, and Tegner scores in the short term. These improvements, however, diminish over time, and treatment failures and degenerative arthritis can be expected in a significant percentage of patients, especially with larger or multiple lesions in older and more active patients [44–46, 54]. However, this may occur with any treatment in this often complex patient population.

Although controversial, in younger patients with symptomatic defects, there may be some downside to microfracturing a lesion when considering future treatment options. Higher-volume ACI surgeons have shown evidence that prior microfracture may adversely affect the outcomes of a secondary ACI procedure [60–62]. This is thought to likely be due to the formation of intralesional osteophytes, which form as a result of disruption of the subchondral plate. Authors who feel ACI may produce a more reliable and durable repair tissue may not microfracture a lesion for this reason. Secondary treatment options utilizing osteochondral grafts should not be affected since the osteochondral unit is replaced in this setting.

Osteochondral Autograft Transfer

Osteochondral autograft transfer/mosaicplasty transfers one or more osteoarticular cylindrical plugs from a lower weight-bearing area of the knee to a symptomatic location [63–65]. This technique has been utilized since the mid-1990s with some variation [63–65]. Some authors have utilized multiple, smaller-diameter plug "mosaic" configurations versus currently, many surgeons prefer to transfer fewer, larger-diameter plugs (Fig. 23.4). This is a good primary or secondary option for symptomatic chondral or osteochondral lesions less than 2.5 cm^2. Delivering the autologous osteochondral plug allows reliable bone-to-bone healing with viable hyaline cartilage usually within 6 weeks of the procedure.

Contact stress studies have been used to help define optimal donor-site locations; however, results and expert opinion vary on the three recognized acceptable harvest-site locations within the knee [63–66]. Potential donor-site morbidity is a concern with this procedure. Hangody, who has the most extensive experience with the procedure, reports a 3–5% incidence of morbidity [67]; however, there are variable rates of reported donor-site morbidity in the literature, and some studies report no donor-site morbidity [68–75]. Bioabsorbable scaffolds and allograft plugs have been used to backfill the donor sites to decrease postoperative hemarthrosis and donor-site morbidity [63]; however, it is unknown if donor-site morbidity is decreased in the long term, and case reports have shown that foreign body reactions can occur following the use of these scaffolds [76, 77]. One large center with prob-

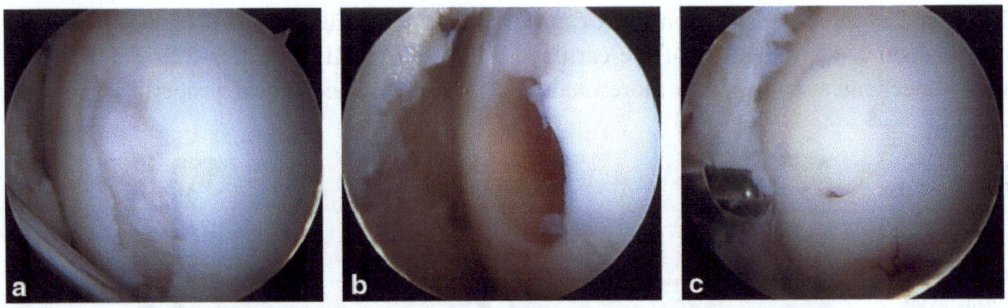

Fig. 23.4 **a** Full-thickness defect of the medial femoral condyle (*MFC*). **b** First recipient site prior to OAT implantation. **c** MFC defect following implantation of two OAT plugs overlapped in a "Mastercard" configuration. *OAT* osteochondral autograft transfer. (With kind permission from Springer Science + Business Media: The Multiple Ligament Injured Knee [31])

ably the greatest experience has published studies revealing remodeling and tissue ingrowth occurs reliably over 2 years but with often poor MRI characteristics prior to that time, while others have not demonstrated synthetic grafts have led to increased bone ingrowth or osteoconductivity [78, 79].

Delivery of the osteochondral plugs can be technically challenging, and placing the graft perpendicular into the recipient's site is critical to the success of the procedure. While this can be performed arthroscopically, surgeons often feel more comfortable using a limited arthrotomy to more reliably deliver plugs perpendicular to the articular surface. Similarly, the superolateral trochlea, which is likely the most popular donor-site location, is often accessed using a small lateral arthrotomy to obtain reproducibly perpendicular donor plugs (Fig. 23.5).

Osteochondral autograft transfer, for a surgeon who is comfortable with the technique, is an option in the acute setting, and should be considered for a younger, active patient with a smaller lesion (<2.5 cm^2). However, given the technical difficulty of the procedure, additional surgical time should be expected, and further morbidity to the joint may occur. It is uncertain at this point if the increased procedural time and trauma make this the most optimal treatment choice in the acute setting, but it is clearly a viable option.

Fresh Osteochondral Allografts

Mutliligament Grade III PCL injuries addressed in the acute setting are often treated within 3 weeks, making it often difficult to obtain a fresh allograft within this limited time frame. Fresh osteochondral allografts are often used to treat larger symptomatic chondral or osteochondral lesions, and the procedure is most often used for the secondary treatment of symptomatic defects. However, if an allograft can be obtained in the acute setting, it may be a reasonable option for certain lesions. Depending on the nature of the lesion, it is often not necessary to obtain a perfect size match for a condylar lesion. We will not uncommonly request a condyle the same size or larger in order to increase the likelihood of obtaining a graft in a timely fashion.

ACI Biopsy

ACI (Carticel; Genzyme Corp, Cambridge, MA) is a two-staged procedure that harvests cartilage during the index procedure and implants cultured cells 4–6 weeks later [61, 80]. ACI is typically used to address persistently symptomatic lesions that have failed primary treatment, but if the surgeon feels that the lesion has a high probability of becoming persistently symptomatic, the index operation to procure the cartilage can be performed in the acute setting. This may be considered in larger-sized defects in a younger, more active patient.

The index biopsy procedure can be done quickly in the acute setting with the goal of minimizing morbidity, and performing the biopsy in the appropriate setting can avoid an additional biopsy procedure in the future. Cartilage is often procured from the lateral side of the intercondylar notch using curettes, and the specimen is sent to the Genzyme Corporation (Cambridge, MA) where the cells are isolated, cultured, and expanded in vitro for use in the second procedure (Fig. 23.6).

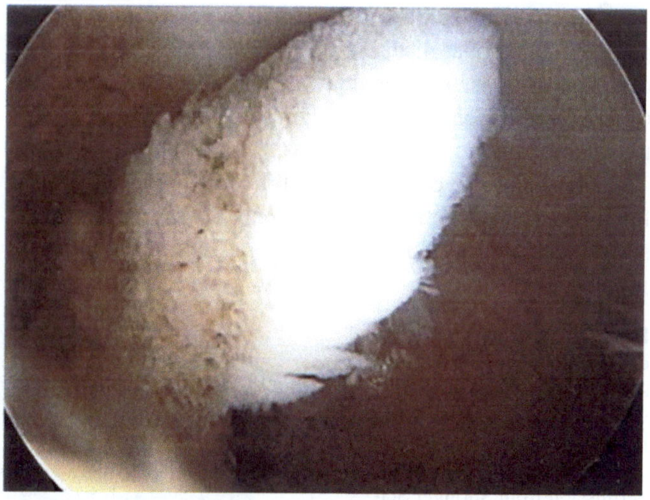

Fig. 23.6 Cartilage biopsy may be obtained at the index procedure if the surgeon feels it may be a future option. (With kind permission from Springer Science+Business Media: The Multiple Ligament Injured Knee [31])

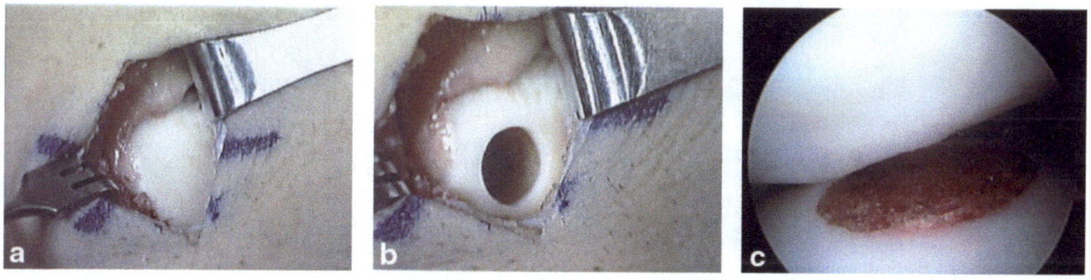

Fig. 23.5 **a** and **b** Superior lateral trochlea visualized thru mini-arthrotomy to harvest OAT donor plug. **c** Donor site (which was backfilled) does articulate under patella. *OAT* osteochondral autograft transfer. (With kind permission from Springer Science+Business Media: The Multiple Ligament Injured Knee [31])

Secondary Treatment for Symptomatic Articular Cartilage Lesions Associated with a PCL Injury

Similar to other articular cartilage treatment algorithms, patient and lesion factors need to be carefully considered when selecting the most appropriate articular cartilage treatment option in the setting of a persistently symptomatic lesion [81, 82]. Patient age, lesion size and location, activity level, and mechanical environment of the involved compartment(s) are factors, which will influence the treatment for these patients [28, 32, 83]. Due to the complexity of many of these patients, it can sometimes be quite difficult to assess the contribution of symptoms resulting from the chondral pathology versus the sequela of the overall joint trauma and altered kinematics, which likely significantly affects the articular cartilage. It is very important, not only in this group but also when treating all patients with articular cartilage pathology with a non-arthroplasty biologic procedure, for the patient and surgeon to have realistic outcome expectations. The goal in the younger patient populations is to significantly improve symptoms and postpone the need for an arthroplasty. However, many of these patients will still have a component of pain and functional disability [28, 32, 61, 83]. Middle-aged or certainly older patients may better be served with non-operative treatment until their symptoms warrant an arthroplasty procedure.

Following recovery from initial treatment including prior ligament reconstruction, patients can be thoughtfully assessed in the office. In addition to an assessment of current complaints, a careful physical exam is essential to ascertain if the patient's complaints and exam correlate to the chondral injury in question. Prior operative reports and arthroscopic pictures are very valuable as well. MRI with cartilage sequences may or may not be helpful depending on the time interval from the initial surgery and the clarity of the problem. Long-alignment films may be required if malalignment is suspected in the involved compartment. Diagnostic intra-articular injections are sometimes useful to differentiate between intra-articular and extra-articular sources of pain in the complicated patient. Unloader braces are occasionally utilized to assist in differentiating pain emanating from the medial tibiofemoral compartment versus other potential etiologies such as pain radiating from the patellofemoral compartment.

The following section of the chapter discusses potential options for the treatment of persistently symptomatic defects associated with a previous PCL or multiligament-injured knee. Special considerations for treatment of symptomatic chondral lesions in this patient population are highlighted in Fig. 23.7. This assumes that malalignment will be concomitantly corrected or was previously corrected. The more diffuse the chondrosis in the involved compartment, the more likely the author favors correcting the malalignment through an unloading osteotomy only. The more focal the defect, the more we tend to favor unloading the compartment and resurfacing the lesion at the same setting. If meniscal deficiency is thought to be a contributing factor, this should also be addressed at the same setting of the chondral resurfacing [84].

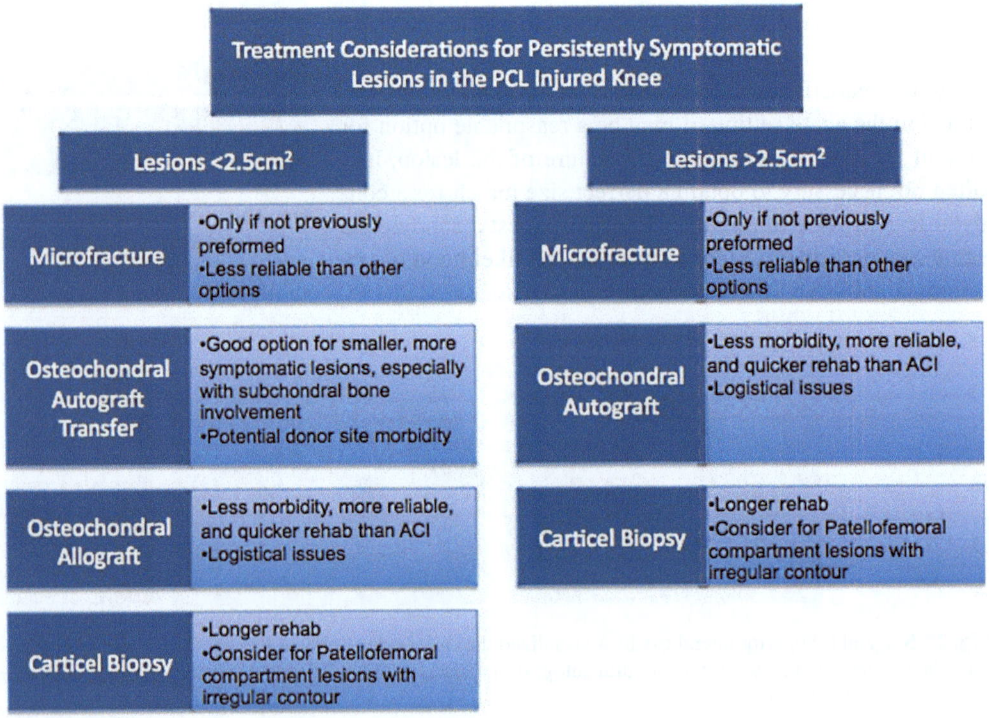

Fig. 23.7 Treatment options and considerations for persistently symptomatic lesions associated with the PCL or multiligament-injured knee. *PCL* posterior cruciate ligament (With kind permission from Springer Science+Business Media: The Multiple Ligament Injured Knee [31])

The younger the patient, the more aggressive we tend to be with biologic alternatives. The opposite is true with individuals who are older and more sedentary or if their pathology is beyond the scope of what can be reasonably addressed with a biologic approach. Unfortunately, many of these patients may be quite young for an arthroplasty, but it still may be their most reliable option when their symptoms justify further intervention.

Microfracture

Microfracture may be considered a viable treatment alternative if the lesion was initially untreated or simply debrided. The results of microfracture are generally considered to be worse with larger defects and patellofemoral lesions, especially in individuals over the age of 35 years. Also, the rate of return to sports when a symptomatic defect is treated may not be as high as with alternative treatment options [41, 58, 85, 86]. In the setting of an individual who has persistent symptoms, thought to be localized to a chondral lesion, in a previous isolated PCL injured or multiligament-injured knee, we tend to opt for other resurfacing alternatives, which may be more reliable or durable. However, microfracture is certainly a reasonable option for certain lesions previously untreated.

Osteochondral Autograft Transfer

OAT procedures have been used with success in the treatment of select chondral defects as outlined previously in this chapter. Advantages include the ability to resurface a defect with autologous viable hyaline cartilage utilizing locally available osteochondral grafts. The dowel grafts are press-fit and heal relatively quickly due to autologous bone-to-bone healing. Recent studies reveal osteochondral autograft transfer outcomes, may be favorable in comparison to microfracture in the athletic population [41, 42, 87]. At 10-year follow up evaluating symptomatic defects in athletes, patients treated with an OAT procedure had better knee scores, lower number of failures, and a lower rate of osteoarthritis development compared to those treated with microfracture. Furthermore, these patients treated with an OAT procedure had a higher rate of return to sports at their pre-injury level and maintained that level of activity longer than the microfracture group [87]. Disadvantages include the potential for donor-site morbidity and limitations on the size and number of grafts available. Typically, this is an option for lesions less than 2.5 cm^2.

Fresh Osteochondral Allografts

Fresh osteochondral allografts have a fairly extensive clinical history, extending over three decades [88–94]. Allograft transplantation is currently gaining in popularity due to increasing appreciation that it reliably restores viable hyaline cartilage with normal architecture when compared to alternative treatment options for larger defects [94, 95]. Although there are logistic issues associated with obtaining allografts, including waiting for an appropriate graft, the procedure itself is not very technically demanding in most cases. The technique can be accomplished with commercially available instrumentation systems versus preparation of a customized "shell" graft (Fig. 23.8). The technical aspects of the procedure have been well described elsewhere and will not

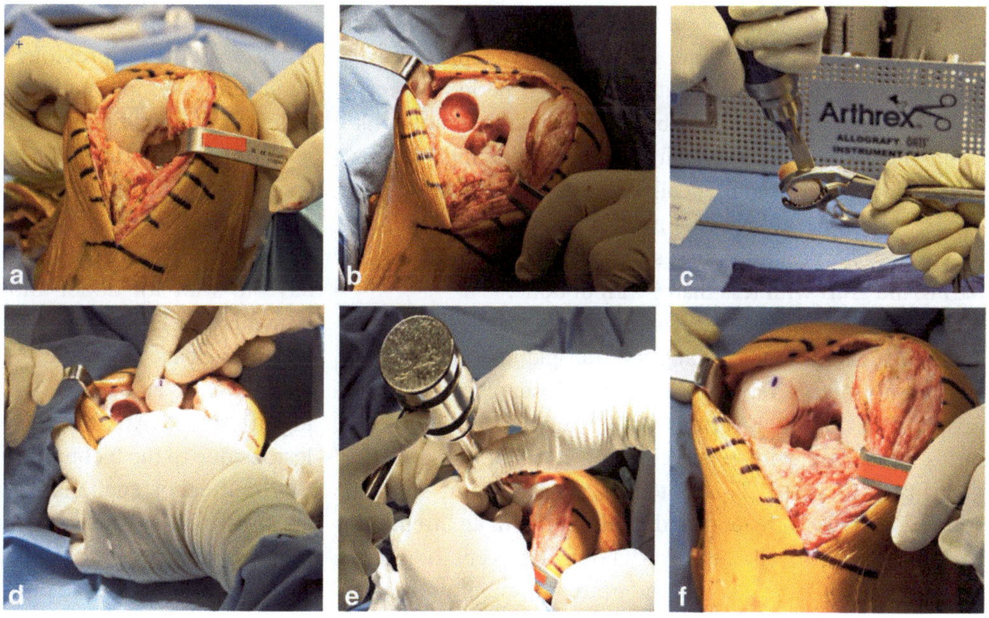

Fig. 23.8 **a** Large chondral lesion of the medial femoral condyle treated with a microfracture at the initial ligament reconstruction. The patient had persistent symptoms medial despite a stable knee. The lesion was revised to a fresh osteochondral allograft. **b** Medial femoral condyle following preparation of recipient site. **c** and **d** Preparation of fresh osteochondral allograft. **e** Gentle impaction of the allograft. **f** Fresh osteochondral allograft seated within the recipient site. (With kind permission from Springer Science+Business Media: The Multiple Ligament Injured Knee [31])

be described here [95]. Fresh allografts are most useful in treating larger chondral or osteochondral lesions (>2.5 cm^2), but can also be utilized for smaller defects in some cases. This is especially appealing in a multiligament-injured knee.

The long-term success of osteochondral allografts is dependent upon preservation of the hyaline cartilage surface, healing of the osseous base to the host bone, and maintenance of structural integrity during the remodeling process [94, 96]. Investigators have shown that chondrocyte viability is paramount in order to maintain the normal extracellular architecture of hyaline cartilage and to prevent the development of degenerative joint disease, but the acceptable degree of chondrocyte viability required is unknown at this time [97, 98]. Although nonviable cartilage will appear grossly normal for a period of time, it will not maintain its histologic, biochemical, or biomechanical properties. As a result, the cartilage will fibrillate, develop clefts, and erode over time [97, 98]. It is important to note that current "fresh" allografts are actually refrigerated for a period of time prior to implantation, in contrast to historical fresh allografts, which were transplanted much closer to time of procurement [99].

Immune compatibility testing and postoperative immunosuppression are not required with osteochondral allograft transplantation despite the fact that chondrocytes and subchondral bone have both been shown to have immunogenic potential [100–103]. Chondrocytes are surrounded by a matrix that isolates them from the host immune cells and makes them relatively "immunologically privileged" [90, 91]. Although donor cells within the osseous component are immunogenic, their immunogenicity is muted and probably not clinically significant in most patients [104, 105]. However, the surgical trauma and the graft itself stimulate a local inflammatory response [106]. This response is primarily directed against the bone constituent of the graft that contains the marrow elements and other immunogenic elements [107]. In general, the osseous component of osteochondral allografts retains its structural integrity and is replaced with host bone via creeping substitution over a period of years [108–111]. If the nonviable bone trabeculae cannot withstand mechanical stresses during the remodeling process, subchondral microfracture, collapse, and fragmentation may occur [94]. Unless there is a need to restore deficient subchondral bone, currently most surgeons have evolved to preparing the graft with less than 6 mm of bone.

Long-term chondrocyte viability and clinical success following osteochondral allograft transplantation has been shown in multiple reports [112–116]. Researchers have biopsied transplants at various time intervals following the index procedure with relatively high rates of chondrocyte viability [113, 116]. This potential for long-term survival supports the use of osteochondral allografts in an attempt to maintain the extracellular matrix and thus prevent long-term articular degeneration within the graft. Although no reports have focused on the PCL or multiligament patient, multiple authors have published on the outcomes of osteochondral allografts in younger patient populations with relatively good success, and a high percentage of patients may be able to return to sport at their pre-injury level, especially in patients <25 years of age with symptoms lasting less than 1 year [95, 110, 111, 113, 115, 117]. New conflicting data, however, suggest that allografts, similar to other treatment options in this often challenging group, are often not successful in getting patients back to their pre-injury level, especially in a population with physically demanding occupations. In a 2013 study looking at active duty military personnel, 42 % of patients were unable to return to active duty following allograft transplantation, and only 5.3 % of patients were able to return to their pre-injury level [118]. Failures do occur with this technique and may increase with follow-up intervals as with any resurfacing procedure. Failures tend to be more related to the osseous component than the cartilage component and may include fragmentation and collapse [94]. Nonunion has not been a significant clinical problem especially with the dowel graft technique. Failure in this difficult patient population can often be the result of progressive overall joint degeneration and not specifically related to graft failure.

There are significant advantages and disadvantages to the use of allograft tissue. Advantages include the lack of donor-site morbidity, the ability to treat large defects including associated subchondral bone deficiency or pathology, and the ability to reliably restore viable hyaline cartilage when compared to alternative treatment options. Disadvantages include the potential for disease transmission, difficulty in attaining a graft, slower healing and incorporation relative to an autograft, and the risk of graft fracture or collapse [94].

Autologous Chondrocyte Implantation

As discussed in a previous section, ACI is an option for a persistently symptomatic lesion that may or may not have failed prior treatment. ACI versus osteochondral allografts may be better choices for larger symptomatic lesions when compared with microfracture or autologous osteochondral transfer. One advantage of ACI over allograft transplantation is availability and surgical scheduling. The patient does not have to wait for donor-allograft availability. Also, disease transmission is obviously not a concern for autologous tissue. In the case of failure, ACI also does not convert a chondral lesion to an osteochondral defect as may occur with allograft failure. ACI may be more optimal for patellofemoral lesions due to the technical difficulty associated with placing a cylindrical osteochondral allograft at these sites. However, approval for isolated patellar lesions can be an issue since ACI was approved by Food and Drug Administration (FDA) for the femoral condyle only [119].

ACI is not without limitation, challenges, and controversy. First, the procedure can be technically difficult at times. Also, the added morbidity of the arthrotomy and periosteal patch harvest (if used) along with the cost of procuring and culturing the cells should be considered. Patients must also be aware and comply with the lengthy rehabilitation period required for this procedure to be effective. The technical difficulty, cost, and some studies questioning whether the ultimate outcome and repair tissue justify these issues are what seem to limit its current use by many surgeons [43, 120]. Still, others advocate that it can more reliably generate higher-quality tissue fill with greater longer-term durability [121, 122].

Increasing evidence supports the use of ACI for the treatment of chondral lesions, and good results have been shown in single-site and multicenter studies [51, 61, 119, 123–127]. Most patients tend to be satisfied following ACI and report reduced pain and improved function [127]. The durability of the procedure is impressive with a survivorship of 71 % after 10 years in a recent review [62]. Younger patients with smaller defects and a shorter duration of symptoms tend to have better results following the procedure [128]. Return to pre-injury function levels, however, should not be expected. This risk of graft failure may be increased with a prior marrow stimulation procedure as well as with very large lesions, which clearly have a worse prognosis [62, 127].

When compared with microfracture, ACI may achieve superior defect fill, especially in larger lesions (Fig. 23.9) [51]. ACI also may produce more durable repair tissue [61, 129]. While some studies suggest that ACI may be better than microfracture, this is certainly controversial and some studies have suggested that this may not be valid [130, 131]. A Cochrane review published in 2010 reported that there was not enough evidence to support the use of ACI over other interventions [131]. A randomized control trial comparing ACI to microfracture showed the two groups had no significant difference in clinical or radiographic results at 5 years, and both groups had a similar rate of failure and development of osteoarthritis [43]. Further complicating the literature, a recent systematic review on articular cartilage surgeries showed the methodologic quality of the studies were poor overall, and while ACI was the most commonly studied technique, only 34 % of these studies denied financial conflicts of interests [132].

Unloading Osteotomies in Articular Cartilage Resurfacing

One would be remiss to discuss the treatment of articular cartilage resurfacing in younger individuals without discussing the role of an unloading osteotomy. Historically, most osteotomies were performed to unload weight-bearing forces from an advanced arthritic compartment to a healthy compartment without performing an "articular cartilage resurfacing" procedure. Currently, altering the biomechanical forces of the joint in the setting of a symptomatic focal defect and malalignment is felt to be important for the long-term success of the resurfacing procedure [36, 133].Debate remains as to the degree of clinical improvement that can be attributed to the unloading osteotomy versus the cartilage resurfacing with these combination cases.

PCL deficiency, which is not corrected, has known consequences to the medial and patellofemoral compartments of the knee. Clearly optimizing joint kinematics back to as close as normal thru PCL reconstruction, when indicated, is more optimal than an unloading osteotomy if the degeneration is not advanced. High tibial osteotomy can be done to unload the medial compartment, while tibial tubercle osteotomy via anteriorization (anteriormedial or straight anterior) can be performed to address the patellofemoral compartment (Fig. 23.10). Unloading both compartments can certainly

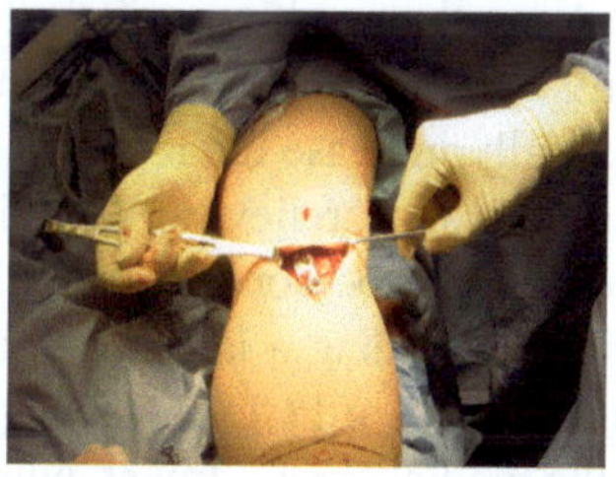

Fig. 23.10 High tibial osteotomy performed in conjunction to OAT of the medial femoral condyle. *OAT* osteochondral autograft transfer

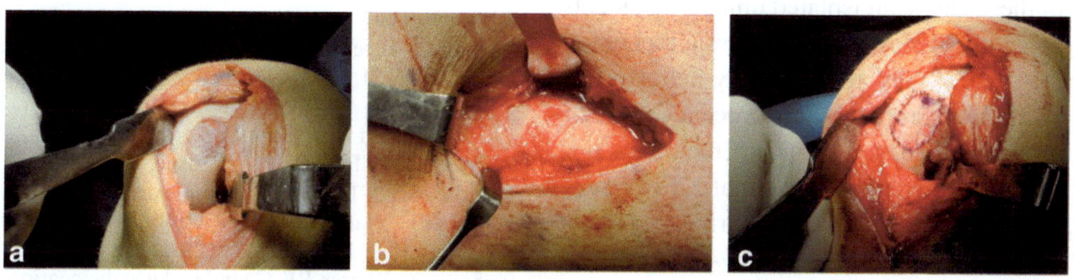

Fig. 23.9 **a** Treatment of a large chondral lesion of the medial femoral condyle with autologous chondrocyte implantation. **b** Periosteum patch harvest site. **c** Periosteal patch sutured onto the defect (just prior to injection of the cells). (With kind permission from Springer Science+Business Media: The Multiple Ligament Injured Knee [31])

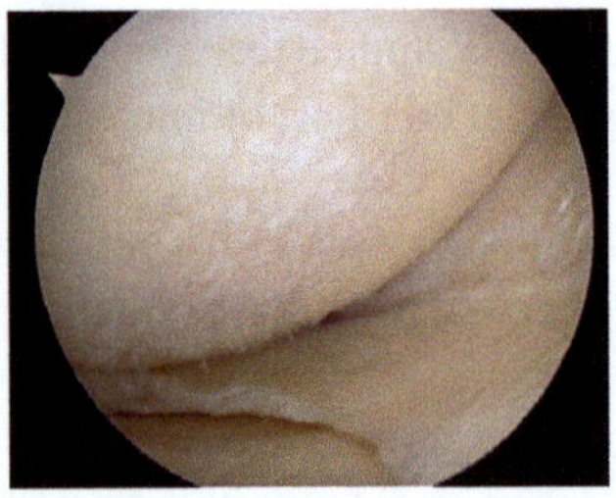

Fig. 23.11 Middle-aged patient with slowly progressive diffuse chondrosis of the medial femoral condyle treated nonoperatively for 10 years following PCL injury. *PCL* posterior cruciate ligament

be considered if indicated; however, this is relatively rare in our experience. Depending on the age of the patient, degree of articular cartilage involvement, and complexity of the overall knee pathology, clearly it may be in the patient's best interest to avoid an osteotomy altogether and to pursue nonoperative or less aggressive measures until they are ready for an arthroplasty procedure (Fig. 23.11).

Patients with a symptomatic articular cartilage defect of the medial femoral condyle as well as a mechanical axis that is medial to the neutral zone (bordered by the tibial spines) should be strongly considered for corrective osteotomy as part of their cartilage restoration treatment [123]. Clearly, the greater the malalignment, the greater the chance of failure of any isolated resurfacing procedure. High tibial osteotomy done in conjunction with a cartilage resurfacing procedure is generally a more limited correction than a traditional unloading osteotomy used to treat diffuse degenerative arthrosis. The goal in most cases is to place the mechanical axis to neutral as opposed to an osteotomy for bipolar arthrosis, which typically places the resulting axis further into the lateral compartment. Additionally, in the setting of PCL laxity, you can potentially increase the resultant posterior tibial slope, which may assist in relieving instability symptoms (the reverse of which can be done for ACL laxity). We are hesitant to consider unloading a lateral defect (distal femoral osteotomy) in the face of PCL deficiency since this will increase load to the medial compartment, which is already at risk of articular contact stress overload.

Patients who develop more diffuse bipolar cartilage degeneration are not optimal candidates for cartilage restoration procedures. In these cases, an isolated unloading osteotomy with an alignment goal similar to the classic technique may be more appropriate if they are not likely better off in the longer term with an arthroplasty. In a recent report of multiligament injuries in athletes, 8 % of the 26 patients underwent an osteotomy by 8 years for symptomatic diffuse degenerative changes. Arthritis and not focal cartilage defects was the clinical issue in this group at follow-up. Unfortunately, this is often the outcome in the multiligament-injured knee. Physicians who treat cartilage lesions should be comfortable with performing osteotomies but at the same time respect their added morbidity and potential complications [77, 134]. Sometimes, despite our drive to avoid arthroplasty in younger individuals for obvious reasons, they may be better served for a longer period of time when a well-performed arthroplasty can be performed with a reliable result.

Future Technologies

Articular cartilage repair is evolving, and new technologies are being explored to increase the treatment options available to surgeons and patients. Some of these new techniques include: next-generation ACI, implantation of particulated autograft or allograft articular cartilage, stem cell therapies, and methods to optimize or augment current marrow-stimulating techniques. These and other technologies are in various investigational stages, and further research will determine which will prove to be more efficacious than conventional options. Optimism surrounding novel technologies must be tempered by the reality that the treatment of articular cartilage defects has been a much more formidable task than perhaps appreciated 20 years ago. As a result of understandable FDA challenges and difficulty in proving superiority of biologic resurfacing options in heterogeneous patient populations, the development of novel treatment options may be more arduous than perhaps appreciated by some. As new techniques are evaluated and potentially become available, treatment algorithms will continue to evolve over time for this challenging patient population.

References

1. Fanelli GC, Edson CJ. Posterior cruciate ligament injuries in trauma patients: part II. Arthroscopy. 1995 Oct;11(5):526–9.
2. Casteleyn PP, Handelberg F, Opdecam P. Traumatic haemarthrosis of the knee. J Bone Joint Surg Br. 1988 May;70(3):404–6.
3. Werner BC, Gwathmey FW Jr, Higgins ST, Hart JM, Miller MD. Ultra-low velocity knee dislocations: patient characteristics, complications, and outcomes. Am J Sports Med. 2014 Feb;42(2): 358–63.
4. Hirschman M, Iranpour F, Muller W, Friederich N. Surgical treatment of complex bicruciate knee ligament injuries in athletes; what long-term outcome can we expect? Am J Sports Med. 2010;Jun;38(6):1103–9.
5. Fanelli GC, Orcutt DR, Edson CJ. The multiple-ligament injured knee: evaluation, treatment and results. Arthroscopy. 2005;Apr;21(4):471–86.
6. Fanelli GC. A practical guide to management. The multiple ligament injured knee. New York: Springer; 2004.
7. Fanelli GC, Edson CJ. Arthroscopically assisted ACL/PCL reconstruction: 2–10 year follow-up. Arthroscopy. 2002;18(7):703–14.
8. Cole BJ, Harner CD. The multiple ligament injured knee. Clin Sports Med. 1999;18:241–62.
9. Sisto DJ, Warren RF. Complete knee dislocation; a follow-up study of operative treatment. Clin Orthop. 1985;198:94–101.
10. Ibrahim SA, Ahmad FH, Salah M, et al. Surgical management of traumatic knee dislocation. Arthroscopy. 2008;24(2):178–87.

11. Chhabra A, Cha PS, Rihn JA, et al. Surgical management of knee dislocations. Surgical technique. J Bone Joint Surg Am. 2005;87(Suppl. 1):1–21.
12. Fowler PJ, Messieh SS. Isolated posterior cruciate ligament injuries in athletes. Am J Sports Med 1987;15:553–7.
13. Geissler WB, Whipple TL. Intraarticular abnormalities in association with posterior cruciate ligament injuries. Am Sports Med 1993;21:846–9.
14. Hamada M, Shino K, Mitsuoka T, Toritsuka Y, Natsu-Ume T, Horibe S. Chondral injury associated with acute isolated posterior cruciate ligament injury. Arthroscopy. 2000 Jan–Feb;16(1):59–63
15. Kaeding CC, Pderoza AD, Parker RD, et al. Intra-articular findings in the reconstructed multiligament-injured knee. Arthroscopy. 2005;21(4):424–30.
16. Granan LP, Bahr R, Lie SA, et al. Timing of anterior cruciate ligament reconstructive surgery and risk of cartilage lesions and meniscal tears: a cohort study based on the Norwegian national knee ligament registry. Am J Sports Med. 2009;37(5):955–61.
17. Slauterbeck JR, Kousa P, Clifton BC, et al. Geographic mapping of meniscus and cartilage lesions associated with anterior cruciate ligament injuries. J Bone Joint Surg Am. 2009;91(9):2094–103.
18. Corten K, Bellemans J. Cartilage damage determines intermediate outcome in the late multiple ligament and posterolateral corner-reconstructed knee: a 5- to 10-year follow-up study. Am J Sports Med. 2008;36(2):267–75.
19. Goyal K, Tashman S, Wang JH, Li K, Zhang X, Harner C. In vivo analysis of the isolated posterior cruciate ligament-deficient knee during functional activities. Am J Sports Med. 2012 Apr;40(4):777–85.
20. MacDonald P, Miniaci A, Fowler P, Marks P, Finlay B. A biomechanical analysis of joint contact forces in the posterior cruciate deficient knee. Knee Surg Sports Traumatol Arthrosc 1996;3: 252–5.
21. Skyhar MJ, Warren RF, Ortiz GJ, Schwartz E, Otis JC. The effects of sectioning of the posterior cruciate ligament and the posterolateral complex on the articular contact pressures within the knee. J Bone Joint Surg Am. 1993 May;75(5):694–9.
22. Van de Velde SK, Bingham JT, Gill TJ, Li G. Analysis of tibiofemoral cartilage deformation in the posterior cruciate ligament-deficient knee. J Bone Joint Surg Am. 2009 Jan;91(1):167–75.
23. Strobel MJ, Weiler A, Schulz MS, Russe K, Eichhorn HJ. Arthroscopic evaluation of articular cartilage lesions in posterior-cruciate-ligament-deficient knees. Arthroscopy. 2003 Mar;19(3):262–8.
24. Shelbourne KD, Gray JS. Outcome of untreated traumatic articular cartilage defects of the knee: a natural history study. J Bone Joint Surg Am. 2003;85-A(Suppl. 2):8–16.
25. Bowers AL, Spindler KP, McCarty EC, et al. Height, weight, and BMI predict intra-articular injuries observed during ACL reconstruction: evaluation of 456 cases from a prospective ACL database. Clin J Sports Med. 2005;15(1):9–13.
26. Hart JM, Blanchard BF, Hart JA, et al. Multiple ligament reconstruction clinical follow-up and gait analysis. Knee Surg Sports Traumatol Arthrosc. 2009;17(3):277–85.
27. Nelson F, Billinghurst RC, Pidoux I, et al. Early post-traumatic osteoarthritis-like changes in human articular cartilage following rupture of the anterior cruciate ligament. Osteoarthr Cartil. 2006;14(2):114–9.
28. Safran MR, Seiber K. The evidence for surgical repair of articular cartilage in the knee. J Am Acad Orthop Surg. 2010;18(5): 259–66.
29. Osti L, Papalia R, DelBuono A, et al. Good results five years after surgical management of anterior cruciate ligament tears, and meniscal and cartilage injuries. Knee Surg Sports Traumatol Arthrosc. 2010;18(10):1385–90.
30. Magnussen RA, Mansour AA, Carey JL, Spindler KP. Meniscus status at anterior cruciate ligament reconstruction associated with radiographic signs of osteoarthritis at 5- to 10-year follow-up: a systemic review. J Knee Surg. 2009;22(4):347–57.
31. Bonner KF, Noel C. Articular cartilage restoration. In: Fanelli G, editor. The multiple ligament injured knee, a practical guide to management. 2nd ed. Philadelphia: Springer; 2013 (Chapter 28).
32. Clancy WG Jr, Shelbourne KD, Zoellner GB, Keene JS, Reider B, Rosenberg TD. Treatment of knee joint instability secondary to rupture of the posterior cruciate ligament. Report of a new procedure. J Bone Joint Surg Am. 1983 Mar;65(3):310–22.
33. Patel DV, Allen AA, Warren RF, Wickiewicz TL, Simonian PT. The nonoperative treatment of acute, isolated (partial or complete) posterior cruciate ligament-deficient knees: an intermediate-term follow-up study. HSS J. 2007 Sep;3(2):137–46.
34. Shino K, Horibe S, Nakata K, Maeda A, Hamada M, Nakamura N. Conservative treatment of isolated injuries to the posterior cruciate ligament in athletes. J Bone Joint Surg Br. 1995 Nov;77(6):895–900.
35. Fanelli GC, Stannard JP, Stuart MJ, et al. Management of complex knee ligament injuries. J Bone Joint Surg. 2010;92A:2235–46.
36. Widuchowski W, Widuchowski J, Koczy B, et al. Untreated asymptomatic deep cartilage lesions associated with anterior cruciate ligament injury: results at 10- and 15-year follow-up. Am J Sports Med. 2009;37:688–92.
37. Aron A, Loken S, Heir S, et al. Articular cartilage lesions in 993 consecutive knee arthroscopies. Am J Sports Med. 2004;32(1):211–5.
38. Hanypsiak BT, Spindler KP, Rothrock CR, et al. Twelve-year follow-up on anterior cruciate ligament reconstruction: long-term outcomes of prospectively studied osseous and articular injuries. Am J Sports Med. 2008;36(4):671–7.
39. Brophy RH, Zeltser D, Wright RW, et al. Anterior cruciate ligament reconstruction and concomitant articular cartilage injury: incidence and treatment. Arthroscopy. 2010;26(1):112–20.
40. Loken S, Heir S, Holme I, et al. 6-Year follow-up of 84 patients with cartilage defects in the knee. Knee scores improved but recovery was incomplete. Acta Orthop. 2010;81(5):611–8.
41. Gudas R, Gudaitė A, Mickevičius T, Masiulis N, Simonaitytė R, Cekanauskas E, Skurvydas A. Comparison of osteochondral autologous transplantation, microfracture, or debridement techniques in articular cartilage lesions associated with anterior cruciate ligament injury: a prospective study with a 3-year follow-up. Arthroscopy. 2013;29(1):89–97
42. Gudas R, Kalesinskas RJ, Kimtys V, Stankevicius E, Toliusis V, Bernotavicius G, Smailys A. A prospective randomized clinical study of mosaic osteochondral autologous transplantation versus microfracture for the treatment of osteochondral defects in the knee joint in young athletes. Arthroscopy. 2005 Sep;21(9):1066–75.
43. Knutsen G, Drogset JO, Engebretsen L, Grøntvedt T, Isaksen V, Ludvigsen TC, Roberts S, Solheim E, Strand T, Johansen O. A randomized trial comparing autologous chondrocyte implantation with microfracture. Findings at five years. J Bone Joint Surg Am. 2007 Oct;89(10):2105–12.
44. Gobbi A, Karnatzikos G, Kumar A. Long-term results after microfracture treatment for full-thickness knee chondral lesions in athletes. Knee Surg Sports Traumatol Arthrosc. 2013 Sep 20;22:1986–8.
45. Goyal D, Keyhani S, Lee EH, Hui JH. Evidence-based status of microfracture technique: a systematic review of level I and II studies. Arthroscopy. 2013 Sep;29(9):1579–88.
46. Bae DK, Song SJ, Yoon KH, Heo DB, Kim TJ. Survival analysis of microfracture in the osteoarthritic knee-minimum 10-year follow-up. Arthroscopy. 2013 Feb;29(2):244–50.
47. Spahn G, Kahl E, Muckley T, et al. Arthroscopic knee chondroplasty using a bipolar radiofrequency-based device compared to mechanical shaver: results of a prospective, randomized, controlled study. Knee Surg Sports Traumatol Arthrosc. 2008;16(6):565–73.
48. Bedi A, Feeley BT, Williams 3rd RJ. Management of articular cartilage defects of the knee. J Bone Joint Surg Am. 2010;92:994–1009.

49. Williams 3rd RJ, Harnly HW. Microfracture: indications, technique, and results. Instr Course Lect. 2007;56:419–28.
50. Mithoefer K, Williams RJ, Warren RF, et al. The microfracture technique for the treatment of articular cartilage lesions in the knee. A prospective cohort study. J Bone Joint Surg Am. 2005;87(9):1911–20.
51. Brown WE, Potter HG, Marx RG, et al. Magnetic resonance imaging appearance of cartilage repair in the knee. Clin Orthop Relat Res. 2004;422:214–23.
52. Ramappa AJ, Gill TJ, Bradford CH, et al. Magnetic resonance imaging to assess knee cartilage repair tissue after microfracture of chondral defects. J Knee Surg. 2007;20(3):228–34.
53. Blackman AJ, Smith MV, Flanigan DC, Matava MJ, Wright RW, Brophy RH. Correlation between magnetic resonance imaging and clinical outcomes after cartilage repair surgery in the knee: a systematic review and meta-analysis. Am J Sports Med. 2013 Jun;41(6):1426–34.
54. Kreuz PC, Steinwachs MR, Erggelet C, Krause SJ, Konrad G, Uhl M, Südkamp N. Results after microfracture of full-thickness chondral defects in different compartments in the knee. Osteoarthr Cartil. 2006 Nov;14(11):1119–25.
55. Mithoefer K, McAdam T, Williams RJ, et al. Clinical efficacy of the microfracture technique for articular cartilage repair in the knee; an evidence-based systematic analysis. Am J Sports Med. 2009;37:2053–63.
56. Steadman JR, Briggs KK, Rodrigo JJ, et al. Outcomes of microfracture for traumatic chondral lesions of the knee; average 11-year follow-up. Arthroscopy. 2003;19(5):477–84.
57. Asik M, Ciftci F, Sen C, et al. The microfracture technique for the treatment of full-thickness articular cartilage lesions of the knee: midterm results. Arthroscopy. 2008;24:1214–20.
58. Gobbi A, Nunag P, Malinowski K. Treatment of full thickness chondral lesions of the knee with microfracture in a group of athletes. Knee Surg Sports Traumatol Arthrosc. 2005;13(3):213–21.
59. Mithoefer K, Williams RJ, Warren RF, et al. High-impact athletics after knee articular cartilage repair; a prospective evaluation of the microfracture technique. Am J Sports Med. 2006;34(9):1413–8.
60. Minas T, Gomoll AH, Rosenberger R, et al. Increased failure rate of autologous chondrocyte implantation after previous treatment with marrow stimulation techniques. Am J Sports Med. 2009;37(5):902–8.
61. Zaslav K, Cole B, Brewster R, et al. A prospective study of autologous chondrocyte implantation in patients with failed prior treatment for articular cartilage defect of the knee. Am J Sports Med. 2009;37:42–55.
62. Minas T, Von Keudell A, Bryant T, Gomoll AH. The John Insall Award: a minimum 10-year outcome study of autologous chondrocyte implantation. Clin Orthop Relat Res. 2014 Jan;472(1):41–51.
63. Levin AS, Angel M, Sgaglione NA. Chapter 10, introduction to osteochondral autograft transplantation. In: Cole BJ, Gomoll AH, editors. Biologic joint reconstruction. Thorofare: Slack Inc; 2008. pp. 93–105.
64. Brown OL, Morgan CD, Leitman EH. Chapter 12, osteochondral autograft transfer. In: Cole BJ, Gomoll AH, editors. Biologic joint reconstruction.Thorofare: Slack Inc; 2008. pp. 119–27.
65. Marcacci M, Kon E, Delcogliano M, et al. Arthroscopic autologous osteochondral grafting for cartilage defects of the knee: prospective study results at a minimum 7-year follow-up. Am J Sports Med. 2007;35(12):2014–21.
66. Hangody L, Kish G, Kárpáti Z, Udvarhelyi I, Szigeti I, Bély M. Mosaicplasty for the treatment of articular cartilage defects: application in clinical practice. Orthopedics. 1998 Jul;21(7):751–6.
67. Hangody L, Vásárhelyi G, Hangody LR, Sükösd Z, Tibay G, Bartha L, Bodó G. Autologous osteochondral grafting—technique and long-term results. Injury. 2008 Apr;39(Suppl. 1):S32–9.
68. Keennedy JG, Murawski CD. The treatment of osteochondral lesions of the talus with autologous osteochondral transplantation and bone marrow aspirate concentrate: surgical technique. Cartilage. 2011;2(4):327–36.
69. Gautier E, Kolker D, Jakob RP. Treatment of cartilage defects of the talus by autologous osteochondral grafts. J Bone Joint Surg Br. 2002 Mar;84(2):237–44.
70. Gobbi A, Francisco RA, Lubowitz JH, Allegra F, Canata G. Osteochondral lesions of the talus: randomized controlled trial comparing chondroplasty, microfracture, and osteochondral autograft transplantation. Arthroscopy. 2006 Oct;22(10):1085–92.
71. Assenmacher JA, Kelikian AS, Gottlob C, Kodros S. Arthroscopically assisted autologous osteochondral transplantation for osteochondral lesions of the talar dome: an MRI and clinical follow-up study. Foot Ankle Int. 2001 Jul;22(7):544–51.
72. Kim YS, Park EH, Lee HJ, Koh YG, Lee JW. Clinical comparison of the osteochondral autograft transfer system and subchondral drilling in osteochondral defects of the first metatarsal head. Am J Sports Med. 2012 Aug;40(8):1824–33.
73. Kim YS, Park EH, Kim YC, Koh YG, Lee JW. Factors associated with the clinical outcomes of the osteochondral autograft transfer system in osteochondral lesions of the talus: second-look arthroscopic evaluation. Am J Sports Med. 2012 Dec;40(12):2709–19.
74. Valderrabano V, Leumann A, Rasch H, et al. Knee-to-ankle mosaicplasty for the treatment of osteochondral lesions of the ankle joint. Am J Sports Med. 2009;37(Suppl. 1):S105–11.
75. Reddy S, Pedowitz DI, Parekh SG, Sennett BJ, Okereke E. The morbidity associated with osteochondral harvest from asymptomatic knees for the treatment of osteochondral lesions of the talus. Am J Sports Med. 2007 Jan;35(1):80–5.
76. Sgaglione NA, Florence AS. Bone graft substitute failure with giant cell reaction in the treatment of osteochondral lesions of the distal femur:a report of 2 cases with operative revision. Arthroscopy. 2009;25(7):815–9.
77. Fowler 3rd DE, Hart JM, Hart JA, Miller MD. Donor-site giant cell reaction following backfill with synthetic bone material during osteochondral plug transfer. J Knee Surg. 2009;22(4):372–4.
78. Bedi AF, Foo LF, Williams RJ III, Potter HG, The Cartilage Study Group. The maturation of synthetic scaffolds for osteochondral donor sites of the knee: an MRI and T2-mapping analysis. Cartilage. 2010;1(1):20–8.
79. Barber FA, Dockery WD. A computed tomography scan assessment of synthetic multiphase polymer scaffolds used for osteochondral defect repair. Arthroscopy. 2011;27(1):60–4.
80. Brittberg M, Lindahl A, Nilsson A, et al. Treatment of deep cartilage defects in the knee with autologous chondrocyte transplantation. New Engl J Med. 1994;331:889–95.
81. Freedman KB, Fox JA, Cole BJ. Chaper 54 knee cartilage: diagnosis and decision making. In: Miller MD, Cole BJ, editors. Textbook of arthroscopy. Maryland Heights: Saunders-Elsevier; 2004. pp. 555–67.
82. Miller M, Cole BJ. Atlas of chondral injury treatment. Oper Tech Orthop. 2001;11:145–50.
83. Bekkers JE, Inklaar M, Saris DB. Treatment selection in articular cartilage lesions of the knee. Am J Sports Med. 2009;37(Suppl. 1):S148–55.
84. Kent R, Kurtz CA, Bonner KF. Meniscus transplantation. In Williams G, Ramsey M, editors. Operative techniques in orthopaedic surgery. Philadelphia: Lippincott Williams Wilkins; 2009.
85. Harris JD, Brophy RH, Siston RA, et al. Treatment of chondral defects in the athlete's knee. Arthroscopy. 2010;26(6):841–52.
86. Namdari S, Baldwin K, Anakwenze O, et al. Results and performance after microfracture in national basketball association athletes. Am J Sports Med. 2009;37(5):943–8.
87. Gudas R, Gudaite A, Pocius A, Gudiene A, Cekanauskas E, Monastyreckiene E, Basevicius A. Ten-year follow-up of a prospective, randomized clinical study of mosaic osteochondral autologous transplantation versus microfracture for the treatment of osteochondral defects in the knee joint of athletes. Am J Sports Med. 2012 Nov;40(11):2499–508.

88. Aubin PP, Cheah HK, Davis AM, Gross AE. Long-term follow up of fresh femoral osteochondral allografts for posttraumatic knee defects. Clin Orthop. 2001;391S:S318–27.
89. Bugbee WD. Seminars Arthroplasty. 2000;11:1–7.
90. Bugbee WD. Fresh osteochondral allografting. Op Tech Sports Med. 2000;8(2):158–62.
91. Garrett J, Wyman J. The operative technique of fresh osteochondral allografting of the knee. Op Tech Orthop. 2001;11(2):132–7.
92. Lattermann C, Romine SE. Osteochondral allografts: state of the art. Clin Sports Med. 2009;28(2):285–301.
93. Branam BR, Johnson DL. Allografts in knee surgery. Orthopedics. 2007;30(11):925–9.
94. Robinson S, Bonner KF. Osteochondral allograft transplantation chapter. In: Insall JN, Scott WN, editors. Surgery of the knee. 5th ed. Maryland Heights: Saunders-Elsevier (Due for publication 2012).
95. Bonner KF, Bugbee WD. Chaper 60 fresh osteochondral allografts in the knee. In: Miller MD, Cole BJ, editors. Textbook of arthroscopy. Maryland Heights: Saunders-Elsevier; 2004. pp. 611–24.
96. Stevenson S, Dannucci GA, Sharkey NA, Pool RR. The fate of articular cartilage after transplantation of fresh and cryopreserved tissue-antigen-matched and mismatched osteochondral allografts in dogs. J Bone Joint Surg Am. 1989;71:1297–307.
97. Simon WH, Richardson S, Harman W, Parsons JR, Lane J. Long-term effects of chondrocyte death on rabbit cartilage in vivo. J Bone Joint Surg. 1976;58A:517–26.
98. Jackson DW, Halbrecht J, Proctor C, et al. Assessment of donor cell and matrix survival in fresh articular cartilage allografts in a goat model. J Orthop Res. 1996;14(2):255–64.
99. LaPrade RF, Botker J, Herzog M, Agel J. Refrigerated osteoarticular allografts to treat articular cartilage defects of the femoral condyles. A prospective outcomes study. J Bone Joint Surg Am. 2009;91(4):805–11.
100. Langer F, Czitrom A, Prizker KP, Gross AE. The immunogenicity of fresh and frozen allogeneic bone. J Bone Joint Surg Am. 1975;57:216–22.
101. Langer F, Gross AE. Immunogenicity of allograft articular cartilage. J Bone Joint Surg Am. 1974;56:297–304.
102. Langer F, Gross AE, West M, Urovitz EP. The immunogenicity of allograft knee joint transplants. Clin Orthop. 1978;132: 155–62.
103. Phipatanakul WP, VandeVord PJ, Teitge RA, Wooley PH. Immune response in patients receiving fresh osteochondral allografts. Am J Orthop. 2004;33(7):345–8.
104. Bugbee WD, Convery FR. Osteochondral allograft transplantation. Clin Sports Med. 1999;18:67–75.
105. Czitrom AA, Keating S, Gross AE. The viability of articular cartilage in fresh osteochondral allografts after clinical transplantation. J Bone Joint Surg Am. 1990;72:574–81.
106. Stevenson S, Horowitz M. Current concepts review: the response to bone allografts. J Bone Joint Surg. 1992;74A:939–50.
107. Sirlin CB, Brossman J, Boutin RD, et al. Shell osteochondral allografts of the knee: comparison of MR imaging findings and immunological responses. Radiology. 2001;219(1):35–43.
108. Burchardt H. The biology of bone graft repair. Clin Orthop Relat Res. 1983;174:28–42.
109. Furukawa T, Eyre DR, Koide S, Glimcher MJ. Biochemical studies on repair cartilage resurfacing experimental defects in the rabbit knee. J Bone Joint Surg Am. 1980;62:79–89.
110. McDermott AG, Langer F, Pritzker PH, Gross AE. Fresh small-fragment osteochondral allografts-long term follow-up study on first one hundred cases. Clin Orthop. 1985;197:96–102.
111. Oakeshott RD, Farine I, Pritzker KP, et al. A clinical and histologic analysis of failed fresh osteochondral allografts. Clin Orthop.1988;233:283–94.
112. Maury AC, Safir O, Heras FL, Pritzker KP, Gross AE. Twenty-five-year chondrocyte viability in fresh osteochondral allograft: a case report. J Bone Joint Surg Am. 2007;89(1):159–65.
113. Williams SK, Amiel D, Ball ST, et al. Analysis of cartilage tissue on a cellular level in fresh osteochondral allografts retrievals. Am J Sports Med. 2007;35(12):2022–32.
114. Gross AE, Kim W, Las Heras F, et al. Fresh osteochondral allograft for post-traumatic knee defects: long-term follow-up. Clin Orthop Relat Res. 2008;466(8):1863–70.
115. Fitzpatrick PL, Morgan DA. Fresh osteochondral allografts: a 6–10 year review. Aust NZJ Surg. 1998;68(8):573–9.
116. Jamali AA, Hatcher SL, You Z. Donor cell survival in a fresh osteochondral allograft at twenty-nine years. A case report. J Bone Joint Surg Am. 2007;89(1):166–9.
117. Krych AJ, Harnly HW, Rodeo SA, Williams RJ 3rd. Activity levels are higher after osteochondral autograft transfer mosaicplasty than after microfracture for articular cartilage defects of the knee: a retrospective comparative study. J Bone Joint Surg Am. 2012 Jun 6;94(11):971–8.
118. Shaha JS, Cook JB, Rowles DJ, Bottoni CR, Shaha SH, Tokish JM. Return to an athletic lifestyle after osteochondral allograft transplantation of the knee. Am J Sports Med. 2013 Sep;41(9):2083–9.
119. Farr J. Autologous chondrocyte implantation improves patellofemoral cartilage treatment options. Clin Orthop. 2007;463:187–94.
120. Mollon B, Kandel R, Chahal J, Theodoropoulos J. The clinical status of cartilage tissue regeneration in humans. Osteoarthritis Cartilage. 2013 Dec;21(12):1824–33.
121. Vavken P, Samartzis D. Effectiveness of autologous chondrocyte implantation in cartilage repair of the knee: a systematic review of controlled trials. Osteoarthritis Cartilage. 2010 Jun;18(6):857–63.
122. Moseley JB Jr, Anderson AF, Browne JE, Mandelbaum BR, Micheli LJ, Fu F, Erggelet C. Effectiveness of autologous chondrocyte implantation in cartilage repair of the knee: a systematic review of controlled trials. Am J Sports Med. 2010 Feb;38(2):238–46.
123. Gomoll AH, Farr J, Gillogly SD, et al. Surgical management of articular cartilage defects of the knee. J Bone Joint Surg Am. 2010;92(14):2470–90.
124. Knutsen G, Engebretsen L, Ludvigsen TC, et al. Autologous chondrocyte implantation compared with microfracture in the knee. A randomized trial. J Bone Joint Surg Am. 2004;86-A(3):455–64.
125. Saris DB, Vanlauwe J, Victor J, et al. Treatment of symptomatic cartilage defects of the knee; characterized chondrocyte implantation results in better clinical outcome at 36 months in a randomized trial compared to microfracture. Am J Sports Med. 2009;37(Suppl. 1):S10–9.
126. Saris DB, Vanlauwe J, Victor J, et al. Characterized chondrocyte implantation results in better structural repair when treating symptomatic cartilage defects of the knee in a randomized controlled trial versus microfracture. Am J Sports Med. 2008;36(2):235–46.
127. Niemeyer P, Porichis S, Steinwachs M, Erggelet C, Kreuz PC, Schmal H, Uhl M, Ghanem N, Südkamp NP, Salzmann G. Long-term outcomes after first-generation autologous chondrocyte implantation for cartilage defects of the knee. Am J Sports Med. 2014 Jan;42(1):150–7.
128. Moradi B, Schönit E, Nierhoff C, Hagmann S, Oberle D, Gotterbarm T, Schmitt H, Zeifang F. First-generation autologous chondrocyte implantation in patients with cartilage defects of the knee: 7–14 years' clinical and magnetic resonance imaging follow-up evaluation. Arthroscopy. 2012 Dec;28(12):1851–61.
129. Mithoefer K, Hambly K, Della Villa S, et al. Return to sports participation after articular cartilage repair in the knee: scientific evidence. Am J Sports Med. 2009 Nov;37;(Suppl. 1):S167–76.
130. Negrin LL, Vécsei V. Do meta-analyses reveal time-dependent differences between the clinical outcomes achieved by microfracture and autologous chondrocyte implantation in the treatment of cartilage defects of the knee? J Orthop Sci. 2013 Nov;18(6): 940–8.
131. Vasiliadis HS, Wasiak J. Autologous chondrocyte implantation for full thickness articular cartilage defects of the knee. Cochrane Database Syst Rev. 2010 Oct 6;(10):CD003323.

132. Harris JD, Erickson BJ, Abrams GD, Cvetanovich GL, McCormick FM, Gupta AK, Bach BR Jr, Cole BJ. Methodologic quality of knee articular cartilage studies. Arthroscopy. 2013 Jul;29(7):1243–52.
133. Behery O, Siston RA, Harris JD, Flanigan DC. Treatment of cartilage defects of the knee: expanding on the existing algorithm. Clin J Sport Med. 2014 Jan;24(1):21–30.
134. Van Den Bekerom M, Patt TW, Kleinhout MY, et al. Early complications after high tibial osteotomy: a comparison of two techniques. J Knee Surg. 2008;21(1):68–74.

24 Meniscus Transplant in the PCL-Injured Knee

Chad A. Haley, Steven J. Svoboda and Brett D. Owens

History of Meniscal Allograft Transplant

The critical function of the meniscus to help preserve cartilage in the knee was first presented by Fairbanks in 1948 when he described the classic radiographic changes associated with osteoarthritis after complete meniscectomy [1, 2]. Thus, the significance of the meniscus in cartilage protection has influenced the current treatment of meniscal injuries with the primary goal of maintaining meniscal integrity and attempting to preserve maximal meniscal tissue. In select patients with complete meniscectomy and symptoms localized to the affected compartment, meniscal allograft transplantation (MAT) surgery is a viable surgical option.

The concept of meniscus replacement can be dated back to 1916 and 1933 when fat interposition was utilized to substitute for the meniscus [3]. In 1908, the first meniscus-transplant surgery was reported in the literature in the setting of limb salvage via complete knee transplantation [4]. More recently, Locht et al. reported the use of massive proximal tibial osteochondral allografts with meniscus allograft to treat chronic tibial-plateau fractures [5]. The short-term success of MAT was shown in animal studies in the 1980s [6, 7]. The first modern MAT was performed in 1984 [3]. Since then, there have been no randomized controlled trials or long-term outcome studies for the procedure.

C. A. Haley (✉) · S. J. Svoboda
Department of Surgery, Keller Army Community Hospital, Building 900 Washington Road, West Point, NY, USA
e-mail: chad.a.haley.mil@mail.mil

S. J. Svoboda
e-mail: steven.j.svoboda.mil@mail.mil

B. D. Owens
USUHS, Bethesda, MD, USA
e-mail: brett.d.owens3.mil@mail.mil

Department of Orthopaedic Surgery , Keller Army Hospital, West Point, NY, USA

G. C. Fanelli (ed.), *Posterior Cruciate Ligament Injuries,*
DOI 10.1007/978-3-319-12072-0_24,

Patient Demographics

It has been estimated that over 850,000 meniscal procedures are performed each year in the USA [8–11]. Males sustain meniscal tears two to four times as commonly as females, and these injuries usually occur in the third decade of life or later [12]. The medial meniscus is more commonly torn in all age groups [1, 13]. MAT is a relatively new procedure with little prospective data, and therefore, there is limited data on the patient demographics as it pertains to MAT.

An early systematic review of the literature on MAT attempted to establish clinical guidelines for surgeons to better understand four very important clinical guidelines: (1) ideal patient for MAT, (2) ideal method of graft sizing, preservation, and implantation, (3) postoperative-rehabilitation guidelines and timing to return to sporting activity, and (4) overall success rate of MAT [14]. The review included 15 studies (3 level III evidence and 12 level IV evidence) and included 516 patients with 547 MATs (263 lateral and 284 medial). The mean patient age in this series was 33.4 (range: 14–55). The procedure was more commonly performed in males (68 %) compared with females (32 %). Mean follow-up time for this series was 55 months (range: 6 months–14.5 years).

A more recent systematic review of 14 articles (1 level III evidence and 13 level IV evidence) published between 2000 and 2007 included seven articles from the aforementioned systematic review and analyzed 352 MAT procedures in 323 patients [15]. The seven studies published between 2005 and 2007 included 160 patients with 161 MATs (69 lateral and 92 medial). The mean patient age was 33.9 (range 14–58). Height, weight, and sex were not addressed in the review of these studies. Based upon these data, the majority of MAT procedures are performed for active patients in their third and fourth decades with a previous history of meniscectomy. There is a trend of MAT more commonly being performed in men and for the medial meniscus.

Meniscus Structure and Function

The menisci are fibrocartilaginous structures with the primary function for load transmission, shock absorption, increasing joint congruity, reducing joint contact stresses, joint lubrication, and nutrition [1, 9, 10, 16–22]. The menisci are primarily composed of water (75 %) and type I collagen (20 %) with smaller proportions of proteoglycans, cells, and types II, III, V, and VI collagen [23, 24]. The function of the meniscus is to convert compressive axial loads across the joint into tensile strain dispersed by the collagen fibers in the meniscus, thereby increasing load-sharing and decreasing point loading across the articular cartilage. Collagen fibers within the meniscus are arranged in a circumferential pattern and are held together by radially oriented collagen fibers arranged to resist hoop stresses, helping to prevent displacement of the menisci during loading [25].

There are several critical differences between the medial- and lateral menisci. First, the lateral meniscus is C-shaped and covers nearly 50 % of the lateral plateau compared with the medial meniscus, which is more oval shaped and covers only 30 % of the medial plateau. Second, the lateral meniscus is much more mobile than the medial meniscus and is more prone to injury in acute traumatic events. Third, the lateral meniscus is an integral structure in the lateral joint space because it helps improve articular conformity of the lateral femoral condyle (LFC) to the relatively convex lateral tibial plateau. Nearly 70 % of load transmitted across the lateral joint space is through the lateral meniscus compared to 50 % for the medial meniscus [26]. Finally, the medial meniscus has the additional role as a secondary stabilizer to anterior tibial translation in an anterior cruciate ligament (ACL)-deficient knee, and the lateral meniscus has no known clear role in knee stability [12, 27].

Effects of Meniscectomy

Biomechanical studies investigating the effects of partial and complete meniscectomy have reaffirmed the importance of maintaining meniscal integrity. Partial meniscectomy is preferable to complete meniscectomy but there still is increased contact stress compared to an uninjured knee and earlier degenerative osteoarthritis results from this condition [28, 29]. Several important points should be made when considering meniscectomy. First, resection of the lateral meniscus has been shown to increase peak joint contact pressures when compared to medial meniscectomy and increase the incidence of osteoarthritis [30]. Therefore, the importance of the lateral meniscus should be stressed, and every attempt should be made to preserve lateral meniscus integrity. Second, radial tears in the central portion of the meniscus may not be amenable to fixation and may be best treated with debridement. Excessive debridement or debridement that extends to the peripheral meniscus completely disrupts the circumferential fibers and this has been shown to be biomechanically equivalent to a complete meniscectomy [31]. Finally, resection of 75 % or more of the posterior horns of the menisci biomechanically functions as a complete meniscectomy [31, 32]. Consequently, not every meniscal tear is amenable to partial meniscectomy and some tears functionally behave like total meniscectomies which may make that patient a candidate for MAT.

Patient subjective outcomes following complete meniscectomy are disappointing in long-term outcome studies [16, 33–36]. Studies have demonstrated the correlation of clinical and radiographic osteoarthritis in patients with a history of previous meniscectomy [1, 37]. A recent systematic review looking at the clinical and radiographic outcomes in patients undergoing meniscectomy described the preoperative and intraoperative predictors of poor outcomes to be total meniscectomy, removal of the peripheral rim of the meniscus, lateral meniscectomy, degenerative meniscal tears, presence of chondral damage, and increased body mass index (BMI) [36]. As a result of the poor outcomes following total meniscectomy, MAT has been an acceptable alternative in a symptomatic and meniscal-deficient knee.

Indications for Meniscal Transplant

The relative indications for meniscal transplantation are variable, however, the following factors are positive: skeletally mature, young and active, prior history of complete- or near-complete meniscectomy, pain localized to affected compartment, normal mechanical alignment and stability, absence of moderate-to-advanced osteoarthritis, and normal range of motion. Concomitant chondral injury, ligamentous instability, or malalignment must be addressed prior to or in conjunction with meniscal transplantation. Although there is no evidence to support prophylactic MAT in asymptomatic patients, young athletes with a complete lateral meniscectomy present a clinical challenge with rapid progression of osteoarthritis commonly experienced. In this highly selected population, early MAT procedure may be a reasonable consideration.

There has been some clinical evidence that the success and rate of healing of the allograft is improved in patients with minimal degenerative changes in the involved joint [38]. Noyes et al. demonstrated that knees with less than Outerbridge grade 3 changes had a complete healing rate of 70 % and a partial healing rate of 30 %. On the contrary, knees with grade 4 changes had a 50 % failure rate.

Advanced arthrosis has also correlated with higher incidence of graft extrusion on MRI and higher risk of failure [39].

The success of MAT depends on ligamentous integrity of the knee. Commonly, MAT is performed with concomitant ACL reconstruction (or revision reconstruction) due to the increased incidence of medial meniscus tears in the chronic ACL-deficient knee. Medial MAT can provide additional AP stability when performing an ACL reconstruction when compared to ACL reconstruction alone in the setting of medial meniscus deficiency [40]. There is insufficient evidence to suggest that ACL reconstruction with MAT prevents the progression of osteoarthritis or decreases pain when compared to ACL reconstruction alone. In contrast to the medial meniscus, lateral MAT has failed to provide additional stability in the ACL-deficient knee [41]. Ligamentous instability should be restored with reconstruction prior to or in conjunction with MAT.

Normal mechanical alignment is critical to the success of MAT and cannot be overstated. Garrett and Stevenson were among the first to report the high failure rate of MAT in extremity malalignment [42]. Malalignment (most commonly the varus type) can create increased contact stress on the allograft tissue and prevent proper revascularization of the allograft from the capsular peripheral blood supply and can lead to graft failure. Good to excellent results in 85 % of patients after MAT have been demonstrated when performed with concomitant realignment osteotomy [43]. There are no prospective trials that compare osteotomy alone or osteotomy with MAT. Therefore, a corrective osteotomy, whether for valgus or varus, should be performed prior to or concomitantly with MAT. In cases of valgus alignment, a varus-producing distal femoral osteotomy should be considered and for a varus-aligned knee, an opening wedge high tibial osteotomy should be considered.

Some additional relative contraindications to allograft transplantation are obesity, infection, and inflammatory arthritis. The ultimate goal of the surgery should be to provide pain relief for the patient during activities of daily living and not return to high-level athletic competition. Therefore, communication with the patient and appropriate preoperative counseling are paramount to the success of the surgery and patient satisfaction. Further research is needed to determine the expected return to high-level sports and long-term outcomes of this procedure to help guide surgeons and patients alike.

Patients who may be candidates for MAT tend to have complex surgical histories [38, 43]. Additionally, patients may have concomitant chondral, ligamentous, or alignment abnormalities that require consideration in their surgical planning. As a result, there are many factors that can affect the long-term success of MAT.

Graft-Specific Factors

Method of preservation, secondary sterilization, and method of graft sizing are critical factors for the success of MAT. There are four methods to preserve grafts once they are harvested: fresh, cryopreserved, fresh-frozen, and freeze-dried or lyophilized.Fresh grafts can be stored at 4 °C for about 1 week. The benefit of fresh grafts is the high percentage of donor cell viability, with the theoretical advantage of better maintenance of the mechanical integrity of allograft tissue [44]. The short period of viability creates difficulty when time is necessary for graft sizing, sterilization, serological testing, and implantation; therefore, fresh allografts are rarely used. Freeze-dried or lyophilized grafts are rarely used due to the biomechanical alteration and shrinkage of the allograft during the freezing and implantation process [3]. Most meniscal allografts are fresh-frozen or cryopreserved. Fresh-frozen grafts are rapidly cooled to −80 °C and maintained at this temperature. The process of freezing is detrimental to cell viability but has no effect on the biomechanical properties of the allograft. Cryopreserved grafts are frozen in a controlled fashion using a cryoprotectant glycerol-based medium to retain cell viability. The expense associated with cryopreservation may not be warranted given evidence to suggest that fresh-frozen grafts clinically have similar results and that cell viability may not be necessary given histological analysis that demonstrates early-graft repopulation with host cells [45, 46].

The implantation of allograft tissue has the potential to transmit bacterial, viral, or fungal infection and secondary sterilization is used to limit this risk. Gamma irradiation was a common means of sterilization of allograft tissue but studies have shown that the dose of irradiation needed to prevent HIV and hepatitis C also caused significant disruption of the mechanical properties of the graft [47, 48]. Ethylene oxide has also been used for sterilization, but its use was discontinued due to the formation of synovitic reactions and effusions. At present, there is no consensus on the best means of sterilization and tissue banks have developed newer sterilization techniques with limited clinical evidence.

Graft sizing is important to match the size of the native meniscus and best restore the normal biomechanics of the knee joint. There are multiple protocols for sizing the meniscus that utilize plain radiographs, MRI, or CT and may utilize the injured or uninjured extremity for measurements [49, 50]. Whichever technique is utilized, the accepted margin of error should be within 5 % or smaller of the native meniscus. Recently, it has been demonstrated that greater than 10 % size mismatch can alter the biomechanics of the joint and place increased stress on the meniscus allograft [51]. The most commonly utilized protocol has been described by Pollard et al. who utilized bony landmarks on AP and lateral plain radiographs [52]. This technique has been associated with some variability of meniscus width and length dimensions. MRI and CT scan measurements were once thought to more accurately predict allograft size, but they have consistently underestimated the size and have not proven to be superior to radiographic measurements [49].

Graft Implantation

MAT can be performed through either an open or arthroscopic approach using several different methods. Two systematic reviews of MAT suggest that there is no one ideal method of surgical approach or fixation [14, 15]. Cadaveric and clinical studies support several basic principles when performing MAT: anatomic meniscal-horn placement, rigid fixation of the meniscal horns, and stable peripheral capsular suturing to allow for revascularization [14, 15, 53].

Attachment of the meniscal horns can be performed with bone-plug fixation, slot technique (bone bridge), or soft tissue suture ligation. Cadaveric biomechanical studies have supported the use of anatomic bone-plug fixation in order to best recreate the normal contact mechanics of the menisci [54–56]. Secure fixation of bone plugs is commonly used for medial MAT to avoid disrupting the native footprint of the ACL, which inserts medial on the tibia between the two horns. Lateral MAT can also be performed with bone plugs but use of a bone-bridge technique has also been described. The proximity of the anterior and posterior horns of the lateral meniscus to each other is a factor cited. The bone-bridge technique avoids the risk of tunnel convergence during transplant surgery; however, given the development of low-profile reamers, it is possible to place separate sockets close to each other and still maintain the proximal tibial-plateau integrity. Animal models have demonstrated decreased tensile strength and increased failure rate with only soft tissue fixation of the meniscal horns [57, 58].

Stable peripheral capsular fixation when performing MAT is critical in order to allow for graft revascularization and healing. Inability to stabilize the periphery of the MAT can lead to a failed allograft transplant. Vertical mattress sutures should be utilized when fixing the allograft to the capsule because of increased tensile and pull-out strength [53].

Perioperative Considerations

Proper patient selection is the most important factor in considering MAT. Meniscal-deficient knees experience abnormal contact forces and may already have advanced degenerative changes. MAT is a technically challenging procedure, and patients with relative contraindications should not be offered this treatment. Risk factors such as high body mass index and tobacco use may be modifiable, but their presence in meniscal-deficient patients may make MAT inappropriate.

Mechanical alignment in the coronal plane is one of the most important factors for successful MAT. If an osteotomy is required to correct mechanical malalignment, this may have significant impact on concomitant and future staged procedures. The authors prefer to perform osteotomies as the initial procedure in malaligned limbs. The osteotomy is usually performed with a concomitant knee arthroscopy to evaluate the meniscal status and condition of the articular cartilage. In acute cases with PCL-based knee injuries, collateral and/or cruciate repairs/reconstructions may be performed early to allow for rehabilitation. In chronic cases, the authors prefer to first ensure proper alignment, and perform any needed collateral reconstructions. After 3–6 months of healing and rehabilitation, we perform a staged MAT along with any necessary cruciate reconstructions. Size-matched meniscus allografts in addition to any chondral grafts can generally be procured during this time period. It also provides for an adequate healing time of the osteotomy site to allow for hardware removal in cases of tunnel obstruction. Cruciate reconstruction is usually performed in conjunction with the meniscus transplantation as an empty notch significantly facilitates this technically challenging procedure.

In almost all cases, the treatment of an acute PCL injury does not involve planning for meniscus transplantation. As previously discussed in other chapters, it is imperative to have a high index of suspicion for a vascular injury. After emergent reduction and confirmation of the patient's vascular status, it is important to define all of the injuries. The presence and management of fractures may dictate the surgical approach, as well as the extent of ligamentous involvement. Meniscal injury has been noted in 50 % of knee dislocations [59]. All peripheral tears as well as meniscocapsular injuries should be repaired. These repairs are usually performed during initial open repair or arthroscopic evaluation. Subtotal or total meniscectomy is rarely necessary, but a thorough documentation of each compartment is important as MAT may be indicated in the future. Since meniscal grafts need to be size-matched, staged transplantation is the approach usually taken and is most appropriate in PCL-based knee injuries as ligamentous stability is the primary goal. Since the meniscus provides additional stability, concomitant meniscal transplantation may be considered in cases of total meniscectomy and cruciate deficiency. However, in the authors' experience, MAT is typically performed in a delayed fashion following initial ligamentous reconstruction. A recent review of our institution's experience revealed that very few meniscal transplantations have been performed in patients that sustained true knee dislocations. In 84 meniscal allograft transplants performed at our institution from 2005 to 2010, only three were multiple-ligament-injured knees, with two undergoing concomitant ACL/PLC reconstructions, and one had a PCL/

PLC reconstruction. Furthermore, we are aware of only one report of a multiple-ligament-injured knee undergoing combined cruciate reconstruction and MAT [60].

Authors' Surgical Technique

As previously mentioned, proper mechanical alignment and ligamentous stability must be considered prior to MAT. While ligament reconstruction may be performed concomitantly with meniscus transplantation, high tibial osteotomy or distal femoral osteotomy should be performed in a staged fashion. Ideally, MAT should be delayed 6 months from the osteotomy to allow for healing and subsequent hardware removal as needed. An arthroscopic evaluation at the time of osteotomy allows for a thorough assessment of the meniscus and cartilage. In cases with neutral alignment confirmed by weight-bearing hip to ankle alignment radiographs, ligamentous deficiencies are confirmed by physical examination and stress radiographs as necessary.

As previously discussed in this chapter, there are several techniques to perform MAT. The authors prefer to use an arthroscopic approach with bone plugs for both medial and lateral transplantation [61]. The bone plugs are fixed into recipient sockets on the tibial plateau.

Surgery begins with graft preparation which is initiated while the patient is being set-up in order to minimize anesthetic time. The free meniscal graft is prepared from the hemi-plateau allograft with attached donor meniscus (Fig. 24.1). The 8 x 10 mm tapered bone plugs are harvested from the hemi-plateau while maintaining their attachment to both the anterior and posterior meniscal roots (Fig. 24.2). A permanent #2 suture is delivered up through a central vertical drill hole in each bone plug and exits on the superior surface of the meniscus. A horizontal-type stitch is delivered through the meniscal root, then the suture is brought back down through the central hole of the bone plug. A second #2 suture, the posterior-horn stitch, is placed in a vertical fashion through the meniscal allograft 1 cm from the posterior-horn bone plug. A third #2 suture, the mid-body stitch, is placed 1 cm from the posterior-horn stitch in a similar fashion (Fig. 24.3). After all sutures are placed, the graft is wrapped in a moist sponge and secured on the back table until the knee is ready for graft passage.

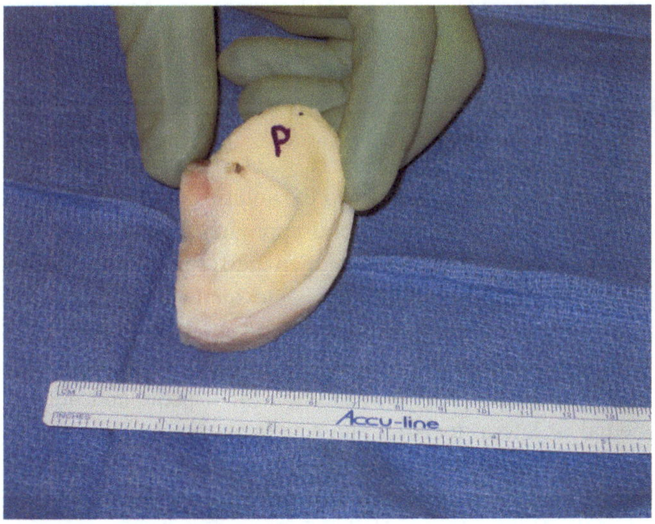

Fig. 24.1 A size-matched fresh-frozen donor hemi-plateau with meniscus is obtained from a tissue bank in order to fashion a free meniscus graft. (With kind permission from Ref. [107])

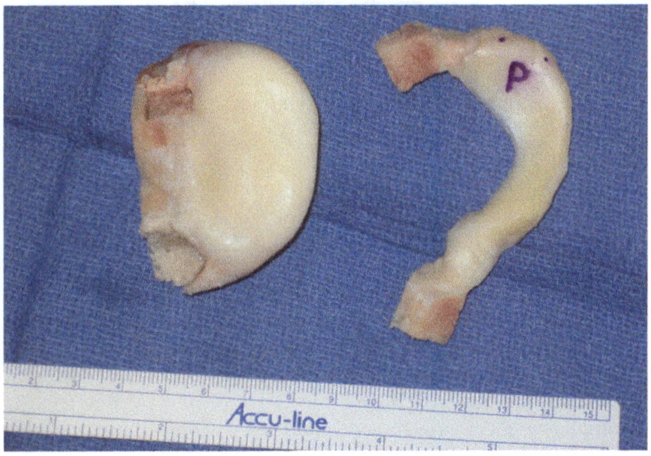

Fig. 24.2 Bone plugs measuring 8 mm diameter by 10 mm long are fashioned to recreate the anterior and posterior meniscal root attachment sites to the tibia. (With kind permission from Ref. [107])

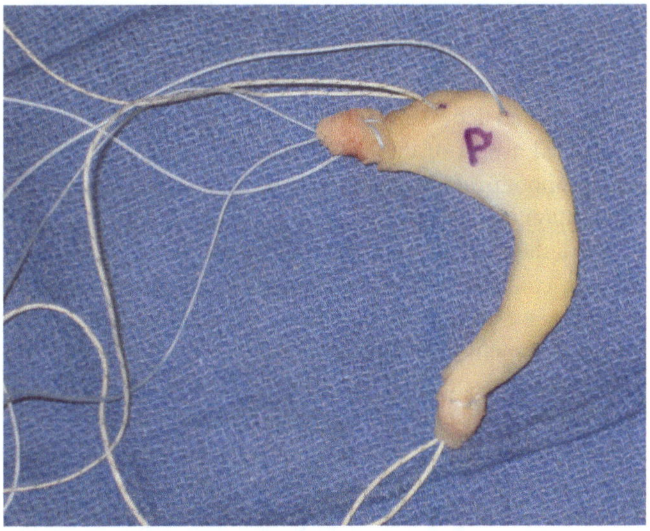

Fig. 24.3 Completed bone-plug meniscal allograft with number 2 permanent sutures passed up central vertical holes in the bone plugs, passed transversely across the root, and back down through the bone plug. Two additional number 2 sutures are placed in the meniscus in the posterior horn and mid-body of the meniscus. (With kind permission from Ref. [107])

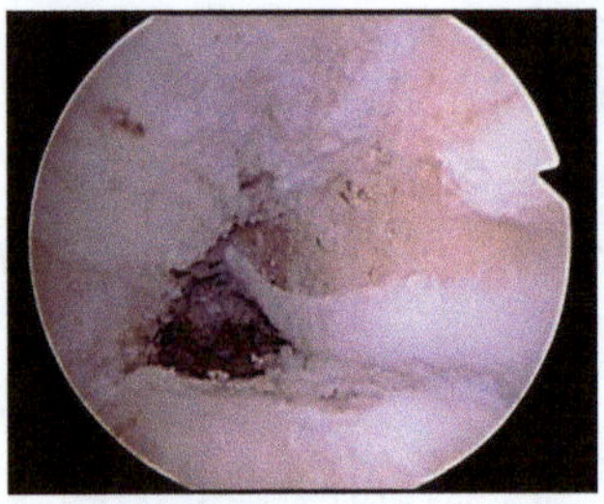

Fig. 24.4 For medial meniscus transplants, a small amount of the PCL posteromedial bundle is debrided along with the extreme lateral aspect of the medial femoral condyle and the medial tibial eminence to facilitate bone-plug passage. *PCL* posterior cruciate ligament. (With kind permission from Ref. [107])

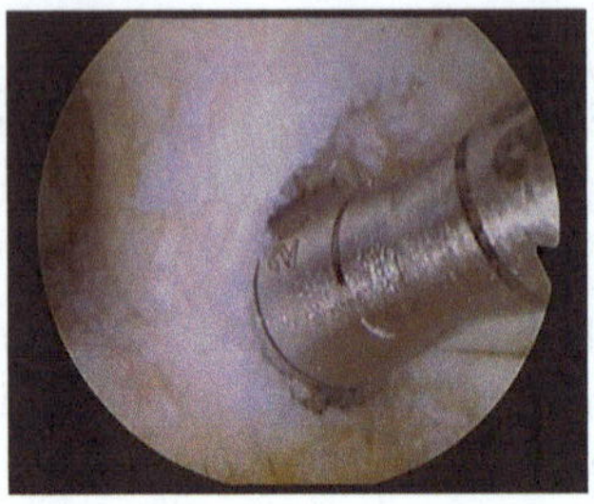

Fig. 24.5 For lateral meniscus transplants, a minimal recession of the ACL posterolateral bundle and debridement of the medial aspect of the lateral femoral condyle and lateral tibial eminence is performed to facilitate bone-plug passage. Successful passage of a 9-mm tunnel dilator confirms that adequate space exists to pass the posterior bone plug. *ACL* anterior cruciate ligament. (With kind permission from Ref. [107])

After diagnostic arthroscopy, the notch is prepared for cruciate reconstruction. In cases of cruciate intact knees, space is cleared to facilitate posterior bone-plug passage through the notch. For medial meniscal transplants, a small amount of the PCL PM bundle is debrided along with the extreme lateral aspect of the medial femoral condyle (MFC) and the medial eminence (Fig. 24.4). Lateral meniscal transplants require minimal debridement of the ACL PL bundle along with the medial aspect of the LFC and lateral eminence. Once a 9-mm smooth dilator can be easily passed (Fig. 24.5), the preparation is adequate.

Next, the meniscal remnant is removed. This is performed using a combination of a radiofrequency probe, meniscal scissors, and an arthroscopic biter to cut along the periphery of the meniscus. The goal is to leave a 1–2-mm rim of meniscal tissue while preserving the chondral surfaces (Fig. 24.6). The insertion of the posterior-horn footprint is cleared of soft tissue and marked with the radiofrequency device (Fig. 24.7). An 8-mm posterior-horn bone tunnel or socket is created. While a traditional tunnel can be used, a reverse-drilled socket is preferable to minimize tunnel convergence which may be a concern in a multiple-ligament-injured knee requiring several tunnels. The authors prefer to use an 8-mm FlipCutter (Arthrex, Naples, FL) through a tibial ACL aiming guide to create an 8 x 10 mm socket at the posterior-horn attachment site (Fig. 24.8). A passing suture is placed through this hole out to the anterior portal.

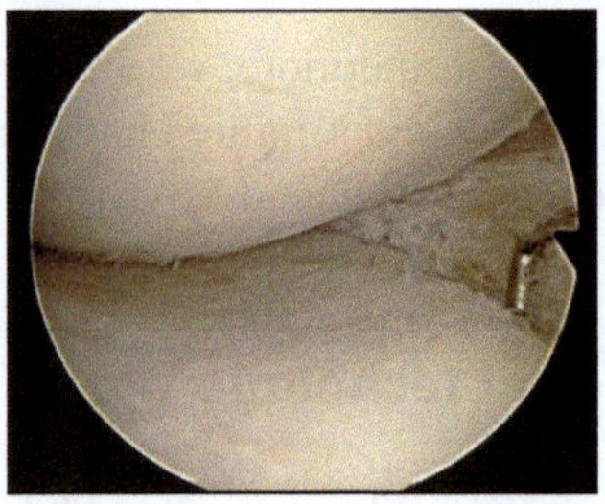

Fig. 24.6 A 1- to 2-mm residual rim of native meniscus is preserved in order to allow secure fixation of the donor meniscus with meniscocapsular suture passage. Extreme care is taken to protect the chondral surfaces during this preparation. (With kind permission from Ref. [107])

Fig. 24.7 The posterior-horn insertion site is cleared of all soft tissue and marked with a radiofrequency device. (With kind permission from Ref. [107])

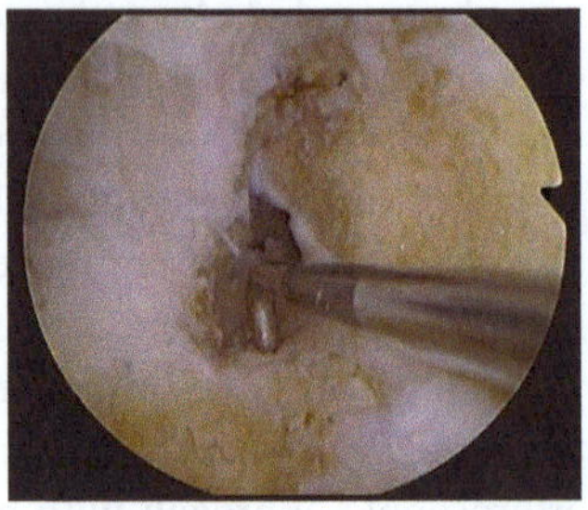

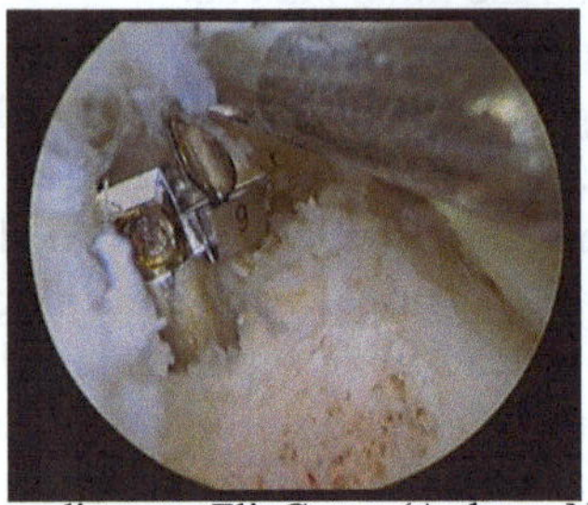

Fig. 24.8 An 8-mm diameter FlipCutter (Arthrex, Naples, FL) is used to create an 8-mm diameter by 10-mm deep socket in the anatomic posterior-horn footprint using a tibial ACL aiming guide. A passing suture will be placed through this hole and socket for passage of the posterior-horn bone plug. (With kind permission from Ref. [107])

A standard medial or lateral approach for the inside-out meniscal repair technique is then performed. The medial or lateral gastrocnemius fascia is elevated and a retractor is placed to protect the vessel. A second suture is placed 1 cm from the posterior root socket using a suture-shuttling device. This suture is passed through the capsule and out the medial or lateral incision and serves as the shuttling suture for the posterior-horn suture in the meniscus (Fig. 24.9). A third passing suture, the mid-body suture, is placed 1 cm from the last one in a similar fashion. Suture management at this point forward is critical to minimize suture entanglement which interferes with graft passage. The authors prefer

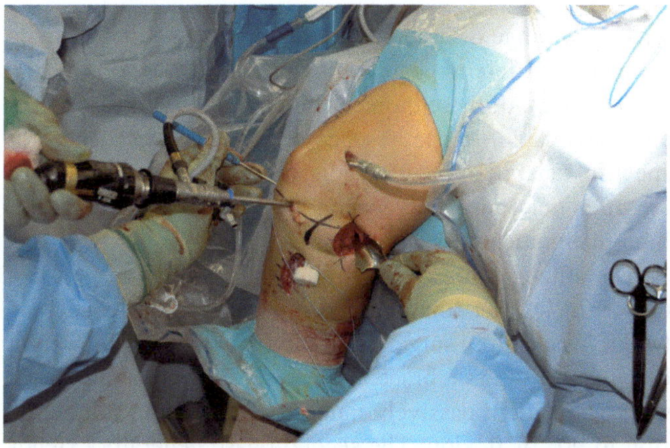

Fig. 24.9 A 90° suture lasso (Arthrex, Naples, FL) is used to place a posterior-horn-passing stitch and a mid-body-passing stitch through the capsule and out the medial or lateral posterior skin incision. After graft passage, the two sutures in the posterior horn and mid-body will be tied to each other over the posterior capsule. (With kind permission from Ref. [107])

to keep the sutures in an ordered fashion with the mid-body suture clamped high on the drape, the posterior-horn suture clamped in the middle, and the posterior root suture clamped low. Again, suture organization is paramount for successful graft passage. At this point, the knee is prepared for meniscus transplantation.

With the camera in the anterior portal opposite the compartment being transplanted, an enlarged ipsilateral portal is created to allow the small finger to freely enter into the joint. Prior to graft passage, a ring grasper is used to "run" the passing sutures from outside to inside the joint to confirm that all three sutures exit the enlarged portal without any soft tissue bridges. The graft is then passed into the knee (Fig. 24.10) by first securing the posterior bone plug into its posterior socket. Next, the posterior horn is passed under

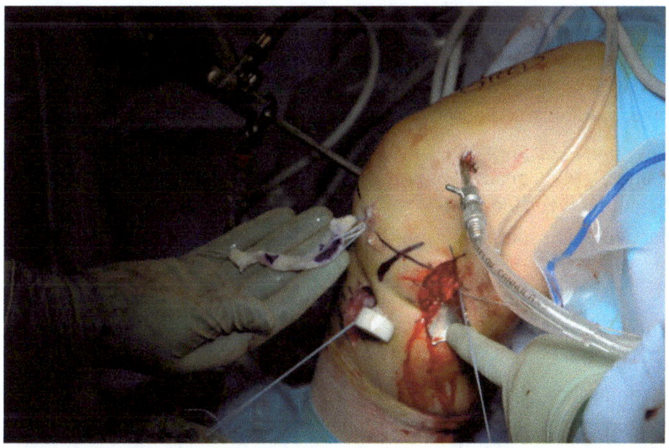

Fig. 24.10 The graft is passed into the knee through the enlarged portal and facilitated by first securing the posterior bone plug into its socket. (With kind permission from Ref. [107])

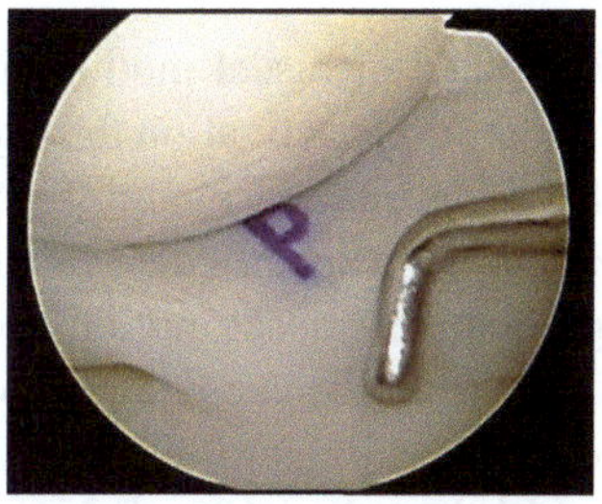

Fig. 24.11 Sequential traction of the posterior-horn and mid-body sutures is used to pass the meniscus beneath the femoral condyle. This may be assisted with appropriate varus or valgus load on the knee and a blunt outflow trocar. (With kind permission from Ref. [107])

Fig. 24.12 Zone-specific cannulas are used to perform a standard inside-out meniscal repair from posterior to anterior. (With kind permission from Ref. [107])

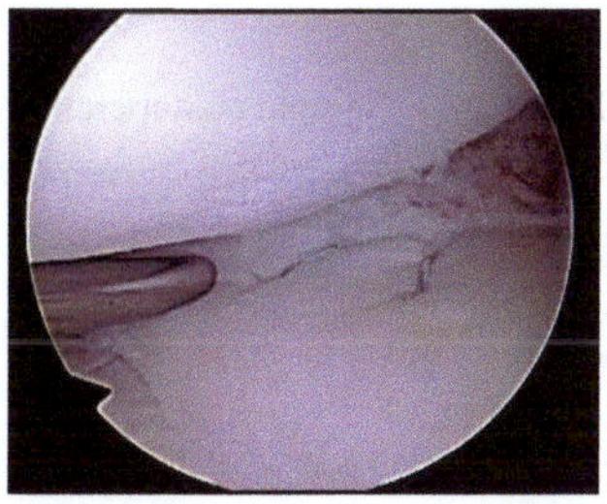

the femoral condyle by pulling on the posterior-horn and mid-body sutures (Fig. 24.11). Passage of the posterior horn can be assisted by varus or valgus stress to open the transplanted compartment and by a blunt outflow trocar to gently direct the meniscus underneath the condyle. The posterior root bone plug is secured by tying its sutures through a button on the anterior cortex. The posterior-horn and mid-body sutures are tied together over the capsule. At this point, an inside-out meniscal repair is performed working from posterior to anterior (Fig. 24.12). The anterior root bone plug is assessed for where it lays in relation to the anterior tibia. An 8 x 10 mm socket is made through the enlarged portal at this position. A guide pin is drilled from the anterior tibial cortex into this socket, and a bent suture passer is used to pass the anterior bone-plug sutures out the tibial cortex. The bone plug is pulled into its socket and the sutures are tied together through a button on the anterior cortex.

When performing concomitant PCL reconstruction, the authors prefer to pass the meniscus graft and secure the posterior bone plug, followed by the mid-body repair. Before we secure the anterior bone plug, we typically pass and fix the PCL on the femoral side. After completing our meniscal transplantation, we then secure the PCL on the tibia using the tensioning boot as covered in other chapters.

Rehabilitation after Meniscal Allograft

Rehabilitation after MAT should allow for healing of the meniscus without exceeding the load-to-failure of the meniscocapsular sutures or meniscal-root fixation. Basic science studies have investigated meniscal motion and loading patterns associated with muscle activation through various knee flexion angles. Meniscal motion is significant during knee flexion and extension [62]. Specifically, flexion greater than 90° results in significant meniscal motion and displacement of the posterior horn from the capsule [25, 63]. In contrast, extension reduces the meniscus to the capsule, and there is minimal motion with less than 60° of flexion [62]. Active and passive knee flexion greater than 60°–90° may stress the meniscocapsular and meniscal root fixation during early healing due to the attachments of the semimembranosus to the medial meniscus and the popliteus to the lateral meniscus [64]. However, case series have shown favorable outcomes with early range of motion protocols [65, 66]. Clinical trials comparing different rehabilitation protocols to determine the clinical effect of these biomechanical studies and case series are unavailable. In the absence of high-level evidence for specific rehabilitation protocols, postoperative restrictions are often determined by concomitant cartilage, ligament, or limb realignment procedures [65].

The authors follow a three-phase rehabilitation protocol (Table 24.1). The first phase is a protective phase and extends 6 weeks from surgery. The patient is kept partial weight bearing and wears a brace at all times locked in full extension. The patient passively ranges the knee from full extension to 90° of flexion. The second phase generally extends

Table 24.1 Sample postoperative protocol for isolated meniscal allograft transplantation (Source: With kind permission from Ref. [107])

Phase I: generally 0–6 weeks post-op	
Phase I goals	ROM: full knee extension, 90° knee flexion
Precautions	Wear brace at all times
	No bending knee with load applied (i.e., squat, leg press, etc.)
Crutches	Begin with touch weight-bearing: progress gradually only when wearing brace locked at 0°
	Weeks 1–2: partial weight-bearing @ 0–25 % body weight
	Weeks 3–4: partial weight-bearing @ 25–50 % body weight
	Weeks 5–6: partial weight-bearing @ 50–75 % body weight
Brace	Locked at 0° extension for 6 weeks
Rehabilitation	Begin patellar mobilizations and scar massage after suture removal
	Calf pumping with tubing
~Weeks 1–2	Heel slides—assisted as needed: within the limits of 0–90°
	Static quad sets, SLRs (in brace)
	Supine passive extension with towel under heel , Gentle HS stretching
~Weeks 3–4	Short arc quads—may add light weights as tolerated
	Seated bilateral calf raises—progress to standing bilateral calf raises
~Weeks 5–6	Hamstring curls—light weight in a painless ROM
	Beginning-level pool exercises: only gait training and deep water jogging
Phase II: generally 7–12 weeks post-op	
Phase II goals	Normal gait and stair ambulation, full knee ROM
Precautions	Continue to wear brace at all times (except while sleeping), no jogging
Crutches	Progress gradually to full weight-bearing during weeks 7–8 post-op
Brace	Open to full ROM
Rehabilitation	
7–8 weeks	Stationary bike, gait training, progressive strengthening
9–10 weeks	Standing balance exercises, progressive strengthening
11–12 weeks	Along with stationary bike, gradually add elliptical for conditioning
Phase III: generally 4–6 months post-op	
Phase III goals	Jog at own pace and distance, ≥90 % quadriceps and hamstring strength, ≥90 % hop for distance compared to the uninvolved side
Precautions	*No* participation in contact/collision sports or military schools
Brace	None required
Rehabilitation	
13–16 weeks	Progressive functional training, strengthening, and balance training
17–26 weeks	Progressive jogging program
Miscellaneous	No return to contact/collision sports or military schools until 9 months
	After 6 months post-op: exercises in phase III are continued, gradually increasing intensity and duration as tolerated with the goal of full return to activity @ ~9 months post-op

ROM range of motion

from weeks 7 through 12 after surgery. This phase focuses on returning full range of motion and achieving a normal gait pattern. The brace is continued but unlocked to allow full range of motion. The patient progresses to full weight-bearing during weeks 7 and 8 and crutches are discontinued when a normal gait pattern is achieved. The third phase goes between 4 and 6 months postoperatively and it is aimed at a return to activity. The brace is discontinued and the focus is on regaining leg strength and a walk to run program. The patient is advised to avoid contact and collision sports for 9 months after surgery at which point they can return to full activities.

Meniscal allografts have a limited life span with deteriorating outcomes over time despite revascularization of the tissue [67, 68]. As a result, the authors do not recommend a return to high-demand activities that involve cutting, pivoting, jumping, or carrying heavy loads. While greater than 60 % of meniscal allograft patients return to some level of sporting activities, the goal of MAT should be a painless knee during activities of daily living [15, 69].

Outcomes

MAT is successful in reducing pain, decreasing effusions, and improving knee function. These clinical improvements are likely due to the improved load transmission characteristics of the meniscal allograft compared to the meniscectomized knee [70]. However, despite improvements in biomechanical function, there is little evidence that MAT slows the progression of cartilage degeneration. Therefore, the goals of this procedure should be to reduce pain, decrease swelling, and improve knee function in the short term while performing activities of daily living.

Despite a high incidence of meniscal injuries after PCL-based knee injuries, very few studies have reported outcomes on MATs with PCL-based knee reconstructions [71]. The literature on PCL-based knee injuries treated with reconstruction and meniscal allograft are limited to individual case reports [50, 60].

The natural history of the meniscectomized knee is consistent cartilage degradation and development of osteoarthritis [1]. Compared to a stable meniscectomized knee, a knee that sustains trauma resulting in PCL injury presumably has cartilage damage and altered mechanics that may hasten the development of arthritis. The goals of MAT in this setting is to provide the meniscectomized knee with tissue that reproduces the improved contact mechanics, reduced peak contact pressures, stabilizing, and chondroprotective effects of the meniscus intact knee.

Prevention of Osteoarthritis

Multiple animal and cadaveric models have evaluated the chondroprotective effects of meniscal allograft transplants. Pressure-sensitive film has been used to evaluate tibiofemoral contact pressures after meniscectomy compared to allograft transplantation in cadaveric models. In lateral meniscal allograft transplants, peak local contact pressures decrease 55–65 % compared to meniscectomy, but contact pressures remain higher than the intact state [70]. After medial meniscal transplantation, maximum and mean contact pressures are reduced 75 % and this contact pressure reduction is closely related to the accuracy of size-matched graft tissue [56]. Peak pressures are restored to near normal after lateral allograft transplantation and bone-plug fixation was found to be superior compared to suture fixation alone [72]. These cadaveric models suggest a chondroprotective effect of MAT through reduction in contact pressures.

A sheep model was utilized by Szomor et al. to evaluate in vivo chondroprotective effects of meniscal transplantation [73]. The area of damaged articular cartilage was reduced by 50 % with meniscal allograft or autograft compared to meniscectomized animals 4 months after surgery. Similarly, Kelly et al. used a sheep model to compare meniscectomized animals with lateral MAT [74]. The cartilage was evaluated at 2, 4, and 12 months with gross inspection, magnetic resonance imaging, T2 mapping, biomechanical testing, and histologic analysis. Significant chondroprotective effects of meniscal allograft transplant were found compared to meniscectomy, but there was still more cartilage damage in the meniscus transplant group compared to the meniscal intact control group. The authors concluded that meniscal allografts provide significant, but incomplete, protection from cartilage degradation in short-term follow-up after meniscectomy.

Rijk et al. utilized a rabbit model to compare radiographic and cartilage cellular activity changes 1 year after meniscectomy or meniscal allograft transplant [75]. No differences in these parameters were found between the meniscectomized animals and the meniscal allograft transplanted animals with the conclusion that transplantation does not prevent degenerative changes with longer follow-up in this rabbit knee model [75, 76].

The chondroprotective effects of meniscal allografts in human subjects have been described only in case series. Ha et al. noted no progression in arthrosis grade in 77.8 % of knees evaluated with magnetic resonance imaging or 64 % of second-look arthroscopies evaluated at relatively short-term follow-up of 31 months [77]. Verdonk et al. reported that 41 % of knees with fresh-meniscal allograft transplants had no further decrease in tibiofemoral joint space width at a minimum of 10 years postoperatively [78]. The authors concluded that the operation had a potentially chondroprotective effect based on the absence of additional joint space narrowing. While this study is compelling by its longer-term follow-up, a randomized trial or prospective comparison to a meniscectomy control group is necessary to define the clinically relevant chondroprotective effects of meniscal allografts compared to meniscectomy.

Healing of Meniscal Allograft

Animal studies have reported healing of meniscal allografts with host cellular repopulation in peripheral meniscal tissue. Fibrovascular scar tissue has been shown in a dog model to be the mechanism of healing to the capsular tissues for cryopreserved menisci [79]. A normal cellular distribution was found, but the allograft cells had a decrease in the number of metabolically active cells. Fresh and cryopreserved menisci showed peripheral healing and revascularization in a goat model, but biochemical changes were noted in the extracellular matrix at 6 months after transplantation [80].

During healing, a transplanted meniscus is revascularized and repopulated with host cells. DNA-probe analysis in a goat model revealed that cells from the meniscus did not survive transplantation, and host cellular DNA was identified completely by 4 weeks [81]. DNA analysis of meniscal allograft tissue retrieved 1 year after transplantation confirmed host repopulation in a patient [46]. Cells derived from the synovial membrane with characteristics similar to synovial cells and fibroblasts repopulate the meniscus in meniscal allograft biopsies 16 months after implantation [82]. The authors in this study also noted cells indicative of an immune response directed at the meniscal allograft, but it did not affect the clinical outcome.

Clinical Outcomes

The clinical evidence for the success of MAT is derived from case series. Comparisons between studies are difficult due to a lack of uniformity on surgical technique, sterilization and preservation methods, outcome measures reported, and patient selection. Furthermore, important characteristics that may affect outcome are not uniformly described including method of size matching, concomitant chondral and ligamentous injury, and limb alignment. With these limitations of clinical outcome comparisons after meniscal transplantation noted, a recent systematic review reported patient satisfaction ranges from 62.5 to 100 % and early failure rates range from 7 to 35 % [15, 83–85]. The early failure rate averaged 10 % when excluding older patients with preexisting osteoarthritis [15].

Milachowski first reported MAT in 1989 and reported an 86 % success rate with 22 meniscal allografts at 14 months after surgery [3]. Noyes et al. reported on 96 fresh-frozen, gamma-irradiated meniscal allografts and noted a 58 % failure rate which has been largely attributed to the gamma-irradiation [38]. Lyophilized meniscus transplants have also had inferior outcomes similar to a meniscectomy control group [68].

Recent series with improved sterilization and preservation methods have shown improved outcomes. A prospective case series of 40 meniscal allografts with anterior and posterior bone-plug fixation had an 86 % success rate and International Knee Documentation Committee (IKDC) scores in the normal or near normal range at 2 years [84]. Cryopreservation was the most common type of graft preparation. Another case series of 40 patients treated with frozen, nonirradiated meniscal allografts implanted with a bone-plug technique, IKDC and Modified Cincinnati scores improved significantly after surgery with reductions in pain, decreased effusions, and improved function [86].

Long-Term Follow-Up

While early results of allograft transplantation have been successful with objective and patient-reported outcome measures, long-term results remain the most important. Van der Wal evaluated 63 cryopreserved meniscal allografts with soft tissue fixation alone at 13.8 years after surgery [67]. A 29 % failure rate and deterioration in patient outcomes over time was noted. Lysholm scores of 79 at 3 years after surgery significantly declined to 61 at final follow-up. There was no difference in Lysholm scores between allograft survivors and those that failed requiring a knee arthroplasty. Wirth et al. reported a decline in Lysholm scores from 84 at 3 years to 75 at 14 years follow-up [68]. A 55 % failure rate at 11.8 years in a recent case series of 22 cryopreserved meniscal allografts was noted. The authors noted improvements in pain and function with only fair results at longer-term follow-up [87]. In contrast to this, a series of 50 cryopreserved meniscal allografts implanted with soft-tissue-only fixation had a 10 % failure rate [88].

Medial Versus Lateral

Outcomes of medial versus lateral MAT have been different in several series [78, 87, 89, 90]. In one study, lateral meniscal allografts had a 76.5 % survival rate at 10 years while medial allografts had a 50.6 % survival rate at 9 years [89]. In contrast, another series had a 25 % medial allograft failure rate compared to a 50 % lateral failure rate at 11.8 years after surgery [87]. Several authors found no significant differences in outcomes between medial and lateral meniscal allografts [66, 91, 92]. The disparity in outcomes may potentially be attributed to differences in ligamentous stability or mechanical alignment. A recent systematic review of MAT found no difference in outcomes between medial and lateral allograft transplants [93].

Preexisting Osteoarthritis

Preexisting knee osteoarthritis portends a worse prognosis after MAT. An 80 % failure rate was noted in knees with advanced arthrosis compared to 6 % in patients with normal articular cartilage or mild arthrosis in an early study of MAT [38, 94]. Improved postoperative Lysholm and Tegner scores in patients with Outerbridge scores of less than 2 have been noted, while patients with Outerbridge scores greater than 3 in any area did not improve with surgery [66]. Evaluation of 29 meniscal allografts using magnetic resonance imaging revealed allograft degeneration was associated with moderate and severe chondral wear and the authors recommended preoperative assessment to identify patients at risk for failure [95].

Defining the optimal time to offer MAT remains difficult. Total meniscectomy results in long-term degradation of articular cartilage [1]. While only limited data are available to support MAT to prevent or slow progression of osteoarthritis, it is currently the only surgical option for young patients with a symptomatic meniscus-deficient knee. Prophylactic meniscal allografts before the onset of symptoms in an attempt to prevent degenerative changes have been reported [96]. Without clinical studies proving chondroprotective benefits, meniscal allografts are not currently recommended for asymptomatic meniscus-deficient patients. Waiting for a patient to develop cartilage degeneration and symptoms may reduce graft survival and symptomatic relief. Given this difficult clinical situation, we recommend yearly follow-up for young patients with meniscus-deficient knees with weight-bearing radiographs to monitor progression of symptoms and joint space narrowing. Future surrogate markers of cartilage degradation (i.e., imaging or biomarkers) may enable earlier detection to help define the appropriate indications for MAT. Little evidence exists supporting the routine use of MRI or bone scanning in such patients and the cost over time obtaining such studies may be prohibitive.

Extrusion

Meniscal allograft extrusion is reported in 40–100 % of patients after transplantation [78, 97, 98]. While some studies have shown inferior clinical outcomes associated with meniscal extrusion, other studies have failed to show meniscal extrusion to be associated with clinical outcomes [95]. Lee evaluated 43 patients treated with a variety of fixation techniques and found that 40 % of grafts extruded an average of 3 mm at 1 year after surgery, but the extrusion did not progress at the 5-year evaluation [98]. The presence of graft extrusion did not correlate with joint space narrowing or clinical outcomes at 5 years.

Ha et al. evaluated 36 patients 31 months after MAT and noted average meniscal extrusion to be 3.9 mm [98]. No correlation with clinical, radiologic, or arthroscopic outcomes and meniscal extrusion were found. Gonzalez et al. noted all 33 patients in a case series of meniscal allografts had meniscal extrusion that averaged 36.3 % of the width of the meniscus [97].

Allograft Tear Rate

The symptomatic tear rate after meniscal allograft transplant ranges from 10 to 36 % and is the most common reason for revision surgery after transplantation [43, 86, 87, 93, 97, 99]. Magnetic resonance imaging of meniscal allografts correlates with arthroscopic findings regarding capsular incorporation and allograft tears [95]. Meniscal allograft tears are treated with partial meniscectomy, revision repair of capsular attachments, or resection in large tears not amenable to repair. There is no literature to guide treatment for allograft tears and the decision to repair or resect is individualized and based on tear pattern, size, and quality of the remaining allograft tissue.

Outcomes Related to Graft Morphology

Sizing characteristics that are most important to clinical outcome and the tolerance of the anatomy to accept deviations from those measurements have not been defined. Cadaveric studies have demonstrated that tibiofemoral contact pressures after meniscal allograft transplant are returned most closely to the native state with appropriately size-matched graft tissue [56]. Meniscal grafts larger than the native meniscus lead to increased forces across the articular cartilage, while smaller grafts result in increased forces across the menisci [51].

Pollard performed a cadaveric study that showed meniscal sizing could be accomplished with standard anteroposterior and lateral radiographs [52]. On anteroposterior films, medial and lateral width could be estimated from the peak of the tibial eminence to the periphery of the tibial metaphysis. Medial and lateral meniscal length was reported to be 80 and 70 % of the tibial plateau on the lateral radiograph, respectively. Shaffer compared radiographic and magnetic resonance imaging to actual meniscus dimensions finding that both modalities were more than 2 mm different than actual dimensions [49]. A recent report found that meniscal sizing based on height, weight, and gender may be more accurate than radiographic measurements [100]. Further research is needed to accurately define the sizing parameters that correlate with outcome and the best methods to match those to the recipient anatomy.

Fixation Method

Numerous techniques have been described for medial and lateral MAT, but studies have drawn a distinction between techniques that employ bony versus soft tissue fixation of the meniscal horns. Successful function of the meniscus demands stable fixation of the meniscal horns. Biomechanically, loss of horn fixation has been shown to be equivalent to a total meniscectomy [70]. Cadaveric studies have shown that stable fixation of the anterior and posterior horns are necessary for the restoration of the load sharing properties of the meniscus [54, 56]. While no clinical study has directly compared different methods of fixation, biomechanical studies have shown tibiofemoral contact mechanics to be superior with use of bone-plug fixation of the meniscal horns [55, 72]. Despite these models, clinical series have shown successful results with soft-tissue-only fixation of the meniscal horns [97, 101]. The authors of the series note the potential for an unexplained in vivo remodeling unaccounted for in cadaveric studies, the immunogenicity of transplanted bone, and technical ease as rationale for soft tissue fixation of the meniscal horns.

Meniscal Allograft with Ligament Reconstruction

In addition to improving contact mechanics, medial MAT can provide secondary stabilization. A cadaveric model showed medial meniscectomy allowed significant displacement of the tibia in ACL-deficient knees, which was restored to normal with MAT [102]. While case series and case-controlled trials are available to evaluate outcomes associated with single ligament reconstruction with meniscal allograft, only individual case reports are available describing multiligamentous knee reconstruction with a meniscal allograft transplant [50, 60].

Wirth et al. reported the first series of ACL reconstructions with concomitant MAT and noted Lysholm knee scores of 75 at 14-year follow-up [68]. Sekiya et al. reported 86 % normal or near-normal IKDC scores 3 years after ACL reconstruction with MAT [103]. Small case series with mean long-term follow-up of 10 and 20 years have corroborated the short-term good results with meniscal allograft and concomitant ACL reconstruction [90, 104]. A case controlled trial of 16 ACL reconstructions with meniscal pathology-matched medial meniscus transplantations with meniscal repair or partial meniscectomy [105]. At 5 years follow-up, the groups had similar IKDC and Lysholm scores with only the meniscal allograft group having more swelling. A recent systematic review revealed no difference in outcomes between isolated MAT and those with concomitant procedures [93].

Meniscal Allograft with Osteotomy

The long-term survival of meniscal transplantation requires appropriate mechanical alignment. Prior reports have documented the importance of normal joint alignment in patient outcomes and survivability of meniscal allografts [39, 101]. A high tibial or distal femoral osteotomy is useful to unload a damaged compartment and to protect the transplanted allograft. In contrast to osteotomy for osteoarthritis, mechanical alignment is adjusted to align with the opposite tibial spine of the transplanted meniscus [106]. A case series of meniscal allograft transplants with concomitant procedures revealed a survival rate to be longer when performed with a high tibial osteotomy [101]. Mean survival time in combination with osteotomy was 13 years, and the 10-year survival rate was 83 %. Cameron and Saha [43] reported on 34 knees that received a tibial or femoral realignment osteotomy and a meniscal allograft with 85 % attaining good-to-excellent results at a mean follow-up of 31 months. A realignment osteotomy can be performed concomitantly or as a staged procedure to restore neutral mechanical alignment, offload damaged articular cartilage, and protect a transplanted allograft.

Conclusion

MAT is a challenging procedure that improves patient satisfaction after subtotal or total meniscectomy. While not proven to be chondroprotective, it can improve patient's subjective outcome scores over the short- to mid-term follow-up period. MAT combined with PCL-based knee reconstruction is uncommon, and limited clinical evidence exists in the literature regarding outcomes for these combined procedures.

References

1. Fairbank TJ. Knee joint changes after meniscectomy. J Bone Joint Surg Br. 1948 Nov;30B(4):664–70.
2. Fauno P, Nielsen AB. Arthroscopic partial meniscectomy: a long-term follow-up. Arthroscopy. 1992;8(3):345–9.
3. Milachowski KA, Weismeier K, Wirth CJ. Homologous meniscus transplantation. Experimental and clinical results. Int Orthop. 1989;13(1):1–11.

4. The classic. Joint transplantation. By Eric Lexer. 1908. Clin Orthop Relat Res. 1985 Jul–Aug;197:4–10.
5. Locht RC, Gross AE, Langer F. Late osteochondral allograft resurfacing for tibial plateau fractures. J Bone Joint Surg Am. 1984 Mar;66(3):328–335.
6. Canham W, Stanish W. A study of the biological behavior of the meniscus as a transplant in the medial compartment of a dog's knee. Am J Sports Med. 1986 Sep–Oct;14(5):376–9.
7. McNickle AG, Wang VM, Shewman EF, Cole BJ, Williams JM. Performance of a sterile meniscal allograft in an ovine model. Clin Orthop Relat Res. 2009 Jul;467(7):1868–76.
8. Greis PE, Bardana DD, Holmstrom MC, Burks RT. Meniscal injury: I. Basic science and evaluation. J Am Acad Orthop Surg. 2002 May–Jun;10(3):168–76.
9. Baker BE, Peckham AC, Pupparo F, Sanborn JC. Review of meniscal injury and associated sports. Am J Sports Med. 1985 Jan–Feb;13(1):1–4.
10. Hede A. Treatment of meniscal lesions in the knee. Epidemiological, clinical and experimental aspects. Dan Med Bull. 1993 Jun;40(3):317–31.
11. Hede A, Jensen DB, Blyme P, Sonne-Holm S. Epidemiology of meniscal lesions in the knee. 1,215 open operations in Copenhagen 1982–84. Acta Orthop Scand. 1990 Oct;61(5):435–7.
12. Levy IM, Torzilli PA, Warren RF. The effect of medial meniscectomy on anterior-posterior motion of the knee. J Bone Joint Surg Am. 1982 Jul;64(6):883–88.
13. Abdon P, Turner MS, Pettersson H, Lindstrand A, Stenstrom A, Swanson AJ. A long-term follow-up study of total meniscectomy in children. Clin Orthop Relat Res. 1990 Aug;257:166–70.
14. Matava MJ. Meniscal allograft transplantation: a systematic review. Clin Orthop Relat Res. 2007 Feb;455:142–57.
15. Hergan D, Thut D, Sherman O, Day MS. Meniscal allograft transplantation. Arthroscopy. 2011 Jan;27(1):101–12.
16. Roos EM, Ostenberg A, Roos H, Ekdahl C, Lohmander LS. Long-term outcome of meniscectomy: symptoms, function, and performance tests in patients with or without radiographic osteoarthritis compared to matched controls. Osteoarthr Cartil. 2001 May;9(4):316–24.
17. Roos H, Lauren M, Adalberth T, Roos EM, Jonsson K, Lohmander LS. Knee osteoarthritis after meniscectomy: prevalence of radiographic changes after twenty-one years, compared with matched controls. Arthritis Rheum. 1998 Apr;41(4):687–693.
18. Accadbled F, Cassard X, Sales de Gauzy J, Cahuzac JP. Meniscal tears in children and adolescents: results of operative treatment. J Pediatr Orthop B. 2007 Jan;16(1):56–60.
19. Cannon WD Jr. Arthroscopic meniscal repair. Inside-out technique and results. Am J Knee Surg. Summer 1996;9(3):137–43.
20. Lohmander LS, Roos H. Knee ligament injury, surgery and osteoarthrosis. Truth or consequences? Acta Orthop Scand. 1994 Dec;65(6):605–9.
21. Bach BR Jr., Dennis M, Balin J, Hayden J. Arthroscopic meniscal repair: analysis of treatment failures. J Knee Surg. 2005 Oct;18(4):278–84.
22. Kalliakmanis A, Zourntos S, Bousgas D, Nikolaou P. Comparison of arthroscopic meniscal repair results using 3 different meniscal repair devices in anterior cruciate ligament reconstruction patients. Arthroscopy. 2008 Jul;24(7):810–6.
23. Cheung HS. Distribution of type I, II, III and V in the pepsin solubilized collagens in bovine menisci. Connect Tissue Res. 1987;16(4):343–56.
24. McDevitt CA, Webber RJ. The ultrastructure and biochemistry of meniscal cartilage. Clin Orthop Relat Res. 1990 Mar;252:8–18.
25. Bullough PG, Munuera L, Murphy J, Weinstein AM. The strength of the menisci of the knee as it relates to their fine structure. J Bone Joint Surg Br. 1970 Aug;52(3):564–7.
26. Walker PS, Erkman MJ. The role of the menisci in force transmission across the knee. Clin Orthop Relat Res. 1975;109:184–92.
27. Shoemaker SC, Markolf KL. The role of the meniscus in the anterior-posterior stability of the loaded anterior cruciate-deficient knee. Effects of partial versus total excision. J Bone Joint Surg Am. 1986 Jan;68(1):71–9.
28. McGinity JB, Geuss LF, Marvin RA. Partial or total meniscectomy: a comparative analysis. J Bone Joint Surg Am. 1977 Sep;59(6):763–6.
29. Ferkel RD, Davis JR, Friedman MJ, et al. Arthroscopic partial medial meniscectomy: an analysis of unsatisfactory results. Arthroscopy. 1985;1(1):44–52.
30. Chatain F, Adeleine P, Chambat P, Neyret P. A comparative study of medial versus lateral arthroscopic partial meniscectomy on stable knees: 10-year minimum follow-up. Arthroscopy. 2003 Oct;19(8):842–9.
31. Lee SJ, Aadalen KJ, Malaviya P, et al. Tibiofemoral contact mechanics after serial medial meniscectomies in the human cadaveric knee. Am J Sports Med. 2006 Aug;34(8):1334–44.
32. Baratz ME, Fu FH, Mengato R. Meniscal tears: the effect of meniscectomy and of repair on intraarticular contact areas and stress in the human knee. A preliminary report. Am J Sports Med. 1986 Jul–Aug;14(4):270–5.
33. Englund M, Roos EM, Roos HP, Lohmander LS. Patient-relevant outcomes fourteen years after meniscectomy: influence of type of meniscal tear and size of resection. Rheumatology (Oxford). 2001 Jun;40(6):631–9.
34. Kim SJ, Chun YM, Jeong JH, Ryu SW, Oh KS, Lubis AM. Effects of arthroscopic meniscectomy on the long-term prognosis for the discoid lateral meniscus. Knee Surg Sports Traumatol Arthrosc. 2007 Nov;15(11):1315–20.
35. Papalia R, Del Buono A, Osti L, Denaro V, Maffulli N. Meniscectomy as a risk factor for knee osteoarthritis: a systematic review. Br Med Bull. 2011 Jan 19;99:89–106.
36. Salata MJ, Gibbs AE, Sekiya JK. A systematic review of clinical outcomes in patients undergoing meniscectomy. Am J Sports Med. 2010 Sep;38(9):1907–16.
37. King AG. Meniscal lesions in children and adolescents: a review of the pathology and clinical presentation. Injury. 1983 Sep;15(2):105–8.
38. Noyes FR, Barber-Westin SD, Butler DL, Wilkins RM. The role of allografts in repair and reconstruction of knee joint ligaments and menisci. Instr Course Lect. 1998;47:379–96.
39. Rodeo SA. Meniscal allografts—where do we stand? Am J Sports Med. 2001 Mar–Apr;29(2):246–61.
40. Garrett JC. Meniscal transplantation. Am J Knee Surg. Winter 1996;9(1):32–4.
41. Shelbourne KD, Gray T. Results of anterior cruciate ligament reconstruction based on meniscus and articular cartilage status at the time of surgery. Five- to fifteen-year evaluations. Am J Sports Med. 2000 Jul–Aug;28(4):446–52.
42. Garrett JC, Steensen RN. Meniscal transplantation in the human knee: a preliminary report. Arthroscopy. 1991;7(1):57–62.
43. Cameron JC, Saha S. Meniscal allograft transplantation for unicompartmental arthritis of the knee. Clin Orthop Relat Res. 1997 Apr;337:164–171.
44. Siegel MG, Roberts CS. Meniscal allografts. Clin Sports Med. 1993 Jan;12(1):59–80.
45. Fabbriciani C, Lucania L, Milano G, Schiavone Panni A, Evangelisti M. Meniscal allografts: cryopreservation vs deep-frozen technique. An experimental study in goats. Knee Surg Sports Traumatol Arthrosc. 1997;5(2):124–34.
46. Debeer P, Decorte R, Delvaux S, Bellemans J. DNA analysis of a transplanted cryopreserved meniscal allograft. Arthroscopy. 2000 Jan–Feb;16(1):71–5.
47. Gibbons MJ, Butler DL, Grood ES, Bylski-Austrow DI, Levy MS, Noyes FR. Effects of gamma irradiation on the initial mechanical and material properties of goat bone-patellar tendon-bone allografts. J Orthop Res. 1991 Mar;9(2):209–18.

48. Schwartz HE, Matava MJ, Proch FS, et al. The effect of gamma irradiation on anterior cruciate ligament allograft biomechanical and biochemical properties in the caprine model at time zero and at 6 months after surgery. Am J Sports Med. 2006 Nov;34(11):1747–55.
49. Shaffer B, Kennedy S, Klimkiewicz J, Yao L. Preoperative sizing of meniscal allografts in meniscus transplantation. Am J Sports Med. 2000 Jul–Aug;28(4):524–33.
50. Veltri DM, Warren RF, Wickiewicz TL, O'Brien SJ. Current status of allograft meniscal transplantation. Clin Orthop Relat Res. 1994 Jun;303:44–55.
51. Dienst M, Greis PE, Ellis BJ, Bachus KN, Burks RT. Effect of lateral meniscal allograft sizing on contact mechanics of the lateral tibial plateau: an experimental study in human cadaveric knee joints. Am J Sports Med. 2007 Jan;35(1):34–42.
52. Pollard ME, Kang Q, Berg EE. Radiographic sizing for meniscal transplantation. Arthroscopy. 1995 Dec;11(6):684–7.
53. Kohn D, Wirth CJ, Reiss G, et al. Medial meniscus replacement by a tendon autograft. Experiments in sheep. J Bone Joint Surg Br. 1992 Nov;74(6):910–7.
54. Chen MI, Branch TP, Hutton WC. Is it important to secure the horns during lateral meniscal transplantation? A cadaveric study. Arthroscopy. 1996 Apr;12(2):174–81.
55. Alhalki MM, Howell SM, Hull ML. How three methods for fixing a medial meniscal autograft affect tibial contact mechanics. Am J Sports Med. 1999 May–Jun;27(3):320–8.
56. Alhalki MM, Hull ML, Howell SM. Contact mechanics of the medial tibial plateau after implantation of a medial meniscal allograft. A human cadaveric study. Am J Sports Med. 2000 May–Jun;28(3):370–6.
57. Gao J, Wei X, Messner K. Healing of the anterior attachment of the rabbit meniscus to bone. Clin Orthop Relat Res. 1998 Mar;348:246–58.
58. Shibuya S. Meniscus transplantation using a cryopreserved allograft. Histological and ultrastructural study of the transplanted meniscus. J Orthop Sci. 1999;4(2):135–41.
59. Owens BD, Neault M, Benson E, Busconi BD. Primary repair of knee dislocations: results in 25 patients (28 knees) at a mean follow-up of four years. J Orthop Trauma. 2007 Feb;21(2):92–6.
60. Lill H, Hepp P, Rose T, Engel T, Kunzel E, Josten C. Fresh meniscal allograft transplantation and autologous ACL/PCL reconstruction in a patient with complex knee trauma following knee dislocation—a case report. Scand J Med Sci Sports. 2004 Apr;14(2):112–5.
61. DeBerardino T. Arthroscopically assisted meniscal allograft transplantation. Op Tech Sports Med. 2005;13:227–32.
62. Thompson WO, Thaete FL, Fu FH, Dye SF. Tibial meniscal dynamics using three-dimensional reconstruction of magnetic resonance images. Am J Sports Med. 1991 May–Jun;19(3):210–5; discussion 215–6.
63. Morgan CD, Wojtys EM, Casscells CD, Casscells SW. Arthroscopic meniscal repair evaluated by second-look arthroscopy. Am J Sports Med. 1991 Nov–Dec;19(6):632–7 (discussion 637–8).
64. Fritz JM, Irrgang JJ, Harner CD. Rehabilitation following allograft meniscal transplantation: a review of the literature and case study. J Orthop Sports Phys Ther. 1996 Aug;24(2):98–106.
65. Rijk PC. Meniscal allograft transplantation—part I: background, results, graft selection and preservation, and surgical considerations. Arthroscopy. 2004 Sep;20(7):728–43.
66. Stollsteimer GT, Shelton WR, Dukes A, Bomboy AL. Meniscal allograft transplantation: a 1- to 5-year follow-up of 22 patients. Arthroscopy. 2000 May–Jun;16(4):343–7.
67. van der Wal RJ, Thomassen BJ, van Arkel ER. Long-term clinical outcome of open meniscal allograft transplantation. Am J Sports Med. 2009 Nov;37(11):2134–9.
68. Wirth CJ, Peters G, Milachowski KA, Weismeier KG, Kohn D. Long-term results of meniscal allograft transplantation. Am J Sports Med. 2002 Mar-Apr;30(2):174–81.
69. Noyes FR, Barber-Westin SD, Rankin M. Meniscal transplantation in symptomatic patients less than fifty years old. J Bone Joint Surg Am. 2004 Jul;86-A(7):1392–404.
70. Paletta GA Jr, Manning T, Snell E, Parker R, Bergfeld J. The effect of allograft meniscal replacement on intraarticular contact area and pressures in the human knee. A biomechanical study. Am J Sports Med. 1997 Sep–Oct;25(5):692–8.
71. Kaeding CC, Pedroza AD, Parker RD, Spindler KP, McCarty EC, Andrish JT. Intra-articular findings in the reconstructed multiligament-injured knee. Arthroscopy. 2005 Apr;21(4):424–30.
72. McDermott ID, Lie DT, Edwards A, Bull AM, Amis AA. The effects of lateral meniscal allograft transplantation techniques on tibio-femoral contact pressures. Knee Surg Sports Traumatol Arthrosc. 2008 Jun;16(6):553–60.
73. Szomor ZL, Martin TE, Bonar F, Murrell GA. The protective effects of meniscal transplantation on cartilage. An experimental study in sheep. J Bone Joint Surg Am. 2000 Jan;82(1):80–8.
74. Kelly BT, Potter HG, Deng XH, et al. Meniscal allograft transplantation in the sheep knee: evaluation of chondroprotective effects. Am J Sports Med. 2006 Sep;34(9):1464–77.
75. Rijk PC, de Rooy TP, Coerkamp EG, Bernoski FP, van Noorden CJ. Radiographic evaluation of the knee joint after meniscal allograft transplantation. An experimental study in rabbits. Knee Surg Sports Traumatol Arthrosc. 2002 Jul;10(4):241–6.
76. Rijk PC, Tigchelaar-Gutter W, Bernoski FP, Van Noorden CJ. Functional changes in articular cartilage after meniscal allograft transplantation: a quantitative histochemical evaluation in rabbits. Arthroscopy. 2006 Feb;22(2):152–8.
77. Ha JK, Shim JC, Kim DW, Lee YS, Ra HJ, Kim JG. Relationship between meniscal extrusion and various clinical findings after meniscus allograft transplantation. Am J Sports Med. 2010 Dec;38(12):2448–55.
78. Verdonk PC, Verstraete KL, Almqvist KF, et al. Meniscal allograft transplantation: long-term clinical results with radiological and magnetic resonance imaging correlations. Knee Surg Sports Traumatol Arthrosc. 2006 Aug;14(8):694–706.
79. Arnoczky SP, Warren RF, McDevitt CA. Meniscal replacement using a cryopreserved allograft. An experimental study in the dog. Clin Orthop Relat Res. 1990 Mar;252:121–8.
80. Jackson DW, McDevitt CA, Simon TM, Arnoczky SP, Atwell EA, Silvino NJ. Meniscal transplantation using fresh and cryopreserved allografts. An experimental study in goats. Am J Sports Med. 1992 Nov–Dec;20(6):644–56.
81. Jackson DW, Whelan J, Simon TM. Cell survival after transplantation of fresh meniscal allografts. DNA probe analysis in a goat model. Am J Sports Med. 1993 Jul–Aug;21(4):540–50.
82. Rodeo SA, Seneviratne A, Suzuki K, Felker K, Wickiewicz TL, Warren RF. Histological analysis of human meniscal allografts. A preliminary report. J Bone Joint Surg Am. 2000 Aug;82-A(8):1071–82.
83. Bhosale AM, Myint P, Roberts S, et al. Combined autologous chondrocyte implantation and allogenic meniscus transplantation: a biological knee replacement. Knee. 2007 Oct;14(5):361–8.
84. Cole BJ, Dennis MG, Lee SJ, et al. Prospective evaluation of allograft meniscus transplantation: a minimum 2-year follow-up. Am J Sports Med. 2006 Jun;34(6):919–27.
85. Graf KW Jr, Sekiya JK, Wojtys EM. Long-term results after combined medial meniscal allograft transplantation and anterior cruciate ligament reconstruction: minimum 8.5-year follow-up study. Arthroscopy. 2004 Feb;20(2):129–40.
86. LaPrade RF, Wills NJ, Spiridonov SI, Perkinson S. A prospective outcomes study of meniscal allograft transplantation. Am J Sports Med. 2010 Sep;38(9):1804–12.

87. Hommen JP, Applegate GR, Del Pizzo W. Meniscus allograft transplantation: ten-year results of cryopreserved allografts. Arthroscopy. 2007 Apr;23(4):388–93.
88. Vundelinckx B, Bellemans J, Vanlauwe J. Arthroscopically assisted meniscal allograft transplantation in the knee: a medium-term subjective, clinical, and radiographical outcome evaluation. Am J Sports Med. 2010 Nov;38(11):2240–7.
89. van Arkel ER, de Boer HH. Human meniscal transplantation. Preliminary results at 2 to 5-year follow-up. J Bone Joint Surg Br. 1995 Jul;77(4):589–95.
90. Farr J, Rawal A, Marberry KM. Concomitant meniscal allograft transplantation and autologous chondrocyte implantation: minimum 2-year follow-up. Am J Sports Med. 2007 Sep;35(9):1459–66.
91. Ryu RK, Dunbar VW, Morse GG. Meniscal allograft replacement: a 1-year to 6-year experience. Arthroscopy. 2002 Nov–Dec;18(9):989–94.
92. Yoldas EA, Sekiya JK, Irrgang JJ, Fu FH, Harner CD. Arthroscopically assisted meniscal allograft transplantation with and without combined anterior cruciate ligament reconstruction. Knee Surg Sports Traumatol Arthrosc. 2003 May;11(3):173–82.
93. Hergan D, Thut D, Sherman O, Day MS. Meniscal allograft transplantation. Arthroscopy. 2011 Jan;27(1):101–12.
94. Noyes FR, Barber-Westin SD. Irradiated meniscus allografts in the human knee. A two to five year follow-up study. Orthop Trans. 1995;417.
95. Potter HG, Rodeo SA, Wickiewicz TL, Warren RF. MR imaging of meniscal allografts: correlation with clinical and arthroscopic outcomes. Radiology. 1996 Feb;198(2):509–14.
96. Johnson DL, Bealle D. Meniscal allograft transplantation. Clin Sports Med. 1999 Jan;18(1):93–108.
97. Gonzalez-Lucena G, Gelber PE, Pelfort X, Tey M, Monllau JC. Meniscal allograft transplantation without bone blocks: a 5- to 8-year follow-up of 33 patients. Arthroscopy. 2010 Dec;26(12):1633–40.
98. Ha JK, Shim JC, Kim DW, Lee YS, Ra HJ, Kim JG. Relationship between meniscal extrusion and various clinical findings after meniscus allograft transplantation. Am J Sports Med. 2010 Dec;38(12):2448–55.
99. Rath E, Richmond JC, Yassir W, Albright JD, Gundogan F. Meniscal allograft transplantation. Two- to eight-year results. Am J Sports Med. 2001 Jul–Aug;29(4):410–4.
100. Van Thiel GS, Verma N, Yanke A, Basu S, Farr J, Cole B. Meniscal allograft size can be predicted by height, weight, and gender. Arthroscopy. 2009 Jul;25(7):722–7.
101. Verdonk PC, Demurie A, Almqvist KF, Veys EM, Verbruggen G, Verdonk R. Transplantation of viable meniscal allograft. Survivorship analysis and clinical outcome of one hundred cases. J Bone Joint Surg Am. 2005 Apr;87(4):715–24.
102. Spang JT, Dang AB, Mazzocca A, et al. The effect of medial meniscectomy and meniscal allograft transplantation on knee and anterior cruciate ligament biomechanics. Arthroscopy. 2010 Feb;26(2):192–201.
103. Sekiya JK, Giffin JR, Irrgang JJ, Fu FH, Harner CD. Clinical outcomes after combined meniscal allograft transplantation and anterior cruciate ligament reconstruction. Am J Sports Med. 2003 Nov–Dec;31(6):896–906.
104. von Lewinski G, Milachowski KA, Weismeier K, Kohn D, Wirth CJ. Twenty-year results of combined meniscal allograft transplantation, anterior cruciate ligament reconstruction and advancement of the medial collateral ligament. Knee Surg Sports Traumatol Arthrosc. 2007 Sep;15(9):1072–82.
105. Rueff D, Nyland J, Kocabey Y, Chang HC, Caborn DN. Self-reported patient outcomes at a minimum of 5 years after allograft anterior cruciate ligament reconstruction with or without medial meniscus transplantation: an age-, sex-, and activity level-matched comparison in patients aged approximately 50 years. Arthroscopy. 2006 Oct;22(10):1053–62.
106. Amendola A. Knee osteotomy and meniscal transplantation: indications, technical considerations, and results. Sports Med Arthrosc. 2007 Mar;15(1):32–8.
107. Fanelli GC. Meniscus transplant in the multiple ligament injured knee. In: Svoboda SJ, et al., editors. The multiple ligament injured knee, a practical guide to management. 2nd ed. Heidelberg: Springer; 2013. pp. 401–19.

Rehabilitation Following PCL Reconstruction: Scientific and Theoretical Basis

25

Craig J. Edson

Introduction

As the techniques to diagnose injuries to the posterior cruciate ligament (PCL) and multiligament injuries have advanced, as well as the knowledge of the sequelae and pathomechanics that occur at the knee if left untreated, surgical procedures to address these injuries continue to evolve. Like its anterior cruciate ligament (ACL) counterpart, the PCL and associated ligament disruption may result in knee pain, instability, and functional impairment if not addressed surgically [1]. Although more technically demanding, PCL reconstruction can result in improved functional stability and greater patient satisfaction when compared to preoperative measures [2]. A significant factor in the outcome is the design and implementation of a rehabilitation program that will allow the patient to return to a satisfactory level of function without jeopardizing the surgical repair. As we continue to treat and follow these patients, many things are clear. First and foremost is that there is great individual patient variance in regard to pain perception, healing response, and outcome expectations. In this regard, although protocols are necessary for providing guidelines, their implementation must have sufficient flexibility to account for patient difference. Second, rehabilitation following these complex procedures cannot be as simple as ACL rehabilitation done backwards. Especially when one considers that is common for multiple ligaments to be involved and that all structures must be protected during the early phase of the rehabilitation process. Finally, the learning curve for designing an extensive and thorough rehabilitation program is very large, and we are far from writing the final chapter.

C. J. Edson (✉)
1250 Broadway Road, Milton, PA 17847, USA

G. C. Fanelli (ed.), *Posterior Cruciate Ligament Injuries*,
DOI 10.1007/978-3-319-12072-0_25, © Springer International Publishing Switzerland 2015

Current Concepts and Theories

There are several chapters in this book that have examined the function and biomechanics of the PCL as well as the other major ligamentous stabilizers of the knee, so it is not necessary to duplicate them for the purpose of this chapter. However, in order to design a rehabilitation program that promotes the restoration of function, while minimizing potentially detrimental forces on the healing graft tissue, it is crucial to understand how various exercises and activities impact these structures following reconstruction. More specifically, what is occurring at the tibiofemoral joint and what effect will this have on the healing tissues. To be fair, it is difficult to determine with any certainty the pure biomechanics in vitro since most studies have utilized physiological models or imaging studies to calculate joint forces [3–7]. Obviously, the implantation of force transducers in vivo to accurately assess ligamentous dynamics as well as joint translation is not practical or feasible at this time. Subsequently, we must take the research that is available and combine this with critical observation when progressing exercises and activities.

In reviewing the literature, most studies have examined the tibiofemoral joint in the isolated PCL or posterolateral corner-deficient knee [3–10]. There are no available studies that examine these forces in the knee that has undergone reconstruction of these structures. Is it realistic that surgical intervention has restored "normal" joint mechanics? Although techniques continue to evolve, it is impractical that the exact biomechanical properties of the native PCL can be duplicated. Conversely, it is reasonable to assume that reconstruction has improved ligamentous integrity of the knee and restored a near physiological and biomechanical equivalent. It would appear that the best course of action would be to apply a combination of the results found in the normal knee and those reported in the ligament-deficient knee when determining the appropriate implementation and timing of various exercises and activities.

In a study by Goyal and colleagues [4], an in vivo analysis of the PCL-deficient knee during functional activities was conducted. Only subjects with isolated grade II PCL injuries were included, and the activities studied were level running and stair ascent. As expected, increased posterior translation on the effected knee with both activities was observed, and this decreased at the point where the greatest degree of quadriceps activity occurred. This happened prior to heel strike in running, but not until late heel strike with ascending stairs. In addition, the velocity associated with the tibia moving from a posterior subluxed position to its normal anterior position was greater during stair ascension, thus creating higher axial joint loading and shear forces. Therefore, in regard to early postoperative rehabilitation, it may be safer to have the patient ascend stairs with the uninvolved leg only, and to take one step at a time. Fortunately, this is the method taught to the majority of patients who ascend stairs during partial weight-bearing (PWB) gait (up with the good and down with the bad) regardless of the injury. In regard to joint forces at various degrees of knee flexion, Eisenhart-Rothe and associates noted minimal posterior translation of the tibia from 0 to 60°, but there was significant anterior tibial translation at 90° as well as a prominent lateral shift of the patella on the femur. Ironically, when subjects performed isometric contraction of the hamstrings at 90°, the anterior translation was greater than in a state of muscle relaxation. These findings, as they relate to tibiofemoral forces, agree with previous studies that have found greater anterior translation at knee angles of 90° or greater. Accordingly, this range of motion (ROM) needs to be avoided during functional activities and rehabilitation exercises during the early phase of graft maturation.

Although these studies give us greater insight into the tibiofemoral kinematics of the PCL-deficient knee, they are limited to single-plane analysis and do not consider the effects of combined ligamentous instability. In addition, there is a dearth of studies that have examined joint forces in the reconstructed knee. Therefore, until these studies are designed and implemented, the best assessment of the effectiveness of any rehabilitation program should be based on patient satisfaction outcomes and objective measurements of ligamentous integrity, both through instrumented and radiological assessment.

Rehabilitation Following PCL and Associated Ligament Reconstruction

Weeks 1–7

As previously stated, it is imperative that rehabilitation programs allow indulgence for individual patient's needs, while still establishing structured benchmarks and guidelines to base recovery and progression. In accordance, there have been modifications made in our current protocols as compared to those we previously presented in the literature. One major change deals with the amount of time the patient remains non-weight bearing (NWB) and the brace is locked in full extension. In the past, this was a 6-week period; however, this made it difficult for a certain percentage of patients to restore a functional range of knee flexion. Although many of these patients were aided by manipulation, this was not successful in all cases. Now, it should be noted that a 10–15° loss of terminal knee flexion can be expected following multiple ligament reconstruction due to graft positioning and tensioning. In fact, our initial 6-week period of immobilization was based on those patients (many of them noncompliant with their postoperative instruction) who attempted to attain full flexion within the early phase of the postoperative period resulting in graft attenuation. It was clear that a delicate balance of early knee flexion had to be weighed against excessive motion (Table 25.1).

Salata and Sekyla [11] described a surgical technique that eliminated the so-called "killer turn" of the PCL graft as it courses over the posterior tibia. They advocated the implementation of immediate weight bearing in full extension and early ROM based on the lack of potential graft stress with this technique. Although this concept has merit, it was based on isolated PCL reconstruction only. In that particular patient population, it would be advisable to allow for early ROM and weight bearing, much like isolated ACL reconstruction. It still may be advisable to introduce these forces in a graded fashion, partial weight bearing initially with progression to full weight bearing over 3–4 weeks, given that the PCL has a greater role in stability during ambulation than the ACL. Early ROM would also be advantageous in the isolated PCL reconstruction patient regardless of the surgical technique; however, it may be prudent to limit this to 70° initially since increased posterior translation has been observed once flexion angles progress beyond this point [12]. In their treatise, the amount of flexion permitted was not discussed, and they had not yet established any long-range outcome studies.

In a majority of the cases, when there has been sufficient energy to cause PCL disruption at the time of injury, it is likely that other structures have also been compromised. At our institution, the number of isolated PCL injuries has been less than 10 %. The associated injuries may include ACL disruption and varying levels of injures to the medial and lateral collaterals. In many instances, there is a rotational component at the time of injury that may result in rotary instability in the absence of pure valgus or varus instability. The degree of collateral ligament injury is crucial in determining the most appropriate surgical correction of laxity; however, it does not have a significant impact on the rehabilitation since these structures must be protected during the early phase of healing. It is with these multiple-ligament-injured patients on which we have designed our rehabilitation practices.

Table 25.1 Rehabilitation guidelines following multiple-ligament reconstruction

2. Rehabilitation following multiple-ligament reconstruction	
3. Phase I surgery to 8 weeks postop	
4. Rehabilitation goals	5. Graft protection
	Control effusion
	Initiate quadriceps strengthening
	Maintain full extension
Guidelines	Brace locked in full extension and intact 24/7 for 3–4 weeks
	Non-weight bearing with crutches for 3–4 weeks
	Brace unlocked 0—full at 3–4 weeks
	Begin PWB gait 25 % per week for 4 weeks at 3–4 weeks
	No isolated hamstring exercises or activities
	Passive ROM only
Therapeutic exercises	Patella mobilization
	Quad sets
	Straight leg raise (SLR) with brace locked
	Ankle DF and PF
	Electrical stimulation to the quadriceps as necessary
	Isometric abdominal exercises
	Upper extremity exercises or UBE as tolerated
	Initiate closed chain exercises in standing with brace
End-phase goals	Full weight bearing (FWB) at end of 8 weeks
	Knee flexion to 90° or greater—full extension
	Quadriceps control during functional activities on level surfaces
	D/C Brace
Phase II (8–16 weeks)	
Rehabilitation goals	ROM: full extension to 125° or greater
	Joint circumference within 2 cm of contralateral limb
	Quadriceps control and during functional movements such as stairs
	Scar mobility
Guidelines	No open chain or isolated hamstring strengthening
	No open chain or isolated quadriceps strengthening if ACL is involved
	Increased flexion should be gradual and patient driven only once 110° is attained
	Gentle hamstring stretching only
Therapeutic exercises	Stationary bike for ROM with gradual addition of resistance
	Progressive–resistive closed-chain strengthening 0–60°
	Double leg with progression to single leg (squats, lunges, leg press)
	Progressive hip and core strengthening
	Balance and proprioceptive training (single leg)
	Isometric quadriceps strengthening at 70°
End-phase goals	Active knee flexion of 110° or greater
	Single-leg stance of 30 s or greater
	Symmetrical LE loading with functional activities
	Resolution of swelling—pain level of 0–2/10 with activities
Phase III (4–8 months)	
Rehabilitation goals	Maximum knee flexion: 10–15° terminal flexion deficit is not unusual
	Quadriceps strength 80–90 % of the contralateral limb
	Straight-line jogging with gradual progression to sprinting (if necessary)
	Sport-specific training toward end of Phase III
Guidelines	Jogging should be performed on a flat, predictable surface. Minimize treadmill running
	No open-chain hamstring strengthening until after postop month 5
	May begin open-chain quadriceps exercises—low resistance
	Single-leg jump equal to 80 % or greater of the contralateral limb before beginning plyometrics

Table 25.1 (continued)

2. Rehabilitation following multiple-ligament reconstruction	
Therapeutic exercises	Progressive–resistive closed-chain quadricep exercises
	Hamstring curls against gravity after postop month 5
	Begin isolated resistive hamstring exercises after postop month 6
	Progressive hip, core, and proprioceptive training—multiple planes
	Plyometric and agility exercises between months 6 and 7 (Jump Program)
	Low-intensity sport-specific training drills after month 7
Precautions	Monitor for anterior knee pain, swelling, or asymmetric landing patterns with increased activity
	Patient education regarding appropriate progression of activity. No sports
End-phase goals	Preparation for more aggressive sport-specific training and drills
	Introduction of multiplane forces with single-limb activities
Phase IV (9 months to 1 year)	
Rehabilitation goals	Quadriceps symmetry
	Completion of "Jump Program" and advanced agility training
	Return to sports if all criteria met
Guidelines	Patient must demonstrate symmetry with single-leg hop test for distance and vertical jump
	Single-leg proprioceptive skills equal to the contralateral limb
	Must be fitted with a functional brace prior to return to sports
Therapeutic exercises	Continuation of strengthening and agility training
	Sport-specific drills at 50 % intensity with progression to full participation
	Aggressive cutting, change of direction, and stop and go activities at end of phase
Precautions	Monitor for pain, swelling, or asymmetric patterns with sport-specific drills
	Assure proper fitting of functional brace
End-phase goals	Safe return to sports without restrictions
	Follow-up with surgeon on an yearly basis for laxity testing, X-ray, and functional outcomes

PWB partial weight bearing, *ROM* range of motion, *DF* dorsiflexion, *PF* plantar flexion, *UBE* upper-body ergometer, *D/C* discontinued, *ACL* anterior cruciate ligament, *LE* lower extremity

Regardless of the presence or absence of ACL reconstruction, the initial phase of the postoperative recovery is the same. This consists of NWB in a long-leg brace locked in extension. The exception to NWB is when the patient is standing in one place. At that time, they are permitted equal weight bearing to promote balance and to decrease the risk of falling that might occur if the patient was attempting to maintain NWB. The brace remains intact for 24 h a day during this initial phase, and they are provided with a knee immobilizer to utilize for showering. Consequently, exercises at this time are limited to those that can be conducted without removing the brace. These include quad sets, patella mobilization, straight-leg raise (SLR) if able, ankle pumps, and scar massage once the incisions are fully healed. It might also be advantageous to utilize a home electrical stimulation unit at this time for quadriceps reeducation. Patient education is critical at this point since, given the limited program, it is often not necessary for the patient to be seen formally in the clinic. The entire rehabilitative program following multiple-ligament reconstruction is oftentimes exhaustive and might involve a protracted period of clinical visits. In these times of limited insurance benefits and coverage, conserving these visits is beneficial. Certainly, if the patient is a scholastic or collegiate athlete and has access to rehabilitation professionals than supervised visits can be advantageous from the standpoint of monitoring the patient's compliance and understanding of this early protective phase. In other instances, the patients may be seen by the therapist during their scheduled postoperative visits with the surgeon to provide instructions and review the key components of the protocol. Again, the time frame for this early protection phase is 3 weeks.

At the end of the third postoperative week, the patient's long-leg brace is opened fully, and the patient is allowed to begin a PWB gait. This phase is 4 weeks in duration, and the patient is advised to progress weight bearing by 25 % each week in a progressive fashion so that they are full weight bearing (FWB) by the end of this phase. It is during this time that it can be beneficial for the patient to begin formal physical therapy primarily to assure that the ROM is progressing adequately. Our goal for the end of this 4-week period is for the patient to attain 90° of knee flexion in conjunction with full extension. Assessment of the patient's tolerance to this early ROM and their willingness to push through potential pain barriers is crucial. This can be an uncertain science, given the individual variances in pain perception, associated injuries, as well as concern by the patient for graft damage if they push themselves too far. It is imperative that flexion is obtained passively to ensure that the patient does not activate the hamstrings. There are several techniques that may be utilized during this time including standing stair stretch and gravity hangs (Fig. 25.1). We have also found success by

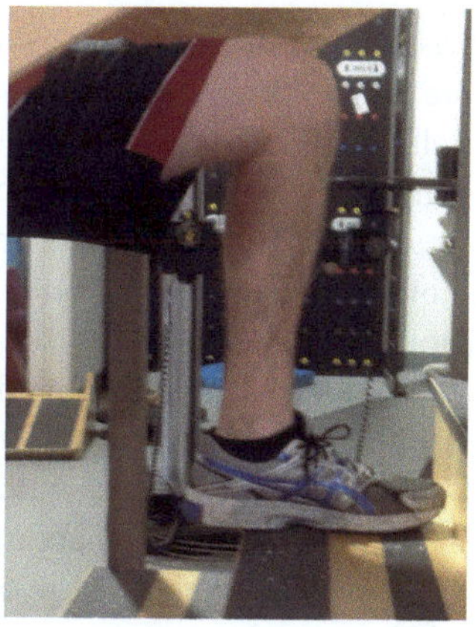

Fig. 25.1 Active flexion stretch on stair

utilizing an isokinetic device with a passive-mode component. The distal pad is placed as proximal as possible to minimize posterior shear forces, and the patient is advised to progress motion gradually (Fig. 25.2). During gravity hangs, when the ACL is involved, the patient is instructed to support the entire weight of the involved leg with the contralateral extremity to avoid quadriceps activation. If the ACL is not involved, then the patient is allowed to involve the quadriceps when flexing (eccentric contraction) and extending the knee. It is also important to avoid any type of rotational, valgus, or varus stretch that might be exerted by the contralateral leg, while supporting the surgical side. Finally, joint mobilization is often instituted at this time although the use of aggressive posterior glides is avoided. Distraction techniques with judicious use of grade II posterior glides are preferable. As knee flexion increases, utilizing a stationary bike in a pendulum-like fashion can also be beneficial for progressing motion. If there is access to a pool, the patient would be able ambulate in the water once they have reached 50% weight bearing on the land and assuming all the incisions are well healed. Short-arc squats could also be performed in the water as well as open-chain knee extension if the ACL is not involved. Isolated hamstring contraction should continue to be avoided.

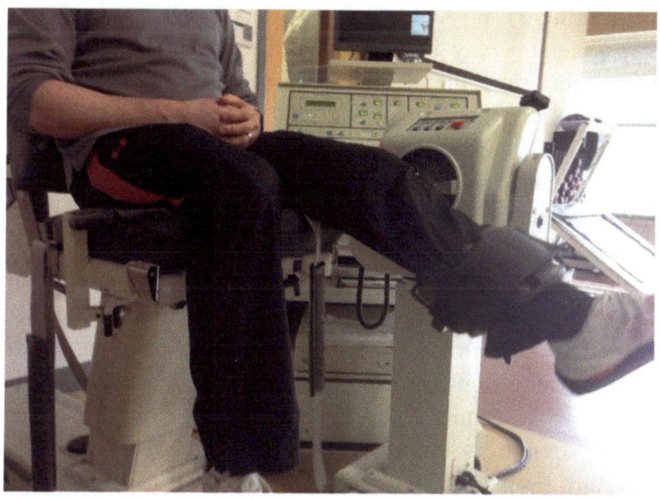

Fig. 25.2 Biodex for passive flexion

Although this phase is 4 weeks, the patient is often reassessed by the surgeon in 2 weeks to assess the ROM status. If the patient appears to have developed early adhesions preventing them from progressing their flexion, this is an opportune time for manipulation of the knee under anesthesia. If this procedure is required, it is vital to begin aggressive passive ROM immediately. In fact, ideally, the patient is seen as soon as possible following the procedure to maximize the effects of the manipulation.

Full extension of the knee is equally important and should be obtained immediately following the surgery. This is accomplished by maintaining the brace in full extension during the initial postoperative period, and the patient is advised to avoid placing any type of support or cushion under the knee during this time. Once the brace is unlocked, the position of the knee will change from one of complete extension at all times, to varying degrees of flexion. Preserving full extension during this phase is vital, and the patient is cautioned about focusing entirely on gaining flexion. The utilization of prone hangs may be utilized for short intervals (3–5 min) while in the clinic to promote hamstring fatigue and gentle prolonged stretching. Extended episodes are not recommended in order to avoid prolonged contraction of the hamstrings. For their home program, the patient is instructed to place a bolster or cushion just proximal to the malleoli in a supine position to achieve passive extension. They are also advised to gauge extension of the surgical side by comparing it to the contralateral knee.

In addition to ROM, quadriceps strengthening is vital at this time. There is significant quadriceps inhibition and atrophy secondary to edema during the period of NWB. The extent of atrophy is also patient dependent and can be impacted by several factors including preoperative muscle strength and tone, level of fitness, age, and degree of swelling. Certain adolescents appear to be susceptible to significant quadriceps inhibition for reasons unknown. Conventional quadriceps strengthening exercises, such as quad sets and SLR, as well as electrical stimulation for muscle reeducation with the knee in full extension are all appropriate at this stage regardless of ACL involvement. If the ACL is not involved, then short-arc quads and multiangle isometrics (0°–60°) may be employed. In addition, if the patient has adequate quadriceps control as demonstrated by an independent SLR without any extension lag, low-intensity closed chain is often initiated. This may occur prior to attaining the FWB status since, as stated earlier, the patient is allowed equal weight on the lower extremities when standing stationary. The degree of flexion permitted is usually limited to 45° to assure patient comfort and minimize patellofemoral forces. This is also beneficial to introduce early proprioceptive training.

In regard to the long-leg brace during this phase, the patient is advised to wear it whenever they are ambulating or standing. They are allowed to undo the brace when they are at rest and discontinue its use during sleep.

Phase II

Weeks 7–16

It is apparent that the initial protection and early ROM phase is the most critical and acts as the building block for maximal recovery and function. Nonetheless, assuring that the patient continues to progress ROM and strength of the knee safely and effectively during the second phase is of equal importance. At this point, the patient will likely discontinue the use of crutches and the long-leg brace assuming that they demonstrate adequate quadriceps control. They must be cautioned that this is not a license to participate in activities and/or exercises outside the scope of the protocol. Persistent quadriceps weakness and limited proprioception place them at continued risk for injury, especially when combined with the lack of any substantial graft maturation or vascularization.

Now that the patient is FWB, closed-chain exercises are introduced and may include light resistance. Lutz et al. [10] reported that there is decreased shear force at the tibiofemoral joint during this type of exercise due to the axial orientation of the applied force in conjunction with muscular co-contraction. This type of exercise also assists with proprioception by assimilating joint mechanoreceptors to compensate for the disruption of the PCL. Katonis et al. [13] identified numerous mechanoreceptors in the native PCL that communicated with the central nervous system, and they determined that the loss of these receptors contributed to muscle dysfunction and joint laxity. A similar phenomenon has been reported following ACL disruption [14] making the training and restoration of proprioception vital, especially when both ligaments are involved. There are several exercises that can facilitate recovery of proprioception and several have been listed in the protocol.

In regard to resistive closed-chain exercises, the amount of knee flexion is limited to 60°. The ratio of quadriceps and hamstring activity has been shown to be equal from 0 to 60°, thus minimizing the degree of tibial translation in anterior and posterior directions [15]. A possible variance with these findings is that the study group consisted of normal subjects. In contrast, quadriceps atrophy and weakness is often greater than the hamstring for several months postsurgically. The majority of postoperative patients do tolerate these exercises without complication; however, static stability should be monitored periodically. Quadriceps weakness and inhibition is a major hurdle in restoring function to the knee. Disuse and the period of NWB in the postsurgical patients are no doubt significant contributors to atrophy. However, Palmieri-Smith and associates [16] also identified arthrogenic muscle inhibition as a major component of quadriceps weakness. They theorized that due to diminished efferent motor drive, a patient would not be able to recruit sufficient motor fibers to promote strength regardless of the amount of resistance applied. To minimize this effect, the use of cryotherapy and neuromuscular electrical stimulation was recommended. Another option for quadriceps strengthening in the early phase of rehabilitation is to incorporate eccentric exercise techniques. These exercises when used in concert with standard concentric strengthening have been shown to cause a twofold greater increase in quadriceps peak cross-sectional area and volume when compared to those patients receiving standard exercises only [17].

In regard to active ROM, the goal for the end of this second phase is 125° or greater. Again, the gradual restoration of this motion in a progressive fashion is preferred and a 10° loss of terminal knee flexion is common following PCL reconstruction. Cardiovascular conditioning is also addressed during this time and a stationary bike can serve to progress ROM and increase heart rate with the incorporation of resistance. In general, the use of elliptical devices is discouraged specifically when the medial and/or lateral structures are involved. This is based on the observation of compensatory valgus or varus as the patient completes a full revolution. There are some devices that, due to a narrower base, do not produce these forces, as the motion is limited to the sagittal plane. If considering a purely cardiovascular exercise, an upper extremity ergometer (UBE) is a viable option.

As the patient progresses through Phase II, single-leg strengthening exercises may be implemented. This may include but is not limited to leg press, step-ups, lunges, and squats. Again, the ROM is limited to 0–70° for reasons previously outlined. As the patient initiates these exercises, they are monitored for any complaints of anterior knee pain. If there is no ACL involvement, open-chain quadriceps strengthening may be initiated judiciously. The ROM for these exercises is the same as for closed-chain strengthening; however, since patellofemoral contact forces are increased from 30°[18], resistance should be nominal. It is often preferable to perform these exercises with ankle weights placed at the proximal tibia versus a leg extension machine. As the patient progresses, a leg extension machine may be implemented although it is preferable for this to be done with both legs initially. It is up to the therapist's discretion and patient response to determine if single-leg exercises on a leg extension machine would be both benign and beneficial. Regardless of what techniques and exercises are employed, quadriceps strength is the key component in allowing patients to return to their desired level of function. It is this process that is the most time consuming and acquiring symmetrical

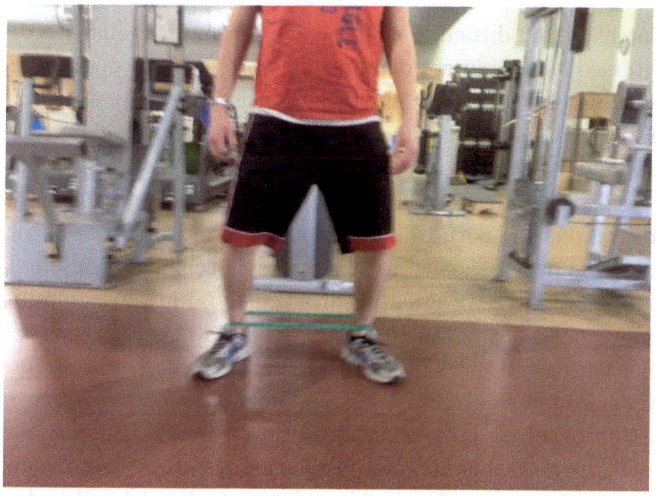

Fig. 25.3 Side shuffles with theraband

strength is the primary criteria for determining return to sports or strenuous activities.

Recently, there has been a greater emphasis on proximal hip and core strength to supplement traditional lower-extremity strengthening [19]. There are many forms of these exercises; however, the avoidance of isolated hamstring activity must be considered when implementing them. An example of this type of exercise is side shuffles against theraband with the knees in slight flexion (Fig. 25.3). The patient is instructed to maintain tension in the band at all times by sustaining a wide stance throughout the exercise. A second activity that utilizes theraband is "monster walks" (Fig. 25.4). In this exercise, the patient is encouraged to take long circular steps with the knee in full extension. This is an excellent method for strengthening of the hip rotators, while side shuffles incorporate the gluteus medius and hip abductors. Planks may also be beneficial for core strengthening

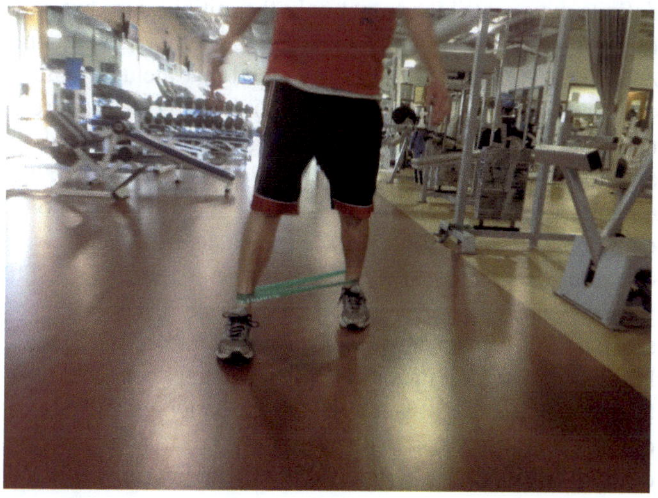

Fig. 25.4 "Monster Walks" with theraband

and, when performed properly, do not elicit excessive hamstring force. As stated, there are many creative methods to incorporate core strengthening that are both challenging and safe at this stage in the postoperative recovery.

Although the patient continues to make progress toward the goal of full functional return, jogging should be avoided during this phase. Of course, there may be exceptions in some cases, and it is at the discretion of the surgeon and therapist to make this decision. If allowed, this should not be permitted until very late into this second phase. Utilizing a treadmill set at various levels of incline at a brisk walking pace is a viable option and may provide an equal amount of cardiovascular conditioning as well as quadriceps strengthening. This phase of the recovery process can become somewhat mundane so a creative approach to the exercises is beneficial, but they must remain aligned with the central principles of graft protection and avoidance of isolated hamstring activity.

Phase III

Postop Month 5–9

This phase begins with the first week of postop month 5 and signals the point where specific activities and exercises may be initiated for the first time, specifically isolated hamstring exercises and straight-line jogging. At the outset, it is preferable to limit isolated hamstring strengthening to gravity-resisted exercises only with gradual progression to resistive exercises as the patient approaches the end of postop month 5. As resistance is added, monitoring PCL integrity through serial, static examination is recommended. It is unlikely that the addition of light resistance would result in any increased posterior translation; however, if suspected, further resisted hamstring exercises should be eliminated. If the static exam proves negative for increased posterior displacement, the exercises are progressed within the patient's tolerance.

Quadriceps strengthening should now consist of progressive isolated, single-leg activities with resistance. The restoration of muscle strength and bulk is the primary goal of this phase and ideally, the surgical leg should be 70–80 % as strong as the contralateral leg prior to initiating continuous jogging. It will also serve to ready the patient for more aggressive agility training. There are no substantial restrictions for quadriceps strengthening at this phase although ROM limits of 0–70° are generally encouraged for PCL protection. Interestingly, Escamilla and associates [3] found that single-leg squat exercises resulted in less tensile force within the PCL than the standard bilateral squat; however, more ACL tensile force was noted. This serves as additional corroboration for emphasizing single-leg exercises in addition to the proprioceptive benefits.

With regard to jogging, the ideal setting would be a flat, predictable surface such as a track. In general, a treadmill is not recommended as modifications in running kinematics have been shown to occur when compared to land running [20]. Assuming that the running kinematics may already be altered when the patient initiates this activity, the potential risk for injury is greater. Another viable option would be to begin the initial course in a pool to minimize impact forces. When available, we have allowed some patients to begin jogging in a pool, earlier in the recovery phase, assuming sufficient quadriceps and proprioception development, as well the absence of any swelling. This decision is based on the patient's goals and the physical requirements basic for the eventual return to competitive or recreational sports. Regardless of the chosen environment, it is recommended that the patient starts with a fast walking pace with gradual progression to a comfortable jogging speed. As the patient begins to fatigue, or if there is a noticeable change in their mechanics, they are advised to resume walking. This procedure is repeated until the patient is able to maintain an efficient jogging pace on a consistent basis. Sprinting is avoided until the beginning of postop month 6 and is only included if integral for return to sports.

At this point, in the rehabilitation process, the inclusion of specific exercises will depend upon the individual patient's goals and needs. A person whose main goal is to return to a physical job would benefit from progressive strengthening as previously described, and this might also include some type of work hardening to simulate their daily occupational requirements. Recreational or high-level athletes will require advanced training to prepare them for the demands of their individual sport. The complexity and intensity of these exercises will again depend on the specific sport and level of participation.

Plyometrics and agility training are commonly introduced at the beginning of the 6th postoperative month. There are a myriad of programs that have been designed to enhance neuromuscular reeducation and dynamic stabilization and although many of these programs were initially designed for ACL injury prevention, they can also serve as an excellent instrument during postsurgical recovery. In 2006, Hewett, Ford and Myer [21] performed a meta-analysis of neuromuscular interventions designed for injury prevention while Barber-Westin and Noyes [22] examined 42 ACL injury prevention programs that were reported in the medical literature. The majority of these programs consist of three basic fundamentals: neuromuscular control, strength training, and plyometrics. Plyometrics consist of exercises that build muscular power and explosiveness through a series of lengthening contractions (eccentric phase) followed immediately by a shortening contraction (concentric phase). Clinically, these consist primarily of jumping and hopping activities and may include steps or barriers to jump from or over. The intensity and difficulty of these activities are gradually progressed as the patient demonstrates proper form during the landing phase, specifically, the absence of any valgus movement upon contacting the ground. Maintaining the knees in a slightly flexed position and landing on the balls of the feet are also encouraged. Verbal cueing is essential to correct any deviations and performing the exercises in front of a mirror can also provide visual feedback. Advancement of these exercises involves progressing from bilateral lower-extremity movements to single-leg activities. Typically, these exercises are performed three times per week for 6 weeks; however, including various components of this exercise type serves as an excellent adjunct to traditional strength training. As mentioned, maintaining the surgical leg in correct alignment during the stance phase of jumping tasks is vital and is dependent on the proper firing sequence of the stabilizers of the hip, knee, and trunk. Therefore, the building blocks for this neuromuscular control occur during the early phase of the rehabilitative process as emphasis is placed on hip and core strengthening. As plyometric and agility activities are introduced, greater demands are placed on these structures. It is imperative that a criteria-based system exists that determines the individual's progression through these more advanced dynamic exercises, specifically quadriceps strength grossly 80 % of the contralateral leg (based on a single-leg hop test), the absence of pain during participation, and demonstrable dynamic neuromuscular control in a single plane.

With regard to the type of plyometric and agility exercises employed, the clinician should be familiar with the specific physical and energy demands of the individual sport. The progression should be from low-velocity, single-plane movements to higher velocity multiplane activities. The ultimate goal of this phase is for dynamic neuromuscular control with these multiplane activities without instability or pain. It is natural for the focus of attention to be on the involved leg; however, there is evidence that contralateral deficits may contribute to not only the initial injury but also to the incidence of reinjury in patients who have undergone ACL reconstruction [21]. It is assumed that including bilateral limb exercises and dynamic training will also address these deficiencies; however, ongoing assessment of pelvic and lower-limb symmetries is crucial to insure desirable outcomes. In addition, although hamstring atrophy is not a common occurrence, the lack of isolated hamstring exercises during the first 5 months postoperatively may result in functional weakness. This may be manifested as excessive landing contact noise during both double- and single-legged landing activities [23]. Thus, as the patient performs these tasks, focus is placed on "quiet" landings and verbal cues, such as "soft as a feather," are utilized to reinforce this concept. To summarize, inclusion of dynamic, sport-specific training exercises that emphasize multiplane neuromuscular control, coactivation of the hamstrings and quadriceps, proprioception, and core stabilization are integral in preparing the patient for return to sport. The successful completion of criteria-based objectives must be met prior to progressing to the next phase of the exercise program.

Prior to the operative procedure, a discussion is held with the patient to inform them that the release to unrestricted sports participation will be 1 year. In very rare instances, patients have returned after postoperative month 10; however, their respective sport lacked the need for dynamic stop and go, change of direction, or jumping and landing. There has been emerging evidence that suggests athletes are at increased risk of a second injury within the first 7 months following ACL reconstruction [23]. No such studies exist for patients undergoing multiligament reconstruction; however, one could surmise that this perilous situation would be longer in duration, given the immobilization and limited strengthening that occurs during the initial postoperative period as opposed to more aggressive postop ACL protocols. Consequently, to give the patient the best prospect of returning to a level of participation that approaches their preoperative level, a 1-year program of intensive rehabilitation and conditioning is compulsory. Once this point has been reached, the determination of the patient's ability to safely return to sports needs to be assessed. There does not appear to be any consensus regarding the most effective means to make this judgment. Several functional tests have been suggested including single-leg hop test for distance, vertical jump, figure-8s over a specified course of time, and isokinetic testing. The inclusion of some or all of these as well as sport-specific tasks will most likely produce the most desirable outcome.

Regardless of the prereturn to sports training or the successful completion of all return to sports criteria, the ability of the athlete to perform at his or her pre-injury level may be compromised. Arden and associates [24] reported two-third of athletes had not attempted a full return to their previous level within 1 year of ACL reconstruction. Of that population, less than 50 % intended to return to sport. The completion of the rehabilitation program is a long and arduous process and oftentimes, the patient is not willing to chance a reinjury or jeopardize further insult to the knee. This is an individual decision, and the patient must understand all of the potential risks involved. Conversely, especially in the younger athlete, the goal of the surgery and the rehabilitation program is to get them to a point where they can safely return to their desired level of function. We have seen many athletes return to full participation in their sporting activity without limitations. In some instances, the ability to replicate their pre-injury level of participation does not occur until their second full season.

For the first season of their return, the patient is required to utilize a multidirectional functional brace. There has been little research that validates the use of functional braces following ACL reconstruction and even less for PCL reconstruction. Jannson and colleagues [25] performed a perspective study on PCL bracing and found little evidence substantiating the biomechanical effectiveness of these devices. No controlled studies were found that evaluated the effectiveness of multidirectional functional braces. Nonetheless, there are anecdotal reports of patients feeling more confident and stable when utilizing a brace just as there are many athletes who find the brace cumbersome and limiting. If some form of protection is afforded against undesirable forces in the frontal and sagittal planes while wearing a brace, the benefits would appear to outweigh the weaknesses.

Finally, outcome studies following multiple-ligament reconstruction are the true indication of successful restoration of stability and function of the knee. At our facility, we utilize KT-1000 measurements, Telos stress X-rays, and three separate outcome measures to determine functional outcomes. The current treatment methodology is based on this introspective review and yearly reassessment of patients following multiple-ligament reconstruction.

References

1. Fanelli GC, Orcutt DR, Edson, CJ. Current concepts: the multiple ligament injured knee. Arthroscopy. 2005;21:471–86.
2. Fanelli GC, Edson CJ. Arthroscopically assisted combined ACL/PCL reconstruction. 2–10 year follow-up. Arthroscopy. 2002;18:703–14.
3. Escamilla RF, Zheng N, Imamura R, Macleod TD, Edwards WB, Hreljac A, Fleisig GS, Wilk KE, MoormanIII CT, Andrews JR. Cruciate ligament force during the wall squat and the one-leg squat. Med Sci Sports Exerc. 2009;41(2):408–17.
4. Goyal K, Tashman S, Wang JH, Li K, Zhang X, Harner, C. In vivo analysis of the isolated posterior cruciate ligament-deficient knee during functional activities. Am J Sports Med. 2012;40(4):777–85.
5. von Eisenhart-Rothe R, Lenze U, Hinterwimmer S, Pohlig F, Graichen H, Stein T, Welsh F, Burgkart R. Tibiofemoral and patellofemoral joint 3D-kinematics in patients with posterior cruciate ligament deficiency compared to healthy volunteers. BMC Musculoskel Disord. 2012;13:231.
6. Gill TJ, Van de Velde SK, Wing DW, Oh LS, Hosseini A, Li G. Tibiofemoral and patellofemoral kinematics after reconstruction of an isolated posterior cruciate ligament injury: in vivo analysis during lunge. Am J Sports Med. 2009;37(12):2377–85.
7. Li G, Pappannagari R, Li M, Bingham J, Nha KW, Allred D, Gill T. Effect of posterior cruciate ligament deficiency on in vivo translation and rotation of the knee during weight bearing flexion. Am J Sports Med. 2008;36(3):474–9.
8. Amis AA, Bull AM, Gupte CM, Hiljazi I, Race A, Robinson JR. Biomechanics of the PCL and related structures: posterolateral, posteromedial and meniscofemoral ligaments. Knee Surg Sports Traumatol Arthrosc. 2003;11(5):271–81.
9. Escamilla RF, Macleod TD, Wilk KE, Paulos L, Andrews JR. Cruciate loading during common knee rehabilitation exercises. Proc Inst Mech Eng. 2012;226(9):670–80.
10. Lutz GE, Palmatier RA, An KN. Comparison of tibiofemoral joint forces during open-kinetic-chain and closed-kinetic-chain exercises. J Bone Joint Surg Am. 1993;20:44–50.
11. Salata MJ, Sekiya JK. Arthroscopic posterior cruciate ligament tibial inlay reconstruction: a surgical technique that may influence rehabilitation. Sports Health. 2011;1:52–8.

12. Escamilla RF, Fleisig GS, Zheng N, Barrwntine AW, Wilk KE, Andrews JR. Biomechanics of the knee during closed kinetic chain and open kinetic chain exercises. Med Sci Sports Exerc. 1998;4:556–69.
13. Katonis P, Papoutsikadis A, Aligizakis A, Tzanakakis G, Kontakis GM, Papaqelopoulos PJ. Mechanoreceptors of the posterior cruciate ligament. J Int Med Res. 2008;36:387–93.
14. Dhillon MS, Bali K, Prabhakar S. Differences among mechanoreceptors in healthy and injured anterior cruciate ligaments and their clinical importance. Muscles Ligaments Tendons J. 2012;7: 38–43.
15. Wilk KE. Rehabilitation of isolated and combined posterior cruciate ligament injuries. Clin Sports Med. 1994;13:649–77.
16. Palmieri-Smith RM, Thomas AC, Wojtys EM. Maximizing quadriceps strength after ACL reconstruction. Clin Sports Med. 2008;27:405–24.
17. Gerber JP, Marcus RL, Dibble LE. Safety, feasibility and efficacy of negative work exercise via eccentric muscle activity following anterior cruciate ligament reconstruction. J Ortho Sports Phys Ther. 2007;37:732–9.
18. Beiser TF, Draper CE, Gold GE, Beaupre' GS, Delp SL. Patellofemoral joint contact area increases with knee flexion and weightbearing. J Orthop Research. 2005;23:345–50.
19. Myer GD, Paterno MV, Ford KR, Hewitt TE. Neuromuscular training techniques to target deficits before return to sport after anterior cruciate ligament reconstruction. J Strength Cond Res. 2008;22(3):987–1014.
20. Sinclair J, Richards J, Taylor PJ, Edmundson CJ, Brooks, D, Hobbs SJ. Three-dimensional kinematic comparison of treadmill and overground running. Sports Biomech. 2013;12(3):272–82.
21. Hewett TE, Ford KR, Myer GD. Anterior cruciate ligament injuries in female athletes. Am J Sports Med. 2006;34(3):490–8.
22. Barber-Westin SD, Noyes FR. Objective criteria for return to athletics after anterior cruciate ligament reconstruction and subsequent reinjury rates: a systematic review. Phys Sportsmed. 2011;39(3):100–10.
23. Hewett TE, Di Stasi SL, Myer GD. Current concepts for injury prevention in athletes after anterior cruciate ligament reconstruction. Am J Sports Med. 2013;41(1):216–24.
24. Arden Cl, Webster KE, Taylor NF, Feller JA. Return to the preinjury level of competitive sport after anterior cruciate ligament surgery: two-thirds of patients have not returned by 12 months after surgery. Am J Sports Med. 2011;39(3):538–43.
25. Jansson KS, Costello KE, O'Brien L, Wijdicks CA, LaPrade RF. A historical perspective of PCL bracing. Knee Surg Sports Trauma Arthrosc. 2013;21(5):1064–70.

26 Brace Considerations for Posterior Cruciate Ligament Injuries of the Knee

Eileen A. Crawford and Edward M. Wojtys

Introduction

Isolated partial and some complete ruptures of the posterior cruciate ligament (PCL) have a high probability of successful treatment using nonoperative means [1–4]. In most cases, patients with these injuries can expect a stable and functional knee because of the superior healing potential of the PCL in comparison to the anterior cruciate ligament (ACL), which has been attributed, in part, to its better synovial coverage and vascularity [1–2]. However, the knee must be allowed to heal in a reduced and stable orientation to minimize the risks of loosening. Achieving this goal has proven challenging, as even surgical reconstruction of the PCL is often associated with residual laxity and rates of osteoarthritis as high as 60 % [1].

Historically, immobilization in a cast was the standard treatment for ligamentous knee injuries [5] to promote healing by limiting stress on the ligament, and maintaining proper knee orientation. Favor has since shifted toward early range of motion, as the knee stability gained by long-term casting is of little worth if the knee is too stiff to be functional for the patient. Many experts continue to treat isolated PCL injuries with initial cast immobilization, but the cast is replaced with a brace after 3–4 weeks to regain knee motion [1, 6].

Although most patients who have posterior laxity from a PCL injury will wear a brace for a portion of their recovery, there has been limited investment by the orthopedic and orthotic communities in the development and evaluation of PCL-specific braces. Most braces that are marketed as PCL braces are simply modified from preexisting ACL braces [2], understandably given the much higher incidence of ACL injuries. Despite the lower numbers of PCL injuries, however, orthopedic sports medicine surgeons will still encounter a number of these injuries in their practice. Understanding the nuances of bracing for PCL injuries is critical for proper management and for providing the best chance for a stable, functional, and pain-free knee in the long term. This chapter reviews such nuances and perhaps stimulate more critical thinking on how to improve the current nonoperative management of PCL injuries.

PCL Biomechanics

Braces intended to protect the PCL while healing must be designed with the complexity of PCL biomechanics in mind. The length and tension of the intact PCL vary throughout the normal arc of motion of the knee [2]. As the knee flexes under a load from 0° to 90–105°, the length of the PCL increases and the in situ force increases [7]. The elongation plateaus between 105° and 120°, and then the PCL shortens from 120° to 135° [2, 8] (Fig. 26.1). The PCL also internally rotates 80–84° around its long axis as the knee flexes from full extension to 90° [7, 8] (Fig. 26.2). This rotation of the PCL fibers increases the in situ axial force of the PCL with increasing flexion. Likewise, the reactive force of the PCL pulling the distal femur posteriorly and proximal tibia anteriorly changes with the degree of knee flexion [2].

The dysfunction and instability seen in the PCL-deficient knee reflect this characteristic of varying force through the arc of motion. When the PCL is sectioned in cadaveric knees, posterior translation increases from 2.4 mm in full extension to 10.1 mm in 90° of knee flexion [9]. For most athletic activities, knee flexion is less than 60°; however, posterior translation still averages 9 mm at 60° of flexion [9]. Indeed, posterior translation typically exceeds 5 mm once the knee flexes to 20–30°, so instability may be experienced even in terminal stance with normal gait [5, 9]. Posterior sag of the tibia in a PCL-deficient knee (Fig. 26.3) also affects the mechanical advantage of the extensor mechanism and may lead

E. M. Wojtys (✉)
Sports Medicine, Orthopedic Surgery, University of Michigan, Ann Arbor, MI, USA
e-mail: edwojtys@umich.edu

E. A. Crawford
Sports Medicine, Orthopedic Surgery, University of Michigan, Ann Arbor, MI 48118, USA
e-mail: ceileen@med.umich.edu

G. C. Fanelli (ed.), *Posterior Cruciate Ligament Injuries,*
DOI 10.1007/978-3-319-12072-0_26,

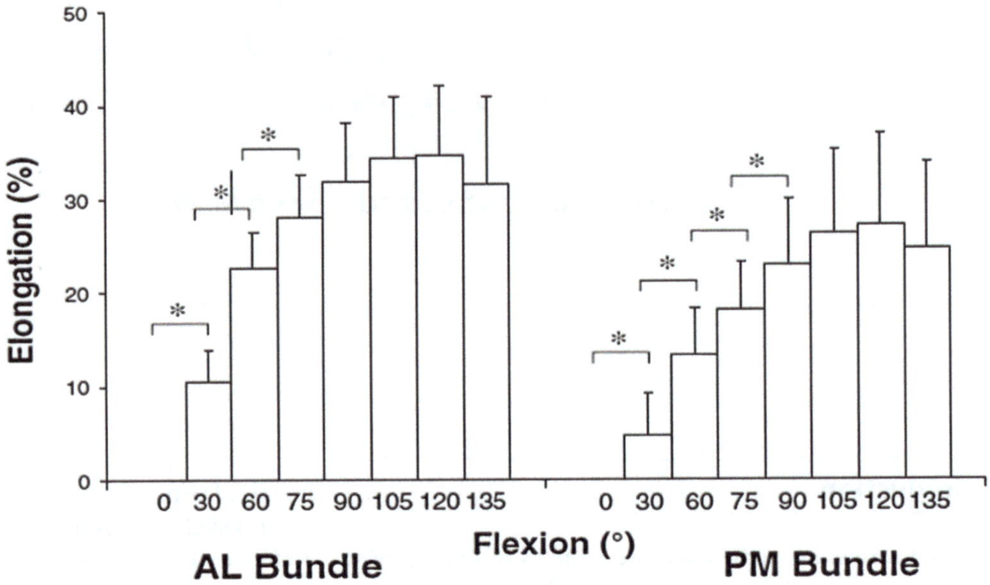

Fig. 26.1 Elongation of the anterolateral (*AL*) and posteromedial (*PM*) bundles of the PCL with weight-bearing knee flexion from 0° to 135°. PCL—posterior cruciate ligament. ([8] Reprinted with permission from SAGE Publications)

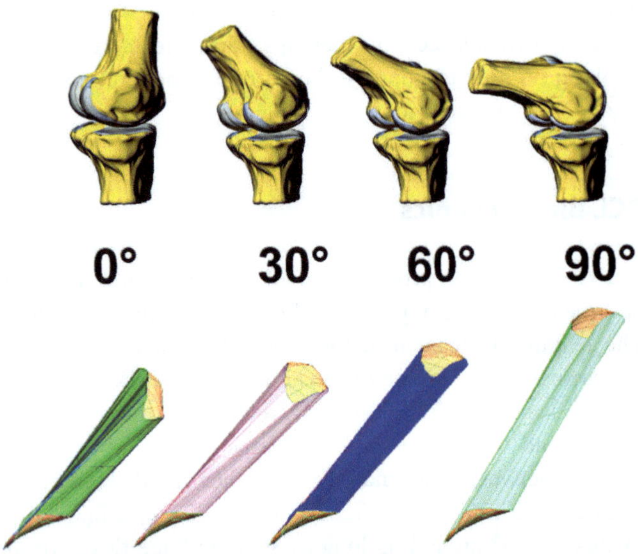

Fig. 26.2 Schematic representation of the relative length and orientation of the PCL with varying degrees of knee flexion. PCL—posterior cruciate ligament ([7] Reprinted with permission from SAGE Publications)

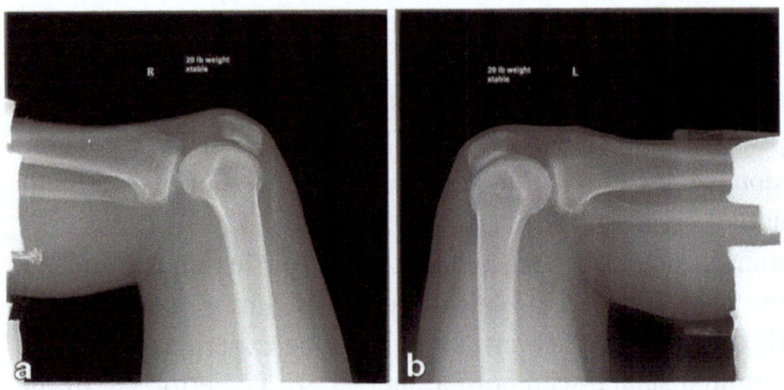

Fig. 26.3 Posterior sag of the right tibia **a** compared to the normal left knee **b** as seen on stress X-ray with a 20 lb. weight placed over the patient's anterior tibia while the hip and knee are each flexed to 90°

to anterior (patellofemoral) knee pain in patients with PCL insufficiency [5].

The ideal brace for PCL-deficient knees would thus provide an anterior force on the proximal tibia that increases in magnitude as the knee flexes to 90°. Similarly, postoperative braces following PCL injury and reconstruction should increase support with increasing knee flexion to relieve strain on the reconstructed ligament as it heals. Braces should be worn for ambulation as well as rehabilitative exercises until the early stages of healing are complete, so comfort and ease of use are also important considerations in brace design.

Indications for Bracing

For all types of orthopedic injuries, bracing falls into different categories. Braces may be rehabilitative, functional, or prophylactic. Rehabilitative braces for PCL injuries are intended to protect the surgically reconstructed ligament or to provide a stable environment for the native torn ligament to heal by limiting tibial translation and rotation. Functional braces may provide external stability in the setting of ligamentous insufficiency allowing patients to complete daily activities and progress to higher-level athletic pursuits. The goal of prophylactic braces is to prevent or limit the severity of future injuries, particularly in knees that have been injured or experience excessive forces with certain activities [2, 5, 10]. Unfortunately, this is still just a theoretical benefit as we have no evidence that bracing for PCL insufficiency reduces the development of osteoarthritis. Osteoarthritis following nonoperative treatment of PCL insufficiency occurs in as much as 78 % of patients, with the medial and patellofemoral compartments most susceptible [2].

Most braces will be prescribed for rehabilitative purposes, for either initial nonoperative treatment or in the postoperative period. These braces should reduce the posterior translation of the tibia, which is created by the pull of the hamstrings and by gravity in the supine position, so that the healing ligament or graft does not elongate [2]. Different methods of bracing and immobilization have been used, but the principle of applying an anteriorly directed force to the proximal tibia remains consistent.

In theory, braces can control anterior–posterior tibial translation and even varus–valgus angulation relatively well as long as the braces are adequately rigid [10]. Internal and external tibial rotation, on the contrary, will not be well controlled without the hip and ankle included in the brace [10]. Therefore, standard PCL braces may not be sufficient when the PCL has associated injuries to the posterolateral corner or other rotational stabilizers of the knee. There is a lack of biomechanical research specifically on PCL braces to support this theory, however. Biomechanical testing of the Lenox Hill brace placed on cadaveric knees with sectioning of the ACL and medial collateral ligament (MCL) demonstrated a 20% reduction in anterior–posterior translation [11]. An in vivo study by Jonsson and Kärrholm [12] also found a reduction in anterior–posterior translation by approximately one third using the Lenox Hill and Ecko braces for ACL-deficient knees. The Lenox Hill brace also controlled external rotatory laxity, but not internal rotatory laxity [12]. Despite these encouraging studies, extrapolating the biomechanical data from ACL bracing studies is inadequate for directing PCL management. Biomechanical testing of PCL braces is needed to understand if the current braces can achieve comparable reductions in abnormal tibial translation and rotation.

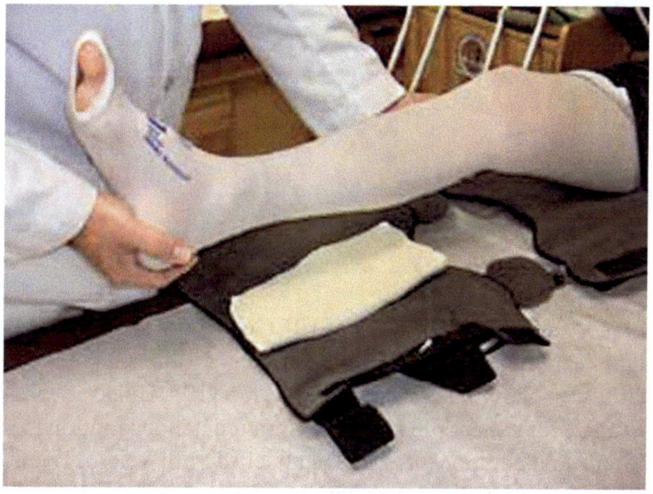

Fig. 26.4 Padding added to the posterior tibial support of a static knee brace. ([21], reprinted with permission from Elsevier Limited)

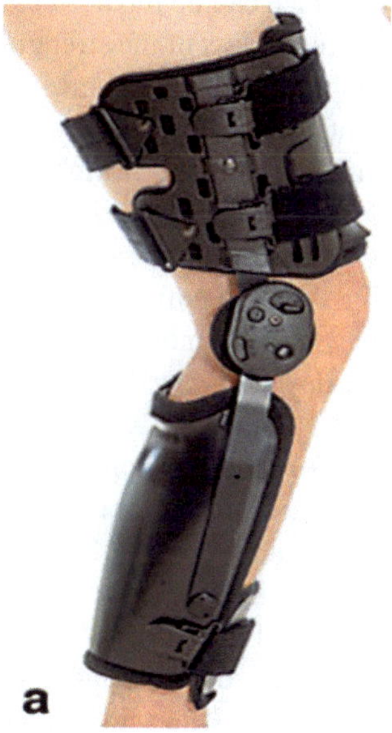

Fig. 26.5 The PCL Jack brace. PCL— posterior cruciate ligament. ([2], Reprinted with permission from Springer)

Brace Specifications

Selecting the proper brace for a patient depends on matching various brace specifications to both the injury and the individual. This thoughtful attention will increase the likelihood of the brace achieving its desired goals.

The first decision is choosing between static and dynamic PCL braces. Static braces rest passively on the leg in a position that resists pathologic motion. Their countering force is only applied when the pathologic motion is encountered [5, 10]. An example of a static brace would be a device that has additional padding between the calf and the posterior tibial support to counteract the posterior translation of the proximal tibia in the supine position (Fig. 26.4). In contrast, dynamic braces are constantly applying a force or preload that resists the undesired motion [5, 10]. This may be accomplished with springs, as with the PCL Jack brace (Albrecht, Stephanskirchen, Germany; Fig. 26.5) [2]. While dynamic braces are considered superior in their ability to resist tibial translation, they may create abnormal forces on the knee [10]. As discussed above, the anterior–posterior translational forces in the knee vary with range of motion. Similar to the PCL, the in situ force on the ACL changes throughout the arc of motion. The ACL experiences its peak force at low flexion angles between 15° and 30°, with a significant drop in force by 45° of flexion [13, 14]. Therefore, a constant anterior force on the proximal tibia from a dynamic PCL brace may increase strain on the intact ACL in a non-physiologic pattern. Whether or not the force generated by the brace is enough to damage the ACL remains to be seen.

The strength and rigidity of the brace will determine the degree of unintended motion and the resistance to high loads, as with a fall. Straps should interlock with the brace struts to provide the best support. Braces with bilateral hinges and hard-shell supports are more rigid than those with unilateral

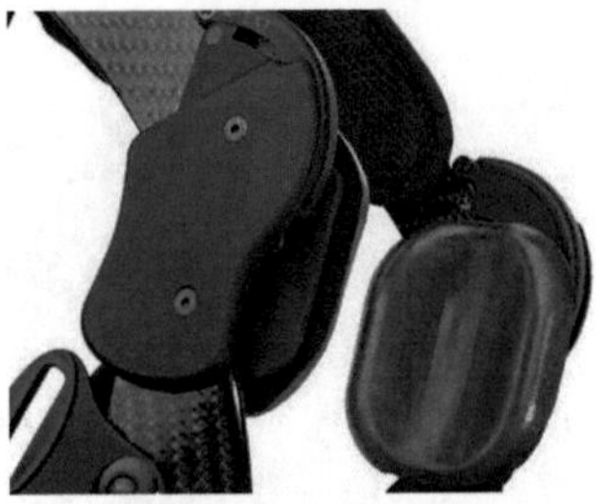

Fig. 26.6 A knee brace with condylar pads. (Image courtesy of Össur, Inc.)

hinges and soft-shell supports [10]. Condylar pads (Fig. 26.6) that keep the hinges centered over the joint line enhance the ability of the hinges to control motion [10]. Hinge mechanisms with a shear pin stop may limit unintended motion [5]. Straps and components may be attached with Velcro, rivets, stitching, or glue, and the quality of these attachments should be inspected prior to use of a particular brace. As PCL braces will typically be worn for several weeks, normal wear and tear of the brace should be expected and monitored so that the brace can be replaced as needed [5].

Regardless of the strength and sophistication of the brace, an improperly fitted brace will not adequately protect the patient's knee. The tightness of fit must be balanced to prevent slippage without compromising circulation and lymphatic drainage. The brace should also be appropriately padded over bony prominences to prevent irritation to the underlying skin and soft tissues [5]. Even with a secure fit, braces tend to allow more motion than indicated by the hinge stops. Cawley et al. [15] found that during ambulation, patients could achieve 15–20° more extension than the amount set by the extension stop. The amount of adipose tissue between the bone and the brace will also affect how well the brace can limit motion [5]. Similarly, as the patient regains muscle girth during rehabilitation, the fit of the brace will need to be adjusted [10].

Finally, comfort and ease of use are important factors to the patient, who will ultimately determine if the brace is to be worn as prescribed. Custom braces may provide a more comfortable fit since they can be specifically contoured to the patient's anatomy. However, they are more expensive and may become loose as swelling subsides or tight as the muscles regain their normal size. Longer braces will provide more leverage for applied forces, but are often less tolerable to the patient and more difficult to achieve a snug fit with rigid struts [10]. Dynamic braces tend to be bulkier and may become too restrictive as the patient progresses in activity level. For example, the PCL Jack brace limits knee flexion from 0° to 90–110°, and hinge mechanisms at both the knee and the ankle make it cumbersome for athletic participation [2].

A single type of rehabilitative brace may not be satisfactory for all patients with PCL injuries, and individual patients may need more than one type of brace over the course of recovery and rehabilitation. However, braces are costly, and more complex designs are not always better. Attention to the needs of the patient and the brace specifications can help to provide optimal chances for successful treatment without incurring unnecessary costs.

Duration of Bracing

There is no clear evidence supporting a particular duration for bracing knees with PCL injuries as part of nonoperative management. Studies on PCL bracing report various length of time in a brace, ranging from 4 weeks to 6 months [2–4]. Some authors report that their selected duration for bracing was chosen somewhat "arbitrarily" [3], though it is based on the current understanding of ligament and soft tissue healing. During the first 2–3 weeks following injury, fibroblasts enter the zone of injury and collagen fibers proliferate [4]. Protection of the healing ligament during this time is critical, so it is necessary to brace or even immobilize the knee in a cast or splint.

For postoperative care of a reconstructed PCL, a total of 6 weeks of bracing has been recommended to allow for sufficient biological healing [2, 16]. However, bracing beyond 6 weeks has been justified by the concept that ligament healing and remodeling continues for over a year [3]. Kim et al. [16] performed a systematic review of studies that described the postoperative rehabilitation protocol following PCL reconstruction. They determined that most authors used a protocol of bracing for the first 6–8 weeks following surgery, with restricted weight-bearing during the first 6 weeks [16].

In both operative and nonoperative situations, bracing must be accompanied by proper rehabilitation. Guided motion should start soon after the injury or surgery to encourage appropriate organization of the collagen fibers, as well as to minimize the negative effects of immobilization on cartilage, muscle, and bone [4]. Within the first 2 weeks, patients may perform range of motion exercises from 0° to 30° with little harm because posterior force is minimal in this arc, especially when exercises are performed in the prone position. At knee flexion angles less than 30°, the anterior force produced by the quadriceps mechanism overpowers any posterior shear force created by the hamstrings [16]. After 2 weeks, a gradual increase of 15° of flexion per week will allow the patient to get to 90° of flexion by 6 weeks [16]. The use of a brace during early mobilization can support proper positioning of the knee, limit excessive motion, and provide some protection against the stresses that the PCL experiences in simple activities of daily living.

The additional support of a brace may be especially important when the quadriceps muscle is weak from immobilization and disuse. The quadriceps mechanism provides a dynamic anterior tibial force that is synergistic with the intact PCL [16]. When the PCL is injured or reconstructed, the quadriceps becomes even more important in counteracting

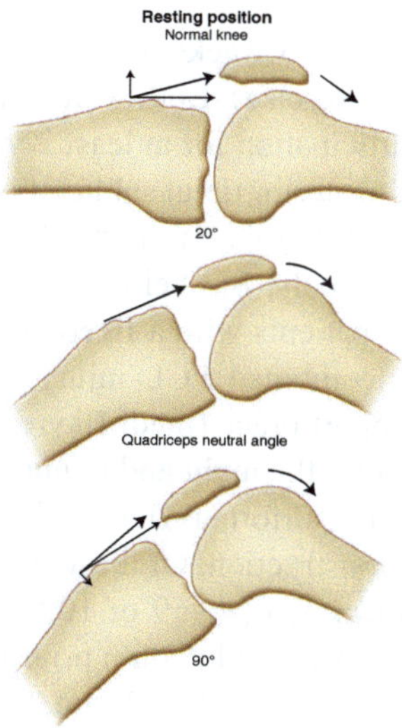

Fig. 26.7 Demonstration of the force vectors created by the pull of the patellar tendon with quadriceps contraction. The quadriceps neutral angle is the knee flexion angle at which there is no force vector perpendicular to the tibial plateau

the posterior forces of the hamstrings and ACL on the proximal tibia. Focused quadriceps strengthening helps to prevent posterior joint subluxation and protect the PCL while it is healing [16]. Quadriceps strengthening exercises should be performed at knee flexion angles less than 70°, the so-called quadriceps neutral angle (Fig. 26.7) [17]. Beyond this degree of flexion, quadriceps contraction creates a *posterior* force on the proximal tibia because of the orientation of the patellar tendon [17].

In setting a plan for the duration of bracing during rehabilitation, the physician must take patient compliance into consideration. Continuous wear of the brace is more critical for PCL injuries than for many other ligamentous injuries. Unstrapping a PCL brace just while lying on the couch will transfer the force of gravity to the healing ligament [3]. Therefore, strict compliance during the early stages of healing may be more important than the overall duration of bracing.

Achieving a high level of compliance depends on the patient understanding the role of the brace, and the potential consequences of not using it properly. The physician or his or her designee should be responsible for communicating this to the patient in terms that he or she can understand. In order to function properly, the brace may feel restrictive, bulky, and uncomfortable to the patient, particularly the more complex dynamic braces [3, 5, 10]. Indeed, if a patient feels comfortable in the PCL brace, the proper functioning and wear of the brace should be investigated [5]. Patients need encouragement to continue to wear the brace despite this, and limiting the duration of bracing can make the process more tolerable.

Tailoring the brace type and specifications to the individual patient can also improve compliance. Older and less active patients will appreciate a lower-profile brace that is easy to apply. Young, active patients will need a more restrictive brace to account for their more physically demanding lifestyle. Either way, patients should understand that bracing is only one part of the recovery process. Without lifestyle modifications and dedicated rehabilitation, bracing will not be sufficient to reach the optimal outcome [5, 10].

Bracing Outcomes

Outcome studies of bracing PCL injuries are rare, and the variety of protocols applied in these studies makes it difficult to form a consensus on how to achieve the best functional results. The primary dichotomy observed in these studies is whether or not there is a period of cast immobilization prior to bracing.

Jung et al. [18] described a long initial period of casting of 6 weeks with acute PCL injuries. The cylinder cast with posterior tibial support was applied once edema from the injury started to resolve, and the cast was changed as needed over the 6 weeks to maintain a good fit. Subjects were then transitioned to a brace with a posterior tibial support for another 6 weeks. They reported very good objective and functional outcomes, with improvement of radiographic posterior translation from 7.4-mm pre-immobilization to 3.5 mm at the minimum 2-year follow-up. Mean KT-1000 scores for side-to-side differences were 6.2 mm pre-immobilization and 2.97 mm at final follow-up. They also reported that 100 % of subjects had a normal or nearly normal International Knee Documentation Committee (IKDC) grade [18].

Ahn et al. [1] reported less favorable outcomes using a protocol of a shorter period of cast immobilization. In this retrospective study of 38 patients with acute isolated PCL injury, subjects were treated with the same protocol: 3 weeks in a long-leg cast once the swelling subsided, followed by a limited-motion brace with a posterior tibial support for 6 weeks with 0–30° of knee flexion permitted and transition to full weight-bearing by 8 weeks from the injury. At a mean of 52 months, they reported that only 29 % of subjects improved a grade of posterior laxity, and the mean KT-1000 posterior translation decreased from 6.7 mm to 5.2 mm. Magnetic resonance imaging (MRI) evidence of ligament continuity with low signal at a minimum of 6 months post-injury correlated with greater improvements in posterior laxity and KT-1000 translation. Functional scores were modest, with 66 % of subjects having a satisfactory IKDC score and an overall decrease in the mean Tegner activity level [1].

Respective times for casting and bracing were further evaluated in a prospective randomized study by Yoon et al. [6]. Patients who had chronic grade III PCL injuries underwent surgical reconstruction of the PCL with postoperative bracing. Both groups were initially immobilized in a splint for 1 week following surgery. The cast group was then placed in a long-leg cast and allowed to put full weight on the operative leg. After 4 weeks in the cast, they were transitioned to a brace for another 7 weeks, and started gradually increasing knee motion. The brace group went from the splint to a brace locked in full extension with no weight-bearing on the operative leg for 2 weeks. Then motion and weight-bearing were gradually increased during the subsequent 9 weeks in the brace, with a goal of reaching full weight-bearing by 6 weeks from surgery. The cast group had better IKDC grade and greater improvement in posterior translation on stress radiographs at 1 and 2 years postoperative. However, there were no differences between groups in range of motion, Lysholm score, overall IKDC score, or Tegner score at 1 or 2 years postoperative [6].

When cast immobilization is used for PCL injuries, the cast should be applied in a prone position to eliminate posterior sag while the cast hardens. A benefit of casting is that it is rigid enough to allow early weight-bearing. Weight-bearing facilitates maintenance of reduction due to the posterior slope of the tibial plateau, which creates an anterior force on the proximal tibia when axially loaded [6]. The downside of prolonged casting is muscle atrophy and interference with activities such as bathing, working, and driving [18]. If a brace is used early in the recovery period, locking the brace in full or near-full extension will limit the stress on the PCL, which increases with flexion up to 90°.

The dynamic brace that has been credited for being well designed for PCL injuries is the PCL Jack brace (Albrecht GmbH, Stephanskirchen, Germany). It has been tested with acute, isolated grade I and II PCL injuries [3]. The brace was worn for 4 months with full weight-bearing and ROM from 0° to 110° allowed from the outset. They reported improvement in posterior sag based on arthrometry, from 7.1 mm at presentation to 2.3 mm at 12 months and 3.2 mm at 24 months from injury. Likewise, the posterior sag measured on radiographs decreased from 8.1 mm to 3.1 mm at 12 months and 3.4 mm at 24 months post-injury. While 95 % of subjects had good or excellent results on Lysholm score, there were small but significant decreases on IKDC, Lysholm, and Tegner scores from pre-injury to 12 and 24 months post-injury. Complications associated with this brace included two minor skin abrasions and one subject experiencing exacerbation of his preexisting patellofemoral osteoarthritis [3].

A couple of smaller series evaluated return to sports in athletes who sustained an acute isolated PCL injury and were treated with bracing only. Parolie and Bergfeld [19] assessed subjects within 24 hours of the injury, placed them in a Lenox Hill brace, and allowed early motion with a vigorous rehabilitation protocol. At a mean of 6.2 years follow-up, all of the athletes returned to full sports participation and were satisfied with the function of their knees [19]. Iwamoto et al. [9] treated two professional baseball players with acute PCL injury by immobilizing them in a brace in full extension for 3 weeks, while focusing on quadriceps strengthening exercises. Both were able to return to their prior level of participation for at least 2 years, although they had 5–8 mm of posterior tibial subluxation and one was still experiencing instability with running [9].

Finally, Strobel et al. [20] studied preoperative bracing for patients with a fixed posterior subluxation from isolated or combined PCL injury. Subjects wore a posterior tibial support brace (medi Bayreuth, GmbH, Bayreuth, Germany) during the night and a functional PCL brace (DonJoy, Carlsbad, California) during the day prior to their surgical PCL reconstruction. Of those who had anterior stress radiographs performed ($n=59$ of 109), 85 % had reduction of the fixed posterior subluxation prior to surgery, and in 59 % it was reduced to less than 3 mm. Subjects who had a grade III fixed posterior subluxation were less likely to achieve reduction with preoperative bracing [20]. Preoperative correction of the fixed posterior subluxation makes anatomic reconstruction of the PCL possible without releasing other tissues.

Summary

Bracing can play a prominent role in the management of PCL injuries. The majority of isolated PCL injuries can be treated nonoperatively, and those that do require surgery will typically need a course of bracing in the perioperative period. Braces used for PCL injuries come in a variety of designs, each with advantages and disadvantages that should be appropriately matched to the individual patient. The existing evidence for the duration of nonoperative bracing and the use of cast immobilization prior to bracing is inconclusive. However, there is agreement among experts that regardless of the bracing protocol used, patient compliance is crucial and dependent on ongoing communication between the patient and the treating physician.

References

1. Ahn JH, Lee SH, Choi SH, Wang JH, Jang SW. Evaluation of clinical and magnetic resonance imaging results after treatment with casting and bracing for the acutely injured posterior cruciate ligament. Arthroscopy. 2011 Dec;27(12):1679–87.
2. Jansson KS, Costello KE, O'Brien L, Wijdicks CA, Laprade RF. A historical perspective of PCL bracing. Knee Surg Sports Traumatol Arthrosc. 2013 May;21(5):1064–70.
3. Jacobi M, Reischl N, Wahl P, Gautier E, Jakob RP. Acute isolated injury of the posterior cruciate ligament treated by a dynamic anterior drawer brace: a preliminary report. J Bone Joint Surg Br. 2010 Oct;92(10):1381–4.
4. Kannus P, Järvinen M. Nonoperative treatment of acute knee ligament injuries. A review with special reference to indications and methods. Sports Med. 1990 Apr;9(4):244–60.
5. Nelson KA. The use of knee braces during rehabilitation. Clin Sports Med. 1990 Oct;9(4):799–811.

6. Yoon KH, Park SW, Lee SH, Kim MH, Park SY, Oh H. Does cast immobilization contribute to posterior stability after posterior cruciate ligament reconstruction? Arthroscopy. 2013 Mar;29(3):500–6.
7. DeFrate LE, Gill TJ, Li G. In vivo function of the posterior cruciate ligament during weightbearing knee flexion. Am J Sports Med. 2004 Dec;32(8):1923–8.
8. Papannagari R, DeFrate LE, Nha KW, Moses JM, Moussa M, Gill TJ, et al. Function of posterior cruciate ligament bundles during in vivo knee flexion. Am J Sports Med. 2007 Sep;35(9):1507–12.
9. Iwamoto J, Takeda T, Suda Y, Otani T, Matsumoto H. Conservative treatment of isolated posterior cruciate ligament injury in professional baseball players: a report of two cases. Knee. 2004 Feb;11(1):41–4.
10. France EP, Cawley PW, Paulos LE. Choosing functional knee braces. Clin Sports Med. 1990 Oct;9(4):743–50.
11. Anderson K, Wojtys EM, Loubert PV, Miller RE. A biomechanical evaluation of taping and bracing in reducing knee joint translation and rotation. Am J Sports Med. 1992 Jul–Aug;20(4):416–21.
12. Jonsson H, Kärrholm J. Brace effects on the unstable knee in 21 cases. Acta Orthop Scand. 1990 Aug;61(4):313–8.
13. Fleming BC, Beynnon BD, Renstrom PA, Johnson RJ, Nichols CE, Peura GD, et al. The strain behavior of the anterior cruciate ligament during stair climbing: an in vivo study. Arthroscopy. 1999 Mar;15(2):185–91.
14. Hosseini A, Gill TJ, Van de Velde SK, Li G. Estimation of in vivo ACL force changes in response to increased weightbearing. J Biomech Eng. 2011 May;133(5):051004-1–9.
15. Cawley PW, France EP, Paulos LE. Comparison of rehabilitative knee braces: A biomechanical investigation. Am J Sports Med. 1989 Mar–Apr;17(2):141–6.
16. Kim JG, Lee YS, Yang BS, Oh SJ, Yang, SJ. Rehabilitation after posterior cruciate ligament reconstruction: a review of the literature and theoretical support. Arch Orthop Trauma Surg. 2013 Dec;133(12):1687–95.
17. Daniel DM, Stone ML, Barnett P, Sachs R. Use of the quadriceps active test to diagnose posterior cruciate-ligament disruption and measure posterior laxity of the knee. J Bone Joint Surg Am. 1988 Mar;70(3):386–91.
18. Jung YB, Tae SK, Lee YS, Jung HJ, Nam CH, Park SJ. Active non-operative treatment of acute isolated posterior cruciate ligament injury with cylinder cast immobilization. Knee Surg Sports Traumatol Arthrosc. 2008 Aug;16(8):729–33.
19. Parolie JM, Bergfeld JA. Long-term results of nonoperative treatment of isolated posterior cruciate ligament injuries in the athlete. Am J Sports Med. 1986 Jan–Feb;14(1):35–8.
20. Strobel MJ, Weiler A, Schulz MS, Russe K, Eichhorn HJ. Fixed posterior subluxation in posterior cruciate ligament-deficient knees: diagnosis and treatment of a new clinical sign. Am J Sports Med. 2002 Jan–Feb;30(1):32–8.
21. Noyes' Knee Disorders: Surgery, Rehabilitation, Clinical Outcomes by Frank R. Noyes, Rehabilitation of posterior cruciate ligament and posterolateral reconstructive procedures, Page 634, © 2009.

Complications and PCL Reconstruction

27

Matthew S. Marcus and Jason L. Koh

Introduction

Posterior cruciate ligament (PCL) injuries and reconstructions are relatively infrequent. The incidence has been reported to be between 1 and 44 % of all acute knee injuries [1]. Therefore, our understanding and experience with the operative treatment of PCL injuries lag that of anterior cruciate ligament (ACL) injuries. This lack of familiarity with the diagnosis, procedure, and rehabilitation, combined with the proximity of neurovascular structures, results in a significantly higher rate of complications (> 20 % of cases) during the treatment of PCL injuries when compared to ACL injuries. This chapter reviews the complications associated with PCL injuries.

Anatomy and Diagnosis

The PCL is an intra-articular, extra-synovial ligament found in the knee. Its femoral attachment is on the medial femoral condyle. On the tibial side, the PCL attaches to a fovea approximately 1.0–1.5 cm below the joint line. The PCL is composed of two bundles: the anterolateral (AL) and posteromedial (PM) bundle, with the AL bundle twice as large as the PM bundle [2]. It receives its vascular supply from the middle geniculate artery, a branch directly off the popliteal artery [3]. The PCL is innervated by the posterior articular nerve, a branch off the tibial nerve [4].

PCL injuries occur usually from an external force. A dashboard injury is the classic mechanism, where the knee is flexed and a posteriorly directed force is transmitted through the proximal tibia. A fall directly onto the knee, with a plantar flexed foot, also can result in a PCL injury. Noncontact PCL injuries can occur with forced knee hyperflexion, which mainly causes a partial tear. Knee hyperextension, combined with a varus or valgus force, results in a multiligamentous knee injury [5]. A careful physical examination and imaging are important to determine if a multiligamentous injury has occurred; a lack of recognition can result in significant complications such as uncorrected laxity or graft failure.

PCL-injured patients do not typically feel a "pop" when the injury occurs, nor do they have a sense of instability. Most patients will have some posterior pain, mild swelling, stiffness, and may lack terminal flexion [6]. The most accurate clinical exam for PCL injuries is the posterior drawer test. Normally, the tibial plateau sits 1 cm anterior to the femoral condyles with the knee flexed to 90°. The PCL injury is graded by the amount of posterior tibial translation in this position. Grade I is increased translation (0–5 mm), but tibia remains anterior to femoral condyles, grade II is with the tibia flush with the femoral condyle (5–10 mm), and grade III is when the tibia is posterior to the femoral condyles (> 10 mm) [5]. Magnetic resonance imaging (MRI) is the diagnostic study of choice for a PCL injury [7].

Initial Injury Complications

Complications can be associated with the initial injury. Most of these complications are a neurovascular injury from a multiligamentous knee injury, not an isolated PCL injury. Overall, there is a 30 % incidence of neurovascular injury with a knee dislocation. A vascular injury occurs 32 % (16–64 %) of the time. The injury severity can range from an intimal tear to a complete transection, requiring vascular surgery intervention [8, 9]. The common peroneal nerve is the site of most nerve injuries. The incidence is 10–40 % with knee dislocations. As with vascular injuries, the injury severity can vary: neuropraxia to complete transection

J. L. Koh (✉)
Orthopaedic Surgery, NorthShore University HealthSystem,
2650 Ridge Ave., Walgreen's 2505, Evanston, IL 60201, USA
e-mail: jkoh@northshore.org; e-mail: DAffinati@northshore.org

M. S. Marcus
40 N. State Street #2304, Chicago, IL 60654, USA
e-mail: Matthew.s.marcus@gmail.com

G. C. Fanelli (ed.), *Posterior Cruciate Ligament Injuries*,
DOI 10.1007/978-3-319-12072-0_27, © Springer International Publishing Switzerland 2015

[9, 10]. Therefore, it is crucial to do a complete neurovascular exam when working up a multiligamentous knee.

Nonoperative Treatment Complications

PCL injury treatment is still controversial; there are no agreed-upon indications for the surgical management or the rehabilitation protocols. With that in mind, most grade-I and grade-II PCL injuries are treated nonoperatively in a knee brace with the knee in the extended position. There is protected weight bearing, advance in range of motion, and quadriceps strengthening. Most patients return to sports in 2–6 weeks. A grade-III PCL injury can also be treated nonoperatively, but the outcomes are less predictable. Complications from nonoperative treatment include laxity, stiffness, knee pain, degenerative joint disease, and reflex sympathetic dystrophy [11–13].

Laxity can persist in a PCL-injured knee treated nonoperatively, particularly the grade-III injuries. Shelbourne et al. prospectively followed nonoperatively treated grade-I and grade-II PCL injuries for 5.4 years. Out of 68 patient cohorts available for complete follow-up, 63 had the same or decreased laxity, while 5 patients had increased laxity. In addition, 46 % of patients had subjective feelings of instability according to the modified Noyes subjective stability scores [14].

Pain also can persist in the nonoperatively treated PCL-injured knee. Keller et al. retrospectively reviewed 40 patients with isolated PCL injuries. They had a mean of 6 years of data for the patients. About 90 % complained of continued pain in their knee, 65 % felt their knee limited their activities, and 43 % had difficulty walking [15].

Even though most studies show good results in patients with PCL-deficient knees, by no means are their knees normal. A PCL-deficient knee has increased contact pressures in the medial and patellofemoral compartments [16–18]. This occurs because of increased posterior translation of the tibia on the femur. The overload in the medial femoral and patellofemoral compartments can be seen with the degenerative changes noted in these compartments in the PCL-deficient knee. Geissler and Whipple looked at associated injuries in acute and chronic PCL-deficient knees. In the acute group, they found 12 % had chondral defects and 27 % had meniscal tears. In the chronic group, they found 49 % had chondral defects and 36 % had meniscal tears, both mostly found on the medial side [19].

Intraoperative Complications

Surgical indications include instability, bony avulsion of PCL, and multiligamentous knees. When the PCL is treated surgically, it is done with the use of autograft or allograft to reconstruct the ligament. Salzler et al. recently looked at the complication rates of six common knee arthroscopic procedures, including PCL reconstruction. They found the overall complication rate for arthroscopic knee surgery was 4.7 %; however, 20.1 % of PCL reconstructions had a complication [20]. Complications that can occur during PCL reconstruction intraoperatively are neurovascular injury, medial femoral condyle osteonecrosis, tibial or patella fracture, compartment syndrome, and tourniquet complications.

The most devastating intraoperative complication is a neurovascular injury. The popliteal artery and tibial nerve lie posterior to the posterior horn of the lateral meniscus, separated from the knee joint by only the capsule. The popliteal artery lies approximately 7–8 mm posterior to the tibial insertion of the PCL [11, 21–23]. This distance decreases with the knee in the extended position, and increases with knee flexion to 9–10 mm [22] (Fig. 27.1). When using the transtibial technique, the guidewire will exit in the PCL fossa, which is subsequently reamed. If one drills or reams a few millimeters too far, the neurovascular structures are in close proximity. They may be in even closer proximity in revision cases where the neurovascular structures can be adherent to

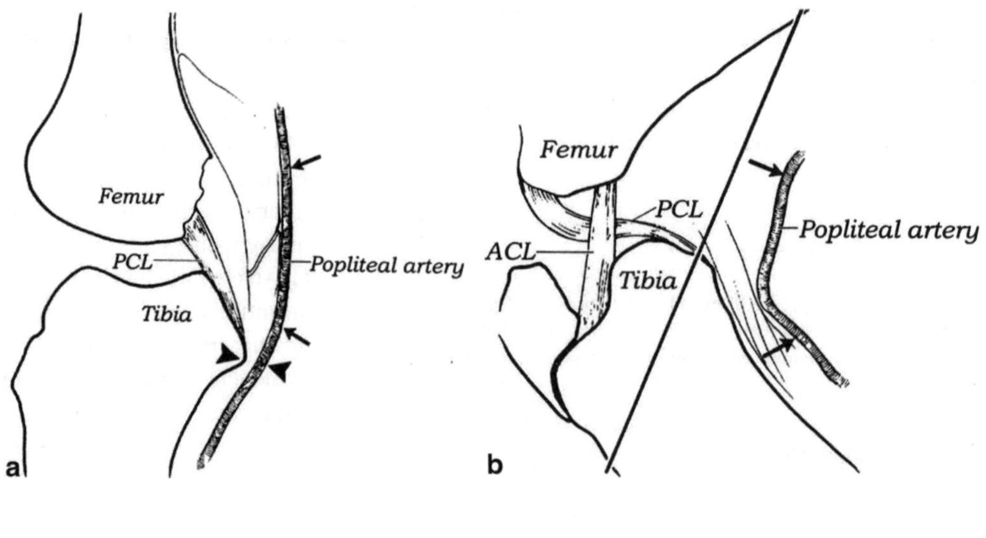

Fig. 27.1 **a** Distance to *popliteal artery* in extension. **b** Increased distance to *popliteal artery* in knee flexion. (From Ref. [22]. Reprinted with permission from Elsevier Limited)

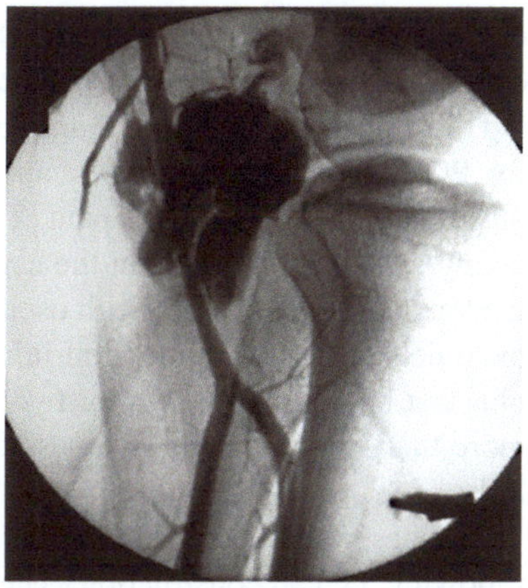

Fig. 27.2 Popliteal artery injury during posterior cruciate ligament reconstruction. (From Ref. [1]. Reprinted with permission from Elsevier Limited)

the posterior capsule. The neurovascular bundle can be directly injured or become entangled with the drill bit. There have been case reports of both popliteal artery laceration [1] (Fig. 27.2) and popliteal artery occlusion [24] during arthroscopic PCL reconstruction.

Several techniques have been developed to decrease the risk of this feared complication. Knee flexion to 100° increases the distance between the posterior tibia and popliteal neurovascular bundle [22]. Posterior capsular release off of the proximal posterior tibia can also increase the distance to the neurovascular structures [25] (Fig. 27.3). Fluoroscopy can be used to monitor the position of the guidewire and reamer [11]. Guide pins can be inadvertently advanced while reaming occurs, so great care should be used to either arthroscopically or radiographically visualize or palpate the guide pin and reamer. The guide pin or reamer can be advanced by hand through the posterior cortex to enter the fossa in a controlled fashion. Specialized guides that have a large backstop to prevent the excessive advancement of the guide pin or reamer can be used to decrease the risk of penetration. Retrograde cutting techniques also decrease the risk of injuring posterior structures, although anterograde drilling remains a part of these procedures. A PM safety incision as described by Fanelli [26] (Fig. 27.4) allows the surgeon to place their fingers extracapsular to protect the neurovascular bundle [11]. Similarly, the open tibial inlay procedure uses a similar interval and retractors to protect the popliteal artery and nerve.

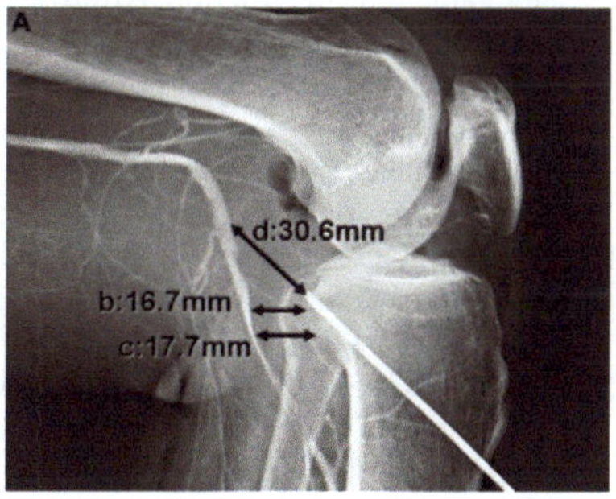

Fig. 27.3 Increased distance after a tibial-side posterior capsule release. (From Ref. [25]. Reprinted with permission from SAGE Publications)

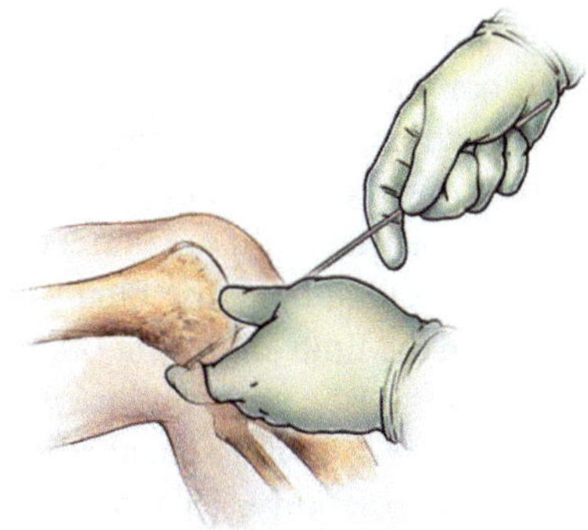

Fig. 27.4 Posteromedial safety incision. (From Ref. [40]. Reprinted with permission from WB/Saunders Co)

Osteonecrosis of the medial femoral condyle has been reported from PCL reconstruction [27]. The extraosseous and intraosseous blood supply to the medial femoral condyle is more tenuous than the lateral femoral condyle [28]. Drilling the femoral tunnel for PCL reconstruction, may cause injury to the single nutrient vessel found in the medial femoral condyle. Osteonecrosis of the medial femoral condyle can lead to continued medial-sided knee pain [11, 27, 28]. Prevention of this complication can be accomplished by leaving a sufficient bone bridge of 8–10 mm between the femoral tunnel and the articular surface of the medial femoral condyle [11].

Tibial fractures are a rare complication of PCL reconstruction. This can occur if the tunnel is too large. It is also seen in double-bundle PCL reconstruction or combined ACL/PCL reconstructions if the tunnels converge. Thus, to prevent this complication, one must have divergent tunnels. In addition, tibial fractures have been reported during hammering a staple for fixation [11, 23]. Patellar or tibial fractures can also occur due to bone–patellar tendon–bone (BPTB) harvesting. The reported rate for fracture during BPTB harvesting during ACL surgery ranges from 0.2 to 2.3 % [29–31].

Other complications that can arise intraoperatively are related to the use of a tourniquet and compartment syndrome. Tourniquets can help provide a bloodless field for operating, but this does not come without potential complications. Muscle injury, nerve injury, metabolic dysfunction, coagulopathy, and deep vein thrombosus have all been reported [32]. Compartment syndrome after knee arthroscopy has been reported and is a rare complication. This can occur by a rent in the capsule, which leads to fluid extravasation in the operative leg [23, 33]. In addition, positioning can result in compartment syndrome of the contralateral extremity, including a case report of gluteal compartment syndrome after PCL reconstruction [23].

Postoperative Complications

There are several complications that can arise is the postoperative period after PCL reconstruction. These include continued laxity, stiffness, anterior knee pain, painful hardware, heterotopic ossification (HO), and infection. A continued laxity after surgical reconstruction of the PCL can be due to both bony and soft tissue problems. A malalignment of the lower extremity with a varus deformity at the knee leads to a lateral thrusting gate. This can have a deleterious effect on a PCL reconstruction if not corrected prior to PCL reconstruction with a high tibial osteotomy [11, 34].

When the limb alignment is normal and there is persistent laxity, soft tissue problems are most likely the culprit. Inaccurate diagnosis of associated ligament injuries can lead to increased instability. This is particularly true with an unrecognized posterolateral corner injury (PLC). When there is a PLC injury and it is not reconstructed with a concomitant PCL injury, the posterior tibial insertion of the PCL rotates medially and anteriorly. This leads to a relative shortening of the distance from the medial femoral condyle to its tibial insertion, resulting is a functionally lax PCL [11]. A missed diagnosis can be avoided by a diligent physical exam and careful review of MRI. Technical errors in the PCL reconstruction is another soft tissue reason for the continued laxity. Early graft loading during rehabilitation can lead to laxity and clinical instability [23]. Femoral tunnels placed too posterior and/or proximal to the femoral isometric point, lead to decreased graft tension in flexion, and thus the knee feels lax [23, 35]. In addition, insufficient graft size and strength and improper graft tensioning can lead to knee laxity [11, 35, 36]. The use of a tensioning boot may avoid excess laxity. Meticulous surgical technique and rehabilitation are key to help avoid these problems.

Loss of flexion after PCL reconstruction is more common than the loss of extension [37]. The loss of flexion becomes functionally limiting when the patient is limited to 110° or less. This can be due suprapatellar adhesions, arthrofibrosis, improper tunnel placement, improper graft tensioning, nonisometric nature of the PCL, multiligamentous procedures, and poor compliance with physical therapy [11, 23]. Suprapatellar adhesion can occur after an arthrotomy or bone-quadriceps tendon autograft harvesting. These adhesions lead to loss of flexion. These patients can be treated with manipulation under anesthesia and arthroscopic lysis of adhesions [11, 23]. Femoral tunnel placement leads to loss of flexion when they are located too anterior and/or distal to the femoral isometric point [23, 35]. Fanelli and Monahan reported on 120 PCL injuries, most of them combined ligament injuries. They found an average of 10° loss of flexion and 5.4% required lysis of adhesions and manipulation [11]. In addition, the inherent nonisometric nature of PCL reconstructions to reproduce the complex arrangement of the PCL fibers leads to the loss of flexion [11, 23].

Anterior knee pain after PCL reconstruction is the result of continued laxity, prominent hardware, or donor-site morbidity. When the reconstructed PCL is lax, there is a continued posterior sag of the knee with patella baja. This will lead to an increase in contact pressure in the patellofemoral joint, causing anterior knee pain [11, 17, 18]. Prominent hardware can cause anterior knee pain. This can be treated by removing the fixation device [11]. If autologous BPTB is harvested for PCL reconstruction, there can be donor-site morbidity presenting as anterior knee pain. This can be prevented by taking a graft no larger than the central third of the patellar tendon, taking bone plugs with oscillating saw instead of osteotomes to minimize chondral injuries, and taking patellar plug not be more than inferior two thirds of patella and not more than one third the thickness of the median ridge [11, 23].

HO has been reported in the literature as a complication following PCL reconstruction. There are rare case reports describing posterolateral capsular HO believed to be the result of femoral tunnel reaming. If the HO is prominent, it can affect a patient's range of motion. In these cases, removing to HO should improve a patient's range of motion [23].

Wound infections and septic arthritis are complications of all operative procedures. In ACL reconstruction, meniscal repair and prior knee surgery were found to increase the risk of infection [38, 39]. Wound dehiscence can occur when large flaps are not raised, specifically during the tibial inlay technique for PCL reconstruction. Prophylactic antibiotics prior to the start of the case, careful soft tissue handling, adequate skin bridges, and thick subfascial flaps can decrease these complications [11].

Conclusion

Overall, our knowledge of PCL reconstruction technique is lacking when compared to ACL reconstruction. Because of this, our complication rate is significantly higher. This chapter was meant to review potential complications we face when treating PCL injuries, both nonoperatively and operatively. As our understanding of the PCL increases in the future, our complication rate will subsequently decrease, evidenced by our improvement in ACL reconstruction.

References

1. Makino A, Costa-Paz M, Aponte-Tinao L, Ayerza MA, Muscolo DL. Popliteal artery laceration during arthroscopic posterior cruciate ligament reconstruction. Arthroscopy. 2005 Nov;21(11):1396.
2. Van Dommelen BA, Fowler PJ. Anatomy of the posterior cruciate ligament. A review. Am J Sports Med. 1989 Jan–Feb;17(1):24–9.
3. Arnoczky SP, Rubin RM, Marshall JL. Microvasculature of the cruciate ligaments and its response to injury. An experimental study in dogs. J Bone Joint Surg Am. 1979 Dec;61(8):1221–9.
4. Kennedy JC, Alexander IJ, Hayes KC. Nerve supply of the human knee and its functional importance. Am J Sports Med. 1982 Nov–Dec;10(6):329–35.
5. Clancy WG, Shelbourne KD, Zoellner GB, Keene JS, Reider B, Rosenberg TD. Treatment of knee joint instability secondary to rupture of the posterior cruciate ligament. Report of a new procedure. J Bone Joint Surg Am. 1983 Mar;65(3):310–22.

6. Wind WM, Bergfeld JA, Parker RD. Evaluation and treatment of posterior cruciate ligament injuries: revisited. Am J Sports Med. 2004 Oct–Nov;32(7):1765–75.
7. Polly DW, Callaghan JJ, Sikes RA, McCabe JM, McMahon K, Savory CG. The accuracy of selective magnetic resonance imaging compared with the findings of arthroscopy of the knee. J Bone Joint Surg Am. 1988 Feb;70(2):192–8.
8. Gray JL, Cindric M. Management of arterial and venous injuries in the dislocated knee. Sports Med Arthrosc. 2011 Jun;19(2):131–8.
9. Rihn JA, Groff YJ, Harner CD, Cha PS. The acutely dislocated knee: evaluation and management. J Am Acad Orthop Surg. 2004 Sep–Oct;12(5):334–46.
10. Peskun CJ, Chahal J, Steinfeld ZY, Whelan DB. Risk factors for peroneal nerve injury and recovery in knee dislocation. Clin Orthop Relat Res. 2012 Mar;470(3):774–8.
11. Fanelli GC, Monahan TJ. Complications in posterior cruciate ligament and posterolateral corner surgery. Oper Tech Sports Med. 2001;9(2):4.
12. Lubowitz JH, Elson W, Guttmann D. Complications in the treatment of medial and lateral sided injuries of the knee joint. Sports Med Arthrosc. 2006 Mar;14(1):51–5.
13. Paulos LE, Wnorowski DC, Beck CL. Rehabilitation following knee surgery. Recommendations. Sports Med. 1991 Apr;11(4):257–75.
14. Shelbourne KD, Davis TJ, Patel DV. The natural history of acute, isolated, nonoperatively treated posterior cruciate ligament injuries. A prospective study. Am J Sports Med. 1999 May–Jun;27(3):276–83.
15. Keller PM, Shelbourne KD, McCarroll JR, Rettig AC. Nonoperatively treated isolated posterior cruciate ligament injuries. Am J Sports Med. 1993 Jan–Feb;21(1):132–6.
16. Logan M, Williams A, Lavelle J, Gedroyc W, Freeman M. The effect of posterior cruciate ligament deficiency on knee kinematics. Am J Sports Med. 2004 Dec;32(8):1915–22.
17. MacDonald P, Miniaci A, Fowler P, Marks P, Finlay B. A biomechanical analysis of joint contact forces in the posterior cruciate deficient knee. Knee Surg Sports Traumatol Arthrosc. 1996;3(4):252–5.
18. Skyhar MJ, Warren RF, Ortiz GJ, Schwartz E, Otis JC. The effects of sectioning of the posterior cruciate ligament and the posterolateral complex on the articular contact pressures within the knee. J Bone Joint Surg Am. 1993 May;75(5):694–9.
19. Geissler WB, Whipple TL. Intraarticular abnormalities in association with posterior cruciate ligament injuries. Am J Sports Med. 1993 Nov–Dec;21(6):846–9.
20. Salzler MJ, Lin A, Miller CD, Herold S, Irrgang JJ, Harner CD. Complications after arthroscopic knee surgery. Am J Sports Med. 2014 Feb;42(2):292–6.
21. Cosgarea AJ, Kramer DE, Bahk MS, Totty WG, Matava MJ. Proximity of the popliteal artery to the PCL during simulated knee arthroscopy: implications for establishing the posterior trans-septal portal. J Knee Surg. 2006 Jul;19(3):181–5.
22. Matava MJ, Sethi NS, Totty WG. Proximity of the posterior cruciate ligament insertion to the popliteal artery as a function of the knee flexion angle: implications for posterior cruciate ligament reconstruction. Arthroscopy. 2000 Nov;16(8):796–804.
23. Zawodny SR, Miller MD. Complications of posterior cruciate ligament surgery. Sports Med Arthrosc. 2010 Dec;18(4):269–74.
24. Wu RW, Hsu CC, Wang CJ. Acute popliteal artery occlusion after arthroscopic posterior cruciate ligament reconstruction. Arthroscopy. 2003 Oct;19(8):889–93.
25. Ahn JH, Wang JH, Lee SH, Yoo JC, Jeon WJ. Increasing the distance between the posterior cruciate ligament and the popliteal neurovascular bundle by a limited posterior capsular release during arthroscopic transtibial posterior cruciate ligament reconstruction: a cadaveric angiographic study. Am J Sports Med. 2007 May;35(5):787–92.
26. Fanelli GC, Edson CJ, Reinheimer KN, Garofalo R. Posterior cruciate ligament and posterolateral corner reconstruction. Sports Med Arthrosc. 2007 Dec;15(4):168–75.
27. Athanasian EA, Wickiewicz TL, Warren RF. Osteonecrosis of the femoral condyle after arthroscopic reconstruction of a cruciate ligament. Report of two cases. J Bone Joint Surg Am. 1995 Sep;77(9):1418–22.
28. Reddy AS, Frederick RW. Evaluation of the intraosseous and extraosseous blood supply to the distal femoral condyles. Am J Sports Med. 1998 May–Jun;26(3):415–9.
29. Lee GH, McCulloch P, Cole BJ, Bush-Joseph CA, Bach BR. The incidence of acute patellar tendon harvest complications for anterior cruciate ligament reconstruction. Arthroscopy. 2008 Feb;24(2):162–6.
30. Stein DA, Hunt SA, Rosen JE, Sherman OH. The incidence and outcome of patella fractures after anterior cruciate ligament reconstruction. Arthroscopy. 2002 Jul–Aug;18(6):578–83.
31. Viola R, Vianello R. Three cases of patella fracture in 1,320 anterior cruciate ligament reconstructions with bone-patellar tendon-bone autograft. Arthroscopy. 1999 Jan–Feb;15(1):93–7.
32. Fitzgibbons PG, Digiovanni C, Hares S, Akelman E. Safe tourniquet use: a review of the evidence. J Am Acad Orthop Surg. 2012 May;20(5):310–9.
33. Ekman EF, Poehling GG. An experimental assessment of the risk of compartment syndrome during knee arthroscopy. Arthroscopy. 1996 Apr;12(2):193–9.
34. Noyes FR, Barber-Westin SD. Posterior cruciate ligament revision reconstruction, part 1: causes of surgical failure in 52 consecutive operations. Am J Sports Med. 2005 May;33(5):646–54.
35. Burns WC, Draganich LF, Pyevich M, Reider B. The effect of femoral tunnel position and graft tensioning technique on posterior laxity of the posterior cruciate ligament-reconstructed knee. Am J Sports Med. 1995 Jul–Aug;23(4):424–30.
36. Ogata K, McCarthy JA. Measurements of length and tension patterns during reconstruction of the posterior cruciate ligament. Am J Sports Med. 1992 May–Jun;20(3):351–5.
37. Irrgang JJ, Harner CD. Loss of motion following knee ligament reconstruction. Sports Med. 1995 Feb;19(2):150–9.
38. Viola R, Marzano N, Vianello R. An unusual epidemic of Staphylococcus-negative infections involving anterior cruciate ligament reconstruction with salvage of the graft and function. Arthroscopy. 2000 Mar;16(2):173–7.
39. McAllister DR, Parker RD, Cooper AE, Recht MP, Abate J. Outcomes of postoperative septic arthritis after anterior cruciate ligament reconstruction. Am J Sports Med. 1999 Sep–Oct; 27(5):562–70.
40. Fanelli GC, Boyd J. How I manage PCL injuries. Oper Tech Sports Med. 2009;17:175–83.

Part VII
Outcomes of Treatment

Results of Treatment of Posterior Cruciate Ligament Surgery

28

Iftach Hetsroni, Samuel A. Taylor and Robert G. Marx

Introduction

Interpreting outcome after posterior cruciate ligament reconstruction (PCLR) is a complex task given that only a subset of all PCLRs is performed in isolation [1]. More commonly, these procedures are performed as combined-ligament (PCL–anterior cruciate ligament (ACL) or PCL-lateral or medial-side) or multiligament (three or more ligaments) knee reconstructions. Postoperative instrumented and non-instrumented knee laxities are therefore influenced by the complex interrelations in multiple planes among several reconstructed ligaments. Moreover, there is inconsistency among authors as to reported outcome scales and a relatively low methodological quality has been demonstrated for the majority of these studies [2]. On the other hand, positive correlation has recently been demonstrated between quality of PCLR outcome studies (as reflected by their methodological score) and the year of publication [2].

In order to summarize current knowledge about outcomes of PCLR in view of the quality of PCLR outcome studies in recent years [2], a PubMed search of the English literature was performed to identify review manuscripts assessing PCLR outcomes that were published between 2010 and December 2013. Related citations of original research that reported posterior laxity at a minimum 2 years follow-up for specific groups of isolated PCLRs or for PCL-based combined- or multiligament reconstructions, and that were published in the past 10 years only (i.e., between 2003 and 2013) were retrieved from these reviews. Studies reporting postoperative posterior laxity in mixed groups of isolated and combined reconstructions or in cases of revision PCL surgeries, and studies that did not report side-to-side posterior laxity outcome by KT-1000/2000 or by posterior stress radiographs were excluded from our review. Outcome measures included: posterior knee laxity, range of knee motion, degree of knee arthritis, and scores of activity level and function.

Posterior Knee Laxity

Table 28.1 summarizes posterior knee laxity outcomes after isolated PCLR, measured with knee arthrometer, stress radiographs, and physical examination. By using knee arthrometer, most studies showed that mean side-to-side differences were below 3 mm [3–12], which is considered within the acceptable range of knee laxity. Nevertheless, mean side-to-side values were above 3 mm in yet a substantial portion of the cases [13–16]. Moreover, some studies demonstrated wide range of side-to-side differences despite the apparently normal mean values [9–11]. In terms of posterior drawer tests, grade-0 (i.e., less than 3 mm) and grade-1 (i.e., 3–5 mm) posterior laxity was achieved in 55–94 % of the cases [3–6, 12, 14, 16–21], but only a small subset of studies showed recreation of grade-0 posterior laxity (i.e., normal laxity) in the majority of their cases [3, 12, 16, 20]. Stress radiographs showed mean side-to-side values of 2–4 mm, but again large ranges or large standard deviations in side-to-side differences were observed in some cases [7, 13, 22, 23]. Of note, in most cases, no significant differences in posterior laxity outcomes were detected among different graft types [9, 18, 22], between transtibial and posterior inlay techniques [15, 18], or between single- versus double-bundle PCLRs [10, 19, 24], although there were some exceptions [23, 24]. Side-to-side posterior laxity findings after PCL-based multiligament reconstructions (Table 28.2) showed posterior laxity less than 3 mm in 55–76 % of the cases [25–28]. Again, similar to

R. G. Marx (✉) · S. A. Taylor
Sports Medicine and Shoulder Service,
Hospital for Special Surgery and Weill Medical College of Cornell University,
New York, NY, USA
e-mail: MarxR@hss.edu

I. Hetsroni
Department of Orthopedic Surgery, Meir General Hospital, Sapir Medical Center, Kfar Saba, Israel

I. Hetsroni
Sackler Faculty of Medicine, Tel Aviv University, Tel Aviv, Israel

G. C. Fanelli (ed.), *Posterior Cruciate Ligament Injuries*,
DOI 10.1007/978-3-319-12072-0_28,

Table 28.1 Posterior knee laxity after isolated PCLR

Author, year	KT-1000/2000	Posterior drawer (%)	Telos, and other comments
Ahn et al. 2005 [22][a]	–	–	2.2 (0–7) vs. 2.9 (1–7) (p=ns)
Chan et al. 2006 [14]	0–2 in 50%; 3–5 in 35%; >5 in 15%	Grade I in 80	–
Chen and Gao, 2009 [3]	1.0±1.0	Normal in 90; Grade I in 5	–
Garofalo et al. 2006 [17]	–	Normal in 20; Grade I in 67	–
Hermans et al. 2009 [5]	2.1±1.6	Normal in 9; Grade I in 68	–
Wong et al. 2009 [11][b]	2.8 (1–6) vs. 3.3 (1–10) (p=ns)	–	–
Jung et al. 2004 [7]	1.8±1.2	–	3.4±2.4 64% had 3 mm increased displacement
Kim et al. 2009 [24][c]	–	–	3.6±1.4 vs. 5.6±2.0 (p<0.03)
Lim et al. 2010 [32]	0–2 in 23%; 3–5 in 68%	–	–
MacGillivray et al. 2006 [15][d]	5.9 vs. 5.5 (p=ns)	Grade I–II in 70	–
Seon and Song, 2006 [18][e]	–	Grade I in 90 vs. 91	–
Wang et al. 2004 [10][f]	2.3 (1–6) vs. 3.1 (0–7) (p=ns)	–	–
Wang et al. 2004 [9][g]	3.2 (1–10) vs. 2.8 (1–6) (p=ns)	–	–
Wang et al. 2003 [20]		Normal in 52	–
Wu et al. 2007 [21]	0–2 in 46%; 3–5 in 18%	Grade I in 73	–
Zhao and Huangfu, 2007 [16][h]	3.7±1.6 vs. 1.7±1.4 (p<0.05)	Normal in 52 vs. 68	–
Zhao et al. 2008 [20]	<3 mm in 94%	Normal in 94	–
Jackson WF et al. 2008 [6]	1.1±1.9	Normal in 36; grade I in 55	–
Deehan DJ et al. 200 [34]	<2 in 74%; 3–4 in 26%	Normal in 50; grade I in 46	–
Shon OJ et al. 2010 [19][i]	–	Normal–grade I in 93 vs. 94	3.0±1.1 vs. 2.6±0.5 (p=ns)
Yoon KH et al. 2011 [23][j]	–	–	4.5±2.3 vs. 3.1±2.4 (p<0.05)
Sekiya JK et al. 2005 [8]	<3 mm in 62%; 3–5 in 31%	–	–
Adachi N et al. 2007 [13]	3.7±2.4	–	3.5±2.7

KT-1000/2000 is presented as mean side-to-side difference in millimeter (± SD, or range) for entire study group or for subgroups
Posterior drawer is presented as percent "normal" and "grade I" (the others were grade II and III)
Telos represents side-to-side posterior displacement on stress radiographs in mm (±SD or range)
SD standard deviation, *PCLR* posterior cruciate ligament reconstruction
[a] Double-loop hamstrings vs. Achilles allograft
[b] Anteromedial tibial tunnel drilling vs. anterolateral tibial tunnel drilling
[c] Tibial inlay Achilles allograft double bundle vs. transtibial Achilles allograft single bundle
[d] Transtibial vs. tibial inlay
[e] Transtibial autologous quadrupled hamstrings vs. tibial inlay autologous bone-patellar tendon-bone
[f] Single-bundle vs. double-bundle autologous hamstrings
[g] Autograft vs. allograft
[h] Four-strand hamstrings vs. seven-strand hamstrings
[i] Single- vs. double-bundle tibial inlay
[j] Single-bundle vs. double-bundle transtibial Achilles allograft

Table 28.2 Posterior knee laxity after PCL-based combined- and multiligament reconstruction

Author, year	KT-1000/2000	Posterior drawer	Concomitant ligaments
Lo et al. 2009 [26]	2.6 (0–7)	Normal in 55%; grade I in 45%	Ligaments reconstructed included ACL and PCL in all 11 patients, PLC in 3 patients, and MCL repair in 4 patients
Strobel et al. 2006 [29]	2 (−4 to 7)	Grade I–II in 88%	Ligaments reconstructed included ACL and PCL and PLC
Zhao et al. 2006 [27]	0–2 in 75%; 3–4 in 25%	–	Ligaments reconstructed included ACL and PCL
Zhao et al. 2008 [28]	0–2 in 16 patients (76%); 3–5 in 4 patients; 6–10 in 1 patient	–	Ligaments reconstructed included ACL and PCL
Fanelli and Edson, 2004 [25]	2.0 (−2 to 7)	Normal in 70%; grade I in 27%	Ligaments reconstructed included PCL and PLC
Khanduja et al. 2006 [30]	–	Normal in 37%; grade I in 58%	Ligaments reconstructed included PCL and PLC

PCL posterior cruciate ligament, *ACL* anterior cruciate ligament, *MCL* medial collateral ligament, *PLC* posterolateral corner isolated PCLR, wide variability in side-to-side posterior laxity values was noticed [25, 26]. From the most current data, it appeared that in the majority of the cases PCLRs produced normal or nearly normal posterior laxity measurements. The wide spread in the values may be related to differences in postoperative rehabilitation, not just surgical technique. The clinical significance of residual posterior laxity remains unclear since patients may function well during activities of daily living and may not be aware of this residual laxity unless they participate in high-level sports.

Range of Knee Motion

After isolated PCLR, limitation in range of knee motion was most commonly encountered during terminal flexion as opposed to terminal extension (Table 28.3). Approximately 10 % of patients undergoing PCLR were affected by some motion limitations [4, 6, 11, 12, 14, 16, 19, 21], but up to 20 % of patients had impaired motion in some reports [4, 17]. When present, knee flexion deficit was usually 5°–10° [3–5, 8, 12, 14, 16, 17, 19, 30], but was reported as high as 25° or more in rare cases [21, 22]. Nevertheless, functional impairment was minimal given the relatively minor loss in terminal flexion (5°–10°) and its minimal impact on activities of daily living and in sports that do not require deep bend or a squatting position. A loss of terminal knee extension was noticed in fewer studies [3, 6, 8, 12, 14, 16]. When reported, some indicated only "loss of hyperextension" but not lacking the ability to straighten the knee to 0° [12, 16]. Rarely did patients require manipulation under anesthesia (MUA) or lysis of adhesions after isolated PCLR (only 4–7 % of cases) [4, 5, 22, 23]. Similarly, with regard to lost range of motion, PCLR in the combined- or multiligament injured knee was generally related to terminal flexion rather than terminal extension (Table 28.4). Compared to isolated PCLR, loss of terminal knee flexion after PCL-based combined- or multiligament reconstruction was as twice as common, involving 12–24 % of the cases [26, 28, 29]. The amount of flexion deficit was also greater after PCL-based combined- or multiligament reconstruction compared to isolated PCLR, ranging between 10° and more than 25° [25, 26, 28, 29]. Severe stiffness that required MUA and lysis of adhesions after PCL-based combined- or multiligament reconstruction were also roughly twice as common as after isolated PCLR, affecting 7–11 % of patients [25, 26, 30]. Of note, in one series of combined PCL–ACL reconstructions, MUA was performed in 67 % of the cases [27]. Limitation in range of motion may be multifactorial. It could be related to tunnel location, amount of tension applied to the graft, knee angle during graft tensioning, other reconstructed ligaments, and arthrofibrosis related to early surgery. Moreover, limitation of knee motion may also be related to postoperative management guidelines such as duration of immobilization. In summary, the current literature suggests that lost terminal flexion is more common than loss of extension, but is relatively uncommon among patients who underwent isolated PCLR. PCL-based combined- or multiligament reconstructions, however, demonstrate lost flexion in more than 10 % of the patients and may be sufficient to necessitate an additional procedure aimed at restoration of motion. No differences in postoperative range of motion deficits are expected among different graft types, and between single- versus double-bundle PCLRs, but this lack of difference should be viewed in light of the very weak statistical power of such a comparison as a result of the small numbers of patients affected by loss of motion in these series [16, 19, 23, 24].

Knee Arthritis

After isolated PCLR, normal joint or minimal (grade I) degenerative changes were reported in 54–100 % of the cases[5, 6, 8–12, 14, 15, 20, 21], leaving up to 46 % of the cases with more significant (grade II–III) degenerative changes that was noticed in a small subset of these reports [6, 8, 15, 20]. No differences in the incidence of knee arthritis were observed between single- versus double-bundle [10] or between allograft versus autograft reconstructions [9]. After PCL-based multiligament knee reconstructions, grade II–III degenerative changes were observed in up to 60 % of the cases [29], which may be explained by the often high-energy mechanism of injury and/or concomitant intraarticular fractures. Some of these patients had chronic knee instability with recurrent giving way necessitating PCLR. These factors may all be closely related to the development of degenerative changes within the knee. The contribution of the PCLR surgery itself to the progression of arthritis is unknown. Moreover, it has been shown that the degree of degenerative changes in the knee in such cases is correlated with the duration between injury and surgery, the degree of ligament laxity, and the duration of follow-up after surgery [20]. When high incidence of significant arthritis was noticed, follow-up after surgery exceeded 10 years [6]. In summary, the majority of knees after PCLR show only minimal degenerative changes at more than 2-year follow-up. Nevertheless, the incidence of significant arthritis increases when the operation involves PCL-based multiligament reconstruction and when follow-up time after surgery exceeds 10 years (Tables 28.5 and 28.6).

Table 28.3 Knee range of motion after isolated PCLR

Author, year	Flexion deficit n. of patients	Extension deficit n. of patients	MUA/adhesiolysis n. of patients	Comments
Ahn et al. 2005 [22][a]	0 [0/18] vs. 1[1/18=6%]	0 [0/18] vs. 0 [0/18]	0 [0/18] vs. 1 [1/18=6%]	One patient in the Achilles group had ROM 0°–90° which required MUA + adhesiolysis
Chan et al. 2006 [14]	2 [2/20=10%]	1 [1/20=5%]	0 [0/20]	Flexion deficit was 3°–5°, whereas extension deficit was 16°–25°
Chen and Gao, 2009 [3]	2 [2/19=11%]	1 [1/19=5%]	0 [0/20]	Flexion deficit was 5°–10°, whereas extension deficit was 5°
Garofalo et al. 2006 [17]	4 [4/15=27%]	0 [0/15]	0 [0/15]	Flexion deficit was 5°–10°
Hermans et al. 2009 [5]	8°±7°	0 [0/22]	1 [1/22=5%]	Flexion deficit is presented as mean ± SD
Wong et al. 2009 [11][b]	–	–	–	NR
Jung et al. 2004 [7]	–	–	–	NR
Kim et al. 2009 [24][c]	4°±2° vs. 3°±1° (p=ns)	0 [0/29]	0 [0/29]	Flexion deficit is presented as side-to-side mean ± SD difference
Lim et al. 2010 [32]	0 [0/22]	0 [0/22]	0 [0/22]	
MacGillivray et al. 2006 [15][d]	–	–	–	NR
Seon and Song, 2006 [18][e]	–	–	–	NR
Wang et al. 2004 [10][f]	–	–	–	NR
Wang et al. 2004 [9][g]	–	–	–	NR
Wang et al. 2003 [20]	–	–	–	NR
Wu et al. 2007 [21]	2 [2/22=9%]	2 [2/22=9%]	0 [0/22]	Flexion deficit was 16°–25°, whereas extension deficit was 3°–10°
Zhao and Huangfu, 2007 [16][h]	2 [2/21=10%] vs. 1 [1/22=5%]	2 [2/21=10%] vs. 1 [1/22=5%]	0 [0/43]	Flexion deficit was 5°, whereas extension loss was described as "loss of 5° hyperextension"
Zhao et al. 2008 [12]	2 [2/18=11%]	1 [1/18=6%]	0 [0/18]	Flexion deficit was 5°, whereas extension loss was described as "loss of 5° hyperextension"
Jackson WF et al. 2008 [6]	2 [2/22=9%]	1 [1/22=5%]	0 [0/22]	Flexion was above 5°, where extension deficit was above 3°
Deehan DJ et al. 2003 [4]	5 [5/24=21%]	0 [0/24]	1 [1/24=4%]	Flexion and extension deficits above 5°
Shon OJ et al. 2010 [19][i]	1 [1/14=7%]vs. 2 [2/16=13%]	0 [0/14] vs. 0 [0/16]	0 [0/14] vs. 0 [0/16]	Flexion deficit was 10
Yoon KH et al. 2011 [23][j]	See comments column	See comments column	1 [1/25=4%] vs. 2 [2/28=7%]	One [1/25=4%] vs. two [2/28=7%] patients had ROM limitations, but direction and degree of limitation not reported
Sekiya JK et al. 2005 [8]	5°± 5° [range, −1° to 18°]	1°±3° [range, −6° to 5°]	0 [0/14]	Only 14 of 21 [67%] patients returned for follow-up examination
Adachi N et al. 2007 [13]	–	–	–	NR

NR Not reported. In this case, the authors did not mention range-of-motion at latest follow-up in any way, and neither in the "complications" section of their manuscript; *ROM* range of motion; *MUA* manipulation under anesthesia; *SD* standard deviation; *CI* confidence interval; *PCLR* posterior cruciate ligament reconstruction

[a] Double-loop hamstrings vs. Achilles allograft
[b] Anteromedial tibial tunnel drilling vs. anterolateral tibial tunnel drilling
[c] Tibial inlay Achilles allograft double bundle vs. transtibial Achilles allograft single bundle
[d] Transtibial vs. tibial inlay
[e] Transtibial autologous quadrupled hamstrings vs. tibial inlay autologous bone-patellar tendon-bone
[f] Single-bundle vs. double-bundle autologous hamstrings
[g] Autograft vs. allograft
[h] Four-strand hamstrings vs. seven-strand hamstrings
[i] Single- vs. double-bundle tibial inlay
[j] Single-bundle vs. double-bundle transtibial Achilles allograft

Table 28.4 Knee range of motion after PCL-based combined- and multiligament reconstruction

Author, year	Flexion deficit n. of patients	Extension deficit n. of patients	MUA/ adhesiolysis n. of patients	Comments and ligaments reconstructed
Lo et al. 2009 [26]	2 [2/11=18%]	1 [1/11=9%]	1 [1/11=9%]	Flexion deficit was 11°–15° in one patient and above 25° in another patient. Extension deficit was 3°–5° in one patient. Ligaments reconstructed included ACL and PCL in all 11 patients, PLC in 3 patients, and MCL repair in 4 patients
Strobel et al. 2006 [29]	2 [2/17=12%]	0 [0/17]	0 [0/17]	Flexion deficit was above 15° in both patients. Ligaments reconstructed included ACL and PCL and PLC
Zhao et al. 2006 [27]	See comments column	0 [0/12]	8 [8/12=67%]	Flexion deficit is not reported. Rather, mean flexion is reported: 143°±3.7° (range, 130°–150°). Ligaments reconstructed included ACL and PCL
Zhao et al. 2008 [28]	5 [5/21=24%]	0 [0/21]	0 [0/21]	Flexion deficit was 10° in one patient, and 5° in four patients. Ligaments reconstructed included ACL and PCL
Fanelli and Edson 2004 [25]	10°	0 [0/41]	3 [3/41=7%]	Flexion deficit is presented as mean terminal flexion loss. Ligaments reconstructed included PCL and PLC
Khanduja et al. 2006 [30]	NR	NR	2 [2/19=11%]	Ligaments reconstructed included PCL and PLC

PCL posterior cruciate ligament, *ACL* anterior cruciate ligament, *MCL* medial collateral ligament, *NR* not reported, *PLC* posterolateral corner

Table 28.5. Knee arthritis after isolated PCLR

Author, year	Normal joint n. of patients	Grade I OA n. of patients	Grade II OA n. of patients	Grade III OA n. of patients	Comments
Ahn et al. 2005 [22][a]	–	–	–	–	NR
Chan et al. 2006 [14]	18/20=90%	2/20=10%	–	–	
Chen and Gao, 2009 [3]	–	–	–	–	NR
Garofalo et al. 2006 [17]	–	–	–	–	NR
Hermans et al. 2009 [5]	9/22=41%	10/22=45%	–	–	OA graded as "normal" in nine patients, "nearly normal" in ten patients, and "abnormal" in three patients
Wong et al. 2009 [11][b]	11/28=39% vs. 11/27=41% p=ns	17/28=61% vs. 16/27=59% p=ns	–	–	–
Jung et al. 2004 [7]	–	–	–	–	NR
Kim et al. 2009 [24][c]	–	–	–	–	NR
Lim et al. 2010 [32]	–	–	–	–	NR
MacGillivray et al. 2006 [15][d]	4/13=31% vs. 5/7=71%	3/13=23% vs. 2/7=29%	6/13=46% vs. 0/7	–	In this study, Grade I is mild degeneration and slightly decreased joint space; grade II is moderate joint space narrowing p=0.06 between groups
Seon and Song, 2006 [18][e]	–	–	–	–	NR
Wang et al. 2004 [10][f]	13/19=68% vs. 11/16=69% p=ns	6/19=32% vs. 5/16=31% p=ns	–	–	–
Wang et al. 2004 [9][g]	13/32=41% vs. 9/23=39% p=ns	19/32=59% vs. 14/23=61% p=ns	–	–	–
Wang et al. 2003 [20]	15/31=48%	11/31=36%	4/31=13%	1/31=3%	In this study, Grade I is mild, grade II is moderate, and grade III is severe degeneration. The patient with severe changes had comminuted intraarticular fracture of the distal femur
Wu et al. 2007 [21]	18/22=82%	4/22=18%	–	–	–
Zhao and Huangfu, 2007 [16][h]	–	–	–	–	NR
Zhao et al. 2008 [12]	18/18=100%	–	–	–	Three patients with grade III–IV cartilage lesions that had PCLR were excluded from the study group

Table 28.5. (continued)

Author, year	Normal joint n. of patients	Grade I OA n. of patients	Grade II OA n. of patients	Grade III OA n. of patients	Comments
Jackson WF et al. 2008 [6]	14/22=64%	–	4/22=18%	4/22=18%	In this study, Grading performed according to the Kellgrene–Lawrence system. Follow-up in this study was at minimum 10 years
Deehan DJ et al. 2003 [4]	–	–	–	–	NR
Shon OJ et al. 2010 [19][i]	–	–	–	–	NR
Yoon KH et al. 2011 [23][j]	–	–	–	–	NR
Sekiya JK et al. 2005 [8]	25%	50%	17%	8%	In this study, grading performed according to the IKDC system: "normal," "nearly normal," "abnormal," and "severely abnormal." Percentages, rather than actual numbers are reported
Adachi N et al. 2007 [13]	–	–	–	–	NR

Arthritis grading is reported according to Ahlback classification, unless stated otherwise
NR not reported, *OA* osteoarthritis, *PCL* posterior cruciate ligament, *PCLR* posterior cruciate ligament reconstruction, *IKDC* International Knee Documentation Committee
[a] Double-loop hamstrings vs. Achilles allograft
[b] Anteromedial tibial tunnel drilling vs. anterolateral tibial tunnel drilling
[c] Tibial inlay Achilles allograft double bundle vs. transtibial Achilles allograft single bundle
[d] Transtibial vs. tibial inlay
[e] Transtibial autologous quadrupled hamstrings vs. tibial inlay autologous bone-patellar tendon-bone
[f] Single-bundle vs. double-bundle autologous hamstrings
[g] Autograft vs. allograft
[h] Four-strand hamstrings vs. seven-strand hamstrings
[i] Single- vs. double-bundle tibial inlay
[j] Single-bundle vs. double-bundle transtibial Achilles allograft

Table 28.6 Knee arthritis after PCL-based combined- and multiligament reconstruction

Author, year	Normal joint n. of patients	Grade I n. of patients	Grade II n. of patients	Grade III n. of patients	Comments and ligaments reconstructed
Lo et al. 2009 [26]	9/11=82%	2/11=28%	–	–	All 11 patients had ACL + PCL reconstruction. Three patients had also PLC reconstruction, and four patients had also MCL repair
Strobel et al. 2006 [29]	1/17=6%	6/17=35%	8/17=47%	2/17=12%	Patients had ACL + PCL + PLC reconstruction. Joint degeneration grading performed according to the Kellgrene–Lawrence system
Zhao et al. 2006 [27]	11/12=92%	1/12=8%	–	–	Patients had ACL + PCL reconstruction
Zhao et al. 2008 [28]	NR	NR	NR	NR	Patients had ACL + PCL reconstruction. Degenerative changes outcome is not reported
Fanelli and Edson, 2004 [25]	NR	NR	NR	NR	Patients had PCL + PLC reconstruction. Degenerative changes outcome is not reported
Khanduja et al. 2006 [30]	NR	NR	NR	NR	Patients had PCL + PLC reconstruction. Postoperative radiographic articular degeneration is not reported. Rather, arthroscopic changes included four cases (4/19=21%) of grade I lesions and two cases (2/19=11%) of grade II articular lesions

PCL posterior cruciate ligament, *ACL* anterior cruciate ligament, *NR* not reported, *MCL* medial collateral ligament, *PLC* posterolateral corner

Activity Level and Functional Outcomes

The single-bundle transtibial PCLR is the most commonly described technique for PCLR. Deehan et al. followed 31 patients who underwent PCLR with a single-bundle transtibial hamstring tendon autograft technique [4]. The median Lysholm score improved from 64 to 94 at final follow-up. Only 63 % of the cohort, however, was able to participate in moderate or strenuous activity following the operation. Ahn et al. reported on 61 patients who underwent single-bundle PCLR with preservation of posterior fibers of the native PCL [31]. The mean Lysholm score improved from 65.8 preoperatively to 92.9 at 41 months follow-up. Ninety-seven percent of patients were rated normal or nearly normal according to International Knee Documentation Committee (IKDC). Other investigators also demonstrated significant improvements in functional outcome measures using single-bundle transtibial PCLR at midterm follow-up. Chan et al. reported prospective findings from 20 patients with hamstring autograft PCLR at 40 months follow-up [14]. Final average Lysholm score improved from 63 to 93 for the cohort overall. Ninety percent of patients had good or excellent results and 85 % of patients were rated as normal or near normal according to IKDC scores. Postoperative functional testing included one-leg hop test in which 55 % of patients were able to achieve 90 % of the total distance of the contralateral uninjured leg. The overall average Tegner score was 6.3, which was significantly improved from 3 preoperatively. Wu et al. published on their 5-year results of isolated PCLR with quadriceps tendon autograft [21]. Significant improvements were noted in Lysholm and Tegner scores from preoperative to postoperative, with final scores 89 and 6, respectively. Eighty-two percent of patients were rated as normal or nearly normal according to IKDC scores. Another study reported functional outcomes for 21 patients who underwent PCLR with single-bundle technique at nearly 6 years mean follow-up [8]. IKDC subjective assessment scores were normal or nearly normal in 57 % of patients and activity scores improved in 62 % of patients.

Long-Term Data

Few long-term studies have demonstrated the very-long-term durability of PCLR surgery. One study reported results after isolated anterolateral bundle reconstruction of the PCL in 25 patients at a mean of 9 years [5]. Both IKDC and Lysholm scores significantly improved from 38 to 65 and from 50 to 75, respectively. Tegner activity score at the final follow-up was 5.7. Nevertheless, while all patients had significant functional improvements in IKDC, Lysholm, Tegner, and visual analog scale (VAS), those with chondrosis had lower subjective outcomes when compared to those with normal articular cartilage. Another study evaluated long-term outcomes following PCLR with single-bundle hamstring autograft in 26 patients [6]. At a mean of 10 years postoperatively, the IKDC score was 87 and Lysholm was 90. Eighty-eight percent of the cohort was able to participate in moderate to strenuous activity and 92 % were self-reported as normal or nearly normal.

Single- Versus Double-Bundle PCLR

Several authors reported results for double-bundle PCLR techniques. Chen and Gao studied 19 patients who underwent arthroscopic four-tunnel double-bundle PCLR using quadrupled semitendinosus and gracilis autografts [3]. Eighteen of 19 patients were graded as normal or near normal and IKDC scores significantly improved from 65 to 92. Lysholm scores showed similar improvement from 63 preoperatively to 92 at final follow-up. Tegner activity score improved from 5.1 to 6.3. Similarly, Lim et al. treated 22 patients with double-bundle PCLR using an Achilles tendon allograft with double cross-pin tibial fixation [32]. At 33 months follow-up, significant improvements were noted with regard to median Lysholm score from 64 before surgery to 88 at final follow-up. Eighty-eight percent of patients were graded as normal or nearly normal according to IKDC scoring. The final Tegner score was 6. Zhao et al. used a double-bundle four-tunnel "sandwich-style" PCLR technique to treat 18 patients with isolated chronic PCL insufficiency [12]. All functional outcome measures improved from the preoperative state. Final Lysholm, IKDC, and Tegner scores were 95, 96, and 7, respectively. Eighty-nine percent of patients were rated as normal, with the remaining 11 % rated as nearly normal. Another study treated 15 patients with isolated PCL tears using a double-bundle PCLR [17]. At 3.2 years follow-up, Lysholm scores were good or excellent in all but one patient. Sixty-one percent of patients were rated as normal or nearly normal. Nevertheless, while Tegner activity score improved significantly following surgery, none of the patients was able to resume preoperative level of sport.

Comparisons of single- versus double-bundle techniques did not demonstrate any consistent advantage of one technique over the other with regard to functional outcomes. Shon et al. did not show any significant differences between single-bundle and double-bundle PCLR techniques with regard to Lysholm and Tegner scores [19]. Wang et al. prospectively studied 35 patients who underwent either single-bundle (19 patients) or double-bundle (16 patients) PCLR with hamstring autograft [10]. At a mean of 41 months follow-up, no significant differences between groups were identified regarding functional outcome measures such as pain, instability, swelling, locking, or squatting pain. Lysholm and

Tegner scores were also similar for the single-bundle (88 and 4.5, respectively) and double-bundle groups (89 and 5.2, respectively). Single-leg hop test was comparable, as were IKDC scores. Yoon et al. performed a prospective, randomized study to compare outcomes of single-bundle (25 cases) versus double-bundle (28 cases) constructs for PCLR at a minimum of 2 years follow-up [23]. They did not find any significant differences between the two groups with regard to Tegner, Lysholm, or IKDC subjective scores. Similarly, Fanelli et al. [33] compared their results of PCLR with single-bundle versus double-bundle constructs and did not find any differences in functional outcomes measured with Lysholm, Tegner, or HSS rating systems.

Combined Versus Isolated PCLR

Several studies reported functional outcomes after PCL-based combined- and multiligament knee reconstructions and showed that while functional improvements were noticed in many cases, results were not as reproducible as for isolated PCLR. Lo et al. studied simultaneous ACL reconstruction and PCLR and found good or excellent results for all but one patient [26]. Functional outcome scores were significantly improved from preoperatively. Another study reported on a similar combined reconstruction [27]. Twelve patients underwent simultaneous ACL reconstruction and PCLR with hamstring autograft. Lysholm score improved from 67 to 92 and final IKDC scores indicated seven patients as normal, and four as nearly normal. Zhao et al. showed significant improvements in Lysholm, Tegner, and Lysholm scores in a series of patients treated with simultaneous double-bundle ACL and double-bundle PCLR [28], but only 19 % of the cohort reported that they were able to resume their preinjury activity levels. Fanelli and Edson also found satisfactory functional outcomes for chronic combined PCL and posterolateral corner reconstructions (PLCRs) using Achilles tendon allograft [25]. Lysholm score was 92 and Tegner score was 5 at latest follow-up. Another study looked at combined reconstructions of the PCL and PLC in 19 patients performed with single-bundle technique and Larson technique, respectively [30]. At 2–9-year follow-up, significant improvements were observed in Lysholm and in Tegner scores (from 41 to 77, and from 2.6 to 6.4, respectively). Strobel et al. reviewed prospective data on 17 patients who underwent one-stage multiligament reconstruction of ACL, PCL, and PLC [29]. A single-bundle transtibial hamstring autograft PLCR was used in all patients. Based on IKDC scores at final follow-up, the majority of patients were rated as abnormal (ten cases) or grossly abnormal (two cases). Average IKDC subjective score was 72.

Graft Choice

Several studies compared functional outcomes among different graft choices. Ahn et al. did not show significant difference in clinical outcomes in a case-control study that compared 18 patients who underwent autologous hamstring PCLR with 18 patients in whom an Achilles tendon allograft was used [22]. No difference was seen between the two groups with regard to IKDC score, but Lysholm score favored the hamstring autograft (90 vs. 85, $P<0.01$). Of note, the clinical significance of such a small difference is questionable. Wang et al. also investigated the clinical impact of graft choice [9]. Two groups of patients (32 autograft cases vs. 23 allograft cases) who underwent arthroscopic single-bundle PCLR were prospectively followed for 34 months. There were no differences with regard to functional outcomes including pain, instability, swelling, locking, or squatting pain. There were also no differences between the groups with regard to Lysholm, Tegner, or IKDC scores. With regard to the potential effect of graft diameter on functional outcomes, Zhao and Huangfu compared functional outcomes after seven-strand hamstring autograft (8–11 mm diameter) versus four-strand hamstring autograft (5–9 mm) and showed IKDC scores were indeed better when using a larger diameter graft [16].

Inlay Versus Transtibial

Several authors compared functional outcomes after posterior inlay versus transtibial PCLR. MacGillivary et al. did not identify a superior technique when looking retrospectively at 20 patients who underwent PCLR by either transtibial or posterior inlay techniques [15]. Final follow-up was on average 5.7 years. At latest follow-up, 90 % of patients were satisfied and Tegner activity scores were identical between the groups. Seon and Song retrospectively compared 21 isolated transtibial PCLR versus 22 tibial inlay PCLR cases and also did not find technique-driven differences with regard to functional outcomes [18]. Kim et al. compared transtibial single-bundle versus arthroscopic single-bundle inlay versus arthroscopic double-bundle inlay techniques in their retrospective review of 29 patients [24]. Lysholm score improved significantly in all three groups without any significant difference identified among groups.

In summary, despite the varying reconstruction techniques and graft choices, a superior procedure for PCLR with regard to activity levels and functional outcomes has not been demonstrated. Significant improvements in function are generally ubiquitous regardless of construct, surgical technique, or graft choice, although return to preinjury activity levels may not be achieved in a significant portion of these patients, and the procedure may be less reproducible in PCL-based multiligament compared to isolated PCLRs.

Summary

It appears that while PCL reconstructive surgery can improve patient-oriented outcome scores and result in nearly normal posterior knee laxity, outcomes are not consistent across all studies. Residual knee laxity in a substantial proportion of these patients after the operation may affect their ability to resume high-level athletic activities. Despite the multiple techniques, different graft types, and a variety of fixation devices used in PCLR, significant differences are not reported among the different surgical options. While significant variety in graft choice, tensioning techniques, concomitant injuries, number of bundles reconstructed, and postoperative rehabilitation protocols make interpretation of outcomes a challenging task, improvements in methodological quality of newer studies in recent years may lead to improved outcome data for PCLR in the future.

Acknowledgments Thank you to Etti Kirschner, BA in Informatics Studies and Librarianship, and Ilana Flatau, Director of Medical Library, at the Meir General Hospital, Kfar Saba, and the Sackler Faculty of Medicine, Tel Aviv University, Tel Aviv, Israel, for their excellent assistance in performing the literature review.

References

1. Fanelli GC, Edson CJ. Posterior cruciate ligament injuries in trauma patients: part II. Arthroscopy. 1995;11:526–9.
2. Watsend AM, Osestad TM, Jakobsen RB, Engebretsen L. Clinical studies on posterior cruciate ligament tears have weak design. Knee Surg Sports Traumatol Arthrosc. 2009;17:140–9.
3. Chen B, Gao S. Double-bundle posterior cruciate ligament reconstruction using a non-hardware suspension fixation technique and 8 strands of autogenous hamstring tendons. Arthroscopy. 2009;25:777–82.
4. Deehan DJ, Salmon LJ, Russell VJ, et al. Endoscopic single-bundle posterior cruciate ligament reconstruction: results as minimum 2-year follow-up. Arthroscopy. 2003;19:955–62.
5. Hermans S, Korten K, Bellemans J. Long-term results of isolated anterolateral bundle reconstructions of the posterior cruciate ligament: a 6- to 12-year follow-up study. Am J Sports Med. 2009;37:1499–507.
6. Jackson WF, van der Temple WM, Salmon LJ, et al. Endoscopically-assisted single-bundle posterior cruciate ligament reconstruction: results at minimum 10-year follow-up. J Bone Joint Surg Br. 2008;90:1328–33.
7. Jung YB, Tae SK, Jung HJ, et al. Replacement of the torn posterior cruciate ligament with a mid-third patellar tendon graft with use of a modified tibial inlay method. J Bone Joint Surg Am. 2004;86A(9):1878–83.
8. Sekiya JK, West RV, Ong BC, et al. Clinical outcomes after isolated arthroscopic single-bundle posterior cruciate ligament reconstruction. Arthroscopy. 2005;21:1042–50.
9. Wang CJ, Chan YS, Weng LH, et al. Comparison of autogenous and allogenous posterior cruciate ligament reconstructions of the knee. Injury. 2004;35:1279–85.
10. Wang CJ, Weng LH, Hsu CC, et al. Arthroscopi single- versus double-bundle posterior cruciate ligament reconstruction using hamstring autograft. Injury. 2004;35:1293–9.
11. Wong T, Wang CJ, Weng LH, et al. Functional outcomes of arthroscopic posterior cruciate ligament reconstruction: comparison of anteromedial and anterolateral trans-tibia approach. Arch Orthop Trauma Surg. 2009;129:315–21.
12. Zhao J, Xiaoqiao H, He Y, et al. Sandwich-style posterior cruciate ligament reconstruction. Arthroscopy. 2008;24:650–9.
13. Adachi N, Ochi M, Uchio Y, et al. Temporal change of joint position sense after posterior cruciate ligament reconstruction using multi-stranded hamstring tendons. Knee Surg Sports Traumatol Arthrosc. 2007;15:2–8.
14. Chan YS, Yang SC, Chang CH, et al. Arthroscopic reconstruction of the posterior cruciate ligament with use of a quadruple hamstring tendon graft with 3- to 5-year follow-up. Arthroscopy. 2006;22:762–70.
15. MacGillivray JD, Stein BE, Park M, et al. Comparison of tibial inlay versus transtibial techniques for isolated posterior cruciate ligament reconstruction: minimum 2-year follow-up. Arthroscopy. 2006;22:320–8.
16. Zhao J, Huangfu X. Arthroscopic single-bundle posterior cruciate ligament reconstruction: Retrospective review of 4- versus 7-strand hamstring tendon graft. Knee. 2007;14:301–5.
17. Garofalo R, Jolles BM, Moretti B, et al. Double-bindle transtibial posterior cruciate ligament reconstruction with a tendon-patellar bone-semitendinosus tendon autograft: clinical results with a minimum of 2 years' follow-up. Arthroscopy. 2006;22:1331–8.e1.
18. Seon JK, Song EK. Reconstruction of isolated posterior cruciate ligament injuries: a clinical comparison of the transtibial and tibial inlay techniques. Arthroscopy. 2006;22:27–32.
19. Shon OJ, Lee DC, Park CH, et al. A comparison of arthroscopically assisted single and double bundle tibial inlay reconstruction for isolated posterior cruciate ligament injury. Clin Orthop Surg. 2010;2:76–84.
20. Wang CJ, Chen HS, Huang TW. Outcome of arthroscopic single bundle reconstruction for complete posterior cruciate ligament tear. Injury. 2003;34:747–51.
21. Wu CH, Chen AC, Yuan LJ, et al. Arthroscopic reconstruction of the posterior cruciate ligament by using a quadriceps tendon autograft: a minimum 5-year follow-up. Arthroscopy. 2007;23:420–7.
22. Ahn JH, Yoo JC, Wang JH. Posterior cruciate ligament reconstruction: double-loop hamstring tendon autograft versus Achilles tendon allograft- clinical results of a minimum 2-year follow-up. Arthroscopy. 2005;21:965–9.
23. Yoon KH, Bae DK, Song SJ, et al. A prospective randomized study comparing arthroscopic single-bundle and double-bundle posterior cruciate ligament reconstructions preserving remnant fibers. Am J Sports Med. 2011;39:474–80.
24. Kim SJ, Kim TE, Jo SB, et al. Comparison of the clinical results of three posterior cruciate ligament reconstruction techniques. J Bone Joint Surg Am. 2009;91:2543–9.
25. Fanelli GC, Edson CJ. Combined posterior cruciate ligament-posterolateral reconstructions with Achilles tendon allograft and biceps femoris tendon tenodesis: 2- to 10-year follow-up. Arthroscopy. 2004;20:339–45.
26. Lo YP, Hsu KY, Chen LH, et al. Simultaneous arthroscopic reconstruction of the anterior and posterior cruciate ligament using hamstring and quadriceps tendon autografts. J Trauma. 2009;66:780–8.

27. Zhao J, He Y, Wang J. Simultaneous arthroscopic reconstruction of the anterior and posterior cruciate ligaments with autogenous hamstring tendons. Arthroscopy. 2006;22:497–504.
28. Zhao J, Huangfu X, He Y, et al. Simultaneous double-bundle anterior cruciate ligament and posterior cruciate ligament reconstruction with autogenous hamstring tendons. Arthroscopy. 2008;24: 1205–13.
29. Strobel MJ, Schulz MS, Petersen WJ, et al. Combined anterior cruciate ligament, posterior cruciate ligament, and posterolateral corner reconstruction with autogenous hamstring grafts in chronic instabilities. Arthroscopy. 2006;22:182–92.
30. Khanduja V, Somayaji HS, Harnett P, et al. Combined reconstruction of chronic posterior cruciate ligament and posterolateral corner deficiency. A two- to nine-year follow-up study. J Bone Joint Surg Br. 2006;88:1169–72.
31. Ahn JH, Yang HS, Jeong WK, et al. Arthroscopic transtibial posterior cruciate ligament reconstruction with preservation of posterior cruciate ligament fibers: clinical results of minimum 2-year follow-up. Am J Sports Med. 2006;34:194–2004.
32. Lim HC, Bae JH, Wang JH, et al. Double-bundle PCL reconstruction using tibial double cross-pin fixation. Knee Surg Sports Traumatol Arthrosc. 2010;18:117–22.
33. Fanelli GC, Beck JD, Edson CJ. Single compared to double-bundle PCL reconstruction using allograft tissue. J Knee Surg. 2012; 25:59–64.

Part VIII

Clinical Case Studies

Selected Case Studies in Posterior Cruciate Ligament Reconstruction

29

Gregory C. Fanelli

Introduction

This chapter presents selected cases in treatment of the posterior cruciate ligament (PCL)-injured knee that are representative of my practice. I have written this section in the first person to provide a more personal approach to presenting these topics. These selected cases represent real-life management examples in the treatment of difficult knee ligament instability problems. The format followed will be the same for each case study to provide consistency in the presentation, and is outlined as follows: history, physical examination, imaging study findings, surgical timing, graft selection, surgical technique (when applicable), postoperative rehabilitation program, and results. Details of the surgical technique will not be presented in this section since the surgical technique was performed as I have described in Chaps. 1, 9, 15, 19 and 21. Specific topics presented in this chapter of selected case studies of PCL reconstruction include nonsurgical treatment, open growth plates, multiple ligament knee injuries in young athletes and middle-aged adults, 15-year postoperative outcomes, extensor mechanism disruption, complex knee ligament instability in the obese patient, revision PCL surgery, and peroneal nerve injury. The purpose of this case study section is for the reader to gain insight into management and treatment strategy decisions in these complex knee ligament injuries.

Case Study 1: Minimally Displaced PCL Tibial Insertion Site Bony Injury

This patient is a 44-year-old manual laborer who had a fall on to the anterior aspect of his flexed knee while working. This was a low-energy injury from a standing height. The patient felt pain but continued to work. The patient developed an effusion and a limp with ecchymosis on the posterior aspect of his popliteal fossa area and calf which caused him to seek medical attention approximately 10 days post injury.

Physical examination of the lower extremities comparing the injured knee to the uninjured knee revealed the neurovascular status and the skin to be intact. A mild effusion was present, and there was no gross deformity of the lower extremity. The tibial step-offs were equal with the knees at 90° of flexion, and the involved knee had approximately 5 mm of increased excursion of the posterior drawer test with a soft end point compared to the normal knee. The anterior cruciate ligament (ACL), the medial and lateral collateral ligaments, the posteromedial and posterolateral corners, and the extensor mechanism were all stable to physical examination.

Plain radiographs obtained in the orthopedic clinic on the day of consultation demonstrated normal alignment of the patellofemoral and tibiofemoral joints, and no evidence of fractures. Magnetic resonance imaging (MRI) of the injured knee demonstrated a minimally displaced tibial avulsion fracture at the PCL insertion, and no other structural injuries in the knee. Venous Doppler studies that were ordered because of the patient's calf pain were negative for deep or superficial venous thrombosis.

This patient had an isolated PCL injury with a minimally displaced fracture at the PCL tibial insertion site. This was a low-energy injury with less than 5 mm of posterior tibial excursion during posterior drawer testing. It was determined that this injury had excellent healing potential, and would be treated nonsurgically. The patient was placed in a hinged range-of-motion brace locked in extension with weight bearing as tolerated for approximately 4–6 weeks. At approximately 8 weeks post injury, the long leg brace was discontinued. Physical examination after completion of brace treatment for the above-described PCL injury revealed a symmetrical knee range of motion compared to the uninvolved knee. Equal tibial step-offs and a negative posterior drawer test. No varus or valgus laxity, and negative Lachman and pivot shift tests. The posteromedial and posterolateral corners were stable. The patient resumed his pre-injury level of activity, with no subsequent knee instability.

G. C. Fanelli (✉)
303 Kaseville Road, Danville, PA 17821, USA

G. C. Fanelli (ed.), *Posterior Cruciate Ligament Injuries*,
DOI 10.1007/978-3-319-12072-0_29, © Springer International Publishing Switzerland 2015

Case Study 2: PCL, Posteromedial, and Posterolateral Instability in a 12-Year-Old Boy with Open Growth Plates

The patient is a 12-year-old boy referred to me 3 weeks after a right-knee injury sustained playing baseball. The patient slid into base and collided with another player and the fixed base with his knee in 90° of flexion. Initial evaluation by another physician revealed a bloody effusion upon aspiration, posterior tibial translation at 90° of flexion, and an MRI study of the right knee demonstrating a PCL tear. The patient was referred to me for evaluation and treatment.

Physical examination comparing the injured right knee to the uninvolved left knee revealed the skin and neurovascular status to be intact. Range of knee motion was symmetrical to the uninvolved left knee. There was no pain or restriction of motion at the hip or ankle on the involved or normal side. The tibial step-offs were decreased, and the posterior drawer test was positive. There were positive posterolateral and posteromedial drawer tests, and the dial test was positive at both 30 and 90°of knee flexion. The knee was stable to valgus stress at 0 and 30° of knee flexion, and there was varus laxity at both 0 and 30° of knee flexion with a soft end point. The hyperextension external rotation recurvatum test was negative, and the heel liftoff test was symmetrical on the injured and noninjured side. The Lachman and pivot shift tests were both negative.

Initial radiographs taken in the orthopedic clinic demonstrated open growth plates on the distal femur and the proximal tibia with no fractures. There was no physeal injury noted on stress radiography, or on MRI. MRI showed a tear of the PCL, and bone marrow edema without fracture in the anterior tibial epiphysis in the midline. There were no articular cartilage injuries or meniscus tears.

KT 1000 arthrometer testing revealed the following side-to-side difference measurements: PCL screen at 90° of knee flexion 6 mm, corrected posterior measurement at 70° of knee flexion 6 mm, corrected anterior measurement at 70° of knee flexion 4 mm, and the 30-pound anterior displacement measurement at 30° of knee flexion was 1 mm. Side-to-side difference on stress radiography at 90° of knee flexion with a posterior displacement force applied to the tibial tubercle area of the proximal tibia using the Telos device comparing the involved to the normal knee was 10 mm.

Preoperative testing with three knee ligament rating scales revealed the following: Hospital for Special Surgery score was 42/100, Lysholm score was 44/100, and the Tegner activity score was 3 (pre-injury, the patient was level 7).

The diagnosis in this patient is a right-knee subacute PCL-based multiple-ligament-injured knee with PCL tear, posteromedial instability type A, and posterolateral instability type B in a patient with open growth plates. The decision was made to proceed with arthroscopic single-bundle transtibial PCL reconstruction using a fresh frozen Achilles tendon allograft combined with fibular-head-based figure-of-eight posterolateral reconstruction using fresh frozen semitendinosus allograft, and posteromedial reconstruction using the posteromedial capsular shift procedure. The PCL reconstruction femoral tunnel crossed the distal femoral physis, and the PCL tibial tunnel was positioned distal to the tibial physis. Cortical suspensory fixation with two stacked polyethylene ligament fixation buttons were used on the femoral side, and a bioabsorbable interference screw and bicortical screw and spiked ligament washer were used on the tibial side fixation. No fixation device crossed the growth plates.

The posterolateral reconstruction was a fibular-head-based figure-of-eight reconstruction using a fresh frozen semitendinosus allograft. The allograft was looped around the common biceps tendon at the fibular head and sewn there using a permanent braided suture. The fibular collateral ligament component was passed medial to the iliotibial band, and the popliteofibular popliteus tendon component passed medial to the common biceps tendon and the iliotibial band. The allograft limbs were crossed in figure-of-eight fashion with the fibular collateral component being lateral to the popliteus tendon component. The graft limbs were sewn into their respective anatomic femoral insertion sites with number 2 braided permanent sutures with a slight valgus applied to the knee to close the lateral compartment with the knee in approximately 90°of flexion. The allograft was then sewn to the deep capsular layers for additional reinforcement, and a posterolateral capsular shift was also performed. There were no drill holes through or around the lateral side growth plates.

The posteromedial reconstruction was performed using the posteromedial capsular shift technique. This was an all-suture posteromedial capsular advancement procedure performed with the knee in approximately 45° of flexion as described in Chap. 15. The PCL reconstruction, the posterolateral reconstruction, and the posteromedial reconstruction procedures were all protective of the growth plates. Postoperatively, the surgical knee was immobilized in a long leg brace locked in full extension, and was non-weight bearing with crutches. Prophylactic preoperative and postoperative antibiotics were utilized. Progressive weight bearing and range of knee motion were gradually initiated according to our postoperative rehabilitation program detailed in Chap. 25.

Six-year follow-up postoperative examination of the patient at the age of 19 reveals equal leg lengths, normal and symmetrical carrying angles, and normal gait during ambulation. Radiographs reveal closed distal femoral and proximal tibial physes that are symmetrical to the normal knee with no malalignment, no evidence of growth arrest, and no degenerative changes. Physical examination of the surgical right knee compared to the normal left knee reveals the posterior drawer is negative, posteromedial and posterolateral drawer tests are negative, and the dial test is symmetrical at 30 and 90° of knee flexion. The Lachman test is negative, the pivot shift test is negative, and the surgical knee is stable to varus and valgus stress throughout the flexion extension arc. The hyperextension external rotation recurvatum and heel liftoff tests are symmetrical compared to the normal knee.

Three-year postoperative KT 1000, stress radiography, and knee ligament rating scale measurements reveal the following. Range of motion is 0–125° on the surgical right knee, and 0–130° on the uninvolved left knee. Side-to-side difference on KT 1000 measurements on the PCL screen, corrected posterior, and corrected anterior measurements are 2.0, 2.5, and −2.0 mm, respectively. Side-to-side difference on the KT 1000 anterior displacement measurement at 30° of knee flexion is 2.0 mm. Stress X-rays at 90° of knee flexion using the Telos device comparing the surgical knee to the normal knee reveal a 1.8-mm side-to-side difference. The Hospital for Special Surgery, Lysholm, and Tegner knee ligament rating scale scores are 98/100, 99/100, and 7, respectively. The patient's pre-injury Tegner score was 7 indicating a return to pre-injury level of function.

Case Study 3: Acute Combined PCL Tear with Posterolateral Instability in a 17-Year-Old Gymnast

The patient is a 17-year-old competitive gymnast who had a missed landing during a gymnastics event injuring her left knee. At the time of injury, the patient had a hyperextension and varus force applied to her knee with the right foot planted firmly on the ground. The patient developed immediate pain and swelling, and was unable to continue participation in the athletic competition. The patient's initial presentation upon reporting to the emergency department included a right-knee effusion with posterior and lateral right-knee pain. Neurovascular status of the involved right lower extremity was intact, and the skin was intact. There was anterior–posterior and varus laxity with guarding by the patient. The patient was referred to me for evaluation and treatment of the knee injury.

Initial evaluation of this patient in our clinic revealed nearly symmetrical range of motion of both knees with minimal effusion of the injured left knee. The neurovascular examination of the involved left lower extremity was symmetrical to the normal right lower extremity, and the skin was intact on both legs. Physical examination comparing the injured left knee to the normal right knee revealed negative tibial step-offs with the proximal tibia dropped back posterior to the distal femur with the knee at 90° of knee flexion, a grade-three posterior drawer test, positive posterior lateral drawer test, and varus laxity at 30 and 0° of knee flexion with 10 mm of increased lateral joint line opening compared to the normal knee, but with a firm end point. The dial test was positive at both 30 and 90° of knee flexion, and the posteromedial drawer test was negative. The knee was stable to valgus stress throughout the flexion-extension arc, and the Lachman and pivot shift tests were negative. The hyperextension external rotation recurvatum and heel liftoff tests were symmetrical. The extensor mechanism was stable.

Plain radiographs demonstrated symmetrical positioning of the tibiofemoral and patellofemoral joints compared to the patient's normal knee. Stress radiography at 90° of knee flexion with a posterior-directed force applied to the proximal tibial comparing the injured left knee to the normal right knee revealed 12 mm more posterior tibial displacement of the injured knee. MRI study of the left knee revealed a medial femoral condyle bone bruise, complete PCL tear, and disruption of the posterolateral structures of the knee.

The diagnosis in this case is an acute PCL tear combined with posterolateral instability type B in a 17-year-old competitive athlete. The plan was to proceed with reconstruction of the PCL, primary repair of the posterolateral structures, and posterolateral reconstruction at approximately 3–4 weeks post injury. Preoperatively, the patient achieved full range of motion of the injured knee. There was a complete disruption of the PCL, and PCL reconstruction was performed using the single-bundle arthroscopically assisted transtibial tunnel technique using an Achilles tendon allograft to reconstruct the anterolateral bundle of the PCL. The injury complex on the lateral side of the knee consisted of femoral insertion site avulsion of the fibular collateral ligament and popliteus tendon, and attenuation of the midlateral and posterolateral capsule. Primary repair of fibular collateral ligament and popliteus tendon injuries was performed combined with a posterolateral capsular shift procedure, and a posterolateral reconstruction using a fibular-head-based figure-of-eight posterolateral reconstruction technique. Postoperatively, the surgical knee was immobilized in a long leg brace locked in full extension, and was non-weight bearing with crutches. Prophylactic preoperative and postoperative antibiotics were utilized. Progressive weight bearing and range of knee motion were gradually initiated according to our postoperative rehabilitation program detailed in Chap. 25.

Ten years postoperatively, the patient's range of motion is 0–135° on the surgical left knee, and 0–150° on the uninvolved right knee. The posterior drawer is negative, posteromedial and posterolateral drawer tests are negative, and the dial test is symmetrical at 30 and 90° of knee flexion. The Lachman test is negative, the pivot shift test is negative, and the surgical knee is stable to varus and valgus stress throughout the flexion-extension arc. The hyperextension external rotation recurvatum and heel liftoff tests are symmetrical compared to the normal knee.

Side-to-side difference on KT 1000 measurements on the PCL screen, corrected posterior, and corrected anterior measurements are 3.5, 2.0, and −2.0 mm, respectively.

Side-to-side difference on the KT 1000 anterior displacement measurement at 30° of knee flexion is 1.0 mm. The Hospital for Special Surgery, Lysholm, and Tegner knee ligament rating scale scores are 94/100, 94/100, and 5, respectively. Five-year postoperative stress X-rays at 90° of knee flexion using the Telos device comparing the surgical to the knee normal knee reveal a 0.5-mm side-to-side difference.

Case Study 4: Acute Combined PCL Tear with Posteromedial Instability in a 52-Year-Old Woman

The patient is a 52-year-old woman who slipped and fell on an icy deck twisting her left knee. The patient was initially evaluated by her primary care doctor who obtained an MRI that was read by the radiologist as a complex lateral meniscus tear, PCL tear, partial ACL tear, and a disruption of the medial collateral ligament with tearing of the medial patellar retinaculum and tear with elevation of the vastus medialis obliques. The patient was referred to me for evaluation and treatment.

Physical examination of the injured left knee compared to the normal right knee revealed a mild effusion, and nearly symmetrical range of motion. The neurovascular examination of the involved left lower extremity was symmetrical to the normal right lower extremity, and the skin was intact on both legs. Comparing the injured left knee to the normal right knee revealed negative tibial step-offs, with the proximal tibia dropped back posterior to the distal femur, with the knee at 90° of knee flexion, a grade-three posterior drawer test, positive posterior medial drawer test, and valgus laxity at 30 and 0° of knee flexion with 10–15 mm of increased medial joint line opening compared to the normal knee with a soft end point. The dial test was positive at both 30 and 90° of knee flexion, with the anteromedial tibial plateau rotating forward and the anterolateral tibial plateau maintaining its normal anatomic relationships. The knee was stable to varus stress throughout the flexion–extension arc, and the Lachman and pivot shift tests were negative. The hyperextension external rotation recurvatum and heel liftoff tests were symmetrical. The extensor mechanism had increased lateral patellar excursion with the knee at 30° of knee flexion. Plain radiographs demonstrated symmetrical positioning of the tibiofemoral joint; however, the injured knee demonstrated lateral patellar tilting on the 30° axial view of the patella compared to the uninjured knee.

The diagnosis in this case is an acute PCL tear combined with posteromedial instability type B/C, lateral patellar subluxation instability, and a lateral meniscus tear in a 52-year-old woman with a physically demanding job. The plan was to proceed with reconstruction of the PCL, primary repair of the posteromedial structures and the extensor mechanism, address the lateral meniscus tear, and perform a posteromedial reconstruction at approximately 4 weeks post injury. Preoperatively, the patient achieved full range of motion of the injured knee. Surgical findings demonstrated a complete disruption of the PCL, and PCL reconstruction was performed using the single-bundle arthroscopically assisted transtibial tunnel technique with an Achilles tendon allograft to reconstruct the anterolateral bundle of the PCL. The injury complex on the medial side of the knee consisted of femoral insertion site avulsion of the deep medial collateral ligament, and the medial patellar retinaculum and medial patellofemoral ligament. Primary repair of the injured medial side structures was performed using suture anchors. The primary medial side repair was combined with a posteromedial capsular shift procedure, and a posteromedial reconstruction using a looped tibialis anterior allograft surgical technique. Postoperatively, the surgical knee was immobilized in a long leg brace locked in full extension, and was non-weight bearing with crutches. Prophylactic preoperative and postoperative antibiotics were utilized. Progressive weight bearing and range of knee motion were gradually initiated according to our postoperative rehabilitation program detailed in Chap. 25.

One year postoperatively, the patient's range of motion is 0–120° on the surgical left knee, and 0 –130° on the uninvolved right knee. The posterior drawer is negative, posteromedial and posterolateral drawer tests are negative, and the dial test is symmetrical at 30 and 90° of knee flexion. The Lachman test is negative, the pivot shift test is negative, and the surgical knee is stable to varus and valgus stress throughout the flexion–extension arc. The hyperextension external rotation recurvatum and heel liftoff tests are symmetrical compared to the normal knee.

Side-to-side difference on KT 1000 measurements on the PCL screen, corrected posterior, and corrected anterior measurements are 2.0, 2.5, and 0.0 mm, respectively. Side-to-side difference on the KT 1000 anterior displacement measurement at 30° of knee flexion is 3.0 mm. Postoperative stress X-rays at 90° of knee flexion using the Telos device comparing the surgical knee to the normal knee reveal a 1.2-mm side-to-side difference. There is no X-ray evidence of degenerative joint disease in the injured knee. The Hospital for Special Surgery, Lysholm, and Tegner knee ligament rating scale scores are 92/100, 99/100, and 4, respectively. The patient has achieved her pre-injury Tegner activity scale level, and has returned to her regular job.

Case Study 5: Acute Combined PCL, ACL, Posterolateral Instability in a 47-Year-Old Man with 15 Year Outcomes

The patient is a 47-year-old man, involved in an all-terrain vehicle (ATV) accident, who is very active in sports, recreational activities, and has a physically demanding occupation.

The patient was initially seen in a community hospital emergency room after his ATV accident, and the diagnosis was made of a multiple-ligament-injured left knee. X-rays obtained upon initial evaluation demonstrated well-aligned tibiofemoral and patellofemoral joints. It is important to recognize that this was a tibiofemoral knee dislocation with spontaneous reduction. Vascular studies demonstrated no injury to the arterial or venous system of the injured left lower extremity, and the patient had no other injuries. The patient was transferred to our facility for evaluation and treatment of a multiple-ligament-injured left knee.

MRI showed tears of the PCL and ACL, and injury to the lateral and posterolateral structures. Physical examination of the injured left knee and lower extremity compared to the uninjured right knee and lower extremity revealed negative tibial step-offs with the proximal tibia dropped back posterior to the distal femur with the knee at 90° of knee flexion. There was a grade-three posterior drawer test, positive posterior lateral drawer test, and varus laxity at 30 and 0° of knee flexion with 10 mm of increased lateral joint line opening compared to the normal knee with a soft end point. The dial test was positive at both 30 and 90° of knee flexion. The knee was stable to valgus stress throughout the flexion-extension arc with a negative posteromedial drawer test. The Lachman and pivot shift tests were positive. The hyperextension external rotation recurvatum and heel liftoff tests were symmetrical. The extensor mechanism was stable to physical examination. Plain radiographs demonstrated symmetrical positioning of the patellofemoral and tibiofemoral joints.

The diagnosis in this case is a left-knee acute PCL and ACL tears combined with posterolateral instability type B in a 47-year-old man with a physically demanding job who is also an avid sportsman and recreational athlete. The plan was to proceed with reconstruction of the PCL and ACL, perform a primary repair of the posterolateral structures, and posterolateral reconstruction at approximately 4 weeks post injury.

Preoperatively, the patient achieved full range of motion of the injured left knee. Surgical findings demonstrated a complete disruption of the PCL and ACL, and PCL reconstruction was performed using the single-bundle arthroscopically assisted transtibial tunnel technique with an Achilles tendon allograft to reconstruct the anterolateral bundle of the PCL. ACL reconstruction was performed using the single-bundle endoscopic transtibial femoral tunnel technique with an Achilles tendon allograft. The injury complex on the lateral side of the knee consisted of attenuation of the fibular collateral ligament, popliteus tendon, and midlateral and posterolateral capsule with proximal and distal insertion sites of these structures remaining intact. Retensioning of the fibular collateral ligament and popliteus tendon was performed in conjunction with a posterolateral capsular shift procedure. In addition, a posterolateral reconstruction was performed using a fibular-head-based figure-of-eight posterolateral reconstruction technique with a semitendinosus allograft. Postoperatively, the surgical knee was immobilized in a long leg brace locked in full extension, and was non-weight bearing with crutches. Prophylactic preoperative and postoperative antibiotics were utilized. Progressive weight bearing and range of knee motion were gradually initiated according to our postoperative rehabilitation program detailed in Chap. 25.

Fifteen-year postoperative follow-up demonstrated that the patient's range of motion is 0–115° on the surgical left knee, and 0–128° on the uninvolved right knee. The posterior drawer is negative, posteromedial and posterolateral drawer tests are negative, and the dial test is symmetrical at 30 and 90° of knee flexion. The Lachman test is negative, the pivot shift test is negative, the surgical knee is stable to varus and valgus stress throughout the flexion-extension arc, and the hyperextension external rotation recurvatum and heel liftoff tests are negative. All physical examination tests are compared to the uninjured knee.

Side-to-side difference on KT 1000 measurements on the PCL screen, corrected posterior, and corrected anterior measurements are 1.0, 3.0, and 2.0 mm, respectively. Side-to-side difference on the KT 1000 anterior displacement measurement at 30° of knee flexion is 2.0 mm. Postoperative stress X-rays at 90° of knee flexion using the Telos device comparing the surgical knee to the normal knee reveal a 0.4-mm side-to-side difference. There is no X-ray evidence of degenerative joint disease in the injured knee. The Hospital for Special Surgery, Lysholm, and Tegner knee ligament rating scale scores are 90/100, 94/100, and 6, respectively. The patient has achieved his pre-injury Tegner activity scale level, and has returned to his regular job as well as all his recreational activities.

Case Study 6: Acute Combined PCL, ACL, Posterolateral Instability, Patella Tendon Rupture in a 21-Year-Old Man

The patient is a 21-year-old male college student who fell from a height and sustained a closed fracture of his right tibia and fibula and a closed patellar tendon rupture, PCL and ACL tears, and posterolateral instability of his left knee. X-rays obtained upon initial evaluation of the left knee demonstrated a reduced tibiofemoral joint, and a high-riding patella consistent with a patella tendon rupture. Vascular studies demonstrated no injury to the arterial or venous system of the multiple-ligament-knee-injured left lower extremity.

The plan was to perform immediate fracture care, and to perform a staged approach to the multiple-ligament-injured knee. The right lower extremity fractures were treated with closed reduction and casting, and the left patella tendon rupture was primarily repaired and augmented with allograft tissue within 24 h of the injury. The left-knee ligament injuries were treated with bracing. The right tibia and fibula fractures and the left patellar tendon augmented primary repair healed uneventfully, and the patient successfully completed rehabilitation programs for the injuries to the right and left lower extremities. Stage two was to return the patient to the operating room for surgical reconstruction of the multiple-ligament-injured left knee.

MRI showed tears of the PCL and ACL, and injury to the lateral and posterolateral structures. Physical examination of the multiple-ligament-injured left knee and lower extremity compared to the uninjured right knee revealed negative tibial step-offs with the proximal tibia dropped back posterior to the distal femur with the knee at 90° of knee flexion, a grade-three posterior drawer test, positive posterior lateral drawer test, and varus laxity at 30 and 0° of knee flexion with 10 mm of increased lateral joint line opening compared to the normal knee with a soft end point. The dial test was positive at both 30 and 90° of knee flexion. The knee was stable to valgus stress throughout the flexion-extension arc with a negative posteromedial drawer test. The Lachman and pivot shift tests were positive. The hyperextension external rotation recurvatum and heel liftoff tests were symmetrical to the normal knee. The extensor mechanism was stable to physical examination, with symmetrical range of motion to the opposite knee, and restoration of active physiologic extension and hyperextension indicating successful extensor mechanism repair. Plain radiographs demonstrated symmetrical positioning of the patellofemoral and tibiofemoral joints compared to the opposite knee. The diagnosis in this case is a left-knee acute PCL and ACL tears combined with posterolateral instability type B complicated by an ipsilateral patellar tendon rupture, and a contralateral fracture of the right tibia and fibula in a 21-year-old man.

Six months post injury, the patient returned to the operating room for surgical reconstruction of the multiple-ligament-injured left knee. Preoperatively, the patient achieved full range of motion of the injured left knee. Surgical findings demonstrated that a complete disruption of the PCL and ACL, and PCL reconstruction was performed using the single-bundle arthroscopically assisted transtibial tunnel technique with an Achilles tendon allograft to reconstruct the anterolateral bundle of the PCL. ACL reconstruction was performed using the single-bundle endoscopic transtibial femoral tunnel technique with an Achilles tendon allograft. The injury complex on the lateral side of the knee consisted of attenuation of the fibular collateral ligament, popliteus tendon, and midlateral and posterolateral capsule with proximal and distal insertion sites of these structures remaining intact. Retensioning of the fibular collateral ligament and popliteus tendon was performed in conjunction with a posterolateral capsular shift procedure. In addition, a posterolateral reconstruction was performed using a fibular-head-based figure-of-eight posterolateral reconstruction technique with an Achilles tendon allograft. Postoperatively, the surgical knee was immobilized in a long leg brace locked in full extension, and was non-weight bearing with crutches. Prophylactic preoperative and postoperative antibiotics were utilized. Progressive weight bearing and range of knee motion were gradually initiated according to our postoperative rehabilitation program detailed in Chap. 25.

Six-year postoperative follow-up evaluation demonstrated the patient's range of motion is 0–110° on the surgical left knee, and 0–130° on the uninvolved right knee. The posterior drawer test is negative, posteromedial and posterolateral drawer tests are negative, and the dial test is symmetrical to the right lower extremity at 30 and 90° of knee flexion. The Lachman test is negative, the pivot shift test is negative, the surgical knee is stable to varus and valgus stress throughout the flexion-extension arc, and the hyperextension external rotation recurvatum and heel liftoff tests are negative. All physical examination tests are compared to the uninjured knee.

Side-to-side difference on KT 1000 measurements on the PCL screen, corrected posterior, and corrected anterior measurements are 2.0, 4.5, and 0.5 mm, respectively. Side-to-side difference on the KT 1000 anterior displacement measurement at 30° of knee flexion is −3.0 mm. Postoperative stress X-rays at 90° of knee flexion using the Telos device comparing the surgical knee to the normal knee reveal a 2.5-mm side-to-side difference. There is no X-ray evidence of degenerative joint disease in the injured knee. The Hospital for Special Surgery, Lysholm, and Tegner knee ligament rating scale scores are 90/100, 94/100, and 4, respectively. The patient has achieved his pre-injury Tegner activity scale level.

Case Study 7: Subacute Combined PCL, ACL, Posteromedial Instability in a 32-Year-Old Woman with a Body Mass Index of 50

The patient is a 32-year-old woman with a body mass index of 50 who was a pedestrian hit by an automobile sustaining an injury to the right knee and right upper extremity. The patient was seen by an orthopedic surgeon who immobilized the knee in full extension with full weight bearing, and referred the patient to me approximately 4 weeks post injury for evaluation and treatment of the right-knee injury. Plain X-rays obtained in the immobilizer at the time of my initial evaluation revealed well-reduced and well-aligned tibiofemoral and patellofemoral joints and no fractures. MRI of the injured right knee was read by the radiologist as having an anterior horn medial meniscus tear, anterior and PCL tear, tear of the medial collateral ligament, and lateral femoral condyle and lateral tibial plateau bone bruising.

My initial physical examination of the injured right knee compared to the normal left knee revealed a very stiff knee since it had been immobilized in extension for almost 5 weeks. There was valgus laxity at full extension; however, the patient was not able to bend the knee enough to assess anterior–posterior tibial translation with respect to the femur. There was no varus laxity on physical examination. The patient was converted to a hinged range of motion brace to provide valgus stability, and physical therapy instituted to achieve range of motion so that an adequate physical examination of the injured knee could be performed and a surgical treatment plan developed.

My second examination of the patient's injured knee compared to the normal knee revealed range of motion from 0 to 115° of knee flexion. The skin was in good condition, and the neurovascular examination was intact and symmetrical to the uninjured left lower extremity. The knee was stable to varus stress at 0 and 30° of knee flexion, and there is valgus laxity at 0 and 30° of knee flexion with 10 mm of medial joint line opening and a firm end point. The posterior drawer test was positive, and the Lachman and pivot shift tests were also positive. The posteromedial and anteromedial drawer tests were positive, but the posterolateral and anterolateral drawer tests were negative. The extensor mechanism was stable. The diagnosis in this patient is subacute PCL and ACL tears combined with posteromedial instability type B in a patient with a body mass index of 50.

The patient's right knee ligament reconstructive surgery was performed approximately 3 months after her initial injury. The surgery consisted of an arthroscopically assisted transtibial tunnel double-bundle PCL reconstruction using an Achilles tendon allograft for the anterolateral bundle, and a tibialis anterior allograft for the posterior medial bundle. The ACL reconstruction was an arthroscopically assisted single-bundle transtibial femoral tunnel technique using an Achilles tendon allograft. The posteromedial reconstruction was performed using a posteromedial capsular shift surgical technique. Postoperatively, the surgical knee was immobilized in a long leg brace locked in full extension, and was non-weight bearing with crutches. Prophylactic preoperative and postoperative antibiotics were utilized. Progressive weight bearing and range of knee motion were gradually initiated according to our postoperative rehabilitation program detailed in Chap. 25.

Eight-year postoperative follow-up evaluation of the patient's surgical right knee demonstrated the patient's range of motion is 0–118° on the surgical right knee, and 0–133° on the uninvolved left knee. The posterior drawer test is negative, posteromedial and posterolateral drawer tests are negative, and the dial test is symmetrical to the normal left lower extremity at 30 and 90° of knee flexion. The Lachman test is negative, the pivot shift test is negative, the surgical knee is stable to varus and valgus stress at 0 and 30° of knee flexion, and the hyperextension external rotation recurvatum and heel liftoff tests are negative, and symmetrical to the uninjured knee. All physical examination tests of the surgical right knee are compared to the uninjured left knee. The patient's body mass index at 8-year follow-up is 53.

Side-to-side difference on KT 1000 measurements on the PCL screen, corrected posterior, and corrected anterior measurements are 2.0, 0.0, and 0.0 mm, respectively. Side-to-side difference on the KT 1000 anterior displacement measurement at 30° of knee flexion is 3.0 mm. Postoperative stress X-rays at 90° of knee flexion using the Telos device comparing the surgical knee to the normal knee reveal a 0.0-mm side-to-side difference. There is X-ray evidence of degenerative joint disease in the injured knee. The Hospital for Special Surgery, Lysholm, and Tegner knee ligament rating scale scores are 60/100, 54/100, and 2, respectively. The patient's knee is functionally and objectively stable; however, she does have knee pain and her knee ligament rating scale scores are decreased secondary to her degenerative joint disease.

Case Study 8: Acute Combined PCL Tear, ACL Tear, Posterolateral Instability, and Peroneal Nerve Injury

The patient is a 30-year-old man who injured his left knee jumping on a trampoline. The mechanism of injury was an out of control landing resulting in a varus stress to the left knee from a forced figure-of-four position of the patient's left lower extremity under the patient's body weight. Evaluation in the emergency department revealed a multiple-ligament-injured left knee with pulses symmetrical to the uninjured lower extremity. Vascular studies confirmed intact arterial and venous systems in the injured lower extremity, and no arterial intimal flap tear. The patient was unable to dorsiflex the toes, foot, and ankle on the injured left lower extremity. Plain radiographs demonstrated the patellofemoral and tibiofemoral joints to be reduced; however, there was widening of the lateral compartment in the anteroposterior radiographic view. MRI study of the injured left knee demonstrated complete tears of the ACL and PCL, posterolateral corner injury with complete disruption of the fibular collateral ligament and biceps tendon at the head of the fibula, and injury to the popliteofibular ligament, midlateral, and posterolateral capsule.

Physical examination of the injured left knee and lower extremity compared to the uninjured right lower extremity revealed the proximal tibial step-offs to be negative accompanied by a grade-three posterior drawer test. The posterolateral drawer test was positive, and the posteromedial drawer test was negative. The dial test was positive at both 30 and 90° of knee flexion, and there was varus laxity at both 0 and 30° of knee flexion with no discernible end point. The knee was stable to valgus stress, the Lachman test positive, the pivot shift test positive, and the extensor mechanism stable. The patient was unable to dorsiflex the toes, foot, and ankle on the injured left lower extremity. The diagnosis in this patient is an acute PCL tear, ACL tear, posterolateral instability type C, and a peroneal nerve injury.

The patient had surgical reconstruction of the PCL and ACL, primary repair and reconstruction of the posterolateral corner structures, and peroneal nerve neurolysis approximately 3–4 weeks post injury. The PCL reconstruction was an arthroscopically assisted double-bundle PCL reconstruction using a fresh frozen Achilles tendon allograft for the anterolateral bundle of the PCL, and a fresh-frozen tibialis anterior allograft for the PCL posteromedial bundle. The ACL reconstruction was an arthroscopically assisted transtibial femoral tunnel reconstruction using a fresh-frozen Achilles tendon allograft.

Before beginning any surgical repair or reconstruction on the lateral side of the knee, a peroneal nerve neurolysis was performed, and the nerve protected throughout the procedure. The peroneal nerve was in continuity; however, it had been severely stretched and was attenuated. The midlateral and posterolateral capsule were avulsed from the proximal tibia, and were primarily repaired using suture anchors. The fibular collateral ligament, popliteofibular ligament, and the common biceps tendon that were avulsed from the fibular head were primarily repaired with number 2 and number 5 permanent braided sutures through the posterolateral reconstruction drill hole made through the head of the fibula. Posterolateral reconstruction was performed with the fibular-head-based figure-of-eight technique using a fresh-frozen semitendinosus allograft tissue to augment and reinforce the lateral posterolateral primary repair.

Postoperatively, the surgical knee was immobilized in a long leg brace locked in full extension, and was non-weight bearing with crutches. Prophylactic preoperative and postoperative antibiotics were utilized. Progressive weight bearing and range of knee motion were gradually initiated according to our postoperative rehabilitation program detailed in Chap. 25. An ankle foot orthosis was used to prevent foot drop, and subsequent heel cord contracture.

There was no recovery of peroneal nerve function documented by physical examination, and by serial electromyograms and nerve conduction studies. Six months post left multiple knee ligament reconstruction, the patient underwent posterior tibial tendon transfer to restore dorsiflexion function to the left foot and ankle that resulted from the peroneal nerve injury.

Two-year postoperative follow-up evaluation of the patient's surgical left knee demonstrated the patient's range of motion is 0–110° on the surgical left knee, and 0–120° on the uninvolved right knee. The posterior drawer test is negative, posteromedial and posterolateral drawer tests are negative, and the dial test is symmetrical to the normal right lower extremity at 30 and 90° of knee flexion. The Lachman test is negative, the pivot shift test is negative, the surgical knee is stable to varus and valgus stress at 0 and 30° of knee flexion, and the hyperextension external rotation recurvatum and heel liftoff tests are negative, and symmetrical to the uninjured knee. All physical examination tests of the surgical left knee are compared to the uninjured right knee. The patient has active dorsiflexion of the left foot and ankle, does not have drop foot, and does not need to use an ankle foot orthosis indicating successful tendon transfer.

Side-to-side difference on KT 1000 measurements on the PCL screen, corrected posterior, and corrected anterior measurements are 3.0, 1.0, and 0.0 mm, respectively. Side-to-side difference on the KT 1000 anterior displacement measurement at 30° of knee flexion is 3.0 mm. Postoperative stress X-rays at 90° of knee flexion using the Telos device comparing the surgical left knee to the normal right knee reveal a 2.9 mm side-to-side difference. There is X-ray evidence of degenerative joint disease in the injured knee. The Hospital for Special Surgery, Lysholm, and Tegner knee ligament rating scale scores are 77/100, 88/100, and 5, respectively. The patient's knee is functionally and objectively stable, and there is good function of the left foot and ankle. The patient has returned to his pre-injury level of activity with respect to work and recreational activities.

Case Study 9: Revision PCL, ACL, and Posteromedial Reconstruction

The patient is a 40-year-old man who sustained a right-knee tibiofemoral knee dislocation with button holing of the medial femoral condyle through the medial capsule in a snow mobile accident. The patient was treated by another orthopedic surgeon who performed open reduction of the knee, primarily repaired the medial capsule, and applied a spanning external fixator. Wound healing occurred uneventfully, and the external fixator was removed 3 weeks after its application, the knee was manipulated to restore range of motion, and the knee placed in a hinged range of motion brace for protection. Physical examination of the knee under anesthesia confirmed the diagnosis of posterior cruciate and ACL tears, posterolateral instability type A, and posteromedial instability type B.

The patient's right knee ligament reconstructive surgery was performed approximately 4–5 weeks after his initial injury. The surgery consisted of an arthroscopically assisted transtibial tunnel double-bundle PCL reconstruction using a fresh frozen Achilles tendon allograft for the anterolateral bundle, and a fresh frozen tibialis anterior allograft for the posterior medial bundle. The ACL reconstruction was an arthroscopically assisted single-bundle transtibial femoral tunnel technique using a fresh frozen Achilles tendon allograft. The posterolateral reconstruction was performed using a fibular-head-based figure-of-eight posterolateral reconstruction technique with fresh frozen semitendinosus allograft. The posteromedial reconstruction was performed using a posteromedial capsular shift surgical technique. Postoperatively, the surgical knee was immobilized in a long leg brace locked in full extension, and was non-weight bearing with crutches. Prophylactic preoperative and postoperative antibiotics were utilized. Progressive weight bearing and range of knee motion were gradually initiated according to our postoperative rehabilitation program detailed in Chap. 25.

Approximately 4 months post reconstruction, the patient was doing heavy manual labor against medical advice and reinjured his knee. This resulted in tears of the PCL, ACL, and posteromedial reconstructions with resultant functional instability. The patient underwent revision PCL, ACL, and medial posteromedial reconstruction 5 months after his primary reconstruction. The surgery consisted of an arthroscopically assisted transtibial tunnel double-bundle PCL reconstruction using a fresh frozen Achilles tendon allograft for the anterolateral bundle, and a fresh-frozen tibialis anterior allograft for the posterior medial bundle. The ACL reconstruction was an arthroscopically assisted single-bundle transtibial femoral tunnel technique using a fresh frozen Achilles tendon allograft. The posteromedial reconstruction was performed using a posteromedial capsular shift surgical technique combined with a fresh frozen tibialis anterior allograft reconstruction of the superficial medial collateral ligament.

No tunnel bone grafting was required in this case since there was no tunnel osteolysis, or tunnel malposition. Cases where either tunnel osteolysis or tunnel malposition exists require bone grafting and a staged revision reconstruction procedure. Postoperatively, the surgical knee was immobilized in a long leg brace locked in full extension, and was non-weight bearing with crutches. Prophylactic preoperative and postoperative antibiotics were utilized. Progressive weight bearing and range of knee motion were gradually initiated according to our postoperative rehabilitation program detailed in Chap. 25.

Eight-year postoperative follow-up evaluation of the patient's surgical right knee demonstrated the patient's range of motion is 0–122° on the surgical right knee, and 0–135° on the uninvolved left knee. The posterior drawer test is negative, posteromedial and posterolateral drawer tests are negative, and the dial test is symmetrical to the normal left lower extremity at 30 and 90° of knee flexion. The Lachman test is negative, the pivot shift test is negative, the surgical knee is stable to varus and valgus stress at 0 and 30° of knee flexion, and the hyperextension external rotation recurvatum and heel liftoff tests are negative, and symmetrical to the uninjured knee. All physical examination tests of the surgical right knee are compared to the uninjured left knee.

Side-to-side difference on KT 1000 measurements on the PCL screen, corrected posterior, and corrected anterior measurements are 3.0, 5.0, and 3.0 mm, respectively. Side-to-side difference on the KT 1000 anterior displacement measurement at 30° of knee flexion is 2.0 mm. Postoperative stress X-rays at 90° of knee flexion using the Telos device comparing the surgical knee to the normal knee reveal a 2.5-mm side-to-side difference. There is X-ray evidence of minimal degenerative joint disease in the injured knee. The Hospital for Special Surgery, Lysholm, and Tegner knee ligament rating scale scores are 74/100, 88/100, and 5, respectively. The patient's knee is functionally and objectively stable; and the patient has returned to his pre-injury level of function both at manual labor in the road construction industry, and his recreational activities.

Summary

This chapter has presented selected cases in treatment of the PCL-injured knee that are representative of my practice. These selected cases represent real-life management examples in the treatment of difficult knee ligament instability problems. The details of the surgical techniques, not presented in this section, are described in Chaps. 1, 9, 15, 19, and 21. The purpose of this case study section has been for the reader to gain insight into management, treatment strategy, and outcomes of treatment in these complex knee ligament injuries.

Index

18 years old and younger, 3, 11, 231, 233, 237

A

Activity level, 94, 95, 101, 139, 255, 271, 284, 286, 324, 325, 337, 343, 344
All-inside, 107, 147, 149, 151–162, 201, 220
Allograft, 6, 15, 103, 106, 187, 220, 287
  tissue, 5–13, 101, 105, 107, 111, 119, 128, 133, 173, 174, 178–182, 233–240, 248, 268, 269, 288, 297, 304, 305, 356
Anatomy, 19, 21–29, 33, 35, 37, 39, 41, 43, 189, 209, 221, 329
Arthrometer, 4, 5, 11–15, 69–72, 116–121, 149, 151, 184–187, 238, 239, 267, 268, 337, 350
Arthroscopic, 3, 4, 12, 118, 173, 233
Arthroscopic tibial inlay, 123, 135, 137–144, 162, 201, 220, 232
Arthroscopy, 4, 6, 7, 12, 60, 112, 121, 125, 133, 135, 137, 140, 144, 149, 166, 170, 171, 175
Articular cartilage, 4, 20, 21, 41, 61, 62, 75, 131, 151, 202, 204, 210, 220, 239, 246, 247, 250, 272, 282–290, 296, 298, 303–306, 343, 350
Autograft, 12, 102, 103, 151, 197, 215, 232, 248, 267, 276

B

Biomechanics, 5, 19, 21, 23–29, 33–43, 61, 124, 134, 143, 150, 189, 211, 275, 297, 321
Brace, 302, 321, 223, 325

C

Cartilage treatment algorithm, 286
Case studies, 349, 351, 353, 355, 357
Chondral, 26, 27, 148, 201, 281, 282, 286, 289, 296, 300, 305
Clinical evaluation, 49, 84
Compass knee hinge (CKH), 220, 227, 228
Cruciate ligament, 9, 37, 38, 56, 168, 187

D

Deep medial collateral ligament, 39, 40, 42, 209, 210, 352
Defects, 6, 75, 282, 284–290, 330
Degeneration, 26–28, 77, 78, 96, 271, 272, 281, 288–290, 303, 305, 341, 342
Double-bundle, 8, 13, 14, 113, 119, 120, 128, 130, 143, 150, 151, 170, 185, 186, 234
Double-bundle PCL graft, 190

E

Examination Under Anaesthetic, 51

F

Fibular collateral ligament, 9, 10, 33–36, 57, 75, 79–81, 179, 192, 195, 198–201, 205, 236, 241, 275, 350–356

G

Graft
  factors, 102
  selection, 101, 103, 105, 107, 111, 150, 173, 174, 233, 248, 349
  sizing, 295, 297

H

High tibial osteotomy, 251, 271, 277, 289, 290, 297, 299, 306, 332

I

Injury, 33, 89, 349
Inside to outside PCL femoral tunnels, 8, 176, 234, 265
Inside-out repair, 250
Instrumented knee testing, 337

K

Killer Turn, 123, 135, 143, 144, 149–151, 155, 232
Kinematics, 25, 36, 71, 72, 137, 143, 144, 189, 190, 192, 204, 207, 212, 213, 271, 278, 281, 289,
Knee arthritis, 337, 339, 341, 342
Knee dislocation, 50, 57, 95, 137, 143, 168, 191, 220, 247
Knee flexion, 4, 9, 10, 12, 14, 22, 24, 29, 35, 41, 42, 55, 62, 70, 83, 92, 111, 114, 116, 118, 120, 125, 148, 150, 154
Knee ligament injury, 3, 11, 111, 115, 183, 237

L

Lateral Collateral Ligament (LCL), 9, 25, 26, 33, 35, 52, 68, 90, 162, 178, 190, 194, 195, 225, 235, 246, 255, 257, 349
Laxity, 4, 14, 26, 29, 36, 42, 43, 52, 55, 57, 61, 65, 69, 70, 91, 92, 95, 111, 116, 118, 120, 128, 143, 148, 157, 165, 171, 173, 184
Lesions, 27, 53, 61, 106, 275, 281, 282, 284, 285, 287–290
Ligament, 3–6, 9–13, 19, 20, 22, 26, 28, 35, 36, 38, 41, 43, 50, 52, 57, 59, 65, 72, 75, 78, 82, 89, 92, 94, 95, 101, 102, 105, 111, 113, 116, 119, 137, 138, 143, 151
Ligament healing, 94, 227, 324
Ligament reconstruction, 5, 38, 71, 101, 128, 133, 174, 193, 220, 227, 231, 238, 271, 289, 306
Long-term follow-up, 95, 135, 149, 150, 158, 304, 306

G. C. Fanelli (ed.), *Posterior Cruciate Ligament Injuries,*
DOI 10.1007/978-3-319-12072-0, © Springer International Publishing Switzerland 2015

M

Magnetic Resonance (MR) Imaging (MRI), 22, 65, 92, 148, 166, 219, 275, 289, 303, 305, 329
Management, 5, 38, 43, 146, 149, 191, 193, 209, 212, 245, 256, 271, 281, 298, 323, 357
Mechanical axis, 37, 43, 57, 58, 251, 272–278, 290
Mechanical graft tensioner, 11, 116, 267
Mechanical graft tensioning, 3, 7, 8, 11–14, 112, 117, 119, 121, 173–174, 184,185, 233, 265, 267–269
Medial Collateral ligament (MCL), 10, 54, 67, 132, 173, 209, 267, 276, 323
Meniscus, 4, 6, 10, 22, 27, 41, 62, 83, 94, 130, 158, 174, 180, 189, 210, 213, 236, 245, 272, 296, 298, 301, 304
Multi-ligament, 49, 50, 57–62, 147, 158, 159, 162
Multiligament complications, 191, 219, 330
Multiligament injury, 281, 282
Multiligament knee, 66, 128, 190–192, 206, 212, 216, 219, 220, 283, 339, 344
Multi-ligamentous injury, 57, 62, 158
Multiple ligament injured knee, 3, 4, 11, 13, 15, 72, 120, 147, 173, 184, 192, 233, 245, 269, 298, 350
Multiple ligament injuries, 103, 219, 222, 225, 249, 258
Multiple ligament knee injury, 3, 147, 191
Multiple-ligament, 65, 71, 119, 151, 173, 185, 239, 269, 299, 314, 320, 353, 355

N

Natural history, 26, 27, 28, 43, 89, 91, 93–95, 148, 189, 281, 282, 303
Neurovascular injury, 90, 133, 134, 139, 170, 329, 330

O

Obesity, 193, 275, 297
Open growth plates, 11, 15, 231–234, 237–243, 349, 350
Open Tibial Inlay technique, 123–128, 132, 134, 135, 144, 159
Osteoarthritis, 35, 36, 49, 75, 82, 93, 149, 169, 248, 287, 289, 295 297, 303–306, 321, 322, 326, 342
Osteotomy, 38, 139, 247, 251, 256, 277, 289, 297, 306, 332
Outcomes, 5, 29, 35, 62, 101, 137, 151, 159, 162, 171, 216, 232, 272, 282, 302, 306, 341, 344

P

Patellofemoral, 4, 22, 26, 28, 93, 94, 138, 174, 190, 233, 263, 274, 289, 314, 349, 354
PCL complications, 3, 95, 133, 134, 143, 191, 219, 245, 257, 329, 330, 332
PCL deficient, 24, 27, 28, 90, 125, 149, 150, 211, 271, 321, 330
PCL Footprint, 19, 127, 133, 140, 160
PCL injury, 19, 27, 60, 89, 95, 137, 147, 211, 233, 271, 321, 330
PCL reconstruction, 7, 8, 11, 14, 95, 102, 112, 120, 124, 150, 155, 162, 174, 220, 234, 263, 331
PCL repair, 165, 166, 170, 213
PCL Surgical Approaches, 124
PCL-based, 3, 4, 111, 120, 185, 231, 298, 303, 339
Pediatric, 231–233, 242
Peroneal nerve injury, 90, 254, 271, 349, 355, 356
Popliteofibular ligament, 9, 33, 78, 80, 190, 225, 226, 355
Popliteus tendon, 9, 33, 78, 81, 179, 196, 201, 236, 241, 256, 350, 354
Posterior Cruciate Ligament (PCL), 49, 111, 123, 137, 189, 245, 277, 281, 311, 329, 349
Posterior cruciate ligament deficiency, 72
Posterior Cruciate Ligament Reconstruction, 337
Posterior knee laxity, 162, 337, 338, 345
Posterior oblique ligament, 39, 41, 42, 55, 83, 209, 210, 220, 254
Posterolateral corner (PLC), 33, 55, 56, 62, 78, 130, 148, 178, 201, 209, 225, 235, 323, 344
Posterolateral instability, 173
Posteromedial corner (PMC), 4, 39, 58, 209, 216, 219
Posteromedial instability, 3, 4, 14, 120, 184, 209, 211, 239, 240, 350, 352, 354–356
Primary repair, 7, 10, 12, 38, 118, 119, 124, 166, 167, 169, 178, 213, 232, 235, 236, 351
Proprioception, 24, 28, 165, 171, 205
Protocol, 1, 67, 75, 89, 107, 142, 191, 193, 205, 228, 229, 254, 257, 258, 275, 276, 297, 302, 311, 324–326, 330, 345

Q

Quadriceps, 27, 28, 69, 92, 102, 128, 142, 147, 190, 220, 247, 315, 318, 325, 326

R

Radiology, 75
Range of knee motion, 238, 239, 241, 337, 339, 350–357
Reconstruction, 8, 9, 11, 12, 97, 201, 222, 253
Rehabilitation, 115, 142, 183, 237, 254
Repair, 38, 43, 66, 147, 165, 166, 167, 170, 171, 180, 194, 219, 236
Restoration, 9, 114, 157, 161, 169, 183, 205, 213, 266, 282, 283, 285, 287–290, 306, 311, 339, 354
Results, 12, 25, 59, 66, 95, 119, 123, 130, 150, 173, 194, 267, 282
Revision
  surgery, 60, 135, 245, 247–249, 251–257, 277, 305

S

Single-bundle, 13, 111, 119, 120, 143, 150, 151, 161, 184, 186, 344
Staged Procedures, 245, 249, 298
Strength, 27, 28
Stress radiograph, 148, 151, 274
Stress Radiography, 11, 12, 14, 57, 58, 66, 72, 116, 118, 184, 186, 267, 268
Subjective survey, 93, 96
Sub-total meniscectomy, 298, 306
Superficial medial collateral ligament, 10, 39–41, 81, 184, 209, 210, 214, 220, 236, 237, 241, 276, 357
Surgical technique, 8, 11, 14, 123, 128, 137, 139, 144, 164, 176, 178, 231, 234, 242, 263, 268, 349

T

Tear, 23, 83, 305
Telos, 13, 58, 68, 120, 185, 186, 239, 267
Tibial artery injury, 247
Tibial Inlay Graft, 124–127, 129–131, 133, 135
Tibial slope, 191, 256, 274, 276–278, 290
Translation, 24, 25, 42, 55, 72, 312
Transtibial PCL and ACL reconstruction, 119, 263
Transtibial PCL reconstruction, 7, 13, 113, 119, 123, 162, 185, 239, 350
Transtibial Tunnel Graft, 124
Transtibial tunnel PCL reconstruction, 7, 11, 14, 102, 111, 116, 120, 186, 267

V

Varus alignment, 38, 56, 272, 277
Vascular Assessment, 5, 50, 139, 147, 212

MIX
Papier aus verantwortungsvollen Quellen
Paper from responsible sources
FSC® C105338

If you have any concerns about our products,
you can contact us on
ProductSafety@springernature.com

In case Publisher is established outside the EU,
the EU authorized representative is:
Springer Nature Customer Service Center GmbH
Europaplatz 3, 69115 Heidelberg, Germany

Printed by Libri Plureos GmbH
in Hamburg, Germany